W9-CDC-437

Anesthesia
and Transplantation

Anesthesia and Transplantation

Edited by

Michael D. Sharpe, M.D., F.R.C.P.C.

Associate Professor, Department of Anaesthesia,
University of Western Ontario Faculty of Medicine, and
Director, W. E. Spoerel Intensive Care Unit,
London Health Sciences Centre, London, Ontario

and

Adrian W. Gelb, M.B., Ch.B., F.R.C.P.C.

Professor and Chairman, Department of Anaesthesia,
University of Western Ontario Faculty of Medicine,
London Health Sciences Centre, London, Ontario

With 63 Contributing Authors

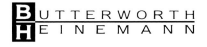

Boston   Oxford   Auckland   Johannesburg   Melbourne   New Delhi

Copyright © 1999 by Butterworth–Heinemann

A member of the Reed Elsevier group

All rights reserved.

No part of this publication may be reproduced, stored in a retrieval system, or transmitted in any form or by any means, electronic, mechanical, photocopying, recording, or otherwise, without the prior written permission of the publisher.

Every effort has been made to ensure that the drug dosage schedules within this text are accurate and conform to standards accepted at time of publication. However, as treatment recommendations vary in the light of continuing research and clinical experience, the reader is advised to verify drug dosage schedules herein with information found on product information sheets. This is especially true in cases of new or infrequently used drugs.

Recognizing the importance of preserving what has been written, Butterworth–Heinemann prints its books on acid-free paper whenever possible.

GLOBAL RELEAF 2000 Butterworth–Heinemann supports the efforts of American Forests and the Global ReLeaf program in its campaign for the betterment of trees, forests, and our environment.

Library of Congress Cataloging-in-Publication Data

Anesthesia and transplantation / [edited by] Michael D. Sharpe, Adrian
    W. Gelb.
        p.   cm.
    Includes bibliographical references and index.
    ISBN 0-7506-9664-8
    1. Transplantation of organs, tissues, etc. 2. Anesthesia.
  I. Sharpe, Michael D. II. Gelb, Adrian W.
    [DNLM: 1. Organ Transplantation--methods. 2. Anesthesia--methods.
    3. Anesthetics. WO 660 A5792 1999]
    RD87.3. T7A544 1999
    617.9'5--dc21
    DNLM/DLC
    for Library of Congress   98-32026
                                                                       CIP

British Library Cataloguing-in-Publication Data
A catalogue record for this book is available from the British Library.

The publisher offers special discounts on bulk orders of this book.
For information, please contact:

Manager of Special Sales
Butterworth–Heinemann
225 Wildwood Avenue
Woburn, MA 01801-2041
Tel: 781-904-2500
Fax: 781-904-2620

For information on all Butterworth–Heinemann publications available,
contact our World Wide Web home page at: http://www.bh.com

10 9 8 7 6 5 4 3 2 1

Printed in the United States of America

In memory of DMS

—MDS

For my family, with love and thanks

—AWG

Contents

Contributing Authors

Cate Abbott, B.A., B.S.W.
Information and Resource Assistant, Multi-Organ Transplant Service, London Health Sciences Centre, London, Ontario

J. Wesley Alexander, M.D., Sc.D.
Professor, Department of Surgery, and Director, Division of Transplantation, University of Cincinnati Medical Center and The Shriner's Burn Institute

Jamal A. Alhashemi, M.B.B.S., F.R.C.P.C.
Fellow, Program in Critical Care Medicine, University of Western Ontario Faculty of Medicine, London, Ontario

Mohammad Al-Sofayan, M.D., F.R.C.S.C.
Transplant Fellow, University of Western Ontario Faculty of Medicine, London Health Sciences Centre, London, Ontario

Angel J. Amante, M.D.
Fellow, Department of Organ Transplantation, Division of Immunology and Organ Transplantation, University of Texas Houston Medical School

Derek C. Angus, M.D., M.P.H.
Associate Professor, Department of Anesthesiology and Critical Care Medicine, University of Pittsburgh School of Medicine

Sami Asfar, M.B., Ch.B., M.D.(U.K.), F.R.C.S. (Edin.), F.A.C.S.
Associate Professor, Department of Surgery, Faculty of Medicine and Health Sciences, Kuwait University, Safat

Lawrence J. Baudendistel, M.D., Ph.D.
Professor and Chairman, Department of Anesthesiology, Saint Louis University School of Medicine

David S. Beebe, M.D.
Associate Professor, Department of Anesthesiology, University of Minnesota Medical School—Minneapolis

Kumar G. Belani, M.D.
Professor, Department of Anesthesiology, and Director, Continuing Medical Education (Anesthesiology), University of Minnesota Medical School—Minneapolis and Fairview University Medical Center, Minneapolis

Thomas P. Beresford, M.D.
Professor, Consultation Liaison Psychiatry, Denver Veterans Administration Medical Center

Arthur J. Boujoukos, M.D.
Assistant Professor, Department of Anesthesiology and Critical Care Medicine, and Medical Director, Ake Grenvik Cardiothoracic Intensive Care Unit, University of Pittsburgh School of Medicine

Roy Y. Calne, F.R.S.
Professor and Head, Department of Surgery, University of Cambridge Clinical School, Cambridge, United Kingdom; Consultant General Surgeon, Professor of Surgery, Addenbrooke's Hospital, Cambridge

B. Cohen, M.S., M.Econ.
Director, Eurotransplant Foundation, Leiden, The Netherlands

R. Duane Davis, M.D.
Assistant Professor and Director of Cardiopulmonary Transplantation, Department of Cardiothoracic Surgery, Duke University Medical Center, Durham, North Carolina

Anthony J. Demetris, M.D.
Director, Division of Transplant Pathology, and Professor, Department of Pathology, University of Pittsburgh Medical Center

David J. Freeman, Ph.D.
Associate Professor, Department of Medicine, Division of Clinical Pharmacology, University of Western Ontario Faculty of Medicine, London, Ontario

Christian L. Freitag, M.S.
Senior Transplant Coordinator, Toronto Region, MORE Program, The Toronto Hospital

Thomas A. Gaisor, M.D.
Associate Professor, Department of Anesthesiology, University of Pittsburgh School of Medicine

Adrian W. Gelb, M.B., Ch.B., F.R.C.P.C.
Professor and Chairman, Department of Anaesthesia, University of Western Ontario Faculty of Medicine, London Health Sciences Centre, London, Ontario

Cameron Ghent, M.D., F.R.C.P.C.
Associate Professor, Department of Internal Medicine, University of Western Ontario Faculty of Medicine, London Health Sciences Centre, London, Ontario

John P. Girvin, M.D., F.R.C.S.C.
Professor and Chairman of Neurosurgery, Department of Clinical Neurological Sciences, University of Western Ontario Faculty of Medicine, London Health Sciences Centre, London, Ontario

David R. Grant, M.D., F.R.C.S.C.
Professor, Department of Surgery, University of Western Ontario Faculty of Medicine, London Health Sciences Centre, London, Ontario

Rainer W. G. Gruessner, M.D., Ph.D.
Associate Professor, Department of Surgery, University of Minnesota Medical School—Minneapolis

Robert M. House, M.D.
Associate Professor and Director, Consultation Liaison Psychiatry, Colorado Psychiatric Hospital, University of Colorado Health Sciences Center, Denver

Sally H. Houston, M.D.
Associate Professor, Department of Medicine, Division of Infectious Diseases, University of South Florida College of Medicine, Tampa

Alan R. Hull, M.D.
Clinical Professor, Department of Internal Medicine, University of Texas Southwestern Medical Center at Dallas Southwestern Medical School

Debra A. Hullett, Ph.D.
Distinguished Scientist, Department of Surgery, Division of Transplantation, University of Wisconsin Medical School, Madison

J. Jastrzebski, M.D., F.R.C.P.C.
Clinical Instructor, Division of Nephrology, Vancouver General Hospital, and University of British Columbia Faculty of Medicine, Vancouver, British Columbia

Rajiv Jhaveri, M.D.
Assistant Professor and Director of Cardiothoracic Transplantation, Department of Anesthesiology, University of Maryland School of Medicine, Baltimore

Barry D. Kahan, Ph.D., M.D.
Professor, Department of Surgery, and Director, Division of Immunology and Organ Transplantation, University of Texas at Houston Medical School

Yoogoo Kang, M.D.
Professor, Department of Anesthesiology, University of Pittsburgh School of Medicine; Director, Hepatic Transplantation Anesthesiology, Presbyterian University Hospital, Pittsburgh

Jeremy Katz, M.D.
Assistant Professor, Department of Anesthesiology, University Hospital, University of Colorado Health Sciences Center, Denver

David M. Kendall, M.D.
Clinical Assistant Professor, Department of Medicine, University of Minnesota Medical School—Minneapolis; Consultant in Endocrinology, International Diabetes Center, Park Nicollet Clinic, Minneapolis

Paul A. Keown, M.B., Ch.B., M.B.A., F.A.C.P., F.A.C.A., F.R.C.P., F.R.C.P.C.
Professor and Director, Department of Immunology, Vancouver General Hospital, and University of British Columbia Faculty of Medicine, Vancouver, British Columbia, Canada

Peter E. Krucylak, M.D.
Assistant Professor, Department of Anesthesiology, and Director, Division of Cardiothoracic Anesthesia, Saint Louis University Health Sciences Center

Judith Kutt, M.D., F.R.C.P.C.
Assistant Professor, Department of Anaesthesia, University of Western Ontario Faculty of Medicine, London Health Sciences Centre, London, Ontario, Canada

Julie A. Larkin, M.D.
Assistant Professor, Department of Medicine, Division of Infectious Diseases, University of South Florida College of Medicine, Tampa

Bruce Leone, M.D.
Assistant Professor, Departments of Anesthesiology and Medicine, Duke University Medical Center, Durham, North Carolina

Adam E. Levy, M.D.
Research Fellow, Department of Surgery and The Shriner's Burn Institute, University of Cincinnati Medical Center

Dilly M. Little, F.R.C.S.I.
Research Associate, Department of Surgery, Division of Transplantation, University of Wisconsin Medical School, Madison

Jonathan Mardirossian, M.D., F.A.C.S.
Attending Surgeon, Department of Ophthalmology, White Plains Hospital, White Plains, New York

Kathryn E. McGoldrick, M.D., F.A.C.A.
Professor, Department of Anesthesiology, Yale University School of Medicine, New Haven, Connecticut; Medical Director, Ambulatory Surgery, Yale–New Haven Hospital, New Haven

Noriko Murase, M.D.
Associate Professor of Surgery, Thomas E. Starzl Transplantation Institute, University of Pittsburgh Medical Center

Howard M. Nathan, B.S., C.P.T.C.
Executive Director, Delaware Valley Transplant Program, Philadelphia

Michael R. Pinsky, M.D.
Professor, Department of Anesthesiology and Critical Care Medicine and Department of Medicine, University of Pittsburgh School of Medicine

Kerri M. Robertson, M.D.
Associate Clinical Professor, Department of Anesthesiology, and Chief, Transplant Services, Duke University Medical Center, Durham, North Carolina

Michael A. Robinette, M.D., F.R.C.S.C.
Associate Professor, Department of Surgery, Division of Urology, The Toronto Hospital, University of Toronto Faculty of Medicine

Marc St. Amand, M.D., F.R.C.P.C.
Assistant Professor, Department of Anaesthesia, University of Western Ontario Faculty of Medicine, London Health Sciences Centre, London, Ontario

John Schweiss, M.D.
Professor Emeritus, Department of Anesthesiology, Saint Louis University Health Sciences Center

Michael D. Sharpe, M.D., F.R.C.P.C.
Associate Professor, Department of Anaesthesia, University of Western Ontario Faculty of Medicine, and Director, W. E. Spoerel Intensive Care Unit, London Health Sciences Centre, London, Ontario

John T. Sinnott, M.D.
Professor, Department of Medicine, and Chief, Division of Infectious Diseases, University of South Florida College of Medicine, Tampa

Hans W. Sollinger, Ph.D., M.D.
Folkert O. Belzer Professor of Surgery and Chairman, Division of Organ Transplantation, Department of Surgery, University of Wisconsin Medical School, Madison

Thomas E. Starzl, M.D., Ph.D.
Professor, Department of Surgery and Thomas E. Starzl Transplantation Institute, University of Pittsburgh School of Medicine

Calvin R. Stiller, C.M., M.D., F.R.C.P.C.
Professor, Department of Medicine, University of Western Ontario Faculty of Medicine, London, Ontario

Carol Stockall, M.D., F.R.C.P.C.
Associate Professor, Department of Anaesthesia, University of Western Ontario Faculty of Medicine, London Health Sciences Centre, London, Ontario

Marc T. Swartz, B.A.
Director of Circulatory Support, Department of Surgery, Saint Louis University School of Medicine

Michael Talamantes, L.C.S.W.
Liver Transplant Social Worker, Department of Social Work and Liver Transplant Surgery, University Hospital, University of Colorado Health Sciences Center, Denver

Barbara Tardiff, M.D.
Assistant Professor, Department of Anesthesiology, Duke University Medical Center, Durham, North Carolina

Edward Thomas, M.D.
Assistant Professor, Division of Critical Care Medicine, Department of Anesthesiology, University of Pittsburgh Medical Center

William J. Wall, M.D., F.R.C.S.C.
Director, Multi-Organ Transplant Program, University of Western Ontario Faculty of Medicine, London Health Sciences Centre, London, Ontario

Phyllis G. Weber, R.N.
Executive Director, California Transplant Donor Network, San Francisco

Celia Wight, S.R.N., H.V. Cert.
Manager, Donor Action Foundation, Cambridge, United Kingdom

Preface

When the medical history of the twentieth century is written, there is little doubt that multiorgan transplantation will be regarded as one of the major achievements. During the 1980s and 1990s, transplantation made the transition from an experimental to a fully accepted form of therapy for many terminal diseases caused by progressive failure of a single organ. This transition has resulted in an exponential increase in the number of transplantations and the number of centers with transplant programs.

We have had the privilege in our capacities as anesthesiologists and intensivists to participate in the growth of multiorgan transplantation at our own institution. In those capacities, we have actively participated in preoperative management, intraoperative care, and postoperative intensive care support of transplant patients. With the growth of programs, we have also seen an increasing number of patients with transplants who present for unrelated surgery. Although review articles and monographs are available, none seem to cover the entire spectrum or the multidisciplinary nature of modern multiorgan transplantation. We have therefore drawn together a unique combination of authors encompassing internal medicine, surgery, anesthesiology, and pharmacology for *Anesthesia and Transplantation*. Our aim is to give the novice and the experienced clinician a complete overview of transplantation. Thus, chapters dealing with a particular organ transplantation are written by internists, surgeons, and anesthesiologists, all of whom are experts in the field. Ethical dilemmas, resource requirements, brain death, transplant-related infections, nutrition, hematologic disorders, psychological considerations, and the use of mechanical devices, all of which pertain to the often complex transplant patient, continue to be important issues and are appropriately reviewed.

Multiorgan transplantation has become an international endeavor. Donor organs are shipped across national borders, and recipients similarly seek out centers of excellence. To reflect this, we have enlisted an international, multidisciplinary group of authors whose expertise and experiences have made significant contributions to transplantation. As such, the book appropriately begins and ends with an overview presented by a transplantation pioneer from each side of the Atlantic.

We gratefully acknowledge the authors whose manuscripts reflect such expertise and significant contributions to the field of multiorgan transplantation. Their patience in the development of multidisciplinary chapters is very much appreciated.

We also wish to extend special thanks to a number of individuals for their invaluable advice and support during the preparation of this book: James MacDonald, C.P.C.; Giep J. Roussow, M.D.; David Colby, M.D.; Collette M. Guiraudon, M.D.; David Pelz, M.D.; Don Lee, M.D.; Allan Fox, M.D.; Robert Reid, M.D.; Calvin R. Stiller, M.D.; William J. Wall, M.D.; and J. Bryan Vaughan, C.M.

Finally, our sincere gratitude to Linda Hunte and Lynn Hinchliffe for their secretarial support and organization, which was crucial to the completion of this project.

Michael D. Sharpe
Adrian W. Gelb

Anesthesia
and Transplantation

Chapter 1

History of Organ Transplantation via the Two-Way Paradigm*

Thomas E. Starzl, Noriko Murase, and Anthony J. Demetris

Chapter Plan

The story of how whole-organ transplantation came to be a clinical discipline has been told elsewhere by many of those who were directly involved.[1] The kidney dominated events through 1959,[2] but in the late 1950s, canine transplant models were developed to study intra-abdominal and thoracic organs. Pig and rodent models came later.

Each organ-defined specialty has had its historians, but they have been preoccupied with a succession of events rather than with the poorly understood biological principles by which all organs can escape rejection. This conventional approach is characterized by noting the first successful allotransplantation of the kidney,[3] liver,[4] heart,[5] lung,[6] pancreas,[7] intestine,[8] multiple abdominal viscera,[9] and bone marrow.[10–12] Such milestones are important, but the concern here is the steps by which organ transplantation was developed empirically and the understanding of what had been accomplished that came only later. Such generic information may be of use to anesthesiologists who care for various organ transplant recipients.

The Immunologic Barrier

In December 1954, Joseph E. Murray unequivocally demonstrated the potential benefit of human whole-organ replacement with an identical twin kidney donor. His achievement was symbolic only, showing with an identical twin organ what was already known to be possible with skin grafts. Seven years later, the father of modern immunology, Macfarland Burnet, wrote in the *New England Journal of Medicine*, "much thought has been given to ways by which tissues or organs not genetically and antigenetically identi-

*Portions of this chapter were previously published in *The Lancet* (TE Starzl, AJ Demetris, N Murase, et al. Cell migration, chimerism, and graft acceptance. Lancet 1992;339: 1579–1582) and the *Journal of the American Medical Association* (TE Starzl, AJ Demetris. Transplantation milestones: viewed with one-and two-way paradigms of tolerance. JAMA 1995;273:876–879).

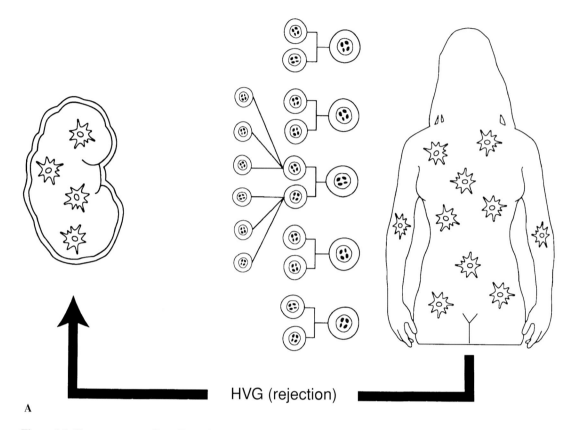

HVG (rejection)

A

Figure 1-1. The one-way paradigm: Transplantation is conceived as involving a unidirectional immune reaction: host-versus-graft (HVG) reaction with whole organs (**A**) and graft-versus-host (GVH) reaction with bone marrow or other lymphopoietic transplants (**B**).

cal with the patient might be made to survive and function in the alien environment. On the whole, the present outlook is highly unfavorable to success."[13]

The One-Way Paradigm

Rejection

What was the genetically determined barrier? Although details are obscure, there was little mystery after 1944 about the general meaning of transplant rejection, after its elucidation by Peter Medawar as an immunologic event.[14] Medawar's contribution created the image of a tissue (or organ) allograft as an island in a hostile recipient sea (Figure 1-1A).

Tolerance

In contrast, how allografts or xenografts can escape rejection with or without the aid of immunosuppression has been one of the most arcane subjects in biology since Billingham, Brent, and Medawar described acquired tolerance in 1953.[15, 16] A simple explanation for the tolerance in their special model was at first beguiling. Immunocompetent adult spleen cells were injected in utero or perinatally into mice that had not yet evolved the immunologic equipment to reject them. The engrafted cells flourished, perpetuated themselves, and, in effect, endowed the recipient with the donor immune system. Thereafter, the chimeric mice failed to recognize donor-strain skin or other donor tissues as alien.

In this second landmark contribution from Medawar's laboratory, tolerance was explained as a

GVH

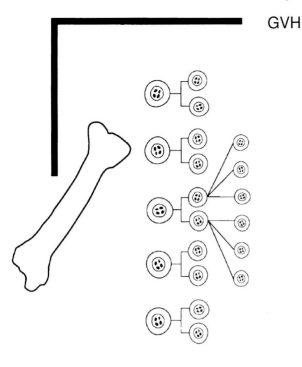

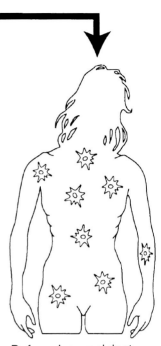

Defenseless recipient
Billingham-Brent-Medawar
Cytoablation (x-ray, drugs)
Parent → offspring F1 hybrid

B

switch in immunologic apparatus. It was consistent with the definition of transplantation immunology as a unidirectional immune reaction (the "one-way paradigm"). Main and Prehn[17] strengthened this view by demonstrating the same tolerance outcome as that of Billingham, Brent, and Medawar in irradiated adult mice. Main and Prehn reconstituted the hematolymphopoietic cells of their cytoablated mice with bone marrow. Hundreds of subsequent tolerance-induction experiments in animals, and eventually clinical bone marrow transplantation, seemed to depend on a similar natural, or iatrogenically imposed, defenseless recipient state (Figure 1-1B).

Graft-versus-Host Disease

The anticipated clinical application of this kind of tolerance induction was temporarily derailed in 1957, when it was realized that an immunologically active graft could turn the tables and reject the recipient (graft-versus-host disease [GVHD]). Billingham and Brent showed in their mouse model[18] and Simonsen in chickens[19] that this risk (also called *runt disease*) was roughly proportional to the extent of the major histocompatibility complex (MHC) barrier. Such disparities became measurable in humans after identification of the HLA by Dausset,[20] Terasaki, and others.[21] For many years, the complication of GVHD in rodent[22] and large animal irradiation chimera models[23–26] forestalled the clinical use of HLA-mismatched bone marrow cells or other mature immunocytes, either for immunologic reconstitution for purely hematologic purposes or as a means of facilitating whole-organ graft acceptance.

Clinical Bone Marrow Transplantation

Nevertheless, a strategy for clinical bone marrow transplantation eventually was assembled directly

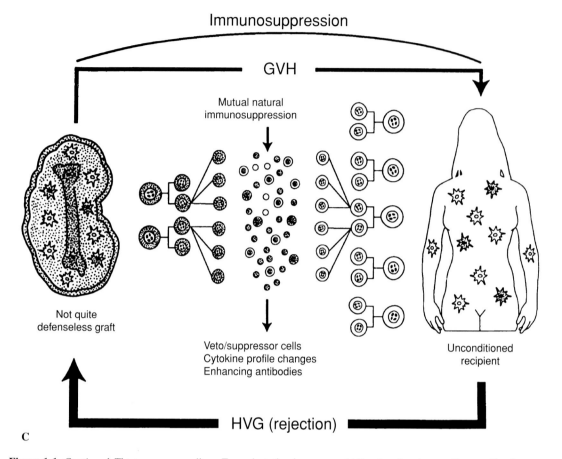

Figure 1-1. *Continued.* The two-way paradigm: Transplantation is seen as a bidirectional and mutually canceling immune reaction that is predominantly HVG with whole-organ grafts (**C**) and predominantly GVH with bone marrow grafts (**D**).

from the rodent experiments, but with similar histocompatibility-imposed restrictions.[23] After recipient cytoablation with total body irradiation (TBI) or cytotoxic drugs, stable chimerism could be induced in humans by the infusion of donor bone marrow if there was a good HLA match. Otherwise, the incidence of GVHD was intolerable. After successful engraftment, maintenance immunosuppression frequently was not needed, mimicking the kind of acquired immunologic tolerance originally described by Billingham, Brent, and Medawar[15, 16] and then by Main and Prehn.[17] The eventual success of clinical bone marrow transplantation[10–12] was a straight-line extension from these rodent models, as Donnel Thomas (1990) has observed.[23]

Clinical Organ Transplantation

Total Body Irradiation

The achievement of clinical bone marrow transplantation effectively detached the surgeons from a scientific base because there was no explanation for successful engraftment. Nevertheless, by the time of the first successful bone marrow transplantation, surgeons had already recorded many successful human whole-organ transplantations (mostly kidneys) under continuous immunosuppression, without dependence on HLA matching or the complication of GVHD, and as it turned out, without host preconditioning. In fact, preconditioning with sublethal TBI was used in the first

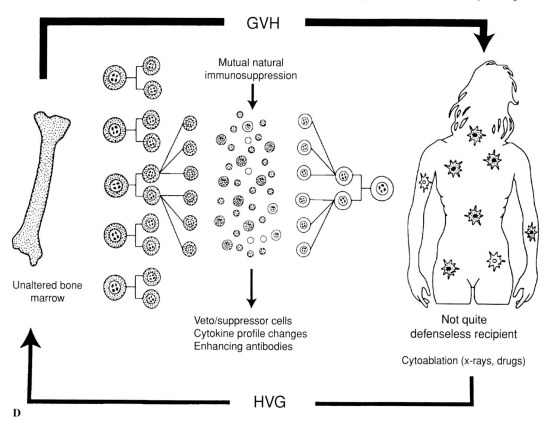

successful renal allotransplantation, described by Merrill et al. in 1960.[3] The kidney recipient, however, whose donor was his fraternal (dizygotic) twin brother, was not given bone marrow, which was a significant departure from the Billingham-Brent-Medawar framework. The recipient's own bone marrow recovered, and the transplanted kidney and patient survived for 20 years. Six additional examples of protracted kidney graft survival (longer than 1 year) after recipient irradiation without marrow were recorded in Paris over the next 36 months.[27, 28] Five of the six donors were more distant relations than a fraternal twin, and two were genetically unrelated.[28] However, these were isolated successes in a sea of failures.

Chemical Immunosuppression

The frustration continued after Murray et al.[29] introduced 6-mercaptopurine and its analogue, aza-thioprine, for human renal transplantation. This followed extensive experimental studies, first with rodent skin transplantation[30, 31] and then with canine kidney transplant models.[29, 32–34] The drugs were originally developed as antileukemic agents by Elion et al.[35] and were first demonstrated to be immunosuppressive by Schwartz and Dameshek.[36] Although the sixth patient treated by Murray with one or the other of these myelotoxic drugs had function of a nonrelated renal allograft for 17 months, the clinical results were poor at first,[29, 37] similar to those with TBI.

The Double-Drug Breakthrough

The tidal wave of whole-organ transplant cases began in 1962, when azathioprine was combined with prednisone to reverse rejection.[38] More important, the subsequent need for maintenance immuno-suppression frequently declined, and in occasional

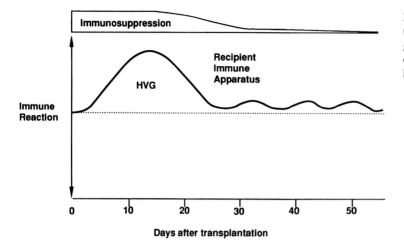

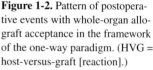

Figure 1-2. Pattern of postoperative events with whole-organ allograft acceptance in the framework of the one-way paradigm. (HVG = host-versus-graft [reaction].)

cases, treatment could be stopped. The same sequence has been shown with all other organs transplanted and with all the immunosuppressive regimens (Figure 1-2). Agents introduced later were more potent and reliable in chaperoning the desired chain of events: antilymphocyte globulin,[39] cyclosporine,[40] and tacrolimus (FK506).[41] Despite their diversity, all these drugs seemed, in a fundamentally similar way, to have allowed something to change in the host, the graft, or both. But what was that something?

The one-way paradigm of transplantation immunology that had gained ascendency nearly a half-century before did not provide answers to that question. The false conception of a unidirectional reaction was never seriously challenged after it was seemingly supported by studies with the one-way mixed lymphocyte reaction introduced in 1963 by Bach and Hirschhorn[42] and Bain et al.[43] These in vitro techniques (so-called minitransplant models) generated thousands of increasingly sophisticated cellular and ultimately molecular studies of unidirectional immunologic reactions. Ironically, the resulting plethora of new information sometimes resembled an exponentially expanding phone book filled with wrong numbers. Most seriously, the flawed context lured successive generations of investigators into the trap of believing that tolerance induction for whole-organ recipients (the "holy grail") lay in variations on the HLA-limiting strategy used for bone marrow transplantation, which included host preconditioning in preparation for a variety of donor leukocyte preparations.

The Two-Way Paradigm

Whole-Organ Transplantation

A plausible explanation for the success of the empirically developed whole-organ transplantation procedures did not emerge until 1992. Then, a study of the surviving pioneer kidney and liver recipients from the earliest clinical trials revealed that donor leukocytes of bone marrow origin, which are part of the structure of all complex grafts (passenger leukocytes[44, 45]), had migrated from the organs to ubiquitous sites in the recipient and survived for up to 30 years.[46, 47] Thus, organ allograft acceptance was associated with the cryptic survival of a small fragment of extramedullary donor marrow, including stem cells (depicted as a bone silhouette encased by the kidney in Figure 1-1C), which was disseminated throughout the recipient after the transplantation and assimilated into the much larger immunologic network of the host. In the meantime, the cells that left the graft were replaced by recipient immune cells moving in the opposite direction. The end result was a small number of residual donor leukocytes (microchimerism) in both graft and host.

From this information, a revision of transplantation immunology was possible. In the new view, the immunologic confrontation after whole-organ transplantation could be seen as bidirectional (GVH as well as HVG) and mutually canceling (Figure 1-3), provided that the participants in the David-and-Goliath mismatch could survive the initial onslaught. In a clinical context, but not in several

Figure 1-3. The pattern of convalescence after organ or bone marrow transplantation in the framework of the two-way paradigm. With bone marrow transplantation, the dominant immune reaction usually is graft-versus-host (GVH) reaction. (HVG = host-versus-graft [reaction].)

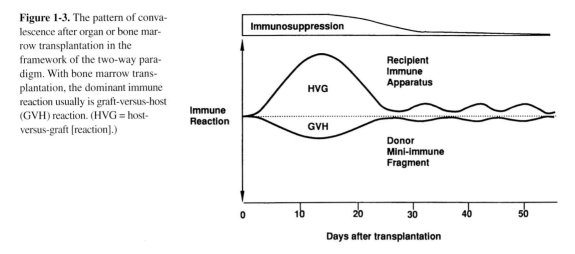

animal models, this survival requires an umbrella of immunosuppression that protects both cell populations equally (see Figure 1-1C). Current research aims at understanding the amplification device that enables a small number of cells to affect so profoundly the immunology of the vast cellular army of the host. Although the chimeric leukocytes are multilineage,[46–49] the antigen-presenting dendritic cells of Steinman and Cohn[50, 51] are thought to be critical because they can modify the expression of cell interaction, MHC, and adhesion molecules, all of which determine how T cells heed antigen signals.[51]

Historic Enigmas

With the two-way paradigm, virtually every previously unexplained experimental or clinical observation after whole-organ transplantation was understood or at least susceptible to experimental inquiry.[46, 47] It was clear why organ grafts are inherently tolerogenic, why HLA matching is so poorly predictive of outcome, and why GVHD does not develop after the transplantation of immunologically active grafts, such as the liver and intestine.

   With the two-way mutual cancellation implicit in this concept, the loss or blunting of an HLA matching effect is easy to understand. With each further level of histoincompatibility, the reciprocal effect is postulated to escalate both ways, providing the process is chaperoned with an effective immunosuppressive umbrella (Figure 1-4). The consequent dwindling of the matching effect as

donor-specific and recipient-specific nonreactivity evolves accounts for blindfolding of the expected HLA effect. In addition to explaining why the HLA matching effect is blindfolded, this bidirectional canceling effect of the two cell populations explains why GVHD does not develop after liver, intestinal, multivisceral, and heart-lung transplantation, despite the heavy lymphoid content of those organs.

Augmentation of Spontaneous Chimerism

Historic efforts to give extra donor antigen in the form of bone marrow[52, 53] or donor blood transfusions[54–56] were hampered in design or execution by the assumption that the infused cells would be destroyed without recipient preconditioning, by the justifiable anxiety about GVHD if the host was preconditioned, and by a lack of information about the appropriate timing of the infusions. The new information that chimerism is a naturally occurring event after whole-organ transplantation[46, 47] exposed a perioperative window of opportunity. In this window, unaltered HLA-incompatible bone marrow or donor-specific blood transfusion was predicted to be safe without recipient preparation or any deviation from the generic practices of immunosuppression for whole-organ transplantation, which had evolved from the original azathioprine-prednisone formula.[38]

   The validity of this strategy was verified in unpreconditioned recipients of cadaveric kidneys, livers, hearts, and lungs who were given $3–5 \times 10^8$

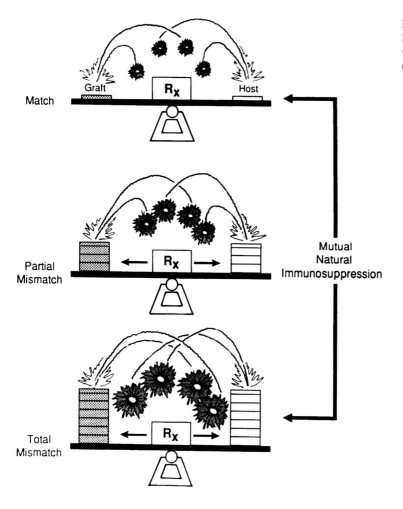

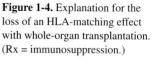

Figure 1-4. Explanation for the loss of an HLA-matching effect with whole-organ transplantation. (Rx = immunosuppression.)

donor bone marrow cells per kg recipient body weight at the same time as organ transplantation under standard FK506-prednisone treatment (Figure 1-5).[57] Chimerism estimated at more than 1,000 times that occurring in conventional whole-organ recipients was reliably and safely produced and sustained. Persistent blood chimerism (usually greater than 1%), a trend toward donor-specific nonreactivity, and a high rate of patient and graft survival has marked these bone marrow–augmented recipients as an advantaged cohort. They are the first patients to undergo HLA-mismatched cadaveric organ transplantation with the reasonable prospect of eventually being drug free. The process of tolerance induction and drug weaning is expected to take 5–10 years in most patients who are given mismatched organs. In some patients, the drug-free state may never be attained.

Whole-Organ Transplantation versus Bone Marrow Transplantation

With the discovery that whole-organ transplantation caused spontaneous chimerism, it was realized that the apparently vast gap between the bone marrow and whole-organ transplantation fields merely reflected entrenched differences of treatment strategy (Figure 1-6). The mutually censoring immunologic limbs were being left intact with organ transplantation, whereas the recipient limb was deliberately removed (cytoablation) in preparation for bone marrow grafting procedures. It is doubtful that it is ever possible (much less desirable) to completely eliminate the entire recipient immune system with the cytoablation techniques of bone marrow transplantation. Although this was long assumed to have occurred in successful cases (see Figure 1-1B),

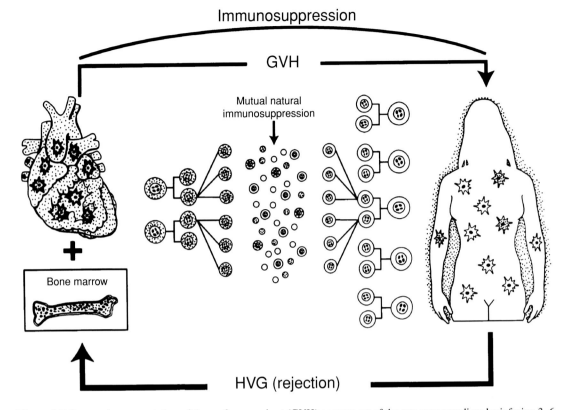

Figure 1-5. Iatrogenic augmentation of the graft-versus-host (GVH) component of the two-way paradigm by infusing 3–6 $\times 10^8$ unaltered donor bone marrow cells per kg recipient body weight at the same time as heart or other whole-organ transplantation. When the recipient is not cytoablated, there is essentially no risk of GVH disease. (HVG = host-versus-graft [reaction].)

a trace population of recipient leukocytes has almost invariably been detected with sensitive techniques in patients previously thought to have complete bone marrow replacement.[58, 59] These bone marrow recipients were mirror images of successfully treated whole-organ recipients, the difference being that their own, rather than donor leukocytes, constituted the trace population. In either kind of recipient (whole-organ or bone marrow), the appearance of MHC-restricted veto and suppressor cells, enhancing antibodies, and changes in cytokine profile could be construed as a by-product of and accessory to the seminal event of mixed chimerism and resulting reciprocal clonal exhaustion and deletion (see Figure 1-1C and D).[46, 47, 60]

Beyond an adjuvant role for whole-organ transplantation, an important question is whether HLA-mismatched bone marrow without an accompanying organ can be engrafted in patients whose disease can be corrected with a minimally chimeric or even microchimeric state, using the same immunosuppression as for marrow-augmented kidney, liver, and heart recipients. The potential list of indications in which complete marrow replacement is unnecessary is a long one, exemplified by the lysosomal enzyme deficiencies.[61] Another look into the future has been provided by the demonstration that xenograft transplantation is followed by the same cell migration process seen with allografts.[62]

Importance of History

The legendary immunologist Melvin Cohn (father of the two-signal concept of self-nonself discrimination) wrote in 1994, "In its recent history, immunology has advanced largely by volume [of

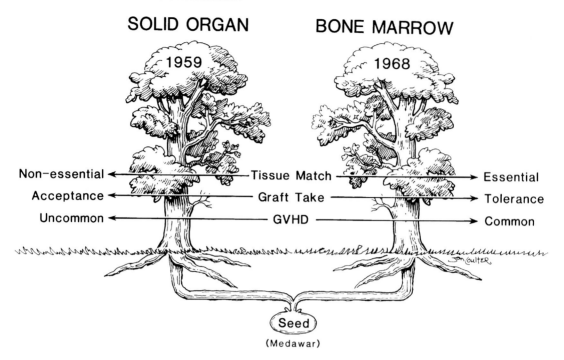

Figure 1-6. The growth of separate disciplines of bone marrow and whole-organ transplantation from the seed planted by Peter Medawar during World War II. It was recognized in 1992 that these seemingly disparate disciplines were mirror images caused by different treatment strategies. (GVHD = graft-versus-host disease.)

publications], complete with waste."[63] In Cohn's opinion, the reason for the slow conceptual advancement in this branch of science has been the immunologists' preference for small theories that explain one or only a few facts (articulated by Mitchison[64]) over the development of generalized principles that explain all facts (coherence of context). It would be hard to find a better way to illustrate the consequences of a small theory than those derived from the durable one-way paradigm, which was blindly accepted despite its failure to explain what was seen daily in every transplantation clinic and laboratory. Virtually no hint of the two-way paradigm can be found in the literature before the description in June 1992 of microchimerism in organ recipients. If the spontaneous development of chimerism after organ transplantation had been recognized 30 years ago, it would have been possible to correctly interpret observations in splenocyte and bone marrow transplant experiments reported in 1960–1962 by Simonsen[65, 66] and Michie, Woodruff, and Zeiss.[67] The hypothesis of these earlier workers—that acquired tolerance must result from a two-way (donor-recipient) immune reaction—resembled the hypothesis that was later used to explain organ graft acceptance. Their great idea was abandoned because it could not be proved, thereby delaying a true understanding of transplantation immunology for a third of a century.

Beacons of understanding shine forward as well as backward. Understanding the history of transplantation in terms of the two-way paradigm provides the intellectual means to devise better treatment strategies, including the achievement of drug-free tolerance and, ultimately, xenotransplantation.

References

1. Terasaki PI (ed). History of Transplantation: Thirty-Five Recollections. Los Angeles: UCLA Tissue Typing Laboratory, 1991.
2. Woodruff WMA (ed). The Transplantation of Tissues and Organs. Springfield, IL: Thomas, 1960.
3. Merrill JP, Murray JE, Harrison JH, et al. Successful homotransplantation of the kidney between non-identical twins. N Engl J Med 1960;262:1251–1260.

4. Starzl TE, Groth CG, Brettschneider L, et al. Orthotopic homotransplantation of the human liver. Ann Surg 1968;168:392–415.

5. Barnard CN. What we have learned about heart transplants. J Thorac Cardiovasc Surg 1968;56:457–468.

6. Derom F, Barbier F, Ringoir S, et al. Ten-month survival after lung homotransplantation in man. J Thorac Cardiovasc Surg 1971;61:835–846.

7. Kelly WD, Lillehei RC, Merkel FK, et al. Allotransplantation of the pancreas and duodenum along with the kidney in diabetic nephropathy. Surgery 1967;61:827–837.

8. Goulet O, Revillon Y, Brousse N, et al. Successful small bowel transplantation in an infant. Transplantation 1992;53:940–943.

9. Starzl TE, Rowe M, Todo S, et al. Transplantation of multiple abdominal viscera. JAMA 1989;261:1449–1457.

10. Bach FH. Bone-marrow transplantation in a patient with the Wiskott-Aldrich syndrome. Lancet 1968;2:1364–1366.

11. Mathe G, Amiel JL, Schwarzenberg L, et al. Haematopoietic chimera in man after allogenic (homologous) bone marrow transplantation. BMJ 1963;(Dec. 28): 1633–1635.

12. Gatti RA, Meuwissen HJ, Allen HD, et al. Immunological reconstitution of sex-linked lymphopenic immunological deficiency. Lancet 1968;2:1366–1369.

13. Burnet FM. The new approach to immunology. N Engl J Med 1961;264:24–34.

14. Medawar PB. The behavior and fate of skin autografts and skin homografts in rabbits. J Anat 1944;78:176–199.

15. Billingham RE, Brent L, Medawar PB. "Actively acquired tolerance" of foreign cells. Nature 1953;172:603–606.

16. Billingham R, Brent L, Medawar P. Quantitative studies on tissue transplantation immunity. III. Actively acquired tolerance. Philos Trans R Soc Lond (Biol) 1956;239:357–412.

17. Main JM, Prehn RT. Successful skin homografts after the administration of high dosage X radiation and homologous bone marrow. J Natl Cancer Inst 1955;15:1023–1029.

18. Billingham R, Brent L. A simple method for inducing tolerance of skin homografts in mice. Transplant Bull 1957;4:67–71.

19. Simonsen M. The impact on the developing embryo and newborn animal of adult homologous cells. Acta Pathol Microbiol Scand 1957;40:480.

20. Dausset J. The HLA Adventure. In PI Terasaki (ed), History of HLA: Ten Recollections. Los Angeles: UCLA Tissue Typing Laboratory, 1990;1–20.

21. Terasaki PI (ed). History of HLA: Ten Recollections. Los Angeles: UCLA Tissue Typing Laboratory, 1990.

22. Trentin JJ. Induced tolerance and "homologous disease" in X-irradiated mice protected with homologous bone marrow. Proc Soc Exp Biol Med 1957;96: 139–144.

23. Thomas ED. Allogeneic Marrow Grafting—A Story of Man and Dog. In PI Terasaki (ed), History of Transplantation: Thirty-Five Recollections. Los Angeles: UCLA Press, 1991;379–394.

24. Mannick JA, Lochte HL, Ashley CA, et al. A functioning kidney homotransplant in the dog. Surgery 1959;46: 821–828.

25. Hume DM, Jackson BT, Zukoski CF, et al. The homotransplantation of kidneys and of fetal liver and spleen after total body irradiation. Ann Surg 1960;152: 354–373.

26. Rapaport FT, Bachvaroff RJ, Mollen N, et al. Induction of unresponsiveness to major transplantable organs in adult mammals. Ann Surg 1979;190:461–473.

27. Hamburger J, Vaysse J, Crosnier J, et al. Renal homotransplantation in man after radiation of the recipient. Am J Med 1962;32:854–871.

28. Kuss R, Legrain M, Mathe G, et al. Homologous human kidney transplantation. Experience with six patients. Postgrad Med J 1962;38:528–531.

29. Murray JE, Merrill JP, Dammin GJ, et al. Kidney transplantation in modified recipients. Ann Surg 1962;156: 337–355.

30. Meeker W, Condie R, Weiner D, et al. Prolongation of skin homograft survival in rabbits by 6-mercaptopurine. Proc Soc Exp Biol Med 1959;102:459–461.

31. Schwartz R, Dameshek W. The effects of 6-mercaptopurine on homograft reactions. J Clin Invest 1960;39: 952–958.

32. Calne RY. The rejection of renal homografts: inhibition in dogs by 6-mercaptopurine. Lancet 1960;1:417–418.

33. Zukoski CF, Lee HM, Hume DM. The prolongation of functional survival of canine renal homografts by 6-mercaptopurine. Surg Forum 1960;11:470–472.

34. Calne RY. Inhibition of the rejection of renal homografts in dogs with purine analogues. Transplant Bull 1961;28:445.

35. Elion GB, Bieber S, Hitchings GH. The fate of 6-mercaptopurine in mice. Ann N Y Acad Sci 1955;60: 297–303.

36. Schwartz R, Dameshek W. Drug-induced immunological tolerance. Nature 1959;183:1682–1683.

37. Murray JE, Merrill JP, Harrison JH, et al. Prolonged survival of human-kidney homografts by immunosuppressive drug therapy. N Engl J Med 1963;268: 1315–1323.

38. Starzl TE, Marchioro TL, Waddell WR. The reversal of rejection in human renal homografts with subsequent development of homograft tolerance. Surg Gynecol Obstet 1963;117:385–395.

39. Starzl TE, Marchioro TL, Porter KA, et al. The use of heterologous antilymphoid agents in canine renal and liver homotransplantation and in human renal homotransplantation. Surg Gynecol Obstet 1967;124:301–318.

40. Calne RY, Rolles K, White DJG, et al. Cyclosporin A initially as the only immunosuppressant in 34 recipients of cadaveric organs: 32 kidneys, 2 pancreases, and 2 livers. Lancet 1979;2:1033–1036.

41. Starzl TE, Todo S, Fung J, et al. FK 506 for human liver, kidney, and pancreas transplantation. Lancet 1989;2:1000–1004.

42. Bach F, Hirschhorn K. Lymphocyte interaction: a potential histocompatibility test in vitro. Science 1964;143:813–814.

43. Bain B, Vas MR, Lowenstein L. The development of large immature mononuclear cells in mixed leukocyte cultures. Blood 1964;23:108–116.

44. Snell GD. The homograft reaction. Annu Rev Microbiol 1957;11:439–458,.

45. Steinmuller D. Immunization with skin isografts taken from tolerant mice. Science 1967;158:127–129.

46. Starzl TE, Demetris AJ, Murase N, et al. Cell migration, chimerism, and graft acceptance. Lancet 1992; 339:1579–1582.

47. Starzl TE, Demetris AJ, Trucco M, et al. Cell migration and chimerism after whole organ transplantation: the basis of graft acceptance. Hepatology 1993;17:1127–1152.

48. Demetris AJ, Murase N, Fujisaki S, et al. Hematolymphoid cell trafficking, microchimerism, and GVHD reactions after liver, bone marrow, and heart transplantation. Transplant Proc 1993;25:3337–3344.

49. Qian S, Demetris AJ, Murase N, et al. Murine liver allograft transplantation: tolerance and donor cell chimerism. Hepatology 1994;19:916–924.

50. Steinman RM, Cohn ZA. Identification of a novel cell type in peripheral lymphoid organs of mice. I. Morphology, quantitation, tissue distribution. J Exp Med 1973;137:1142–1162.

51. Steinman RM. The dendritic cell system and its role in immunogenicity. Annu Rev Immunol 1991;9:271–296.

52. Monaco AP, Clark AW, Brown RW. Active enhancement of a human cadaver renal allograft with ALS and donor bone marrow: case report of an initial attempt. Surgery 1976;79:384–392.

53. Barber WH, Mankin JA, Laskow DA, et al. Long-term results of a controlled prospective study with transfusion of donor specific bone marrow in 57 cadaveric renal allograft recipients. Transplantation 1991;51:70–75.

54. Salvatierra O Jr, Vincenti F, Amend WJ, et al. Deliberate donor-specific blood transfusions prior to living related renal transplantation. A new approach. Ann Surg 1980;192:543–552.

55. Anderson CB, Sicard GA, Etheredge EE. Pretreatment of renal allograft recipients with azathioprine and donor-specific blood products. Surgery 1982;92: 315–341.

56. Sollinger HW, Burlingham WJ, Sparks EM, et al. Donor-specific transfusions in unrelated and related HLA-mismatched donor-recipient combinations. Transplantation 1984;38:612–615.

57. Fontes P, Rao A, Demetris AJ, et al. Augmentation with bone marrow of donor leukocyte migration for kidney, liver, heart, and pancreas islet transplantation. Lancet 1994;344:151–155.

58. Przepiorka D, Thomas ED, Durham DM, Fisher L. Use of a probe to repeat sequence of the Y chromosome for detection of host cells in peripheral blood of bone marrow transplant recipients. Hematopathology 1991;95: 201–206.

59. Wessman M, Popp S, Ruutu T, et al. Detection of residual host cells after bone marrow transplantation using non-isotopic in situ hybridization and karyotype analysis. Bone Marrow Transplant 1993;11:279–284.

60. Starzl TE, Zinkernagel RM. Antigen localization and migration in immunity and tolerance. N Engl J Med (in press).

61. Starzl TE, Demetris AJ, Trucco M, et al. Chimerism after liver transplantation for type IV glycogen storage disease and type I Gaucher's disease. N Engl J Med 1993;328:745–749.

62. Starzl TE, Fung J, Tzakis A, et al. Baboon to human liver transplantation. Lancet 1993;341:65–71.

63. Cohn M. The wisdom of hindsight. Annu Rev Immunology 1994;12:1–62.

64. Mitchison NA. Better to Confess Ignorance. In Answer to Melvin Cohn. In MM Burger, B Sordat, RM Zinkernagei (eds), Cell to Cell Interaction. Switzerland: Basel Karger 1990;232–234.

65. Simonsen M. On the acquisition of tolerance by adult cells. Ann N Y Acad Sci 1960;87:382–390.

66. Simonsen M. Graft versus host reactions. Their natural history, and applicability as tools of research. Prog Allergy 1962;6:349–467.

67. Michie D, Woodruff MFA, Zeiss IM. An investigation of immunological tolerance based on chimera analysis. Immunology 1961;4:413–424.

Chapter 2

Organ Resources and Consent for Donation

Michael A. Robinette and Christian L. Freitag
(Canadian Perspective)
Celia Wight and B. Cohen (European Perspective)
Alan R. Hull, Phyllis G. Weber, and Howard M. Nathan
(American Perspective)

Chapter Plan

Canadian Perspective

Canada is the second largest country in the world but has a relatively small population of 30.3 million. By contrast, California, a small fraction of the size of Canada, has a population of 30.9 million. Significant cultural, ethnic, and economic differences exist within Canada, but common to all inhabitants of the 10 provinces and two territories is a universal health care system, developed and gradually introduced during the 1950s and 1960s. By 1972, all Canadians were covered by a health care system funded equally by the federal and provincial (or territorial) governments. All legal Canadian residents, regardless of age, health, or economic status, have universal access to hospitals and physicians. Each province administers its own health plan, which shares five basic principles:

1. Universal coverage
2. Comprehensive benefits
3. Portability (between provinces or territories)
4. Nonprofit administration (by government)
5. Accessibility

Patients receiving an organ transplant in Canada have all their medical, surgical and pharmaceutical costs covered, including all expenses involved in organ retrieval. All Canadian organ procurement organizations (OPOs) and transplant programs are hospital based and fully funded provincially, based on the number of transplants performed and on a predetermined amount for each organ. Funding flows through each hospital's global budget; consequently, along with other hospital-based programs, organ retrieval and transplantation are similarly vulnerable to staff reductions and limitations on hospital resources resulting from government-imposed budget decreases.

In contrast to the United States, hospitals are not compensated for expenses related to organ retrieval, nor are recipients billed for any service related to transplantation. For example, there is no listing fee, there are no organ acquisition costs, and there are no charges between Canadian provincial programs, except for ground transportation and organ shipping costs, which are paid by the transplant program receiving the organ. When a patient receives a transplant in another province, the institution performing the transplant is reimbursed by the recipient's provincial government health plan. The amount depends on the organ and is calculated according to an agreement reached among the provinces.

Historic Aspects

Renal transplantation began in Canada in the late 1950s with occasional living transplants between HLA-identical twins.[1] Cadaveric renal transplantation programs were established in several hospitals in the late 1960s. By the 1980s, 25 centers were performing renal transplants, the same number that currently exists.

In the early days of renal transplantation, the activity level of each transplant program depended on the number of kidney donors referred by local intensivists and neurosurgeons, usually within the same hospital. This was an informal process very dependent on staff friendships and collegiality with members of the transplant team.

Coordinated and organized organ retrieval began in the mid-1970s out of an increasing need to improve the supply of kidneys for transplantation. Metro Organ Retrieval and Exchange (MORE) in Toronto was the first such Canadian program. A 24-hour hotline was established to give medical staff prompt access to potential donors. A procedural manual outlining steps involved in donor identification and management was distributed to all hospitals for use in their intensive care units (ICUs) and emergency departments; also, a program of education for health care professionals and the public was implemented. Within a year, the

Table 2-1. Organ Procurement Organizations (OPOs) in Canada

Province	OPO
Newfoundland	Organ Procurement and Exchange of Newfoundland and Labrador
New Brunswick	New Brunswick Organ/Tissue Procurement Program
Nova Scotia	Nova Scotia Organ Procurement
Quebec	Quebec Transplant
Ontario	MORE of Hamilton
	MORE of Kingston
	MORE of London
	MORE of Ottawa
	MORE of Toronto
Manitoba	Manitoba Organ Procurement
Saskatchewan	The Saskatchewan Transplant Program
Alberta	HOPE of Calgary
	HOPE of Edmonton
British Columbia	BC Transplant Society

MORE = Multiple Organ Retrieval and Exchange; HOPE = Human Organ Procurement and Exchange.
Source: Adapted from Canadian Organ Replacement Register. Annual Report 1996, Volume 2: Dialysis and Transplantation. Ottawa: Canadian Institute for Health Information, March 1996.

program was expanded to include the remaining provincial transplant centers in Ontario (Hamilton, Kingston, London, and Ottawa).

With initiation of extrarenal transplants (liver, heart, and lung) in the early 1980s, all organs were retrieved through MORE, and its name was changed to Multiple Organ Retrieval and Exchange. During the late 1970s and early 1980s, similar OPOs were established nationally, each one provincially funded and hospital based. Currently, there are 14 Canadian OPOs (Table 2-1) employing 43 procurement coordinators (PCs), 25 full-time and 18 part-time; the latter usually share the remainder of their activities with recipient-related work (i.e., part-time transplant coordinator [TC] or administrative responsibilities). The OPOs provide donor hospitals with complete coordination of all organ donation activities, and they provide transplant programs with all services related to organ acquisition, storage, and distribution. Other services provided by the OPOs include data collection and analysis related to organ donation and transplantation, education programs for health care professionals and the public, and assistance with research programs.

Table 2-2. Transplantation in Canada, 1982–1997[a]

Year	Kidney	Liver	Kidney (Pancreas)	Heart	Heart/ Lung	Lung	Bowel	Total	Donors (RPMP)
1997	996	352	30 (3)	164	7	79	3	1,634	440 (14.8)
1996	952	354	19 (3)	166	4	72	3	1,573	426 (14.4)
1995	921	328	17	183	8	72	1	1,530	425 (14.3)
1994	923	305	8	171	6	65	6	1,484	407 (13.9)
1993	897	295	6	172	8	59	3	1,440	409 (14.2)
1992	755	223	3	122	10	51	0	1,164	330 (12.0)
1991	853	225	7	150	10	67	3	1,315	355 (15.5)[b]
1990	837	192	0	161	11	52	0	1,253	359 (15.6)[b]
1989	858	147	0	160	17	24	0	1,206	360 (16.3)[b]
1988	901	129	1	184	6	16	1	1,238	383 (17.4)[b]
1987	826	106	0	134	8	14	0	1,088	350 (16.1)[b]
1986	871	65	0	121	6	4	0	1,067	383 (17.2)[b]
1985	738	37	0	60	6	2	0	843	316 (14.7)[b]
1984	661	21	0	18	2	1	0	703	292 (13.2)[b]
1983	642	5	1	17	1	1	0	667	268 (12.9)[b]
1982	501	2	0	10	0	0	0	513	212 (10.2)[b]

RPMP = rate per million population.
[a]1991–1997 transplant numbers were audited and revised by Canadian organ procurement organizations.
[b]Calculated value from renal transplant number and RPMP.
Source: Adapted from Canadian Organ Replacement Register. Annual Report 1998, Volume 2: Dialysis and Transplantation. Ottawa: Canadian Institute for Health Information, June 1998.

Provincial programs collaborate informally to exchange and update waiting lists, to facilitate placement of organs into high-priority patients, and to place organs that are not used locally. Canada does not have a national organ retrieval program or agency. Organs not transplanted locally are first offered regionally, then nationally, and then, by way of the United Network for Organ Sharing (UNOS), to the United States or occasionally elsewhere in the world.

Organ Donation in Canada: Current Activity

The chronic shortage of organs that has developed globally is also a problem in Canada. The demand for organs has far outpaced the supply, with the result that waiting lists have grown progressively larger. The donation rate per million population (PMP) in Canada has remained static since the late 1980s (approximately 14 donors PMP, Table 2-2) and is clearly inadequate to meet the requirements of Canadian transplant programs[2] (Table 2-3). This is considerably less than Spain's experience (25 donors PMP), which has the highest donor rate per capita worldwide. The United States also experiences a higher donation rate compared to Canada (Figure 2-1). Although strategies have been introduced to improve the organ donor supply, the chronic shortage of organs remains the most pressing problem in transplantation today.

The majority of patients on the list are waiting for a renal transplant. This is attributable mainly to the rapid growth of dialysis programs across the country (Table 2-4), less rigid criteria for entering the renal transplant program as a potential recipient (e.g., the upper age limit has been raised from 60 to 75 years or older), and the yearly addition to the waiting list of patients with a failed transplant, usually from chronic rejection (approximately 240 Canadian patients per year since 1990).[3] Once placed on a cadaveric waiting list, renal patients are not usually transplanted for several months or even years, depending on their blood group. Of those transplanted in Toronto in 1996, the average wait was 877 days.[4] In contrast to renal failure patients, who can be maintained alive and relatively healthy on dialysis while waiting for a transplant, those

Table 2-3. Waiting List for Transplantation in Canada

Organ	Year					
	1991	1992	1993	1994	1995	1996*
Kidney	1,606	1,823	1,904	1,865	2,126	2,303
Liver	64	89	81	110	149	169
Heart	78	72	86	99	98	94
Lung	52	61	81	53	81	75
Heart/lung	4	13	14	11	14	15
Kidney/pancreas	23	15	13	17	23	29
Other	3	3	5	0	1	1
Total	1,830	2,076	2,184	2,155	2,492	2,686

*As of September 30, 1996.

Source: Adapted from Canadian Organ Replacement Register. Annual Report 1996, Volume 2: Dialysis and Transplantation. Ottawa: Canadian Institute for Health Information, March 1996.

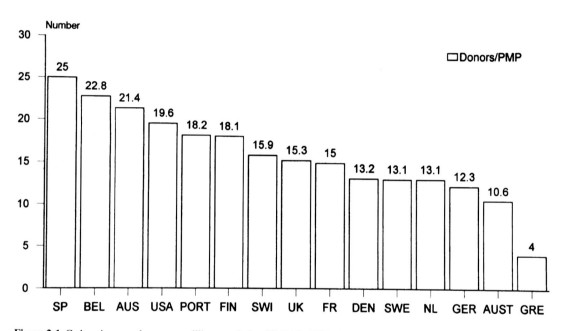

Figure 2-1. Cadaveric organ donors per million population (PMP) in 1994. (SP = Spain; BEL = Belgium; AUS = Austria; USA = United States of America; PORT = Portugal; FIN = Finland; SWI = Switzerland; UK = United Kingdom; FR = France; DEN = Denmark; SWE = Sweden; NL = the Netherlands; GER = Germany; AUST = Australia; GRE = Greece.) (Adapted from data from the Australia and New Zealand Organ Donation Registry, Etablissement Français des Greffes, Eurotransplant Foundation, Hellenic Transplant, Organización National de Transplantes, Scandia Transplant, United Kingdom Transplant Support Service Authority, and United Network for Organ Sharing.)

waiting for an extrarenal transplant (liver, heart, or lung) have no similar artificial organ that can sustain life long term. Therefore, death while waiting is inevitable unless a suitable organ becomes available in time. In 1996, approximately 141 patients died in Canada while waiting for an extrarenal organ transplant (MORE Program, unpublished data).

Compared to dialysis, renal transplantation not only provides significant advantages in quality and length of life and an improved sense of well-being, it also provides a clear financial benefit. The cost of maintaining a patient on dialysis is approximately $50,000 per year (less for home-based peritoneal dialysis). A successful transplant costs $20,000 plus

Table 2-4. Growth in Renal Failure Programs in Canada

Year	Total Patients	Alive with Functional Transplant	Total Dialysis	New Renal Failure Patients	Total Transplants (Cad/LR)
1996	19,424	8,937	10,487	3,322	963 (697/266)
1995	18,129	8,332	9,797	3,223	964 (739/225)
1994	16,730	7,652	9,078	3,093	923 (708/215)
1993	15,413	7,148	8,265	2,902	897 (720/177)
1992	14,211	6,664	7,547	2,748	755 (606/149)
1991	13,123	6,313	6,810	2,640	853 (722/131)
1990	11,986	5,914	6,072	2,299	837 (719/118)
1989	11,211	5,637	5,574	2,126	858 (720/138)
1988	10,313	5,192	5,121	1,954	901 (762/139)
1987	9,303	4,544	4,759	1,838	826 (701/125)
1986	8,637	4,177	4,460	1,734	871 (766/105)
1985	7,804	3,501	4,303	1,571	738 (635/103)
1984	7,305	3,256	4,049	1,455	661 (585/76)
1983	6,640	2,866	3,774	1,312	642 (537/105)
1982	5,916	2,403	3,513	1,265	501 (424/77)

Cad = cadaveric; LR = living-related.
Source: Adapted from Canadian Organ Replacement Register. Annual Report 1998, Volume 2: Dialysis and Transplantation. Ottawa: Canadian Institute for Health Information, June 1998.

$6,000 per year thereafter, which is equivalent to $50,000 over 5 years.[5] Provincial governments have been very supportive of the organ retrieval programs because they know that (applying the numbers above) 100 successful renal transplants save the provincial health care budget approximately $20 million. Although costs may vary from country to country, it is apparent that renal transplantation is a cost-effective exercise. Cost effectiveness is not as readily demonstrated for other organ transplants, however, but the ability to restore an individual's health with a successful transplant and return him or her to his or her regular occupation and family is clearly a desirable objective.

Organ Donation Process

The organ donation process consists of a sequence of steps, in which each step depends on the successful completion of the one preceding (Figure 2-2).[6] A breakdown can occur at any step, resulting in failure to convert a potential donor into an actual donor. The most critical step, and the one that is probably most often missed, is donor identification, which results in a failure to approach the family for consent. These components of the organ donor process are germane to the transplant program in Canada as well as those in the United States and Europe (see Appendix 2A).

Future Considerations

It is clear that current demands by transplant programs are not being met by the supply of organ donors. In Canada, the projected increase in end-stage renal disease (ESRD) incidence and prevalence will continue to average 8.4% per year. By the end of 2005, the number of patients receiving renal replacement therapy will have climbed to 36,748 from 15,602 (at the end of 1994).[7] The current shortfall of dialysis facilities will continue to be a problem, and the demand for donated organs will increase significantly. Several initiatives are being implemented in an effort to increase the number of organ transplants.

Encourage Living-Related Transplants

The only increase occurring in renal transplantation in Canada since the mid-1980s has been the number of living-related transplants, and the poten-

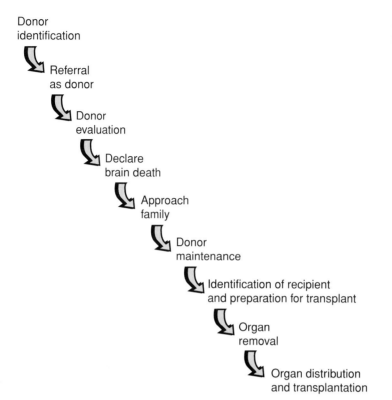

Donor
identification

Referral
as donor

Donor
evaluation

Declare
brain death

Approach
family

Donor
maintenance

Identification of recipient
and preparation for transplant

Organ
removal

Organ distribution
and transplantation

Figure 2-2. The organ donor process.

tial exists to expand this even further. By 1996, at the Toronto Hospital in Ontario, living-related transplants increased to 43% of all kidneys transplanted (83% genetically related and 17% emotionally related), as a result of an active program encouraging family members, spouses, or even friends to donate.

These recipients are transplanted sooner than they would have been if placed on the waiting list for a cadaveric transplant, and graft survival results are better, even in the genetically unrelated group.[8] Living-related liver, lung, and pancreas transplants are being successfully performed in the United States and are now also beginning in Canada.

Improved Hospital Organization

Although ongoing education of health care professionals about donor identification is important, more is required. Government cutbacks in health care have imposed heavier workloads on nurses and physicians working in ICUs and emergency departments, with the result that there is an increased need to designate an individual in each hospital as a donor coordinator. When a potential donor is identified, the donor coordinator, together with the regional OPO PC, can assume the responsibility of the donation process and thereby minimize disruption for the attending staff. The donor coordinator can also arrange an effective tracking mechanism for neurosurgical patients who are referred for evaluation but are returned to the referring hospital for chronic care when they are found to be inoperable but not yet brain dead. Thus, if their conditions deteriorate, these patients may become actual donors. Establishing a network of trained coordinators in appropriately sized hospitals in Spain resulted in an increase in the donor rate from 14.3 PMP in 1989 to 21.7 donors PMP by 1992.[9] The donor rate continued to increase to 27.0 PMP in 1995. A similar program of designated donor coordinators (referred to as *regional communication coordinators*) has been introduced in Ontario through the MORE program. In larger hospitals and those with neurosurgical units, the coordinator is part-time, whereas in smaller centers, a shared on-call system is used, and all coordinators assume a donor advocate and educational function in their hospitals. The result is more donor referrals and donated organs from those hospitals; consequently, this program is gradually expanding to more hospitals.[4]

Hospitals providing organ donation incur expenses in the process, especially extra ICU time for donor maintenance and operating room time, which is often several hours for multiple-organ donors. This extra financial burden is becoming an increasing inhibiting factor in Canada, where there is no cost reimbursement to the donor hospital. In Quebec, a hospital reimbursement system was introduced in the early 1990s with payment of $500 per donor referred and $4,500 per donor retrieved. Initial results revealed an increase from 9.6 to 15.5 donors PMP between 1992 and 1996. Consequently, this policy is being reviewed for possible implementation in other provinces.[10]

Heightened Public Awareness

In spite of a generally high level of support for organ donation (documented in various government-run and private polls), there is still a disturbingly high level of consent refusal (31% in MORE in 1995). Approaches to lowering this percentage include ongoing public awareness campaigns, training in improved techniques for those who ask for consent, and targeting religious and ethnic groups to correct their misconceptions about the appropriateness of organ donation.

European Perspective

As renal transplantation developed in Europe, the need for a central organization to coordinate organ donation and transplantation became evident, particularly with the emergence of nonrenal transplant programs. This development of a central organization resulted in two major benefits:

1. *Reduction in the wastage of available donor organs.* The need and criteria for suitable donor organs varied widely among transplant centers. Small, local waiting lists often led to no suitable recipients being identified. It was recognized that the best possible usage of donated organs depended on the size of the geographic area or the pool of transplant candidates to be served. The greater and more diverse the waiting list, the higher the chance of ultimately using the available organs and thus reducing the wastage.

2. *Optimal use and transparent allocation of donor organs.* Organ allocation policies should concentrate primarily on achieving the best match between donor and recipient and identifying the patients in most urgent need of transplantation. These allocation policies should also be seen to be fair to patients on the waiting lists.

Historic Aspects

The structure of the current organ exchange organization (OEO) is a result of evolution rather than design. Historic bonds, national culture and character, geographic and demographic characteristics, medical and immunologic progress, changes in political and government control, and developments in managerial approach have all contributed to the current OEO. With the addition of improved telecommunications and computer networks, a wide spectrum of models has developed. Most OEOs operate on a national basis, which was established at the time of its initial development (1969 in France) or evolved over time (1986 in the United States). For others, cooperation was always international (i.e., Eurotransplant Foundation [ET, 1967]) in Austria, Belgium, Germany, Luxembourg, and the Netherlands; United Kingdom Transplant Support Service Authority (UKTSSA, 1972) for the United Kingdom and Republic of Ireland; Scandiatransplant (1969) for Denmark, Finland, Iceland, Norway, and Sweden. In contrast, in Italy, several regional organizations continue to operate independently.

The OEOs generally started as a private initiative based on the recognition of the special benefits that widespread professional collaboration could achieve in transplantation. The voluntary, cooperating transplant programs were comparable to members of a club who agree to abide by rules set by the members. As the official of the club, the OEO was the custodian of the rules. It had to strike a delicate balance between satisfying the demands of the individual transplant programs and maintaining the integrity of an organization that represented all its members equally.

Since the late 1980s, donation systems, transplant programs, and OEOs have received increasing attention from governments, particularly ministries of health. This attention has resulted from the increasing demands organ transplantation has made on health care systems; the constitutional rights of citizens to medical care; the shortfall of cadaveric organs; and allegations of organ trading, transplant "tourism," and transplant centers' noncompliance with the organ allocation rules.

In some countries (e.g., the United Kingdom), OEOs were already attached to the Department of Health. In other countries, governments took the opportunity to create formal, national OEOs (e.g., Spain, France). Yet other countries (e.g., Austria, Belgium, Denmark, Sweden) have introduced legislative measures on the diagnosis of brain death, the consent process, organ procurement and transplantation, and (in the Netherlands) decrees concerning authorization of centers to perform transplantation. Nonetheless, most of these OEOs continue to operate with the free will and consensus of the participants, thus achieving a true international collaboration.

Role of the Transplant Coordinator in Organ Procurement

The need for local as well as national organization of organ transplantation led to the introduction of TCs. TCs first appeared in the United States during the 1970s. They were typically renal technicians and nurses already working in the transplant unit. As the demand for transplants grew, their responsibilities expanded into the area of organ procurement. TCs were increasingly appointed in a full-time capacity and began to concentrate more on the elaborate donation and procurement process, including community and professional education.[11] This initiative was quickly adopted in Europe, where the first TCs were appointed in the late 1970s. All European countries with transplant programs now employ TCs.

TCs are instrumental in developing professional links between the transplant units and surrounding ICUs, establishing hospital protocols and procedures for organ donation, and helping the staff with the time-consuming tasks involved in the process of organ donation, often including the approach to bereaved relatives for permission to remove organs for transplantation. TCs have become a focus for professional and, to a lesser extent, public information on organ donation and transplantation and are skilled in the complex process of organ donation (see Appendix 2A).

TCs are responsible for the local organization of organ donation and communicate closely with the OEO during the process. Many TCs travel to the donating hospital on notification of a potential donor. To determine organ suitability, they carefully examine the past medical history. The current medical situation is also evaluated, which often leads to further medical investigations. Once collected, all the relevant information is relayed to the OEO, who will eventually allocate the available organs to patients according to nationally agreed criteria. Any transplant center that needs additional information contacts the local TC.

Once a diagnosis of brain death is confirmed, and there is no objection to organ donation, the local TC arranges a mutually convenient time for organ removal. During this time, patient care changes to donor maintenance aimed at achieving optimal organ function for recipient patients (see Chapter 4). This change in emphasis can be distressing for ICU staff. Donor management can be difficult, costly, and time consuming. Organs can be "lost" at this stage, and a continuing high standard of medical and nursing care is essential. Procurement TCs often take responsibility for donor management.

The Spanish Model

Spain developed a national organ procurement network rather late and differently from other countries.[12] Organización Nacional de Transplantes (ONT) was founded in 1989 under the direction of a national coordinator. Regional TCs have been appointed in the 17 health regions of Spain. The regional TCs are accountable to the national coordinator and administratively responsible for the success or failure of organ and tissue donation activities in their health region. The national and regional coordinators are all medically qualified (usually anesthetists or nephrologists). Local coordinating teams have been established in all hospitals with ICU facilities and are completely separate

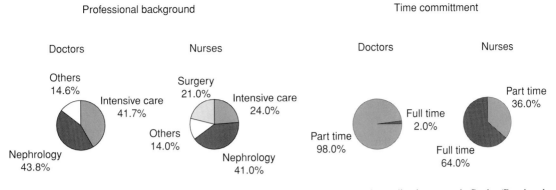

Figure 2-3. The professional background and time devoted to organ donation of local coordinating teams in Spain. (Reprinted with permission from R Matesanz, B Miranda, C Felipe. Organ procurement and renal transplants in Spain: the impact of transplant coordination. Clin Transpl 1994;8:283.)

from the transplant units. The teams are made up of senior medical and nursing staff already employed in the hospital (Figure 2-3). The majority of the doctors work as TCs on a part-time basis, usually for 2–3 years. Organ donation takes absolute priority over other duties, but, when not involved with a donation, these doctors continue with their original professional responsibilities. The medical TCs return to their full-time specialty after a period as a part-time TC. The rationale behind this arrangement is to avoid the "burnout" syndrome, frequently seen in the United States and increasingly in Europe. In contrast, the majority of the nurses working with the medical staff in the local coordinating teams work full-time.

The local coordinating teams are responsible for the whole process of organ donation in the hospital, from the "detection" of a potential donor to the referral of available organs and tissues to ONT for distribution to the appropriate transplant centers. The teams also stay in close contact with all local public agencies that have potential influence on organ donation and transplantation. The TCs are provided with excellent training and support from ONT and are accountable to hospital administration and the national coordinator through the regional coordinators.

Since 1989, Spain has managed to increase the renal transplant rate dramatically, to 42 PMP in 1994, and to provide more donors per capita than any other country (see Figure 2-1). This has been achieved despite a continuing fall in deaths from

road traffic accidents and is attributed to the coordination system and the support and training provided for TCs.[12]

Organ Donation in Europe: Current Activity

Today, European OEOs have developed into an alliance between donor hospitals ("input") and transplant programs ("output"), together with their accompanying tissue-typing laboratories. They are nonprofit bodies that act as service agencies to both donating hospitals and transplant units. All follow the same set of general policies, operating procedures, and organ allocation rules.

In general, OEOs have developed a hierarchic decision-making process. Medical advisory committees, typically related to various organs, histocompatibility testing, and the organization of organ procurement, are the cornerstones in the process. An equal representation of the diverse geographic regions and transplant programs is safeguarded. These committees make recommendations on changes in existing policies for approval by the OEO board and government.

The main functions of OEOs are these:

- Maintain patient waiting lists for all varieties of organ and tissue transplantation
- Participate in tissue bank and bone marrow donor registries
- Allocate available organs and tissue to the appropriate recipient patients according to

medically agreed criteria that take into account clinical urgency and waiting time

- Cooperate with other OEOs during clinical emergencies or if no suitable recipient can be found in the country of donation
- Maintain records on the source and destination of all organs and tissues
- Collect data on postoperative course after transplantation and act as a data reference center
- Carry out research and quality control
- Reimburse costs to donating hospitals
- Support and promote initiatives to increase organ donation

The service areas of the European OEOs vary widely:

ET: 3.2×10^6 sq km with a population of 113×10^6

Spain: 1.5×10^6 sq km with a population of 38×10^6

North Italy: 0.4×10^6 sq km with a population of 1.8×10^6

ET, the largest OEO in Europe, provides its services to the transplant community in 65 renal transplant centers, 34 heart transplant centers, 15 lung transplant centers, 28 liver transplant centers, and 22 pancreas transplant centers.

Organ Allocation

The OEO plays various roles in organ matching and allocation. Some OEOs (e.g., Scandiatransplant) have opted for an organ-matching and allocation procedure totally initiated and executed by the donor center. Thus, no central office is involved. The participation of an OEO depends on mutual agreement on allocation policies by their transplant community. Two models have developed in Europe. In the first, the central allocation office of the OEO coordinates the matching and allocation completely (e.g., ET). In the second model, the OEO assists with organ placement only when needed (e.g., France). In addition, the OEO often arranges the shipment of donor organs between donor and transplant centers or the transportation of complete donor surgical teams.

It is generally accepted that organ allocation should be equitable. The two principles of primary importance are medical criteria and justice. Patient selection based on medical criteria aims at the best predicted long-term result. Selection based on justice aims to give a chance to the sickest patients. Strictly speaking, these principles conflict with each other. Faced with a shortage of donor organs and in an attempt to address the problems of equitable allocation, the medical advisory committees of the OEOs have developed organ-specific allocation criteria. These criteria differ slightly from country to country, but all aim to give the best and fairest chance to the most patients.

Another consideration in organ allocation is geographic area. Should the donor hospital be rewarded for its efforts by giving regional recipients (i.e., those associated with the donor hospital) priority over nonregional recipients, as happens in renal transplantation in Spain? Such local priority can be defended by the argument that a short cold ischemic time may improve the outcome of the transplant. Furthermore, the financial expenses associated with distant organ exchange and increased budgetary constraints increasingly oblige OEOs to account for geographic factors. Many allocation protocols now include geographic considerations. Despite these problems, if no suitable national recipient can be found, the movement of organs across boundaries presents no problems, and there is close cooperation between all the European OEOs. Thus, taking into account the mutually agreed allocation rules, donor organs are often allocated locally, then regionally, nationally, and, finally, internationally.

In all allocation models, the final decision to use an allocated organ remains with the transplant surgeons and physicians responsible for the patient's care.

Role of the Media

The media have an increasing influence on international donation rates. The attention that organ and tissue donation and transplantation has received in the European media is thought to be a crucial factor in organ availability. News outlets have published stories on the following topics:

- The kidnapping of children for organs and tissues
- The use of organs from executed prisoners
- Commercialism of kidney transplantation
- The unknown origin of donor organs and tissues
- The transmission of infectious diseases, such as human immunodeficiency virus
- Sale of tissues after autopsy to pharmaceutical companies
- Removal of donor corneas without permission
- Renewed discussions of brain death

It is not surprising that these stories have a very negative impact on the public attitude toward organ donation. TCs report increasing refusal rates among the relatives of potential donors, and relatives often state that negative press coverage of organ transplantation has influenced their decision. Germany and France were particularly affected by negative media attention in 1993 and 1994, and, as a result, both countries experienced serious decreases (15–20%) in organ donation.

Media stories may have contributed to the introduction of legislation such as the Human Organs Transplant Act in 1990 in the United Kingdom and a complete reorganization of organ and tissue procurement and allocation in France (law number 94-654, 29 July 1994).[13]

The media are often effective watchdogs, and they can create positive public attitudes toward organ donation. This occurred in the United Kingdom in the 1980s. The plight of a child in urgent need of a liver transplant received huge media attention. Consequently, a suitable donor was immediately identified, and pediatric transplantation became permanently established in the United Kingdom. In 1995, similar sympathetic media coverage of organ donation after the murder of an American child in Italy led to an immense increase in the Italian public's support for organ donation, which itself resulted in increased professional enthusiasm.

The transplant community has recognized the need to be open and proactive in its relationships with the media. Some OEOs (e.g., ET, Etablissement Français des Greffes, UKTSSA, ONT) have established publicity offices to respond to the media on a 24-hour basis. Some of the national TC organizations (e.g., the United Kingdom) facilitate media training for their members.

Future Considerations

Xenotransplantation

Since the 1980s, organ transplantation has provided a revolutionary, spectacularly effective therapy for end-stage organ failure. The desperation of patients waiting for a suitable organ for transplantation justifies the efforts of those who would improve the rate of organ donation. Some people believe that, even with an impossible 100% retrieval of all available organs for transplantation, demand would continue to outstrip supply. One possible solution to this dilemma is the use of organs from animals instead of humans. Given the constraints of anatomy, physiology, size, numbers, and ethics, the animal most favored as a suitable donor for humans is the pig. At present, any attempt to use pig organs as a substitute for human organs is prevented by the immunologic barriers that exist between the species. However, research undertaken by groups around the world holds out the hope that such transplants may be possible in the future. This research is based on the novel concept that the immune barrier may be breached by changing the pig rather than treating the recipient. Thus, research groups from Australia to England are genetically engineering pigs in a variety of ways to make their organs compatible with humans. Clearly, success from such an endeavor would radically change the whole practice of organ transplantation. Although this new science of xenotransplantation (cross-species transplantation) is making rapid progress, it is generally agreed that xenotransplantation will not be widely available for many years.

Increasing the Donor Pool

Many initiatives to increase organ donation have been introduced throughout Europe, including transplant legislation, publicity campaigns, distribution of donor cards, appointment of TCs, implementation of donor protocols in hospitals, reimbursement of procurement costs, and educational programs. Although all these initiatives may help to increase organ donation, none has been sufficient to make a significant impact on the supply of donor organs.[14] Until alternative forms of treatment become available, the overall aim of professionals involved in organ donation and transplantation must be to come together in an international effort to share initiatives aimed at optimizing the donation and transplant process. An example of effective international cooperation is the Donor Action Programme. This recent collaboration between groups in North America and Europe who are committed to alleviating the donor shortage has led to the development in 1995 of a program designed to help hospitals improve or establish their own tailor-made policies and procedures to optimize the donation process. Donor Action also provides the relevant professional staff with the training and support necessary for successful organ donation. Such a cooperative effort could help to alleviate the organ shortage and to provide the best possible chance of treatment for this group of patients.

Acknowledgments

The authors would like to thank Dr. David White, Department of Surgery, University of Cambridge, and Dr. Johan De Meester, of ET, Leiden, for their considerable contributions to this chapter.

American Perspective

Organ donation has evolved differently in Canada, Europe, the United States, and other areas of the world. The differences are many, but the major one is the greater American dependency in kidney transplantation on living donors (LD), both living-related (LR) and living-unrelated (LU), although the Canadians are also increasing the number of LR transplants. This practice has substantially increased the total number of kidney transplants performed (Table 2-5). In addition, the United States is experimenting with LD in two other organ systems, the pancreas and liver. These efforts, although controversial, have produced acceptable organs for children. At the moment, it must be considered an experimental effort, with considerable debate as to its ethics and hence its future. Throughout this section, we highlight the independent American approach, which was notably described by de Tocqueville. This approach to life and government may be the foundation for how the U.S. consent process has evolved, and it may also be the major obstacle to certain successful approaches used in Europe (e.g., presumed consent).

Historic Aspects

Early on, transplant centers developed primarily from a local initiative generally begun by an individual, who was often a transplant surgeon. As these pioneers showed that transplantation could be a successful form of therapy, they began to ask various colleagues to help in the donation process. This approach resulted in colleagues at local hospitals recognizing potential donors, whereas at other hospitals, donors were not referred and the family was never approached. By the early 1970s, many cities had a local network that produced the necessary number of kidneys. In 1973, support for ESRD included transplantation of kidneys; it soon became apparent that local efforts were insufficient. Until the mid-1970s, LR donors were the backbone of the U.S. transplantation effort, a fact that was probably due to two things: (1) These donations were relatively easy to obtain from the families who demanded treatment, and (2) they were successful (this cannot be overemphasized). For example, before the appearance of cyclosporine in 1983, 1-year primary cadaveric kidney graft survival was just under 50%, with some centers reporting mortality rates up to 20%.

As more patients went on dialysis, it became evident that there were fewer LR donations from the lower socioeconomic population. This trend coexisted with an increase in new renal failure patients from this population, and so there was a much greater need for cadaveric donors. The technique of flushing the kidney with Collins solution, thus preserving the organ longer, resulted in a larger number of viable organs suitable for transplantation. Consequently, organs were shipped to farther destinations with greater success. The availability of cyclosporine in 1983 also had a significant impact on the success of transplantation. By the late 1980s, the outlook for transplantation looked excellent, with the increasing incidence of patients going on dialysis (9% per year) matched by the increasing number of donor organs available.

In 1986, this trend ceased. The number of donors plateaued, and the number of patients going on the waiting list has continued to soar.[15] The reasons for this are many, but one major factor was that 40–50% of the potential donor population would say no when asked. In the early years, the families solicited for donation were well selected, and the affirmation rate was high. With the development of the OPO, more potential donors were

Table 2-5. United Network for Organ Sharing Numbers of U.S. Transplants by Organ and Donor Type

Organ	Donor Type	1988	1989	1990	1991	1992	1993	1994	1995	1996
						Year				
Kidney	Cadaveric	7,231	7,087	7,783	7,731	7,697	8,170	8,383	8,599	8,558
	Living	1,812	1,903	2,094	2,393	2,534	2,850	3,007	3,288	3,481
	Total	9,043	8,990	9,877	10,124	10,231	11,020	11,390	11,887	12,039
Liver	Cadaveric	1,713	2,199	2,676	2,931	3,031	3,404	3,593	3,878	4,012
	Living	0	2	14	22	33	36	60	44	50
	Total	1,713	2,201	2,690	2,953	3,064	3,440	3,653	3,922	4,062
Pancreas	Cadaveric	244	413	526	530	554	772	840	1,021	1,011
	Living	5	4	2	1	3	2	2	6	10
	Total	249	417	528	531	557	774	842	1,027	1,021
Heart	Cadaveric	1,669	1,696	2,096	2,121	2,170	2,295	2,338	2,360	2,342
	Living	7	9	12	4	1	2	3	0	1
	Total	1,676	1,705	2,108	2,125	2,171	2,297	2,341	2,360	2,343
Lung	Cadaveric	33	93	202	401	535	660	708	848	796
	Living	0	0	1	4	0	7	15	23	9
	Total	33	93	203	405	535	667	723	871	805
Heart-Lung	Cadaveric	74	67	52	51	48	60	70	70	39
	Living	0	0	0	0	0	0	0	0	0
	Total	74	67	52	51	48	60	70	70	39
Intestine	Cadaveric	0	0	5	12	22	34	23	44	43
	Living	0	0	0	0	0	0	0	1	2
	Total	0	0	5	12	22	34	23	45	45
Total	Cadaveric	10,964	11,555	13,340	13,777	14,057	15,395	15,955	16,820	16,801
	Living	1,824	1,918	2,123	2,424	2,571	2,897	3,087	3,362	3,553
	Total	12,788	13,473	15,463	16,201	16,628	18,292	19,042	20,182	20,354

Source: Adapted from U.S. Scientific Registry for Transplant Recipients. 1997 Annual Report; Organ Procurement and Transplantation Network. Transplant data: 1988–1996. Richmond, VA: United Network for Organ Sharing; and Division of Transplantation, Bureau of Health Resources Development, Health Resources and Services Administration. Rockville, MD: U.S. Department of Health and Human Services.

solicited. In 1994, with nearly 40,000 patients on a national transplant waiting list, organs were recovered from only 5,100 donors. Since 1993, the number of organ donors has remained relatively static. Estimates of organ donor potential throughout the United States vary, but it is widely believed that the potential ranges from 10,000 to 15,000 donors per year. This gap between the potential and actual donor supply is best understood by evaluating the complex medical, legal, and social interactions that are involved in the organ donation process.

Organ Donation in the United States: Current Activity

The U.S. organ donor program is a voluntary system that relies on altruism.[16] As early as 1968,

Congress passed enabling legislation with the Uniform Anatomical Gift Act. This law, which was adopted by all 50 states, allows individuals to state their intent to donate by signing an organ donor card. The total impact of the donor card is unknown. It may be hindered to some extent by the practice of most organ donation programs of obtaining consent from the next of kin despite the knowledge that a legally executed document (i.e., donor card) exists.

Combining the forces of organ donor programs and organ transplant centers was facilitated by the 1984 adoption of the National Organ Transplant Act, PL 98-507, an amendment to the Public Health Service Act. This law directed the secretary of health and human services to contract for the establishment of the Organ Procurement and Transplantation Network (OPTN); to establish and direct a task force on

Table 2-6. Organs Recovered and Organs Transplanted versus Wait List Patients, 1988–1996

	1988	1989	1990	1991	1992	1993	1994	1995	1996
Organs recovered	12,161	12,883	15,013	15,602	16,024	18,082	19,223	19,727	19,652
Wait list patients*	27,805	31,719	36,925	41,223	46,408	52,309	57,612	65,448	72,386
Organs transplanted	10,964	11,555	13,340	13,777	14,057	15,395	15,955	16,820	16,801
Wait list at year end	16,026	19,095	21,914	24,719	29,415	33,352	37,609	43,983	50,169

*Patients listed at any time during the year.
Source: Adapted from U.S. Scientific Registry for Transplant Recipients. 1997 Annual Report; Organ Procurement and Transplantation Network. Transplant data: 1988–1996. Richmond, VA: United Network for Organ Sharing; and Division of Transplantation, Bureau of Health Resources Development, Health Resources and Services Administration. Rockville, MD: U.S. Department of Health and Human Services.

organ transplantation, to study and make recommendations to improve the field of transplantation; to direct OPOs to distribute organs equitably among waiting recipients; and to prohibit the sale of organs. Subsequently, UNOS was awarded the federal contract to administer the OPTN, and the task force recommendations were incorporated into the Omnibus Budget Reconciliation Act of 1986. These recommendations required (1) all hospitals participating in Medicare and Medicaid to establish written protocols for identifying potential donors and to ensure that families are aware of the option to donate organs, (2) the designation of one OPO per service area, (3) OPOs to meet standards and qualifications to receive payment from Medicare and Medicaid, and (4) OPOs and transplant centers to allocate organs in accordance with established medical criteria and OPTN requirements.[17]

Despite the increase in total number of organs transplanted (from 12,788 in 1988 to 20,354 in 1996; see Table 2-5), there is a growing disparity between organs recovered and number of patients on the transplant waiting list (Table 2-6). Furthermore, the number of patients who died while waiting for an organ transplant has also increased (Table 2-7). (See Appendix 2A.)

Public Attitudes toward Organ Donation

Public attitude surveys consistently confirm support for organ donation. The most recent large study, conducted by Gallup in 1993, found that nearly 9 of 10 Americans support the concept of organ donation, but less than half have made a personal decision about donation of their organs, and only 28%

of the respondents had signed an organ donor card.[18] Support for organ donation correlated positively with higher levels of education and was somewhat lower among nonwhite than white respondents. Because OPOs obtain consent from the next of kin despite the presence of a donor card, the results of this survey suggest that public education efforts should reinforce the need to obtain information about donation, to make an informed decision, and to share this decision with family members.[19]

Many factors have been suggested as barriers to support for organ donation. Among them are religious beliefs, the fear that not everything will be done to save a person's life before organs are removed for transplants, and the concern that organ donation may interfere with a regular funeral service.[20]

Other systems to improve donation have been debated. At least 13 European countries have adopted a presumed consent policy. Practicing under such conditions, physicians are theoretically free to recover organs for transplantation without explicit consent, unless the potential donor expressed an objection before death. A slight variation of presumed consent—mandated choice—has been proposed by the Council on Ethical and Judicial Affairs of the American Medical Association.[21, 22] Under mandated choice, individuals would be required to state their preferences about organ donation when they renew their driver's license, file income tax forms, or perform some other task mandated by the state. To date, no state has passed such legislation or implemented such a plan.

Financial incentives for donor families, ranging from assistance with funeral expenses to tax cred-

Table 2-7. Patients Who Died on the Wait List by Organ, 1988–1996

	1988	1989	1990	1991	1992	1993	1994	1995	1996
Kidney deaths	732	749	921	982	1,055	1,286	1,312	1,494	1,797
Liver deaths	195	284	318	435	493	562	658	799	953
Pancreas deaths	5	21	19	36	34	2	8	3	3
Heart deaths	494	518	612	779	779	761	722	769	744
Lung deaths	16	38	50	137	218	250	283	340	386
Heart/lung deaths	62	74	66	41	43	51	47	28	48
Kidney/pancreas deaths	0	0	0	0	14	59	69	83	91

Source: Adapted from U.S. Scientific Registry for Transplant Recipients. 1997 Annual Report; Organ Procurement and Transplantation Network. Transplant data: 1988–1996. Richmond, VA: United Network for Organ Sharing; and Division of Transplantation, Bureau of Health Resources Development, Health Resources and Services Administration. Rockville, MD: U.S. Department of Health and Human Services.

its, have also been proposed, but there is no consensus on the issue among transplant professionals, health care workers, donor families, or the general public.

The Role of Organ Procurement Organizations

Throughout the United States and Puerto Rico, 66 OPOs play a central role in coordinating all aspects of organ donation (Table 2-8). The majority of OPOs are independent, nonprofit organizations; a smaller number of agencies are based at a single transplant hospital and generally serve only that transplant center. Funding for OPOs is generated through a fee-for-service system. When a medically suitable organ is recovered, the OPO bills a standard organ-acquisition charge to the transplant center. The transplant center then invoices the primary insurance carrier of the transplant recipient. Additionally, OPOs may receive funding from Medicare as a condition of coverage for patients with ESRD.

OPO effectiveness is usually measured by the number of donors from whom organs are recovered per population. In 1994, the Association of OPOs reported a range of donors per population, from 10.8 to 33.9 donors PMP. The variations between countries are not entirely understood, but they may reflect a similar rate of medically suitable potential donors throughout the country and variances in consent rates among different ethnic groups.

The staff at OPOs must generate and sustain enthusiasm among the public and health care pro-

Table 2-8. Organ Procurement Organization Responsibilities

1. Educate health care professionals about donation criteria so that all potential organ donors are identified.
2. Evaluate the suitability of organ donors referred.
3. Discuss the options of organ donation with family members of potential donors.
4. Manage the care of the potential donor to ensure viability of organs to be recovered.
5. Coordinate the allocation of organs to waiting patients.
6. Assist with the recovery, preservation, and transportation of organs.
7. Provide reimbursement to the hospital for costs incurred during the donor evaluation, management, and organ recovery.
8. Provide outcome information to donor families and health care professionals involved with the donor process.

fessionals in support for organ donation. The ability to accomplish these tasks may also contribute to explaining the wide range of performance.

Future Considerations

Donor Organ Acceptance Criteria

Significant changes in donor organ acceptance criteria have occurred to counteract the growing disparity between available organ donors and number of patients on the transplant waiting lists. These include the following:

Table 2-9. Organs Recovered versus Organs Transplanted per Cadaveric Donor, 1988–1994

	1988	1989	1990	1991	1992	1993	1994
Organs recovered per donor	2.98	3.20	3.33	3.44	3.54	3.72	3.77
Organs transplanted per donor	2.73	2.92	3.00	3.10	3.17	3.25	3.22

Source: Adapted from U.S. Scientific Registry for Transplant Recipients. 1997 Annual Report; Organ Procurement and Transplantation Network. Transplant data: 1988–1996. Richmond, VA: United Network for Organ Sharing; and Division of Transplantation, Bureau of Health Resources Development, Health Resources and Services Administration. Rockville, MD: U.S. Department of Health and Human Services.

1. *Acceptance of older donors, who have many inherent problems.* This raises the question of how long these organs will last in a younger recipient (e.g., does a 60-year-old kidney live another 50 years in a 20-year-old recipient?).
2. *Acceptance of marginal donors (e.g., non–heart-beating cadavers).* This would appear, at least in kidney transplants, to mean functioning organs with a lower glomerular filtration rate compared with heart-beating cadaver organs.
3. *Promotion of LR and LU donors.* This is still a fertile area in the United States, with some larger centers doing 40–50% of their kidney transplants with this approach.
4. *Usage of all possible organs from each donor.* From 1988 to 1994, the number of organs transplanted per donor increased from 2.73 to 3.22 (Table 2-9).

Minority Donations

Minority donation in the United States was below the national average (i.e., blacks comprise 12% of the U.S. population, but this group contributed less than 12% of the organs donated in 1990). Blacks were disproportionately over-represented in the dialysis population, but donor numbers lagged far behind. Because of public education programs and the hiring of more minority coordinators, the number of minority donors has increased, and it now approaches the percentage of blacks in the population at large.

Living Donation

In the United States, living donors (both LR and LV) have a real potential for a significant contribution above the current 20% of kidney transplants. A poll of transplant physicians and surgeons suggested that there is a potential to double the number of LR donors; yet, their actual professional practice does not reflect this attitude.[23] Furthermore, not all transplant centers support LV donation, but where it is practiced, the number of LV donors has steadily increased (30% per year), and they accounted for 14% of all LDs in 1996. Although this percentage increase is impressive, it accounted for only 453 kidney donors. The 3-year survival rates for spousal and LV kidney donors are encouraging and will, it is hoped, promote increased transplant activity from this donor population.[8]

Presumed Consent

As noted in the European section of this chapter, it is not always clear when presumed consent is a significant factor. The results in the U.S. surveys make presumed consent an unlikely future approach to organ donation. The Kidney Foundation, UNOS, and the Partnership for Organ Donation surveys of the population at large suggest that 80% of Americans favor donation of a loved one's organs, approximately 50% donate when faced with the actual decision, 30% would support a presumed consent law, and 45% of the population ages 18–30 years favor presumed consent.[24] Nonetheless, presumed consent does not appear to be a viable approach to increased organ donation in the United States because many Americans seem to interpret it as an infringement on their individual freedom.

Financial Incentives

A Kidney Foundation poll indicated that approximately 50% favored a trial of some form of financial incentive.[24] The incentive would be in the form of a burial-type allowance that one could apply for, comparable to the current military practice, which offers a $1,000 allowance to cover some burial expenses. This incentive may range from $1,000 to $2,000. Most families who consented to donate the organs of a family member saw this allowance as an affront to their altruism. Financial incentives therefore would probably play a minimal role in the United States. Approximately 10% of people surveyed in the Kidney Foundation poll were vehemently against any financial incentive.

Conclusions

At this time, we must continue to use every source available to increase the number of donors. This includes public education for both cadaveric and living donors. Currently, the mean in the United States is 20 donors PMP. The first step toward increasing the number of donors would use all means available to make the average the minimum. In other words, if every OPO produced 20 donors PMP, a significant increase in number of organs transplanted would result. Furthermore, it seems reasonable to assume that if some areas can find 35 donors PMP, then all areas should be able to reach an average of 30 donors PMP. It may also be possible to double the number of living donors in the United States. This would amount to approximately 20,000 kidneys and 5,000–6,000 hearts and livers transplanted annually. Although this would not solve the problem, it would help to reduce the number of patients on the transplant waiting list. It is hoped that this change also would reduce the number of patients who die while waiting for a transplant, while scientists solve the problems of xenotransplantation.

Until cures are found for the underlying diseases that destroy organs and thus require replacement with a transplant, or until xenografting is introduced using genetically modified animal organs as a donor source, we must continue to rely on cadaveric (and, when possible, living genetically or emotionally related) organ donation. To improve the supply of organs for transplantation, ongoing public awareness programs are essential. Hospital policies and procedures encouraging organ donation should be expanded, with an individual in each hospital designated as a donor coordinator. The role of this person is to act as a donor advocate, ensuring that families of dying patients have an opportunity to consent to organ or tissue donation. Consent is most likely to be given if the person requesting permission for organ donation has developed a good rapport with the family and discusses the issues clearly, simply, and with compassion.

References

1. Dossetor JB. Transplantation: A Canadian Career-Giving Experience. In PI Terasaki (ed), History of Transplantation: Thirty-Five Recollections. Los Angeles: The Regents of the University of California, 1991.
2. Canadian Organ Replacement Register. Annual Report 1996, Volume 2: Dialysis and Transplantation. Ottawa: Canadian Institute for Health Information, March 1996.
3. Canadian Organ Replacement Register. Annual Report 1998, Volume 1: Dialysis and Transplantation. Ottawa: Canadian Institute for Health Information, June 1998.
4. MORE Program. Annual Report 1996. Toronto: MORE Ontario, 1996.
5. Barrable B, Ferguson B. A model of mixed-market health care delivery: the British Columbia Transplant Society. Leadership 1995;4:18–23.
6. Robinette MA, Marshall WJS, Arbus GS, et al. The donation process. Transplant Proc 1985;17(6 Suppl 3):67–69.
7. Desmeules M, Schaubel D, Fenton S, Mao Y. New and prevalent patients with end-stage renal disease in Canada. A portrait of the year 2000. ASAIO J 1995;41:230–233.
8. Terasaki PI, Cecka JM, Gjertson DW, Takemoto S. High survival rates for kidney transplants from spousal and living unrelated donors. N Engl J Med 1985;333:333–336.
9. Matesanz R, Miranda B, Felipe C. Organ donation and renal transplants in Spain: the impact of transplant coordination. Nephrol Dial Transplant 1994;9:475–478.
10. Quebec Transplant. Annual Report 1996, Montreal, Quebec, Canada, 1996.
11. Elick BA. Transplant Coordinators. In JR Chapman, MH Deierhoi, C Wight (eds), Organ and Tissue Donation for Transplantation. London: Oxford University Press, 1997.
12. Matesanz R, Miranda B, Felipe C. Organ procurement and renal transplants in Spain: the impact of transplant coordinators. Clin Transpl 1994;8:281–286.
13. Houssin D. L'etablissement Français des greffes. Entente 1995;1:3.
14. Cohen B. Finding a cure to dramatic fall in organ procurement rates. Nephrol News & Issues 1994;2:21–22.
15. Evans RW, Orians CE, Asher NL. The potential supply of organ donors. An assessment of the efficiency of organ procurement efforts in the United States. JAMA 1992;267:239–246.
16. Siminoff LA, Arnold RM, Caplan AL. Asking for altruism when death occurs: who asks for organ donation and why? Transplant Proc 1996;28:3632–3638.

17. U.S. General Accounting Office. Increased effort needed to boost supply and ensure equitable distribution of organs. Washington, D.C.: GAO/HRD, 1993;39–56.

18. The Gallup Organization. Highlights of Public Attitudes toward Organ Donation and Transplantation. Princeton, NJ: The Gallup Organization, March 1993; 1–8.

19. Siminoff LA, Arnold RM, Caplan AL, et al. Public policy governing organ and tissue procurement in the United States. Ann Intern Med 1995;123:10–17.

20. Youngner SJ, Arnold RM. Ethical, psychological, and public policy implications of procuring organs from non–heart-beating cadavers. JAMA 1993;269:2769–2774.

21. Spital A. Mandated choice, the preferred solution to the organ shortage? Arch Intern Med 1992;152:2421–2424.

22. Council on Ethical and Judicial Affairs, American Medical Association. Strategies for cadaveric organ procurement: mandated choice and presumed consent. JAMA 1994;272:809–812.

23. Beasley CL, Hull AR, Rosenthal JT. Living kidney donation: a survey of professional attitudes and practices. Am J Kidney Dis 1997;30:549–557.

24. National Kidney Foundation. Public and Professional Reaction to Xenotransplantation and Other Options to Increase Organ Availability. New York: National Kidney Foundation (in preparation).

Appendix 2A
Organ Donation Process

Plan

Donor Identification
Referral and Evaluation
Consent
    Presumed Consent "Opt Out"
    Informed Consent "Opt In"
Declaration of Brain Death
Donor Management
Follow-Up

Donor Identification

The crucial initial step of identifying donors is still a problem despite considerable efforts to increase awareness and participation of health care professionals working in intensive care units (ICUs), neurosurgical units, and emergency departments. In a study of Canadian physicians' attitudes toward organ donation,[1] although 95% supported organ donation and 63% had signed an organ donor card, only 55.4% indicated that they knew how to refer potential donors. In the same study, 57% said they did not like to become involved in organ donation, most often (75%) because of the associated emotional strain. Almost 75% of physicians expressed reluctance to approach the relatives of a potential organ donor despite having generally positive attitudes toward organ donation. Failing to initiate the donation process has several explanations, such as the associated emotional strain, the time commitment involved, and a reluctance to acknowledge failure in a patient's resuscitation while advocating organ donation. The next of kin of potential donors sometimes themselves raise the possibility of organ donation with the health care team.

All organ donors have experienced some form of irreversible brain damage, usually because of hypoxia, intracerebral hemorrhage, trauma, or nonmetastasizing primary brain tumor. With the dramatic increases in seat belt use in Canada (90% compliance in 1994) because of laws passed in the late 1970s and early 1980s (depending on the province), deaths from motor vehicle accidents (MVAs) have significantly decreased (Figure 2A-1). In Ontario from 1988 to 1994, the number of donors from MVAs declined from 58 to 33 (a decrease from 30% to 24% of total donors).[2] Another problem for Canadian organ donor programs is that, because the number of hospital beds has decreased, patients with irreversible brain damage referred to neurosurgical units, who after investigation (by computerized tomography scan or magnetic resonance imaging) are found to have inoperable conditions but are not yet brain dead, are no longer admitted to the neurosurgical units. Instead, they are returned to the referring center for their terminal care. As their condition deteriorates, respiratory or cardiac arrest occurs, but organ donation has rarely been planned.

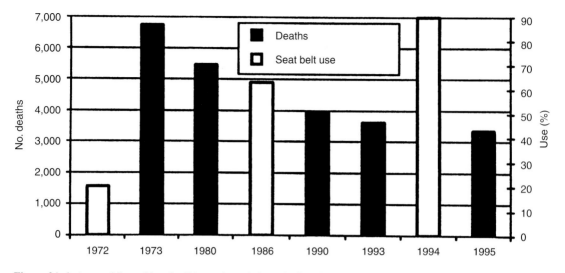

Figure 2A-1. Automobile accident fatalities and seat belt use in Canada. (Adapted from Canadian Motor Vehicle Traffic Collision Statistics: 1995. Ottawa: Transport Canada, 1995.)

Referral and Evaluation

Once a suitable donor has been identified, a physician or nurse in the unit calls the regional organ procurement organization (OPO), and the procurement coordinator (PC) on call obtains the relevant clinical and biochemical information over the phone. A determination is made that the organs are healthy and that the potential organ does not have untreated sepsis or a potentially transmittable disease, such as human immunodeficiency virus infection or hepatitis B. Patients with cancer (except those having nonmetastasizing biopsy-proved primary brain tumors or basal cell carcinomas) are also excluded. A history of hypertension, diabetes, or hepatitis C is not an absolute contraindication but requires further consideration. When conditions preclude organ donation, arrangements for donation of the cornea and other tissues (e.g., bones, heart valves) are made. Otherwise, the PC provides some general advice on management and helps to arrange the next steps.

Consent

In Canada, organ donation is voluntary, with consent required from the next of kin even in the presence of a signed organ donor card or driver's license (both of which are considered legally binding documents). Registering a commitment to donate one's organs at death is encouraged in three ways: on part of the driver's license in all 10 provinces; when obtaining a government health card (provision for organ donation is part of the card in only four provinces); and by various organizations that provide organ donor cards. To ensure that organ donation occurs, those who sign are advised to discuss their wishes with their families.

A 1994 unpublished survey by the Mutual Group revealed that 77% of Canadians were willing to donate organs, but only 58% had signed an organ donor card. Previous survey results have suggested several reasons for the discrepancy between people's positive attitudes and their behavior: superstition (e.g., signing a card might hasten one's death), fear or mistrust (e.g., after trauma, patients with a signed card might be managed differently in the emergency department), religion (an erroneous view that certain religions forbid organ donation), and procrastination (they never got around to signing a card).[3]

In prior surveys and focus groups,[4] Canadians were generally opposed to presumed consent because organ donation represented the final government tax, topping off many years of taxation. A review of organ donor rates in various countries that compared those with and without presumed consent suggests no correlation of improved donation with presumed consent. Even in countries having presumed consent, permission from the next of kin for organ donation is still usually requested.[5–8]

Consent is usually obtained from the physician caring for the patient in the ICU or neurosurgical

Table 2A-1. Principles Useful in Obtaining Consent

Provide a private and comfortable room for discussion
  with the patient's relatives.
Review the circumstances leading to brain death and its
  clinical aspects with the family.
Use simple, nontechnical language.
Show compassion and sympathy.
Provide time between notification of brain death and the
  request for organ donation.
Emphasize the benefits that occur from organ donation and
  the future consolation that some good resulted from the
  family's tragedy.
Avoid such terms as *procurement* and *harvesting*.
Accept a positive consent with personal thanks and gratitude on behalf of the transplant programs and recipients;
  inform donor's family that a follow-up letter of appreciation will be sent.
Accept consent refusal politely and with thanks for the time
  spent to consider organ donation during such a difficult
  time.

unit. Approaching the next of kin for organ donation has become part of the job description and
training of PCs in Canada, with the result that they
are gradually participating in this responsibility.
There is good evidence that the type of approach
used in obtaining consent determines outcome.[9]
Therefore, this important task should always be
assigned to someone who is experienced and who
applies techniques that are likely to result in an
affirmative response (Table 2A-1).

In Europe, despite evidence of considerable public support for organ donation, many countries still
report significant refusal rates. In 1994, data from
United Kingdom Transplant Support Service Association (UKTSSA) and Organización Nacional de
Transplantes revealed national refusal rates of 26%
and 23.6%, respectively. Where European legislation allows postmortem removal of organs for transplantation, methods of establishing no objection to
donation from either the donor or the donor's relatives are classified as either presumed consent "opt
out" or informed consent "opt in."

Presumed Consent "Opt Out"

Individuals can register their objection to organ
donation. This can range from a verbal declaration
(e.g., France) to registration on a central computer

(e.g., Austria, Portugal). This register may even be
linked to all transplant units (e.g., Belgium). In all
cases in which no objection is confirmed, it is not
usually legally necessary to inform relatives of the
intention to remove organs and tissue. However,
practice differs between countries. Much interest has
been shown in the presumed consent system.
National registries for the public to lodge their
wishes seem sensible, although only Belgium (population 10.1 million) has relatively long-term experience. In 1987, Belgium implemented "opting-out"
legislation and, in 1988, introduced a central registration system. Every citizen can register his or her
objection (or consent) to organ donation in his or her
local town hall. Consultation with the database is
mandatory before any organ or tissue removal, but
there is no obligation to inform the donor's relatives.
Between 1988 and May 1995, 194,362 citizens registered their will to be an organ donor. Of these,
1.9% of the total population explicitly objected,
whereas only 0.05% used the facility to explicitly
consent to organ donation. The law resulted in an
immediate increase in organ procurement.[10]

Presumed consent legislation has successfully
increased organ donation. However, caution must be
used in comparing organ donation figures between
European countries that appear to have a presumed
consent system and those that do not. Many differences exist in how hospitals and doctors in charge
of potential donors implement these regulations.[11]
European procurement data reveal that in 1994, for
example, Spain had the highest number of donated
organs per million population (PMP), even though
Spain is a presumed consent country that chooses
not to use the legislation. Presumed consent in countries such as Austria, Belgium, and France, however,
has not resulted in comparable donation rates. On
the contrary, donation figures in these countries have
fallen sharply or plateaued, indicating that neither
public nor professionals automatically accept presumed consent legislation.[12]

Informed Consent "Opt In"

Individuals can carry a signed donor card to indicate
their wish to be an organ donor. In the absence of a
card, relatives are approached to establish that there
is no objection to organ donation. Even if a donor
card is found, in most instances, relatives are
approached for their views. This system relies heavily

on the communication of wishes between family members. The United Kingdom (population 58.3 million), an "opt-in" country, introduced a central register in 1994 for members of the public who want to donate. Registration can be made by post, by driver's license, and through general practitioners' surgeries. The register is maintained by UKTSSA, and transplant coordinators have 24-hour access to the computer, but it is still mandatory to consult the donor's relatives. By April 1, 1995, more than one million applications had been received. Other "opt-in" European countries are closely watching the results of this initiative with a view to introducing a similar system.

Families refuse to donate organs for many reasons, but wide differences in refusal rates between and within all countries suggest that the method and timing of the request might well influence a family's decision.

The Eurotransplant Foundation, concerned about the rise in refusals of organ donation, has taken the initiative in addressing this particular issue. The European Donor Hospital Education Programme (EDHEP) was created in 1991 to meet the widely perceived need to help health professionals feel effective in dealing with bereaved relatives and in requesting organ donation. Their highly interactive skills and awareness workshops are moderated by qualified trainers. The workshops are available for critical care staff who wish to sharpen their communication skills, heighten their sensitivity to the needs of bereaved relatives, and learn ways of making the donation request. The workshops end with guidance to participants in establishing hospital protocols for the care of the bereaved and making requests for organ donation. EDHEP has now been translated into 17 languages and is used in more than 30 countries,[13] thereby demonstrating the need for this kind of professional training. Several countries are now beginning to incorporate EDHEP into national medical and nurse training.

Declaration of Brain Death

In Canada, each province has a Human Tissue Gift Act, which allows for organ donation when brain death has occurred. Declaration of this state is determined by any two physicians, providing they are not part of the transplant team. Hospitals participating in organ donation have developed guidelines to assist in the determination of brain death, based on the recommendations of the Canadian Neurological Society.[14] Comparable guidelines are also applied in Europe and the United States (see Chapter 3, Declaration of Brain Death).

Donor Management

Several hours are usually necessary to arrange for various tests to determine suitability for transplantation of each organ, to declare brain death, and to permit time for some retrieval teams to travel from distant centers. During this time, the donor must be carefully managed to optimize organ function (see Chapter 4, Management of the Organ Donor). The PC from the regional OPO often travels to the donor hospital to provide guidance and advice for the attending staff. During this time, location and preparation of suitable recipients are initiated to minimize the time between organ removal and transplantation (cold storage time). When possible, tissue typing is begun to identify the best HLA match among the potential renal recipients.

Removal of donated organs usually takes place in the donor hospital, but sometimes the donor is transported to the regional transplant center, usually because of lack of availability of operating facilities in the donor hospital. Storage times vary for each organ, but generally, transplantation is arranged as soon as possible to minimize ischemic damage. Organs are distributed according to algorithms predetermined by the transplant surgeons and physicians involved with each organ group. Kidneys are allocated to local patients according to ABO compatibility, a negative cross-match test, best HLA match (patients having a zero mismatch with the donor at the B and DR loci are given priority), and length of time on the waiting list. If no suitable recipient is located locally, the kidney is offered to other regional programs in the province. If no recipient is found in the province, other centers across Canada are contacted.

Similarly, in the United States, organ allocation begins when the OPO coordinator contacts the United Network for Organ Sharing (UNOS) organ center. Based on the donor's variables (e.g., height, weight, age, sex, blood group), a national computer matching program is run for each organ donated. Patients listed with the transplant centers served by the original OPO have local priority. If the organs cannot be placed locally, the organs are offered to programs in a larger region, then nationally.

Due to the size of the waiting lists for kidney transplants, most kidneys are transplanted locally: This concept occurs in most transplant programs worldwide. High-priority patients then take precedence for extrarenal organs; otherwise, these organs are allocated locally according to size, state of health of the recipient, and length of time on the waiting list. Organs not placed in Canada are distributed to UNOS for transplantation in the United States or elsewhere in the world.

Follow-Up

A telephone call is made to the donor family the next day. The director of the OPO and the PC write a bereavement letter extending consolation to the donor's family and expressing appreciation on behalf of the transplant recipients, their families, and the transplant team. Letters are also sent to the donor hospital's nursing and medical staff, thanking them for their participation in the donation process, emphasizing the enormous benefit to the recipients through their efforts, and encouraging them to continue to help in the future. Most transplant recipients write their own personal letters of thanks, which, to maintain confidentiality, are sent by the OPO to the donor's family.

References

1. Molzahn AE. Knowledge and attitudes of physicians regarding organ donation. Ann RCPSC 1997;30: 29–32.
2. Canadian Motor Vehicle Traffic Collision Statistics: 1995. Ottawa: Transport Canada, 1995.
3. The Gallup Organization. Highlights of Public Attitudes toward Organ Donation and Transplantation. Princeton, NJ: The Gallup Organization, March 1993;1–8.
4. Corlett S. Public attitudes to organ transplantation. Transplant Proc 1985;17(6 Suppl 3):103–110.
5. Michielsen P. Organ shortage—what to do? Transplant Proc 1992;24:2391–2392.
6. Land W, Cohen B. Postmortem and living organ donation in Europe: transplant laws and activities. Transplant Proc 1992;24:2165–2167.
7. Kittur DS, Hogan MM, Thukral VK, et al. Incentives for organ donation? The United Network for Organ Sharing Ad Hoc Donations Committee. Lancet 1991; 338:1441–1443.
8. Randhawa G. Improving the supply of organ donors in the UK: a review of health policies. Health Education Journal 1995;54:241–250.
9. Garrison RN, Bently FR, Raque GN, et al. There is an answer to the shortage of organ donors. Surg Gynecol Obstet 1991;173:391–396.
10. Roels L, Deschoolmeester G, Vanrenterghem Y. A profile of people objecting to organ donation in a country with a presumed consent law: data from the Belgian National Registry. Transplant Proc 1997;29:1473–1475.
11. Cohen B. Finding a cure to dramatic fall in organ procurement rates. Neph News & Issues 1994;2:21–22.
12. Wight C. Dying for a transplant. Br J Cardiol 1995; 2:33-34.
13. Wight C, Jager K, Blok G, et al. Overview of the European Donor Hospital Education Program. Transplant Proc 1996;28:422–423.
14. Canadian Congress of Neurological Sciences. Guidelines for the diagnosis of brain death. CMAJ 1987;136: 200A–200B.

Chapter 3
Declaration of Brain Death

John P. Girvin

Historic Perspective

Before the middle of the twentieth century, prolonging life in people without normal respiratory movements was extremely difficult. Anesthetists manually ventilated patients in deep stages of anesthesia, during the triage of acutely traumatized patients with readily reversible lesions, and for patients who required additional gas exchange transiently because of a compromised respiratory state. Patients who lost their natural spontaneous respiratory function for prolonged periods through compromise of the respiratory anterior motor neurons or brain stem were relegated to an external mechanical ventilating device. Although a number of such positive-pressure external devices were used earlier in the twentieth century, particularly by surgeons, the poliomyelitis epidemics necessitated their use for long-term ventilation. In North America, Drinker and McKhann developed an "iron lung."[1] (See the review by Masferrer, Dolan, and Ward for an authoritative history.[2]) Around midcentury, the only monitoring of blood gases during surgery under general anesthesia consisted of drawing arterial or venous blood. The anesthetist and surgeon would wait for tens of minutes and sometimes an hour or longer for the return of the laboratory assessment of blood carbon dioxide and oxygen! At approximately this time, automatic ventilators were introduced that could be easily used with endotracheal intubation.[2]

With the rapidly increasing technology of the 1950s and 1960s, it became possible to sustain life in the absence of a normal functioning respiratory center (brain stem). The cardiovascular system could be supported by a plethora of cardiovascular drugs, which allowed, at least transiently and, albeit artificially, the adequate perfusion of tissues and organs. Thus, during the 1960s, people with compromised respiratory and cardiovascular systems could be kept alive for hours, days, and even weeks.

With this new ability came the evolution of human organ transplantation, which was mainly renal transplantation at first. It was suspected that transplantation was more likely to be successful with the use of kidneys that were perfused until the time of harvesting rather than cadaver kidneys. Furthermore, neurologists and neurosurgeons knew that, with the aid of respirators, some patients could sustain massive destructive lesions of the brain (e.g., trauma, intracerebral hemorrhage) that were clearly incompatible with survival.

These developments led to a number of new logistical and bioethical dilemmas. In earlier times, once it had been shown that patients had these lesions, which were usually intracranial space-occupying lesions, the manual ventilating of such emergently intubated patients simply ceased, and patients were pronounced dead. With the advent of respirators, these patients could be sustained for reasonable periods. The definitions of reasonable period and irreversibility were suddenly of profound practical importance. Apart from the ethical question of defining brain death, economics began to be a factor as more such individuals were kept alive by artificial means in the most expensive beds in hospitals: the intensive care unit.

Thus, brain death had to be redefined to accommodate patients who lacked the normal spontaneous respiratory and cardiovascular activity (e.g., brain stem activity) to sustain life and whose brain injury was incompatible with survival.

Initial Criteria for Determination of Brain Death

In 1968, a landmark article appeared in the *Journal of the American Medical Association*, "A Definition of Irreversible Coma," written by an ad hoc committee at Harvard Medical School.[3] It was the first attempt at defining the neurologic findings in a comatose patient that were considered incompatible with survival. They included the absence of (1) response to external stimuli, (2) respirations, (3) reflexes, and (4) electroencephalographic (EEG) activity (Table 3-1). Neurologically, the Harvard criteria specified that there be no response to any type of external stimuli (e.g., pain, tracheal tug, touch applied to the back of the throat), no evidence of any type of spontaneous respiratory activity, and no evidence of reflex activity. Additionally, there must be no evidence of any type of electrocerebral activity,

Table 3-1. Harvard Criteria for Brain Death

1. Absence of response to external stimuli
   Total unawareness
   No response to intensely painful stimuli
2. Absence of respirations
   Observations over at least a 1-hour period by a physician
   Absence of spontaneous breathing after turning off the respirator for 3 minutes, provided the patient had been breathing room air for at least 10 minutes before
3. Absence of reflexes
   Absence of elicitable reflexes
   Pupils fixed and dilated, no response to light
   Blinking absent
   No ocular movement with head turning and cold-water calorics
   Corneal and pharyngeal reflexes absent
   No evidence of postural activity
4. Absence of electroencephalographic activity
   Flat or isoelectric electroencephalogram (EEG) (EEG not essential, as of 1969)

as determined by the recording of the EEG under rigid criteria governing the application of electrodes to the scalp and the adjustment of EEG parameters.[4-6] These criteria had to be satisfied on at least two occasions separated by a minimum of 24 hours.

In the same year, the Canadian Medical Association published its statement on brain death,[7] and the World Medical Assembly, at its meeting in Sydney, proposed the acceptance of the concept that brain death in fact represented whole-body death.[8]

Modifications to the Definition of Brain Death

After the 1968 publication of the Harvard committee, the "Harvard criteria" of brain death were used throughout the Western world in varying degrees. Initially, in the late 1960s and early 1970s, these criteria were used religiously in the pronouncement of death. In some jurisdictions before 1968 or soon after publication of the Harvard criteria, organs were harvested just before turning off a respirator, usually after many days of its use. Once the Harvard criteria became known in a given jurisdiction, they were used as early as possible in the course of potential cases of irreversible coma. This was especially true when organ procurement was under consideration, with the presumption that organs taken then were more satisfactory than those taken after prolonged survival under artificial conditions.

Most patients who satisfied the criteria for brain death were neurosurgical patients. These patients had a variety of lesions, but the majority fell into the categories of progressive and irreversible increasing brain swelling from trauma, hemorrhagic diseases (e.g., ruptured aneurysms, ruptured arteriovenous malformations, spontaneous intracerebral hemorrhages), or large infarcts of the brain. Later, many physicians urged dropping the rule of two examinations 24 hours apart in cases with obvious irreversible brain damage.[9–13] Thus, in cases with obvious irreversible brain compression, a single neurologic and EEG examination was considered sufficient to determine brain death.

It was also soon appreciated that individuals who satisfied the brain stem criteria for brain death might nevertheless show some spinal reflexes.[14–16] Initially, this was evident in abortive reflexes involving the neck musculature. Ivan labeled these intersegmental tonic neck reflexes *neck-arm flexion, neck-hip flexion*, and *neck-abdominal reflexes*.[15] It also became apparent that segmental (tendon) reflexes may persist in brain death.[14, 15, 17] Thus, the presence of spinal reflexes, very frequently abortive or rudimentary, were ignored, providing that all the criteria for brain stem death were present.

Thus began a series of modifications and refinements of the Harvard criteria, which have led to the currently accepted criterion for the declaration of brain death. In 1969, the EEG was abandoned as a necessary criteria for brain death.[18] Since then, various modifications have been made in different jurisdictions.[19, 20] Slightly different wording of the criteria emerged in different countries, such as Australia,[21, 22] Germany,[23] Denmark,[24] Sweden,[11] Japan,[12, 25] and the United Kingdom.[26] Even in the United States, criteria were independently modified in various states, and two groups developed national criteria, the Harvard criteria and the criteria established by the National Institute of Neurological Diseases and Stroke (i.e., Collaborative Study Group of Cerebral Survival).[27–31]

Nearly all jurisdictions have passed legislation on considerations of either the definition of death or the procurement and harvesting of organs for human transplantation. Before this, the legal definition of death, according to *Black's Law Dictionary* (1951), was "The cessation of life, ceasing to exist, defined by a physician as a total stoppage of blood and cessation of animal and vital functions consequent thereof, such as respirations, pulse, etc."[32] Kansas was the first state in the United States (1971) and Manitoba the first province in Canada (1974) to enact statutes that recognized brain death as equivalent to whole-body death. By 1981, more than half the states had enacted such statutes.[31]

The 1981 report of the Law Reform Commission of Canada to Parliament recommended the acceptance of whole-brain death as equivalent to human death. These legislative decisions reflect the views of Pope Pius XII,[33] who in 1957, a decade before the Harvard criteria, acknowledged to an International Congress of Anesthesiology that the declaration of death in a given patient was the responsibility of the attending physicians. Referring to the artificial, cardiopulmonary preservation of life in irreversible coma, he said, "since these forms of treatment go beyond the ordinary means to which one is bound, it cannot be held that there is an obligation to use them. . . . It remains for the doctors to give a clear and precise definition of death."

Canadian Criteria for Declaration of Brain Death

Canadian neurologists and neurosurgeons, under the auspices of the Canadian Congress of Neurological Sciences, published a series of papers leading to the currently accepted guidelines on the declaration of brain death.[34–36] These criteria include (1) the establishment of a cause for brain death, (2) deep coma with the absence of any type of coordinated movement and response to pain, (3) the absence of brain stem reflexes, and (4) the absence of spontaneous respiration (Table 3-2).

1. Establishment of the cause of brain death. Generally, a cause compatible with brain death is established relatively easily. In cases in which no cause is established (i.e., when the patient has coma of undetermined etiology), it is much more complex to establish cessation of brain activity and irreversibility. The patient's core temperature must be close to normal and certainly above 32.2°C. There must be evidence, either historically or by blood studies, to rule out the simulation of brain death through an overdose of drugs. When the patient has

Table 3-2. Canadian Guidelines for the Diagnosis of Brain Death

An etiology of brain death is established, and potentially reversible conditions are excluded (i.e., drug intoxication, particularly with barbiturates, sedatives, and hypnotics; treatable metabolic disorders; hypothermia [core temperature <32.2°C]; shock; and peripheral nerve or muscle dysfunction due to disease or neuromuscular blocking drugs).

Patient is in deep coma and shows no motor response to stimuli applied to any body regions in the cranial nerve distribution. There is absence of movements, such as cerebral seizures, dyskinetic movements, and decorticate or decerebrate posturing.

Brain stem reflexes are absent.

  Pupils are midsize or larger and unreactive to light (in the absence of atropine or related drugs that may block the pupillary response).

  Corneal reflex is absent.

  Vestibulo-ocular reflex is absent. This reflex should be tested with caloric stimulation while the patient's head is 30 degrees above the horizontal plane. In adults, a minimum of 120 ml of ice water should be used.

  Pharyngeal reflexes are absent (i.e., grimacing or other motor response to pharyngeal or tracheal suctioning).

The patient is apneic when taken off the respirator and $Paco_2$ levels are allowed to increase (apnea test) to elicit an appropriate respiratory stimulus (pH <7.3).

The conditions listed above persist when the patient is reassessed; depending on the etiology, this interval may range from 2–24 hours. Observation for at least 24 hours is recommended to confirm brain death due to anoxia or ischemia.

Source: Adapted from Canadian Congress of Neurological Sciences. Guidelines for the diagnosis of brain death. CMAJ 1987;136:200A–200B.

not been seen immediately before the coma-producing ictus or in circumstances compatible in any way with the ingestion of excessive amounts of sedative drugs, a reasonable period is required for "washout" of any such drug. Under these circumstances, the patient should be examined and, sometimes, additional confirmatory tests should be made at 24-hour intervals and perhaps even longer.

2. *Deep coma with the absence of any type of coordinated movement and response to pain.* There must be deep coma, in which there is no response whatsoever to pain applied to the trigeminal area of the head or any response of a coordinated type to

pain applied elsewhere in the body. Postures such as the decerebrate or decorticate must not be present in any form, abortive or otherwise. Thus, although there may be some evidence of spinal reflexes (see below), there must be no evidence of complex postures, which require the anatomic substrate of the brain stem for their appearance.

3. *Absence of brain stem reflexes.* Brain stem reflexes must be entirely absent. Any suggestion of an abortive brain stem reflex precludes the satisfaction of this criterion and thereby precludes the declaration of brain death. Thus, there must be the absence of the pupillary light, corneal, vestibulo-ocular (e.g., doll's head maneuvers and caloric responses), gag, and tracheal tug or suction reflexes.

4. *Absence of spontaneous respiration.* One of the most difficult criteria to satisfy for the determination of brain death was the absence of spontaneous respiration. At one time, this criterion was satisfied by the simple removal of ventilatory support, a practice that seems barbaric and physiologically foolhardy when compared to the present practice. This withdrawal, which would often take as long as 5–10 minutes, resulted in the patient being subjected to the additional insults of hypoxia and respiratory acidosis. These would certainly aggravate any condition of raised intracranial pressure and, more important, might convert a reversible brain lesion into an irreversible one. Furthermore, it was apparent to most that the viability of potential harvested organs from such a patient might well be compromised (a fact that has now been confirmed).[37, 38]

Apnea Test

Currently, the apnea test is almost universally accepted to determine the viability of the respiratory center. The patient is preoxygenated with 100% oxygen for 10 minutes before the test, thus ensuring the highest possible concentration of oxygen in the blood at the time of testing. If the blood carbon dioxide level is at least 40 mm Hg, the patient is disconnected from the ventilator, a catheter is inserted into the endotracheal tube, and oxygen (fraction of inspired oxygen of 1.0) is delivered at the rate of 6 liters per minute for 10 minutes to maintain arterial oxygen saturation. During the apneic period, the arterial carbon dioxide concentration in the blood is expected to rise approximately 2–3 mm Hg per minute over 10 minutes.[39–43]

The arterial carbon dioxide concentration must reach a critical level, at which there is maximal physiologic drive of the respiratory center. This must be at least 50 mm Hg,[13, 21, 44] although some think that 60 mm Hg is a better figure.[31, 40, 45–49] According to the Canadian guidelines,[34] 50–55 mm Hg is sufficient to stimulate the brain stem respiratory center. This corresponds to an arterial pH below 7.30, assuming a normal range of serum bicarbonate. In the situation of a "CO_2 retainer," in whom serum bicarbonate levels are chronically elevated, the arterial carbon dioxide must be raised even further so that the patient is given an adequate respiratory drive. In the absence of any respiratory effort, gases are drawn at the end of the apneic period to confirm that an adequate respiratory drive exists (pH less than 7.30). The patient is then considered to have satisfied the criteria of the absence of spontaneous respiration.

Potential Confounding Variables in Determination of Brain Death

Many extenuating circumstances may interfere with the physical examination involved in the determination of brain death, and other factors may influence the patient's response to this examination (Table 3-3). Most of these relate to trauma, hypothermia, drug intoxication, metabolic and endocrine causes of coma, and the application of adult brain death criteria to children. These factors may have been of more concern in the 1960s and 1970s, when clinical experience and the sophistication of brain imaging were less well developed. Nevertheless, they deserve mention.

Recognition that brain death could be simulated in cases of hypothermia and drug intoxication was widespread enough when the Harvard criteria were developed that an important criterion was the certainty of an etiology for brain death. The temporal separation of examinations (24 hours apart) reflected the need to make certain that body temperature was normal and that any type of drug intoxication was identified and had in fact lessened.

Hypothermia

It has been known for many years that severe hypothermia results in the loss of normal neurologic

Table 3-3. Confounding Variables in Determination of Brain Death

Metabolic
  Hypothermia (core temperature <32.2°C)
  Drug intoxication (particularly barbiturates, diazepam, meprobamate, methaqualone, trichloroethylene)
  Hypoglycemia, hyperglycemia, ketoacidosis
  Uremia
  Hepatic failure
  Hyponatremia
  Hypercalcemia
  Myxedema
  Adrenal cortical failure
  Panhypopituitarism
  Reye's syndrome
  Shock
  Unrecognized muscle paralysis due to neuromuscular disease or neuromuscular blocking agents
Anatomic
  Ocular trauma (traumatic mydriasis)
  Previous anterior chamber surgery
  Artificial globe or contact lenses
  Middle ear injury
  Cervical spine injury (limits cervical spine manipulation)
  High cervical spinal cord injury

signs and indeed simulates the neurologic criteria of brain death. Electrocerebral silence may also be seen in deep hypothermia. This became more important after the introduction of the concept of brain death because of many patients with clinical criteria of brain death who demonstrated complete reversibility of cerebral depression after elevation of body temperature.[50–54] Accordingly, the Canadian Congress of Neurological Sciences recommends a core temperature above 32.2°C to apply clinical criteria of brain death.[35]

Drug Intoxication

Severe drug intoxication is known to be associated with the clinical findings of apparent death.[55, 56] The picture was much more confused many years ago, when blood levels of many potentially intoxicating drugs could not be estimated. Thus, unlike body temperature, the presence of drug intoxication can never be completely evaluated when the etiology of coma is uncertain. Under these circumstances, therefore, a greater temporal separation of the examinations certifying brain death is required to allow for washout of the drug. When the drug is clearly identified, non–coma-producing levels of the drug must be obtained before clinical examination becomes valid.

Anatomic Variables

Trauma to the eyes or previous anterior chamber surgery may interfere with testing of the pupillary reflex. The presence of an artificial globe, contact lenses, or Bell's palsy can interfere with the corneal reflex. The vestibulo-ocular reflexes elicited through doll's head maneuvers may be affected by middle ear injuries and cannot be carried out in the presence of a potential cervical spinal injury. Diseases or injuries affecting motor neurons (i.e., high, complete cervical cord transection) preclude motor responses to painful stimulation and apnea testing. Such instances are rare, and in the hands of an experienced clinician, these individual exceptions usually do not interfere with the determination of brain death. In some of these instances, however, ancillary tests are required to supplement historic and clinical examination.

Declaration of Brain Death in Children

There was early recognition that the clinical criteria used for the declaration of brain death in adult patients might not be applicable to children. Ashwal and Schneider noted that the EEG was less accurate in infants than in adults in disclosing electrocerebral silence in terminal coma.[57] In fact, in North America, the American Uniform Death Act cautioned against the uncritical application of the adult criteria to children.[31] The Canadian Medical Association took a similar position, as recommended by the Canadian Congress of Neurological Sciences.[34–36]

The concerns and potential difficulties with the declaration of brain death in children have been addressed in a number of publications.[58–63] Since the early 1990s, evidence has increased that the adult guidelines can be applied to most children, which leaves the uncertainty largely with neonates and very young infants.[64–66]

Given the importance of the procurement and harvesting of healthy hearts for transplantation to infants born with aplastic hearts, brief mention should be made of what constitutes brain death in the case of the anencephalic infant. The use of anencephalic infants as a resource for such hearts has been the subject of two conferences.[67, 68] Most of the controversy around the use of such infants' organs has centered on the bioethical issues about the definition of life. The question of what constitutes personhood, however, and whether their use would lead to the use of other hopelessly mentally compromised human beings has made it important that these infants do not satisfy the current criteria for whole-brain death in either adults or children. The question remains whether the adult criteria should be modified specifically to deal with the anencephalic infant.[69, 70]

Supplemental Confirmatory Tests of Brain Death

Electrical

With the Harvard criteria, the EEG came to be of primary importance in the determination of brain death. Although some have expressed concern about inconsistencies in the terminal EEG,[71–73] many of the apparent inconsistencies of so-called electrocerebral silence were attributed to the failure to apply the rigidly defined criteria for recording the EEG in such cases.[14] In general, however, when the EEG is carried out with religious adherence to the details of technical recording, it is a very important confirmatory test of brain death. In 1970, Shalit and colleagues[74] showed that the EEG was perhaps the best criterion of brain death. They examined the cerebral metabolic rate of the dying brain with coincident neurologic and EEG examination. The last sign of brain function to disappear was electrical activity. In addition to the EEG, various types of evoked responses have similarly been used (e.g., auditory[75–77] and somatosensory[76, 78, 79]).

Cerebral Angiography

It is not difficult to make a comfortable diagnosis of death when the clinical criteria for the declaration of brain death are satisfied and when an obvious, irreversible, intracranial structural lesion exists. During the 1960s and 1970s, angiography in such patients failed to disclose evidence of intracranial

Figure 3-1. Lateral radiographs of common carotid artery show no blood flow to the brain. **A.** Early phase shows filling of external carotid artery (*closed arrows*) and filling of internal carotid artery to the level of base of the skull (*open arrow*).

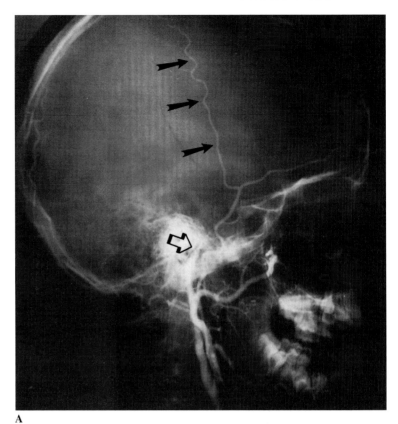

A

circulation. Thus, the absence of intracranial blood flow demonstrated by cerebral angiography became an important confirmatory adjunct to the clinical examination (Figure 3-1).[80–90]

Radioisotope Brain Scan

The refinement of the gamma camera in the 1970s and the introduction of the radiopharmaceutical technetium-99m for labeling hexamethylpropyl-eneamine oxime (^{99m}Tc-HMPAO) in the 1980s provided the basis for the nonangiographic measurement of cerebral blood flow. Correlative studies with cerebral angiography in brain death disclosed the efficacy of radioisotopic cerebral angiography.[89, 91] Thus, this method for determining the absence of intracranial blood flow became an established laboratory test of brain death.[23, 89, 92–96] A particular advantage was that it could be carried out at the bedside (Figure 3-2).[97–99] In North America, the determination of the absence of cerebral blood flow became a more important test than cerebral angiography in the 1980s. Other investigative modalities

also appeared in the 1980s, such as magnetic resonance imaging (Figure 3-3). Monsein[100] has written an in-depth review of the use of ancillary tests in the determination of brain death.

Transcranial Doppler

Transcranial Doppler signals from the pulsating arteries in the intracranial cavity have been used to measure a number of parameters of cerebral blood flow. It has been used as a confirmatory test but has not gained widespread acceptance because of interpretive problems, particularly in inexperienced hands. Nevertheless, it is effective in the hands of the experienced ultrasonographer (Figure 3-4).[101–103]

Timing of Brain Death Determination

There is debate about when the examination should be carried out. It is obvious that an examination immediately after an ictus that ultimately results in brain death is not acceptable. This is pri-

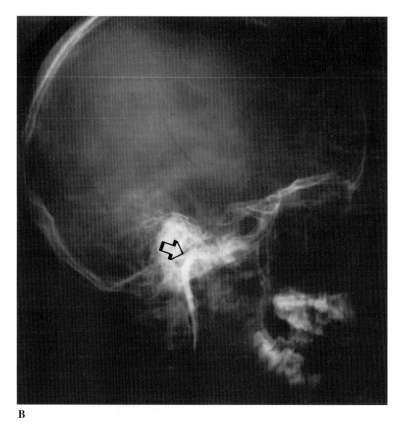

B

Figure 3-1. *Continued.* **B.** Late phase shows persistent filling of the internal carotid artery to the level of the base of skull (*open arrow*) and dissipation of dye in the external carotid artery system. (Courtesy of Dr. Allan Fox, London Health Sciences Centre, London, Ontario, Canada.)

marily an academic point, however, because there is usually a significant interval between an ictus and the initial examination. Certainly, most would agree that a minimum of 2–3 hours should elapse before the initial examination to determine brain death. The etiology of coma also influences the timing interval for the second examination. For example, in the case of massive head trauma, a 2-hour interval would appear to suffice. In the case of cerebral anoxia or ischemia, however, a mini-mum of 24 hours is recommended. Wijdicks and Dobb and Weekes have written two excellent clinical articles on the clinical confirmation of brain death.[104, 105]

Acknowledgment

I would like to thank Mrs. Willa Harding for her typing of the manuscript and for laborious research of the literature.

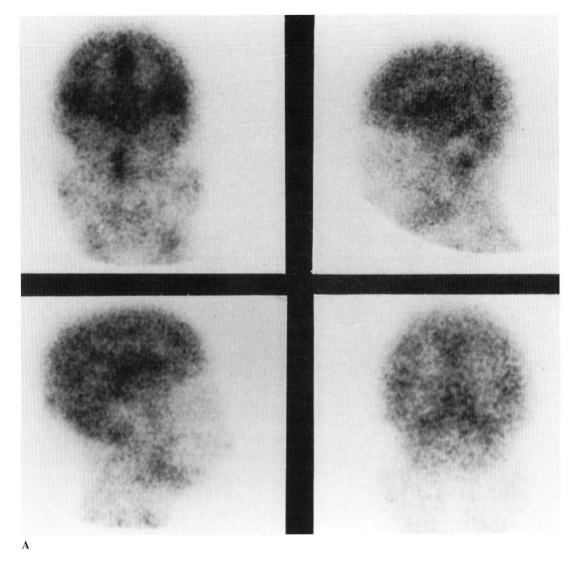

A

Figure 3-2. A. Static planar images in multiple projections (*clockwise from top left: anterior, left lateral, posterior, and right lateral*) minutes after intravenous technetium-99m hexamethylpropyleneamine oxime in a patient without evidence of brain death showing cerebral and cerebellar uptake of the tracer.

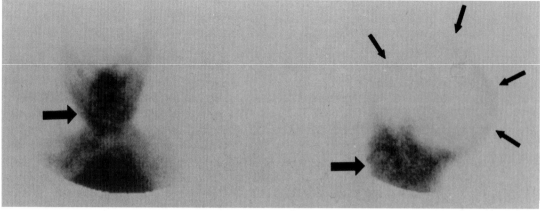

B

Figure 3-2. *Continued.* **B.** Images demonstrate normal extracranial activity (*small arrows*), no intracranial activity, and normal basal nonbrain activity (*large arrows*), indicating nonperfused brain. (Courtesy of Dr. Robert Reid, London Health Sciences Centre, London, Ontario, Canada.)

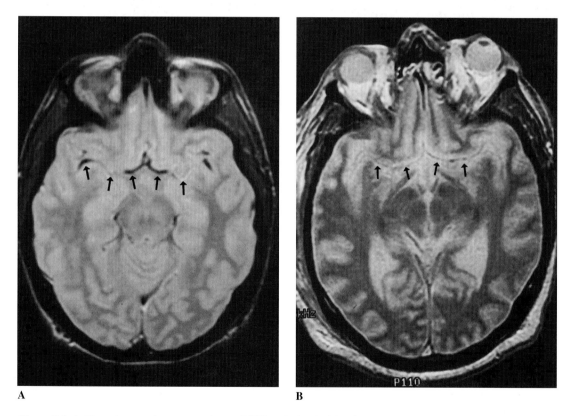

A   B

Figure 3-3. A. Normal magnetic resonance image (MRI) at the level of the circle of Willis shows normal flow signal voids (*arrows*) in the circle of Willis. **B.** MRI at similar level in brain-dead patient shows loss of flow signal voids (*arrows*). (Courtesy of Dr. David Pelz, London Health Sciences Centre, London, Ontario, Canada.)

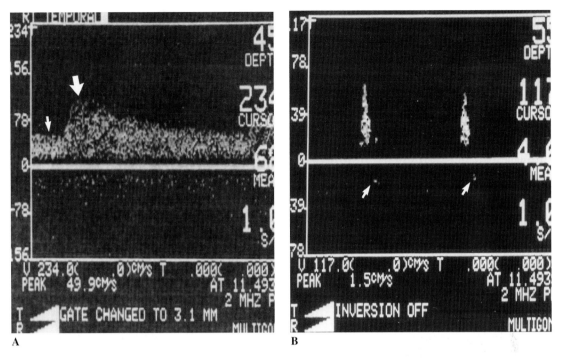

A   B

Figure 3-4. Transcranial Doppler (TCD) images at the level of the middle cerebral artery. **A.** Normal TCD showing diastolic flow pattern (*small arrow*) with systolic peak (*large arrow*). **B.** Typical stump flow pattern with reversible flow (*arrows*), indicating brain death. (Courtesy of Dr. Don Lee, London Health Sciences Centre, London, Ontario, Canada.)

References

1. Drinker PA, McKhann CF. Landmark perspective: the iron lung. First practical means of respiratory support. JAMA 1929;92:1658–1660.
2. Masferrer R, Dolan GK, Ward JJ. History of the Respiratory Care Profession. In GG Burton, JE Hodgkin, JJ Ward (eds), Respiratory Care: A Guide to Clinical Practice. Philadelphia: Lippincott, 1991;3–17.
3. Ad Hoc Committee of the Harvard Medical School to examine the definition of brain death. A definition of irreversible coma. JAMA 1968;205:337–340.
4. Grass ER. Technological aspects of electroencephalography in the determination of death. Am J EEG Technol 1969;9:70–90.
5. Silverman D, Saunders MG, Schwab RS, Masland RL. Cerebral death and the electroencephalogram. JAMA 1969;209:1505–1510.
6. Silverman D, Maslen RL, Saunders MG, Schwab RS. Irreversible coma associated with electrical silence. Neurology 1970;20:525–533.
7. Canadian Medical Association. The Canadian Medical Association statement on death. CMAJ 1968;99: 1266–1267.
8. World Medical Assembly. Sydney, Australia, 1968.
9. Becker DP, Robert CM, Nelson JR, Stern WE. An evaluation of the definition of cerebral death. Neurology 1970;20:459–462.
10. Mohandas A, Chou SN. Brain death. A clinical and pathological study. J Neurosurg 1971;35:211–218.
11. Ingvar DH, Widen L. Brain death. Summary of a symposium. Lakartidningen 1972;69:3804–3814.
12. Ueki K, Takeuchi K, Katsurada K. Clinical study of brain death [paper]. Tokyo: Japan Congress of Neurological Surgery, 1973.
13. Conference of Medical Royal Colleges and their Faculties in the United Kingdom. Diagnosis of brain death. BMJ 1976;2:1187–1188.
14. Ivan LP. Irreversible brain damage and related problems: pronouncement of death. J Am Geriatr Soc 1970;18:816–822.
15. Ivan LP. Spinal reflexes in cerebral death. Neurology 1973;23:650–652.
16. Ivan LP. Brain death in the infant and what constitutes life. Transplant Proc 1988;20(Suppl 5):17-22.
17. Miyazaki, J. Neurology and cerebral death—definitions and differential diagnosis. Trans Am Neurol Assoc 1975;100:210–212.
18. Spoor MT, Sutherland FR. The evolution of the concept of brain death. Annals RCPSC 1995;28:30–32.

19. Walker AE. The Status of Brain Death in the Nations of the World. In AE Walker (ed), Cerebral Death. Baltimore: Urba and Schwarzenberg, 1985;157–195.
20. Diringer M, Steiner T, Angstwurn H. Diagnosis of Brain Death. In W Hacke (ed), Neurocritical Care. New York: Springer-Verlag, 1994;219–234.
21. National Health and Medical Research Council of Australia. An Australian Code of Practice for Transplantation of Cadaveric Organs and Tissues. Canberra, Australia: Australian Government Publishing Service, 1990;23–24.
22. Pearson IY. Australia and New Zealand Intensive Care Society statement and guidelines on brain death and model policy on organ donation. Anaesth Intensive Care 1995;23:104–108.
23. Brock M, Schurmann K, Hadjidimos A. Cerebral blood flow and cerebral death. Acta Neurochir (Wien) 1969;20:195–209.
24. Juul-Jensen P. Criteria of Brain Death. Copenhagen: Munksgaard, 1970.
25. Miyazaki Y, Takamatsu H, Tanaka Y, et al. Criteria of cerebral death. Acta Radiol Diag 1972;13:318–328.
26. Conference of Royal Colleges and Faculties of the United Kingdom. Diagnosis of brain death. Lancet 1976;2:1069–1070.
27. Walker AE, Molinari GF. Criteria of cerebral death. Trans Am Neurol Assoc 1975;100:29–35.
28. National Institute of Neurological Diseases and Stroke. An appraisal of the criteria of cerebral death. A summary statement. JAMA 1977;237:982–986.
29. Black PM. Brain death (Part 1). N Engl J Med 1978;299:338–344.
30. Black PM. Brain death (Part 2). N Engl J Med 1978;299:393–401.
31. Presidential Commission for the Study of Ethical Problems in Medicine and Biomedical and Behavioral Research. Guidelines for the determination of death. JAMA 1981;246:2184–2186.
32. Black's Law Dictionary (4th ed). St. Paul, MN: West Publishing, 1951;1882.
33. Pius XII. The prolongation of life (address of Pope Pius XII to the International Conference of Anaesthesiologists, November 24, 1957). Pope Speaks 1958;4:393–398.
34. Canadian Congress of Neurological Sciences. Guidelines for the diagnosis of brain death. Can J Neurol Sci 1987;14:653–656.
35. Canadian Congress of Neurological Sciences. Guidelines for the diagnosis of brain death. CMAJ 1987;136:200A–200B.
36. Canadian Congress of Neurological Sciences. Death and brain death: a new formulation for Canadian medicine. CMAJ 1988;138:405–406.
37. Cooper DKC, Novitsky D, Wicomb WN. The pathophysiological effects of brain death on potential donor organs, with particular reference to the heart. Ann R Coll Surg Engl 1989;71:261–266.
38. Power BM, Van-Heerden PV. The physiological changes associated with brain death—current concepts and implications for treatment of the brain dead organ donor. Anaesth Intensive Care 1995;23:26–36.
39. Pitts LH, Kaktis J, Caronna J, et al. Brain death, apneic diffusion oxygenation and organ transplantation. J Trauma 1978;18:180–183.
40. Schafer JA, Caronna JJ. Duration of apnea needed to confirm brain death. Neurology 1978;28:661–666.
41. Ropper AH, Kennedy SK, Russel L. Apnea testing in the diagnosis of brain death. J Neurosurg 1981;55:9 42–946.
42. Marks SJ, Zisfein J. Apnea oxygenation in apnea tests for brain death. Arch Neurol 1990;47:1066–1068.
43. Ebata T, Watanbe Y, Amaha K, et al. Haemodynamic changes during the apnoea test for diagnosis of brain death. Can J Anaesth 1991;38:436–440.
44. Pallis C. Diagnosis of brain stem death—II. BMJ 1982;285:1641–1644.
45. Jennett B. Brain death. Br J Anaesth 1981;53:1111–1119.
46. Belsh JM, Blatt R, Schiffman PL. Apnea testing in brain death. Arch Intern Med 1989;146:2385–2388.
47. Benzel EC, Grose CD, Hadden TA, Kesterson L, Landreneau MD. The apnea test for the determination of brain death. J Neurosurg 1989;71:191–194.
48. Darby JM, Stein K, Grenvik A, Stuart SA. Approach to the management of the heart beating "brain dead" organ donor. JAMA 1989;261:2222–2228.
49. Al-Jumah M, McLean DR, Al-Rajeh S, Crow H. Bulk diffusion apnoea test in the diagnosis of brain death. Crit Care Med 1992;20:1564–1567.
50. Kvittingen TD, Naess A. Recovery from drowning in fresh water. BMJ 1963;1:1315–1317.
51. Siebke H, Rod T, Breivik H, Link B. Survival after 40 minutes: submersion without cerebral sequelae. Lancet 1975;1:1275–1277.
52. Montes JE, Conn AW. Near-drowning: an unusual case. Can Anaesth Soc J 1980;27:172–174.
53. Sekar T, MacDonnell K, Namsirikul P, Herman RS. Survival after prolonged submersion in cold water without neurologic sequelae. Report of two cases. Arch Intern Med 1980;140:775–779.
54. Young RS, Zalneraitis E, Dooling EC. Neurological outcome in cold water drowning. JAMA 1980;244:1233–1235.
55. Plum F, Bird TV. Recovery from barbiturate overdose coma with a prolonged isoelectric electroencephalogram. Neurology 1968;18:456–458.
56. Masland R. In discussion of paper by Walker and Molinari, 1975.
57. Ashwal S, Schneider S. Failure of electroencephalography to diagnose brain death in comatose children. Ann Neurol 1979;6:512–517.
58. American Academy of Pediatrics Task Force on Brain Death in Children. Guidelines for the determination of brain death in children. Pediatrics 1987;80:298–300.
59. Coulter DL. Neurologic uncertainty in newborn intensive care. N Engl J Med 1987;316:840–844.
60. Volpe JJ. Brain death determination in the newborn [commentary]. Pediatrics 1987;80:293–297.

61. Freeman JM, Ferry PC. New brain death guidelines in children: further confusion. Pediatrics 1988;81:301–303.

62. Shewmon DA. The probability of inevitability: the inherent impossibility of validating criteria for brain death or "irreversibility" through clinical studies. Stat Med 1987;6:535–553.

63. Shewmon DA. Commentary on guidelines for the determination of brain death in children. Ann Neurol 1988;24:789–792.

64. Ashwal S, Schneider S. Pediatric brain death: current perspectives. Adv Pediatr 1991;38:181–202.

65. Lynch J, Eldadah MK. Brain-death criteria currently used by pediatric intensivists. Clin Pediatr 1992;31:457–460.

66. Parker BL, Frewen TC, Levin SD, et al. Declaring pediatric brain death: current practice in a Canadian Pediatric Critical Care Unit. CMAJ 1995;153:909–916.

67. Stiller CR. Anencephalic donors. Transplant Proc 1988;20:(Suppl 5)83.

68. Bailey LL. Critical issue debates: intervention for infants with fatal heart disease, xenografting, and brain death criteria for anencephalic infants. J Heart Lung Transplant 1993;12(No. 6, Part 2):S351–S378.

69. Girvin JP. Brain death criteria—current approach to the non-anencephalic. Transplant Proc 1988;20(Suppl 5):26–30.

70. Girvin JP. The use of anencephalic infants for organ procurement. J Heart Lung Transplant 1993;12:S369–S374, S376–S378.

71. Deliyannakis E, Ioannou F, Davaroukas A. Brain stem death with persistence of bioelectric activity of the cerebral hemispheres. Clin Electroencephalogr 1975;6:75–79.

72. Korein J, Maccario M. On the diagnosis of cerebral death: a prospective study on 55 patients to define irreversible coma. Clin Electroencephalogr 1971;2:178–199.

73. Grigg MA, Kelly MA, Celesia GG, et al. Electroencephalographic activity after brain death. Arch Neurol 1987;44:948–954.

74. Shalit MN, Beller AJ, Feinsod M, et al. The blood flow and oxygen consumption of the dying brain. Neurology 1970;20:740–748.

75. Starr A. Auditory brain-stem responses in brain death. Brain 1976;99:543–554.

76. Goldie WD, Chiappa KH, Young RR, Brooks EB. Brainstem auditory and short-latency somatosensory evoked responses in brain death. Neurology 1981;31:248–256.

77. Hall JW, Mackey-Hargadine JR, Kim EE. Auditory brain-stem response in determination of brain death. Arch Otolaryngol 1985;111:613–620.

78. Anziska BJ, Cracco RQ. Short latency somatosensory evoked potentials in brain dead patients. Arch Neurol 1980;37:222–225.

79. Stohr M, Riffel B, Trost E, Ullrich A. Short-latency somatosensory evoked potentials in brain death. J Neurol 1987;234:211–214.

80. Bes A, Arbus L, Lazorthes Y, et al. Hemodynamic and metabolic studies in "coma dé pasé." A search for a biological test of death of the brain. In M Brock et al (eds), Cerebral Blood Flow. New York: Springer-Verlag, 1969;213–215.

81. Von Bucheler E, Kaufer C, Dux A. Zerebrale Angiographi zur Bestimmung Des Hirntodes. Fortschr Geb Roentgenstr 1970;113:278–296.

82. Vlahovitch B, Frerebeau P, Kuhner A, et al. Les angiographies sous pression dans la mort du cerveau avec arrete circulatorie encephalique. Neurol Med Chir 1971;17:81–96.

83. Bergquist E, Bergstrom K. Angiography and cerebral death. Acta Radiol 1972;12:283–288.

84. Vlahovitch B, Frerebeau P, Kuhner A, et al. Arrêt Circulatoire Intracraniaen Dans La Mort du Cerveau. Acta Radiol 1972;13:334–349.

85. Cantu RC. Brain death as determined by cerebral arteriography [letter]. Lancet 1973;1:1391–1392.

86. Greitz T, Gordon E, Kolmodin G, Widen L. Aortocranial and carotid angiography in determination of brain death. Neuroradiology 1973;5:13–19.

87. Bradac GB, Simon RS. Angiography and brain death. Neuroradiology 1974;7:25–28.

88. Rosenklint A, Jorgensen PB. Evaluation of angiographic methods in the diagnosis of brain death. Correlation with local and systemic arterial pressure and intracranial pressure. Neuroradiology 1974;7:215–219.

89. Kricheff I, Braunstein P, Korein J, et al. Isotopic and angiographic determination of cerebral blood flow. Correlation in patients with cerebral death. Acta Radiol 1975;347(Suppl):119–129.

90. Kricheff I, Pinto RS, George AE, et al. Angiographic findings in brain death. Am N Y Acad Sci 1978;315:168–183.

91. Korein J, Braunstein P, George A, et al. Brain death: I. Angiographic correlation with the radioisotopic bolus technique for evaluation of critical deficit of cerebral blood flow. Ann Neurol 1977;2:195–205.

92. Schwartz JA, Baxter J, Brill DR. Diagnosis of brain death in children by radionuclide cerebral imaging. Pediatrics 1984;73:14–18.

93. Galaske RG, Schober O, Heyer R. 99mTc-HM-PA and 123I-amphetamine cerebral scintigraphy: a new, noninvasive method in determination of brain death in children. Eur J Nucl Med 1988;14:446–452.

94. Pattel YP, Gupta SM, Batson R, Herrera NE. Brain death: confirmation by radionuclide cerebral angiography. Clin Nucl Med 1988;13:438–442.

95. Laurin NR, Dreidger AA, Hurwitz GA, et al. Cerebral perfusion imaging with technetium-99m HM-PAO in brain death and severe central nervous system injury. J Nucl Med 1989;30:1627–1635.

96. Reid RH, Gulenchyn KY, Ballinger JR. Clinical use of technetium-99m-HM-PA0 for determination of brain death. J Nucl Med 1989;30:1621–1626.

97. Braunstein P, Korein J, Kricheff I. Bedside assessment of cerebral circulation. Lancet 1972;1:1291–1292.

98. Korein J, Braunstein P, Kricheff I, et al. Radioisotopic bolus technique as a test to detect circulatory deficit associated with cerebral death. 142 studies on 80 patients demonstrating the bedside use of an innocuous

IV procedure as an adjunct in the diagnosis of cerebral death. Circulation 1975;51:924–939.

99. Goodman JM, Heck LL, Moore BD. Confirmation of brain death with portable isotope angiography: a review of 204 consecutive cases. Neurosurgery 1985;16:492–497.

100. Monsein LH. The imaging of brain death. Anaesth Intensive Care 1995;23:44–50.

101. Ropper AH, Kehne SM, Wechsler L. Transcranial Doppler in brain death. Neurology 1987;37:1733–1735.

102. Powers AD, Graeber MC, Smith RR. Transcranial Doppler ultrasonography in the determination of brain death. Neurosurgery 1989;24:884–889.

103. Petty GW, Mohr JP, Pedley TA, et al. The role of transcranial Doppler in confirming brain death: sensitivity, specificity, and suggestions for performance and interpretation. Neurology 1990;40:300–303.

104. Wijdicks EFM. Determining brain death in adults. Neurology 1995;45:1003–1011.

105. Dobb GJ, Weekes JW. Clinical confirmation of brain death. Anaesth Intensive Care 1995;23:37–43.

Chapter 4
Management of the Organ Donor

Kerri M. Robertson

Chapter Plan

Organ transplantation is a multidisciplinary specialty that has seen remarkable advances. The standardization of the surgical technique for multiple-organ procurement, significant advances in donor care, the development of more effective preservation solutions that can extend the ischemia time for procured organs, and the introduction of improved immunosuppressant therapy have made organ transplantation an acceptable solution to end-organ failure. As a result, the need for transplantable organs has increased beyond the numbers available.

Since 1992, strategies designed to increase the number of donors have been largely unsuccessful. With an ever-increasing need for transplantable organs, we are limited to optimizing the use of the currently available potential donor pool. Optimal early graft function in the recipient depends on an understanding of the criteria for donor identification and organ suitability coupled with the adoption of a comprehensive donor management strategy and knowledge of retrieval and preservation techniques. Implementing an

Table 4-1. Numbers of U.S. Organ Donors by Organ and Donor Type

Organ	Donor Type	Year										
		1988	1989	1990	1991	1992	1993	1994	1995	1996	1997	1998
Kidney	Cadaveric	3,876	3,810	4,306	4,268	4,276	4,608	4,797	4,999	5,038	5,076	1,664
	Living	1,812	1,902	2,097	2,393	2,535	2,851	3,008	3,297	3,574	3,660	1,107
	Total	5,688	5,712	6,403	6,661	6,811	7,459	7,805	8,296	8,612	8,736	2,771
Liver	Cadaveric	1,833	2,372	2,868	3,165	3,334	3,763	4,095	4,321	4,460	4,577	1,468
	Living	0	2	14	22	33	36	60	47	53	68	14
	Total	1,833	2,374	2,882	3,187	3,367	3,799	4,155	4,368	4,513	4,645	1,482
Pancreas	Cadaveric	577	799	951	1,066	1,004	1,243	1,361	1,279	1,297	1,314	425
	Living	5	4	2	1	3	2	2	8	13	7	1
	Total	582	803	953	1,067	1,007	1,245	1,363	1,287	1,310	1,321	426
Heart	Cadaveric	1,784	1,781	2,167	2,198	2,246	2,441	2,526	2,497	2,475	2,424	815
	Living	7	9	12	4	1	2	3	0	1	0	0
	Total	1,791	1,790	2,179	2,202	2,247	2,443	2,529	2,497	2,476	2,424	815
Lung	Cadaveric	130	191	275	395	526	790	919	889	758	835	240
	Living	0	0	1	4	0	12	31	41	35	31	10
	Total	130	191	276	399	526	802	950	930	793	866	250
Total	Cadaveric	4,080	4,011	4,509	4,526	4,520	4,860	5,099	5,359	5,420	5,475	1,818
	Living	1,824	1,917	2,126	2,424	2,572	2,903	3,102	3,385	3,663	3,760	1,132
	Total	5,904	5,928	6,635	6,950	7,092	7,763	8,201	8,744	9,083	9,235	2,950

Source: United Network for Organ Sharing National Organ Procurement and Transplantation Network. Data as of August 31, 1998 (http://www.unos.org).

aggressive approach to donor management has been reported to increase the donor retrieval rate by 30% without prejudicing outcome.[1]

Organ Procurement

The adoption of the Uniform Anatomical Gift Act by the U.S. Congress in 1973 legally recognized organ donation as a voluntary gift. The Omnibus Budget Reconciliation Act of 1986 stipulated that hospitals would receive no reimbursement from Medicare or Medicaid unless they established written protocols for the identification of potential organ donors.

The United Network for Organ Sharing (UNOS) was awarded a U.S. government contract in 1986 to operate the National Organ Procurement and Transplantation Network (OPTN). The OPTN was established by a federal task force to improve effectiveness of organ procurement and distribution, increase patient access to technology, improve the organ sharing system, operate a national computer listing of patients, and establish quality control. In 1987, UNOS was granted a separate contract to establish and operate a posttransplant recipient data-

base, the Scientific Registry of Transplant Recipients. Both contracts were renewed in 1990, 1993, and again in 1996, for an additional 3-year term. The policies and standards established by UNOS pertain to human organ donation, procurement, preservation, transplantation, and histocompatibility testing; and member institutions are guaranteed equitable access to available donor organs. Revisions of these policies and by-laws were to be adapted by UNOS in 1998.

Table 4-1 summarizes the numbers of U.S. organ donors by organ and donor type (cadaveric, living, and total) for 1988–1998.[2] Since 1990, the rate of cadaveric organ donation has remained relatively stable at approximately 4,500 per year. In fact, the number of potential donors may be declining due to traffic safety laws, improved trauma and stroke care, and the prevalence of transmissible infectious disease (e.g., human immunodeficiency virus [HIV]). In reality, only 3–4% of hospital deaths result in a potential organ donor, and only 15–20% of these become actual donors.[3, 4] This falls far short of the potential size of the donor pool, which is estimated to be between 5,000 and 29,000 patients each year.[5] The number of waiting recipients has grown by approximately 15–20% per year, with nearly 59,000 names on the UNOS national patient waiting list at the end of August 1998.[2] By year-end 1997, 4,331 registrants had died before a suitable donor organ could be found. Waiting-list deaths for each organ included heart-lung (23.7%), heart (19.8%), lung (15.4%), liver (11.7%), kidney (5.2%), kidney-pancreas (7.6%), and pancreas (3%). With achievement of an organ donor rate of 50 per million population per year, representing a pool of 10,000–15,000 per year, most of the patients on the list could receive their transplants.[6, 7] Therefore, a shortage of organs caused by failure to identify suitable donors remains a major limiting factor in meeting the demand for transplantation.

Identification of the Organ Donor

Living, non–heart-beating, and heart-beating donors are currently the only recognized sources of organs for procurement.

Living Donors

Although the total number of donors has grown every year, from 5,908 donors in 1988 to 9,235 donors in 1997, growth since 1990 has been due primarily to the increased use of living donors (see Table 4-1). Organs obtained from living donors are the kidney, segmental liver, segmental (lobar) lung, partial small bowel, partial pancreas, and bone marrow. Living donors, usually healthy adults, require routine vigilant intraoperative care to optimize end-organ function and minimize any perioperative morbidity. Despite the ethical considerations surrounding living donation, this procedure currently accounts for approximately 25–35% of transplanted kidneys in the United States. Potential risks to the donor of unilateral nephrectomy include short-term surgical or anesthesia-related morbidity (0.23–2.50%), long-term risks of impaired renal function and hypertension (nil, small, or unknown), loss of time and money, adverse psychological effects, and death (0.03–0.06%).[8, 9] The evaluation and selection of living kidney donors is discussed in detail in other texts.[9] Long-term risks to living pancreas donors are greater than those for kidney donors. Both endocrine and exocrine function of the donor may be compro-

mised, and the donor may also have to undergo splenectomy.[10] Living-related partial liver donation has been used in a limited capacity for children and small adults with end-stage liver disease. Ethical considerations include weighing donor perioperative morbidity (estimated as high as 7%) and mortality against a reduction in recipient waiting time, high graft viability, superior immunohistocompatibility, and accurate preoperative assessment of size match.[11] Donor complications may include pulmonary embolism, bile leak, transient jaundice, splenectomy, duodenal ulcer, and wound infection. The mortality risk of hepatic resection in noncirrhotic individuals is extremely low, apparently at least as low as that for a live kidney donor.[12] At present, lobar pulmonary transplantation is technically feasible in children and small adults, with prolonged air leaks in right lower lobe donors reported as the most frequent complication.[13]

Non–Heart-Beating Donors

Strategies for increasing the organ donor pool include the use of *controlled* non–heart-beating donors (NHBDs), for whom the patient's family decides to withdraw life support in the absence of brain death determination, and the use of NHBDs in an *uncontrolled* setting, such as patients who are asystolic as a result of trauma or myocardial infarction. Retrieval in a controlled setting implies withdrawal of support in the operating room (or surgical intensive care unit [ICU]) followed by cardiac arrest, declaration of death by an anesthesiologist, and immediate en bloc organ removal. Before extubating the patient, the surgeons will request intravenous administration of phentolamine (10–20 mg), heparin (10,000–20,000 U), and mannitol (12.5–25.0 g). The usual operating time is less than 15 minutes, with an additional 60–90 minutes required for back-table dissection. Uncontrolled circumstances require the rapid infusion of cold preservation solutions into the femoral artery and peritoneum until consent for organ donation can be obtained from family members. Some estimates indicate that an increase of 20–25% in organ donors could be realized if NHBDs were used routinely,[14] but a higher incidence of acute tubular necrosis (ATN), vascular complications, and mortality in kidney recipients should temporize uncritical enthusiasm for this practice.[15, 16] Although several centers are now using kidneys from NHBDs, the question of tolerance to warm ischemia has created a general reluctance to use extrarenal organs from these donors. There are isolated case reports of using the liver, pancreas, and lung from an NHBD.[17] The inherent interval of warm ischemia time imposed by defining death principally as cardiac death and the requirement for immediate graft function to sustain life may prohibit successful recovery of the hypoxically arrested, asystolic heart. Liver allografts from uncontrolled NHBDs have a high incidence of hepatic artery thrombosis and primary nonfunction, which necessitates urgent retransplantation.[15] In contrast, the incidence of primary nonfunction in livers from pediatric patients who died from anoxia does not appear to be increased.[18]

Brain-Dead Heart-Beating Donors

Vital, perfusable organs, including the liver, heart, heart-lungs, kidneys, small bowel, and pancreas, are recovered from a brain-dead donor who is under the care of an anesthesiologist. Tissue recovery may take place immediately after removal of the organs or within 24 hours of cardiac death.

General Criteria

In general, brain-dead donors are previously healthy individuals who have an irreversible, catastrophic structural or metabolic brain injury of known etiology, and the organs being considered for donation have no history of disease, trauma, or dysfunction. Early recognition of the potential multiorgan donor is important because any unnecessary delay may result in rapid physiologic deterioration or complications arising from ventilation and prolonged supportive medical care, which reduces the availability and suitability of potentially transplantable organs. Table 4-2 lists general suitability criteria.

Ideally, brain-dead donors should exhibit cardiovascular stability requiring minimum inotropic support, with no episodes of prolonged hypotension, ischemia, hypothermia, hypovolemia, or cardiac arrest in excess of 30 minutes. Laboratory evaluation of the donor includes the determination of blood group, tissue typing, biochemical assessment of individual organ function, hematology panel, and a

Table 4-2. General Suitability Criteria for Organ Donation

No evidence of generalized atherosclerosis (age older than 70 years, untreated hypertension, juvenile-onset diabetes mellitus or vasculitis)

No overwhelming or untreated systemic infection

No transmissible disease: negative carrier state for hepatitis B, hepatitis C, or human immunodeficiency virus (negative serology or history for high-risk behavior)

No history of visceral malignancy (other than primary intracranial, cervical, or nonmelanotic skin tumors)

No known disease, trauma, or dysfunction of donor organ(s) under consideration

Irreversible brain injury of known etiology

microbiological and serologic evaluation (hepatitis C and B, syphilis, tuberculosis, and HIV) to prevent transmission of infectious diseases to the recipient. Despite the efforts of screening by history and serologic testing, both HIV and hepatitis B have been transmitted to the recipient by donated organs and are likely to run a fulminant course in the immunosuppressed patient. The risk of viral transmission with transfusion of blood products is currently estimated at 1 in 103,300 for hepatitis C, 1 in 63,000 for hepatitis B, 1 in 1 million for hepatitis A, and 1 in 493,000 for HIV.[19, 20] Controversy and ambiguity persist over the practices of transplant centers regarding hepatitis C–seropositive candidates and donors due to an indeterminant risk of viral transmission. This creates uncertainty regarding a possible negative impact on donor graft or end-organ function in the recipient. Blood, sputum, and urine cultures are necessary as indicated by history and clinical presentation or if hospitalization exceeds 72 hours. A potential donor with overwhelming sepsis is ineligible, especially in the presence of disseminated viral infections or with organisms such as *Candida albicans*, *Pseudomonas aeruginosa*, and other gram-negative bacteria that have been highly correlated with life-threatening infections in the recipient posttransplant.[21, 22] Organs from a donor with gram-positive bacteremia are often used, given that the recipient is treated prophylactically for 10 days with sensitivity-specific antibiotics, starting in the immediate postoperative period. A history of high-risk behavior, including homosexuality, intravenous drug use, tattoos, skin piercing, and treatment with human pituitary extracts or blood product transfusions, may preclude organ donation, even with a negative HIV screen. This is due to the latency of seroconversion of HIV after the primary infection. During this "window," infection is present and transmissible, but the serology is not yet positive. Although earlier studies indicated that HIV-1 antibody appeared as late as 6 months after infection, most investigators now agree that, with the current testing methods, seroconversion usually occurs within 6–8 weeks. This interval decreases to 3 weeks when the enzyme-linked immunosorbent assay is used.[20] In addition, antibody titers against HIV may be diluted by resuscitative efforts with large volumes of blood products, and blood products may themselves transmit infection to the donor. HIV antigen testing using an antigen capture assay for the viral p24 antigen received U.S. Food and Drug Administration approval in 1996, effectively further reducing the window period to 18 days. Given the relatively low prevalence of HIV in the donor population, the potential for high false-positive rates, and the high cost of testing and training specialized personnel, it is unlikely that adoption of this test will improve transfusion safety.[20] In addition, many centers prefer to match the donor and recipient with respect to cytomegalovirus or toxoplasmosis serology. *Toxoplasma gondii* seems to have a particular predilection for cardiac allografts because of its affinity for myocardial tissue.[23] Recipient-donor matching for ABO blood groups and approximate body size is a prerequisite. Determination of HLA compatibility is also required for kidney transplantation.

Specific Criteria

Table 4-3 lists the relative contraindication criteria for individual organ donation.[3, 24–26] Because of the critical shortage of donor organs, very few rules are now absolute. Several centers have therefore expanded their criteria for donor acceptance with respect to age, allowable cold ischemia time, inotropic requirements, hemodynamic stability, size mismatching, cause of death, and infection in the donor. Analysis of the UNOS database of 953 donors, of which 16% were considered "expanded donors," showed that significant risk factors for graft loss at 1 year included donor age older than 50 years (kidney), norepinephrine use and female sex (liver), and prolonged hypotension or clinical

infection in the donor (heart). Findings were inconclusive as to whether "expanded" donor factors significantly compromised graft survival.[27]

A standardized cadaveric whole-donor and organ-specific scoring system was developed to objectively convey a comprehensive summary of the clinical and laboratory information needed by most transplant surgeons to decide whether an organ is suitable for procurement. This two-part evaluation system also proved to be highly predictive of immediate graft function, which is 93% for each of the extrarenal organs.[28]

Care of the Donor

When brain death has occurred, the physician assumes the responsibility of serving the needs of the patient, who may have indicated his or her wish to donate; of the family, who may obtain some solace and comfort in their grief and loss by agreeing to donation; and finally, of the prospective recipient candidates. The organs from a single donor may be distributed to as many as 15 recipients; therefore, all therapeutic intervention, no matter how costly, should be as aggressive as that afforded the recipient. Failure to ensure optimum function of perfusable donor organs may result in subsequent primary nonfunction or poor initial function of the graft in the recipient.

Basic management includes continuing care of the brain-dead patient's pre-existing condition, with a shift in primary emphasis from cerebral resuscitation (osmotic diuresis, fluid restriction, and hyperventilation) to donor organ protection. Therapy is aimed at achieving optimal organ perfusion and cellular oxygenation, minimizing ischemic injury, and anticipating the normal physiologic sequelae leading to somatic death. Common problems in the care of the organ donor include hypotension, anemia and transfusion morbidity, coagulopathies, arrhythmias, hypothermia, endocrine abnormalities (e.g., diabetes insipidus, adrenal crisis, low free triiodothyronine [T_3]), and pulmonary injury (Table 4-4).[3, 29–56]

Hemodynamic Sequelae

Brain stem death results in the breakdown of effective central neurohumoral regulatory mechanisms.

Table 4-3. Contraindications for Individual Organ Donation

Heart

Adult donor: men, physiologic age >45–60 years; women, physiologic age >50–60 years

History of pre-existing heart or coronary artery disease, major cardiac structural abnormalities, cardiac trauma (including open cardiac massage, prolonged closed cardiac massage >30 minutes within 24 hours of retrieval)

Prolonged hypotension

Prolonged or high-dose inotropic support

Abnormal investigational studies: echocardiogram (ECG), cardiac catheterization, chest x-ray, PaO_2 <50 mm Hg for 4 hours, pathologic Q waves on the ECG (cardiac isoenzymes have a low sensitivity and specificity in the diagnosis of myocardial contusion in trauma victims[a])

("High-risk" donors for patients in urgent need of cardiac transplantation have been defined as >40 years of age, ischemia time >5 hours, weight <20% of the recipient, requirement for high-dose inotropes, or the presence of systemic infection.[b] By defining which dysfunctional donor hearts may be suitable, a 15% increase in the donor pool could be realized.[c])

Evaluate: possible ischemic injury related to carbon monoxide poisoning, intractable ventricular arrhythmia, arterial saturation <80% on ventilatory support, previous myocardial infarction[d]

Relative contraindications: recurrent supraventricular arrhythmia, severe left ventricular hypertrophy, noncritical coronary disease[d]

Heart-lungs and single lung

Adult donor: men, physiologic age >40–55 years; women, physiologic age >50–55 years

Pre-existing primary pulmonary disease (acute or chronic, including asthma) or surgery

History of heavy cigarette use (>20 pack-years)

Evidence of direct injury (contusion, laceration, bronchial trauma, pneumothorax) or indirect injury (aspiration, pulmonary edema, infection, prolonged ventilation)

Abnormal investigational studies: serial chest x-rays, bronchoscopic examination, sputum culture, excessive alveolar arterial oxygen gradient (PaO_2 <60 mm Hg [300 mm Hg] with FIO_2 ≥0.4, and positive end-expiratory pressure of 5 cm H_2O)

Matching of CMV-negative donor to CMV-negative recipient required (institution specific)

Liver

No age limitation

Abnormal serial liver function tests: serial liver enzymes, bilirubin, coagulation studies (especially prothrombin time refractory to vitamin K and fresh frozen plasma administration)

History of liver disease, injury, or surgery or severe steatosis on liver biopsy

Resuscitated from cardiac arrest or hypotension (same criteria as for heart; center specific)

A history of prolonged or heavy consumption of alcohol (a relative consideration)

A history of gallstones (requires further evaluation)

Kidney

Physiologic age >55–80 years

History or evidence of acute or chronic renal disease, nephrotoxic conditions, or sickle cell or other hemoglobinopathies

Preterminal oliguria <0.5 mg/kg/hr, unresponsive to therapy

Abnormal investigational studies: pathologic urine analysis, abnormal elevation of serum urea nitrogen, and creatinine concentrations on admission

A history of active cocaine abuse (a relative consideration)

Pancreas

History of diabetes mellitus, types 1 and 2

Physiologic age restricted for type 1 to 45–60 years

History of chronic or recurrent acute pancreatitis

Direct trauma or previous duodenal or pancreatic surgery

Alcohol abuse

Resuscitated from cardiac arrest (center specific)

Small bowel

Penetrating abdominal injury

Peritonitis

CMV = cytomegalovirus.

[a]WH Frist, WJ Fanning. Donor management and matching. Cardiol Clin 1990;8:55–71.

[b]MS Sweeney, DE Lammermeier, OH Frazier, et al. Extension of donor criteria in cardiac transplantation: surgical risk versus supply-side economics. Ann Thorac Surg 1990;50:7–10.

[c]MM Boucek, CM Mathis, MS Kanakriyeh, et al. Donor shortage: use of the dysfunctional donor heart. J Heart Lung Transplant 1993;12(Suppl):186–190.

[d]JC Baldwin, JL Anderson, MM Boucek, et al. Task Force 2: Donor guidelines. J Am Coll Cardiol 1993;22:15–20.

Table 4-4. Normal Physiologic Sequelae of Brain Death

Sequela	Cause	Management

Hypotension	Neurogenic shock, hypovolemia, hypothermia, electrolyte disorders, endocrine abnormalities, myocardial dysfunction	Goal: systolic BP >100 mm Hg
		Maintain intravascular volume:
		  CVP <10 mm Hg, PCWP <10 mm Hg
		  SVR <1,000 dynes/sec^{-5}
		Inotropic support in order of preference (in μg/kg/min)
		  Dopamine <10
		  Dobutamine <15
		  Epinephrine <0.1
		  Norepinephrine and renal-dose dopamine

Anemia	Hemorrhage, hemodilution	Transfuse to keep the hematocrit >24%
Coagulopathies	DIC, fibrinolysis, dilutional, hypothermia	Factor replacement, transfusion, rewarming, early organ retrieval
Arrhythmias	Central nervous system injury (loss of neurohumoral regulatory systems and autonomic storm), electrolyte and arterial blood gas disorders, hypothermia, myocardial ischemia	Atropine-resistant resuscitation according to advanced cardiac life support protocols; may be refractory to therapy
Hypothermia	Loss of hypothalamic, neural, or endocrine regulation; resuscitation with cold fluids or blood products	Early aggressive warming to maintain the temperature above 35°C At <30°C may be unresponsive to drug therapy, defibrillation, or pacing Bretylium may prove beneficial
Endocrine abnormalities	Disruption of the hypothalamic-pituitary axis, resulting in adrenal insufficiency, hypothyroidism, or diabetes insipidus	Volume replacement; correct electrolytes; inotropic support Steroid administration: hydrocortisone 250 mg or methylprednisolone 15 mg/kg T_3 4-μg bolus and 3 μg/hr Vasopressin 0.1 μg/kg/min Desmopressin 0.3 μg/kg every 6–8 hrs to maintain the urine output at 3 ml/kg/hr
Hypoxemia	Central, cardiac, or pulmonary	Pao_2 100–150 mm Hg $Paco_2$ 35–45 mm Hg pH 7.35–7.45 PEEP <7.5 cm H_2O Fio_2 <0.40 (heart-lungs)

BP = blood pressure; CVP = central venous pressure; SVR = systemic vascular resistance; DIC = disseminated intravascular coagulation; T_3 = triiodothyronine; PEEP = positive end-expiratory pressure; PCWP = pulmonary capillary wedge pressure; Fio_2 = fraction of inspired oxygen.

In 80% of adult donors, despite maximum physiologic support, cardiac death usually occurs within 48–72 hours of declaring brain death.[57] For children, this interval may be prolonged, with isolated case reports of 70–201 days. Brain-stem injury due to a sudden increase in intracranial pressure and "coning" produces a sequence of hemodynamic events referred to as the *autonomic storm*. Critical ischemic injury of the cerebrum, progressing in a rostrocaudal fashion to include the pons, medulla oblongata, and spinal cord, causes initial vagal activation followed by the classic Cushing's response of hypertension, bradycardia, and an irregular breathing pattern. Subsequent involvement of the entire brain stem culminates in a short "explosive" period of hypertension, tachycardia, and vasoconstriction due to unopposed sympathetic stimulation, with a massive outpouring of catecholamines.[58] This sympathetic storm that occurs in the agonal period of brain death appears to be a common response to brain injury, whether from a mechanical, ischemic, electrical, or traumatic insult.[59]

An attempt to reduce blood pressure in these circumstances may be detrimental and is usually not recommended.[60] Advocates of instituting antihypertensive therapy recommend a titratable infusion of nitroprusside, esmolol hydrochloride, labetalol hydrochloride, or calcium channel blockers to prevent the development of subendocardial injury and subsequent pulmonary edema. Some studies concluded that the early transient hyperdynamic response that follows brain death can be attenuated by beta-adrenoreceptor blockade with propranolol or atenolol; however, the subsequent deterioration of cardiac function does not appear to involve sympathetic or parasympathetic innervation.[61]

After this hypertensive phase, and with the destruction of the pontine and medullary vasomotor structures, an insidious or abrupt onset of hypotension should be anticipated in all organ donors. Contributing factors include derangements of vasomotor control mechanisms, hypovolemia, hypothermia, electrolyte disorders, endocrine abnormalities, and myocardial dysfunction.

Neurogenic shock results from destruction of the central vasomotor control structures, with subsequent progressive loss of systemic vascular resistance (SVR), arterial vasodilatation, and pooling of the intravascular volume in the venous capacitance vessels.

Causes of hypovolemia include therapeutic dehydration to decrease cerebral edema, incomplete resuscitation after trauma and hemorrhage, inadequate replacement of essential and third-space fluid losses, diarrheal losses in children resulting from bowel ischemia,[62] uncontrolled diabetes insipidus, or an osmotic diuresis induced by hyperglycemia, mannitol, or systemic radiocontrast dyes.

As the body temperature decreases below 30°C, hypotension may result from a reduction in cardiac output and arterial pressure, bradycardia, ventricular arrhythmias, and cardiac arrest refractory to drug therapy and defibrillation. Active rewarming may require aggressive fluid replacement to compensate for peripheral vasodilatation.

Metabolic and electrolyte abnormalities may cause rhythm disorders, reduce myocardial contractility, alter responsiveness of the myocardium and vasculature to catecholamines, and increase pulmonary vascular resistance. Avoidance and correction of hyperosmolarity, hyperglycemia, hypernatremia, hypokalemia, hypocalcemia, hypophosphatemia, acidosis, hypoxemia, and hypercarbia are essential.

It has been proposed that disruption of the brain stem results in interruption of the control of endocrine function by the hypothalamic-pituitary axis. A deficiency in anterior pituitary hormones may cause depletion of thyroid hormones and depressed adrenocortical function, resulting in cardiac instability and deterioration in renal function.

Significant biventricular dysfunction has been shown to develop after induction of acute brain death, with the decrease in contractility of the right ventricle being more predominant than that of the left.[63, 64] Potential causes of myocardial dysfunction in donors include

1. Centrally mediated "sympathetic storm" with release of circulating catecholamines causing nonphysiologic extremes in pressure and wall stress, peripheral vasoconstriction, direct myocardial injury, coronary vasospasm, and possibly overall downregulation or uncoupling of the myocardial beta-adrenergic receptor system
2. Stimulation of the cardiac sympathetic plexus with release of endogenous catecholamines resulting in increased calcium uptake by the myocardial cells (cytosolic calcium overload, membrane permeability alteration, and subendocardial impairment of capillary blood flow), which induces myocyte necrosis[65–67]
3. Vascular regulatory injury with progressive vasodilatation, hypotension, and decreased organ perfusion leading to anaerobic metabolism, acidosis, and ischemia
4. Endocrine disturbances; most important, a reduction in free T_3 and cortisol, causing disruption of mitochondrial function, leading to anaerobic glycolysis, lactic acidosis, and eventual cardiac and peripheral circulatory failure
5. Myocardial contusion, thoracic trauma (tamponade, disruption of great vessels, hemo- or pneumothorax), or subendocardial infarction from prolonged external cardiac massage
6. Hypoxemia (cardiac, neurogenic, or pulmonary)
7. Loss of temperature-regulating mechanisms resulting in hypothermia
8. Electrolyte-induced cardiac arrhythmias or myocardial depression

9. Inotropic support resulting in catecholamine depletion of the myocardium, cardiomyopathy, arrhythmia, tachycardia, increased myocardial O_2 requirements, vasoconstriction (coronary, pulmonary, peripheral), acidosis, depletion of high-energy phosphates, and depression of myocardial beta-adrenergic receptors[68]

10. Cerebral resuscitation measures, including hyperventilation (peripheral vasoconstriction and compensatory metabolic acidosis) and fluid restriction with diuresis (hypovolemia, hypokalemia, hypernatremia)

11. Dysrhythmias

To ensure adequate perfusion of transplantable organs, initial therapy should be directed toward aggressive restoration and maintenance of the intravascular volume and the temporary use of vasoactive drugs, as needed. Goals for volume expansion and replacement of urinary losses include maintaining a minimum systolic blood pressure of 90–100 mm Hg (mean arterial pressure [MAP] of 60 mm Hg) and a central venous pressure (CVP) of 8–10 mm Hg (maximum 12 mm Hg), with a normal sinus rhythm of less than 100 beats per minute.

The choice of crystalloid- or colloid-containing solutions for perioperative fluid management depends on institutional preference.[69] When only the kidneys are to be removed, the donor can be maximally fluid-loaded; otherwise, overhydration must be avoided because it may precipitate cardiac decompensation, pulmonary insufficiency, congestion of the liver, or interstitial edema impairing systemic oxygenation and causing ischemic cellular injury during cold storage. The liver and lungs are especially sensitive to low osmotic pressure–mediated tissue edema.[70] Therefore, for lung or heart-lungs retrieval, infusion of colloid is recommended,[71] the use of crystalloid is minimized, high filling pressures are avoided (maintain CVP below 8 mm Hg, MAP above 70 mm Hg, systolic blood pressure above 85 mm Hg), and inotropic support is initiated early.[72] Fresh frozen or banked plasma should never be used for volume expansion. The use of dextran 40 has several proposed benefits, including rapid expansion and prolonged maintenance of the plasma volume, moderate hemodilution, improved microcirculation and tissue oxygenation, and a decreased risk of thromboembolic complications.[69, 73, 74]

Hydroxyethyl starch-based solutions may reduce the incidence of reperfusion injury[75] but have been implicated in causing osmotic nephrosis–like lesions in kidney transplant recipients.[76] In addition to measuring cardiac filling pressures and urine output, serial measurements of the serum osmolarity and colloid oncotic pressure may be useful in assessing the degree of hydration and choice of fluid replacement. Deleterious tissue edema is preventable if serum albumin levels are 25 g per liter or greater.[70]

Use of vasopressors may be required temporarily to maintain an adequate blood pressure during fluid resuscitation, but ideally they should be discontinued before organ retrieval to avoid peripheral vasoconstriction and disruption of regional blood flow with possible ischemic end-organ injury. In order of preference, the choice of agent for inotropic support of the myocardium is dopamine (less than 10 µg/kg/minute[77]), dobutamine (less than 15 µg/kg/minute), epinephrine (less than 0.1 µg/kg/minute), and, when the need is critical, an infusion of norepinephrine with low-dose dopamine (2–4 µg/kg/minute) for protective renal vasodilation.[78, 79]

Dopamine is usually the preferred vasopressor because at low infusion rates (under 5 µg/kg/minute), it increases the glomerular filtration rate and dilates renal, mesenteric, and coronary vasculature, causing less ischemia than other sympathomimetic agents.[47, 80] Generally, doses of 3–10 µg/kg per minute predominantly stimulate the beta-adrenergic receptors, resulting in an increase in cardiac output and a slight increase in heart rate, without marked peripheral vasoconstriction or an increase in the pulmonary artery pressure. Doses greater than 10 µg/kg per minute cause generalized vasoconstriction. Infants may require significantly larger doses of dopamine than adult donors do, presumably because of the immaturity or deficiency of catecholamine receptors.[81] At these higher doses (15 versus 5 µg/kg/minute in infants and adults, respectively), no adverse effects on the glomerular filtration rate or urine output are apparent.[82] Several groups have reported no significant difference in the incidence of ATN in allografts receiving dopamine support, but they found a significant difference in graft survival at 6 months posttransplantation.[83–85] Others report an increased risk of ATN, with no subsequent adverse impact on long-term graft survival.[86] It is conceivable that the cause of the unstable hemodynamic state, rather than the administration of dopamine per se, may account for any adverse affects on renal function.[87] At a dose of 15 µg/kg per minute, dopamine impairs liver metabolism, despite increased portal and hepatic arterial blood flow,[88, 89] and may increase the incidence of primary graft failure.[90]

Dopamine is not preferred by some institutions[85, 91, 92] because of two theoretical concerns: catecholamine depletion of the myocardium and catecholamine-induced cardiomyopathy. Because dopamine modulates presynaptic norepinephrine release, prolonged dopamine infusion may cause depletion of norepinephrine stores in the heart, resulting in decreased myocardial contractility and an attenuated response to subsequent catecholamine exposure. This may render the heart unsuitable for transplantation or increase the incidence of primary nonfunction or initial poor function of the graft in the recipient. During the agonal period, the release of endogenous catecholamines within the myocardium and peripheral vessels is induced by a period of accelerated sympathetic activity, leading to direct myocardial injury, coronary vasospasm, or downregulation of beta-adrenergic receptor sites. The use of inotropic agents may augment this process; therefore, these agents should be either avoided or titrated to the minimum effective dose.[68] In addition, it is known from animal experiments that exogenous catecholamines reduce subsequent myocardial ischemic tolerance.[93] The mechanism for cellular injury during ischemia and reperfusion involves the disruption of calcium homeostasis, which may be augmented by catecholamine activation of intracellular processes that increase calcium entry into cells or calcium release from intracellular organelles.[94]

Dobutamine primarily stimulates the beta-adrenergic receptors, increasing myocardial contractility and heart rate, but its vasodilatory effects may be deleterious. No direct effects on renal, splanchnic, or hepatic blood flows occur, although an increase in cardiac output may produce a secondary increase in renal blood flow. At doses greater than 15 µg/kg per minute, several undesirable effects can occur. Tachycardia, dysrhythmias, excessive increases in blood pressure, and a decrease in SVR are possible, and these may be poorly tolerated.[95] An increase in myocardial contractility and oxygen consumption may adversely affect a heart that is already stressed.[96]

Use of isoproterenol as a beta-adrenergic agonist in adult donors is limited by the resultant tachycardia, which may induce myocardial ischemia and vasodilatation, possibly exacerbating diastolic hypotension and leading to coronary insufficiency.[97] On the other hand, increasing the heart rate may be especially useful in infant donors because of their fixed stroke volume and rate-dependent cardiac output.

Epinephrine has both alpha- and beta-stimulating properties, with the latter predominating at low infusion rates. Its vasoactive effects are dose-dependent, and at high concentrations, it causes peripheral vasoconstriction, aggravating tissue hypoperfusion and lactic acidosis. Marked histopathologic changes associated with renal dysfunction have been described from brain-dead patients treated with vasopressin and epinephrine.[98] Others have found that the use of epinephrine to maintain a systolic blood pressure above 80 mm Hg did not increase the frequency of ATN.[94] To protect renal, hepatic, and pancreatic (mesenteric) blood flow, an infusion of low-dose dopamine is often used in conjunction with "alpha" pressor infusions of epinephrine and norepinephrine. The efficacy of this practice has not been confirmed. Potentially, a manageable diuresis secondary to diabetes insipidus may be aggravated by the use of a renal vasodilator dose of dopamine in conjunction with the osmotic effects of hyperglycemia induced by catecholamine infusions. Use of predominantly alpha-adrenergic vasopressors, such as metaraminol, phenylephrine, or norepinephrine, should be reserved for the rare situation when only the heart is to be removed. Otherwise, they should be avoided because they may cause severe peripheral vasoconstriction.[99] Their efficacy lies in maintaining coronary perfusion pressure and limiting the increase in myocardial oxygen consumption and the change in coronary artery flow induced by changes in heart rate.

Experimental protocols for providing hemodynamic support of donors up to 14–23 days include the addition of arginine vasopressin (AVP) to a continuous infusion of low-dose epinephrine.[100–102] In the state of brain death, pressor sensitivity to vasopressin is greatly enhanced.[103] A synergistic effect exists between these two drugs, with vasopressin potentiating pressor responses to catecholamines, thereby reducing the total catecholamine requirement necessary for "pressor" support.[104] This regimen has been recommended for maintenance of optimum liver graft viability.[105] In an experimental model, a similar enhanced sensitivity in pressor response was reported with the combination of norepinephrine and antidiuretic hormone (ADH) at physiologic doses.[103] These investigational studies indicate preservation of renal, hepatic, and pancreatic blood flow, with no deleterious effects on subsequent function in the recipient.

Transfusion Requirements

An adequate flow of oxygenated blood to perfusable organs depends on the arterial oxygen content, cardiac output, and regional distribution of blood flow. Transfusion requirements are determined by matching this oxygen-carrying capacity and blood flow relative to changes in viscosity with the estimated oxygen demands of the donor. Most transplant centers recommend transfusion of packed red blood cells (pRBC) to achieve a hematocrit of 25–30%.[106, 107] The debatable efficacy of setting these particular transfusion guidelines is supported in theory by the application of basic science principles aimed at maximizing oxygen supply to the tissues. The risks of blood product use include the possibility of infectious disease transmission, metabolic disturbances, transfusion reactions, coagulopathy, hypothermia, and difficulty in matching histocompatibility. The knowledge that acquired immunodeficiency syndrome can be transmitted via blood transfusion has intensified public and peer-review scrutiny of transfusion practices in general. Therefore, the appropriate choice of a transfusion threshold for donors, based on practical and educated judgment, might be a hematocrit of 24%. This guideline assumes a normovolemic state because the oxygen extraction reserve is easily exhausted in the presence of hypovolemia combined with reduced hemoglobin levels.[108] Four units of pRBC (2 units pRBC in children), cross-matched and compatible with the donor's cytomegalovirus status, should be readily available at all times for transfusion. One may anticipate requirements of more than 6 units of pRBC in 25% of solid-organ donors.[51] Multiple donor transfusions before retrieval seem to have a favorable effect on graft outcome, presumably due to a nonspecific effect that modifies the antigenic presentation of donor cells.[109]

Coagulopathy

A bleeding diathesis may be initiated by the release of tissue thromboplastin or plasminogen activators into the systemic circulation from an ischemic or necrotic brain. Other factors, such as severe tissue injury, shock, multiple transfusions, hypothermia, fat embolism, extensive burns, and nontraumatic causes, such as subarachnoid hemorrhage, are associated with the development of severe coagulopathies.[110] Disseminated intravascular coagulation (DIC) is evident in up to 90% of patients with lethal head injuries.[111–113] This is an exceedingly difficult problem to manage, and despite attempts at factor replacement with fresh frozen plasma and platelets, primary fibrinolysis or DIC may persist, necessitating early organ retrieval. The use of antifibrinolytic therapy (e.g., aprotinin, epsilon-aminocaproic acid, tranexamic acid) is not recommended due to the potential for inducing microvascular thrombosis in donor organs. The impact of donor DIC on the subsequent function of transplanted organs is essentially unknown. Platelet-rich microthrombi have been found in organs of patients with acute DIC, more often in the lungs and kidneys than in the liver. Subsequent vasoconstriction and microvascular thrombosis is thought to ensue, resulting in ischemia and end-organ dysfunction. Of the few reports using kidneys from donors with DIC, Shamash cited a 25% overall graft failure rate, whereas Ngheim and others recommend keeping kidneys that have excellent terminal function and flush well at the time of organ retrieval.[114–116] No adverse affects of donor DIC have been observed on graft function or patient outcome in pancreas[117] and liver transplant recipients.[110]

Arrhythmias

Changes in ST and T waves may be seen in patients with intracranial injury. Although these findings are usually of no pathologic significance, coronary vasospasm has been described in animal models during the early phase of brain death, when levels of epinephrine and norepinephrine are increased.[96] Experimentally, beta-blockers have been used successfully to treat catecholamine-mediated hypertension during early brain herniation.[91] Prior sympathectomy and beta-blockade prevent the early myocardial changes associated with experimental brain death; therefore, therapy using a short-acting beta-blocker (such as esmolol hydrochloride) may prevent histopathologic changes to the myocardium and lungs.[91] The preoperative administration of calcium channel blockers in both the donor and recipient has reduced the incidence of delayed graft function after transplantation of the cadaveric kidney.[118] The rationale for the use of calcium antagonists includes the proposed attenuation of the ischemic insult induced by excessive intracellular entry of calcium into vascular smooth muscle cells and evidence of the role played by calcium in the pathogenesis of ischemia-reperfusion syndrome.

Atrial and ventricular arrhythmias, as well as conduction defects, occur frequently as terminal rhythms in the organ donor.[119] Contributing factors include ventricular irritability with increased levels of circulating catecholamines, electrolyte and arterial blood gas disorders, brain herniation, drug therapy, myocardial ischemia, hypothermia, and cardiac contusion. Appropriate therapeutic intervention should be implemented. Bradycardia is not a problem unless it contributes to hypotension, and it can be treated with isoproterenol, epinephrine, or temporary venous pacing. The donor should be resistant to the chronotropic effects of atropine.[120]

Despite aggressive therapeutic efforts, all brain-dead patients eventually undergo terminal arrhythmias that resist therapy. Bradycardia and asystole are the most common terminal cardiac rhythms in children, whereas ventricular fibrillation is more common in adults. This tendency may be due to the immature autonomic nervous system and smaller muscle mass in the younger age group.[121] In the event of cardiac arrest, immediate resuscitation should proceed according to standard cardiopulmonary resuscitation and advanced life support protocols. Intracardiac injections, which may damage the heart and potentially disqualify it for donation, should be avoided. Cardiopulmonary resuscitation maneuvers have been reported to cause cyanotic congestion and hypoperfusion of the liver because of a partial venous outflow blockage of the abdominal viscera.[122] An estimated 15–20% of organ procurement operations in adult donors are abandoned each year due to hypotension or cardiac arrest occurring at some stage between acceptance of the donor and start of the donor operation.[51, 71, 123] Boucek and col-

leagues reported a 72% incidence of pediatric heart donors having a similar history.[124] Despite a documented arrest as long as 30 minutes and arterial pH as low as 6.5, with dopamine infusions of up to 30 μg/kg per minute, the long-term graft survival rate in 25 infant recipients was 84%.[124] In the pediatric porcine model, after brain death, function of the left ventricle, beta-adrenergic receptors, and adenylate cyclase enzyme system was preserved, in contrast to a deterioration observed in the adult porcine myocardium.[125] Therefore, a history of severe chest trauma, prolonged cardiac arrest, or requirement of aggressive inotropic support in the pediatric donor should not necessarily preclude heart donation.[126, 127]

Hypothermia

The loss of hypothalamic temperature regulation, with failure to compensate for heat loss by neural (shivering or vasoconstriction) or endocrine responses, and administration of large volumes of cold intravenous fluids or blood products often result in profound hypothermia. With a relatively larger body surface area facilitating rapid evaporative, conductive, and radiant heat losses, temperature instability is often one of the first clinical signs in children with severe neurologic injury progressing to brain death.[62] Although a mild degree of hypothermia may be beneficial to organ protection and preservation, a core temperature less than 32°C could result in significant morbidity that compromises organ function (Table 4-5).[128] Hypothermia further complicates the process of certification of brain death, which requires the core temperature to be greater than 35°C. After cardiac arrest, postresuscitation hyperthermia above 39°C is an early predictor of brain damage culminating in subsequent brain death.[129]

Therapeutic intervention to maintain a core temperature above 35°C should be early and aggressive. Such intervention involves the use of external warming devices that blow warm air over the patient through a porous plastic mattress, warming blankets (especially in children weighing less than 10 kg), and warmed intravenous fluids. Head draping and wrapping the extremities with aluminum foil (Mylar) reduces radiant heat loss. Active internal rewarming techniques, such as heated humidification of inspiratory gases to 42°C, pleural or

Table 4-5. Consequences of Hypothermia in the Donor

Arrhythmias
  Progressive bradycardia
  Ventricular arrhythmias or ventricular fibrillation
  Cardiac arrest (often refractory to therapy)
Myocardial depression
Hypotension
Left shift in the oxyhemoglobin dissociation curve (reduced
  O_2 availability)
Decrease in the glomerular filtration rate
Decrease in the renal tubular concentration gradient (cold
  diuresis)
Coagulopathy, hemolysis
Pancreatitis, hyperglycemia

peritoneal lavage, and extracorporeal rewarming with partial bypass may result in injury to the lungs or intra-abdominal viscera. The hypothermic heart may be unresponsive to cardiotonic drugs, pacemaker stimulation, and defibrillation and exquisitely sensitive to mechanically or reflex-induced arrhythmias, such as those seen during pulmonary artery catheter (PAC) insertion or nasogastric intubation.[128,130] Management of hypothermic cardiac arrest includes rapid core rewarming, cardiopulmonary resuscitation, three shocks for ventricular fibrillation or ventricular tachycardia to determine fibrillation responsiveness, and cautious administration of antiarrhythmic drugs (e.g., epinephrine, lidocaine, magnesium sulfate, procainamide) until the core temperature rises above 30°C.[131] Bretylium tosylate given as a 5-mg/kg intravenous push, repeated in 5 minutes at 10 mg/kg, may prove beneficial in treating refractory ventricular fibrillation by raising the fibrillation threshold.[132, 133] There is some evidence that increasing the ventilation to induce a mild degree of respiratory alkalosis, particularly in patients with a core temperature of less than 34°C, reduces the threshold for ventricular fibrillation.[134–136]

Endocrine Abnormalities

The possibility that endocrine dysfunction may contribute to the hemodynamic deterioration of the donor has been a topic of interest to researchers since its conceptualization by Drs. Novitzky, Wicomb, and Cooper in the early 1980s. Significant neuroendocrine changes have been shown to occur in previously healthy individuals who had an acute major stress, required aggressive therapeutic support, and ultimately succumbed to the insult.[137, 138] Disruption of the hypothalamic-pituitary axis could result in adrenal insufficiency or clinical hypothyroidism, which may then lead to functional instability in many organ systems.

Clinical Hypothyroidism

In animal models, a rapid depletion of ADH, circulating cortisol, insulin, thyroxine (T_4), and free T_3 has been found after brain death. A similar reduction in free T_3 and T_4 has been found in human organ donors.[139, 140] Alterations in cardiovascular function induced by a reduction in free T_3 have been attributed to changes in peripheral vascular resistance,[141] metabolic demand,[142] and depressed myocardial contractility[143] secondary to impairment of calcium homeostasis, sodium-potassium-adenosine triphosphatase (ATPase) activity, myosin ATPase, coronary flow, and myocardial energy status.[61] Hypothyroidism, induced by thyroidectomy, has been shown experimentally to produce no impairment of the heart's tolerance to hypothermic ischemic storage.[61]

The administration of T_3 or T_4 to human donors has been claimed to offset the natural course of metabolic deterioration in the brain-dead patient and to improve cardiac and renal functional stability in the recipient.[144–147] These observations probably explain why more than 50% of surgical groups administer thyroid hormones to hemodynamically "rescue" unstable donors in an attempt to increase the size of their potential pool for multiorgan retrieval and promote a better clinical outcome for the transplant recipient.[148] Evidence from clinical and experimental studies supporting T_3 therapy includes a proposed cause-and-effect relation between the lack of myocardial intracellular thyroid hormone and myocyte injury; clinically significant improvement, both hemodynamic and metabolic, in myocardial function with donor and recipient treatment[149–152]; reversal of renal graft dysfunction[87, 153]; and significantly higher intracellular adenine nucleotide stores, measured as an index of cell viability, found in the kidneys and pancreas.[154] A need for increased mean dosage and duration of inotropic support to maintain an adequate arterial blood pressure has been recorded in patients receiving hearts from thyroid hormone–depleted donors.[155]

These investigators recommend treating heart and kidney donors, who, despite adequate volume resuscitation and pressor support, give evidence of anaerobic metabolism or hemodynamic instability, with a hormonal supplement cocktail consisting of T_3 (2 µg), cortisol (100 mg), and insulin (10–20 IU). This therapy is repeated at hourly intervals, depending on the condition of the donor and response to therapy, until the heart is excised.[156, 157] Intensivists at Papworth Hospital have developed a "hormone package," with the goal of providing physiologic resuscitation of the donor with hormonal replacement therapy in the face of possible reductions in serum free T_3, cortisol, AVP, and insulin (Table 4-6).[158] In March 1989, the Colorado Organ Recovery Systems successfully instituted a T_4-based protocol to "rescue" hemodynamically unstable donors. They have subsequently shown an increase in the long-term survival of T_4-treated liver and heart grafts.[159]

Steroid administration (hydrocortisone 250 mg intravenously, followed by 5 mg per hour) for stress coverage and replacement of a presumed deficiency in adrenocorticotropic hormone (ACTH)-cortisol is recommended in the hemodynamically unstable donor, already fluid-loaded and receiving high doses of inotropes.[61] The rationale for cortisol therapy is supported by the findings of Bittner and colleagues, in which plasma levels of ACTH and cortisol decreased significantly 15 and 45 minutes after the induction of brain death in a canine model, with levels undetectable by 7 hours.[160]

Although several studies have substantiated the reduction in free T_3,[156, 161–163] the physiologic significance of this finding is uncertain. Investigators have found no correlation between a reduction in

free T_3 and the need for inotropic support in the donor,[161, 164–169] the pressor requirements in the cardiac transplant recipient,[170] or the incidence of ATN in the renal transplant recipient.[170] Most likely, the acute changes seen in the thyroid profile represent a stress response, termed the *sick euthyroid syndrome*, rather than a deficiency in thyroid-stimulating hormone causing truly functional hypothyroidism.[164, 165, 171] Therefore, the proposed beneficial effects reported from T_3 replacement therapy may represent a pharmacologic effect independent of the actual physiologic status of the donor.

The indications for substitutional T_3 or T_4 therapy, its mechanism of positive inotropic effect, and efficacy for pressor support in the donor and recipient are still debated and continue to be under investigational review. Difficulty in correlating experimental and clinical studies lies in the fact that T_3 possesses no intrinsic inotropic activity in normal hearts.[172] In animal studies, infusion of T_3 improves myocardial function within 15 minutes, but only after severe global ischemic injury.[172–175] Novitzky et al. showed a decreased need for inotropic support after "T_3-pressor therapy" in clinical studies of donors, cardiac recipients, and patients undergoing open-heart surgery.[145, 149] Corroboration of the proposed role of T_3 as an effective inotropic agent after cardiopulmonary bypass has been unsuccessful. Most recently, perioperative administration of T_3 in patients undergoing coronary artery bypass surgery who are at high risk for myocardial ischemia resulted in no dramatic effect on cardiac function, no alteration in the need for support with inotropic and vasodilator drugs in patients with impairment of ventricular function, or no improvement in outcome.[176–178] The extent to which low T_3 and T_4 may play an interactive role in altering adrenergic receptor response and adrenal steroid hormone status also remains to be clarified.[167, 179] Concerns have been raised about possible adverse effects of T_3 administration to euthyroid donors, including tachycardia, supraventricular arrhythmias, hyperthermia, metabolic acidosis, and oxygen wasting. T_3 replacement therapy has been shown in tissue slices to have a detrimental effect on liver energy status.[180]

Proposed subcellular effects of T_3 that could have acute inotropic and vasodilative effects are shown in Figure 4-1.[181] T_3 effects on myocytes include augmentation of active ion transport systems, sensitization of beta-adrenergic pathways,

Table 4-6. Papworth Hospital "Hormone Package"

Invasive monitoring
Bolus steroids
    Methylprednisolone 15 mg/kg
Insulin (and dextrose)
    Aim for normoglycemia
    Minimum 1 U/hr
Arginine vasopressin
    1-U bolus and 1.5 µ/hr infusion
Triiodothyronine
    4-µg bolus and 3 µg/hr infusion

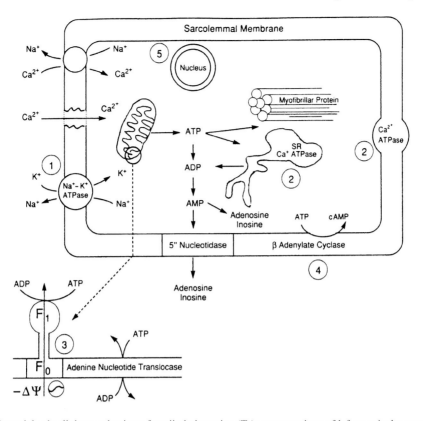

Figure 4-1. Potential subcellular mechanisms for triiodothyronine (T_3) augmentations of left ventricular systolic function. Numeric labels indicate potential sites of action of T_3: (1) T_3 increases bursting of cardiac sodium channels, resulting in increased Na^+ entry into the cell; (2) T_3 increases Ca^{2+} adenosine triphosphatase (ATPase) activity in the plasma membrane and sarcoplasmic reticulum (SR); (3) mitochondrial adenine nucleotide translocase, situated on the inner mitochondrial membrane, regulates the entry of adenosine diphosphate (ADP) into the mitochondrial cytosol for phosphorylation and is activated by thyroid hormone; (4) T_3 may increase adenylate cyclase activity, thereby increasing the concentration of the second messenger, cyclic adenosine monophosphate (cAMP); and (5) T_3 nuclear receptors and effects on synthesis are well established, although unlikely to account for an acute (within minutes) increase in contractile function. (ATP = adenosine triphosphate.) (Reprinted with permission from CM Dyke, T Yea Jr, JD Lehman, et al. Triiodothyronine-enhanced left ventricular function after ischemic injury. Ann Thorac Surg 1991;52:14.)

and increased transcription of messenger ribonucleic acid (mRNA) resulting in protein synthesis. In Figure 4-1, T_3 binding to the myocyte plasma membrane or sarcoplasmic reticulum receptors increases calcium-ATPase activity, activates adenylate cyclase, and increases sodium channel activity. Each upregulation at a membrane ion pump may increase intramyocardial calcium and cardiac contractility. In addition, T_3 activation of mitochondrial adenine nucleotide translocase stimulates oxidative phosphorylation and may be important in metabolic recovery after ischemic injury. T_3 may also reduce the breakdown of catecholamines and

activate conversion of alpha-receptors to beta-receptors,[182] thereby potentiating the effects of endogenous or exogenous inotropes. Delayed nuclear effects, mediated by the transcription of mRNA, can alter myosin isomer expression and increase production of sarcoplasmic calcium-ATP, which may improve diastolic relaxation.[183]

Diabetes Insipidus

Clinical evidence of diabetes insipidus occurs in the vast majority of brain-dead patients, with a reported incidence of up to 85%.[3, 33, 184] Posterior pituitary or hypothalamic dysfunction with lack of central production or release of ADH results in an inappropriate and frequently massive urine output that bears no relation to the intravascular fluid volume. Worsening hypernatremia in conjunction with a low urinary sodium and osmolality is strongly suggestive of diabetes insipidus rather than a diuresis secondary to fluid loading, diuretics, mannitol, or hyperglycemia, in which the urinary sodium is usually greater than 40 mmol/liter. If the diabetes is left untreated, hemodynamic instability may then occur as a result of hypovolemia or electrolyte imbalances. A common presentation of diabetes insipidus includes alterations in urinary and serum sodium and osmolality (comprising the diagnostic criteria),[185] as well as complications of the uncontrolled physiologic process and therapeutic intervention (Table 4-7). A triad of clinical signs, including central diabetes insipidus, low glucose demand, and low CO_2 production, has been referred to in children as *Turner's triad*.[186]

Because polyuria may be multifactorial, the urinary losses should be replaced with crystalloid on a volume-for-volume basis, with the solution composition determined by serum electrolyte and osmolality measurements every 4–6 hours. Usually, a hypotonic solution, such as half normal saline or dextrose in water, is indicated in an amount sufficient to replace urinary losses, meet daily fluid requirements, avoid hyperglycemia, and maintain the serum sodium at less than 155 mmol/liter. Frequently, adequate volume replacement is technically difficult due to the inability to obtain sufficient venous access in children or the problem of inducing hyperglycemia with the rapid infusion of large volumes of glucose-containing fluids in a patient who is glucose intolerant.[62]

Twenty mmol of potassium chloride is added to each liter of intravenous solution given, with additional supplements as required to maintain the serum potassium level above 3.5 mmol/liter. Because hypophosphatemia often occurs as a physiologic consequence of brain death, it seems prudent to use potassium phosphate for simultaneous potassium replacement and phosphorus loading. Maintenance of normal phosphate homeostasis is required for skeletal and respiratory muscle function, hemostasis, red cell integrity and function, oxygen delivery, myocardial contractility, and responsiveness to catecholamines. Clinically, there

Table 4-7. Diabetes Insipidus

Diagnosis
    Hypotonic polyuria: urine output >4 ml/kg/hr
    Hypernatremia
    Urinary sodium <10 mmol/liter
    Urine specific gravity <1.005
    Plasma osmolality >300 mOsm/liter
    Urine osmolality <300 mOsm/liter
Complications
    Metabolic
        Hypovolemia
        Hyperosmolality
        Hypernatremia
        Hypomagnesemia
        Hypokalemia
        Hypophosphatemia
        Hypocalcemia
    Therapy-related
        Volume-replacement
            Hypothermia
            Hyponatremia
            Hyperglycemia
            Nephrogenic diabetes insipidus
            Diuresis secondary to fluid loading or osmotic
                effects
        Vasopressin or desmopressin
            Vasoconstriction
            Hypophosphatemia
            Hyponatremia

appears to be no correlation between plasma phosphate concentration and left ventricular function or oxygen delivery and consumption after brain death. Acute hypophosphatemia secondary to volume expansion and intracellular shift of phosphates, with no significant decrease in intramyocardial stores, could explain these findings.[187]

If the urine output consistently exceeds 5 ml/kg per hour and, most important, if adverse effects of infusing large volumes of crystalloid become evident, vasopressin should be started. A controlled intravenous low-dose infusion of AVP, starting at 0.05–0.1 U/kg per minute (or 2 U/liter of crystalloid, infused to match the previous hourly urine output[188]), or bolus doses of desmopressin acetate (DDAVP) 0.3–0.4 µg/kg every 6–8 hours (pediatric dose 0.025 µg/kg, maximum 1 µg per dose), may be efficacious in increasing water and sodium reabsorption from the distal tubule and titrating the urine output to 2–3 ml/kg per hour. Intramuscular or subcutaneous administration is discouraged because it results in variable absorption and cumulative effects. Early intervention is best because persistent polyuria managed with large quantities of crystalloid infusions may wash out the renal countercurrent system, reducing the kidney's responsiveness to vasopressin. This necessitates the infusion of higher doses of vasopressin to achieve the desired antidiuretic effect, which increases the risk of ischemic injury to transplantable organs or uneven distribution of the preservation solutions during flushing.

The use of AVP or desmopressin to limit the morbidity of polyuria and hemodynamic instability in a brain-dead organ donor is a controversial subject. The hemodynamic effects of AVP are dose dependent and include generalized systemic vasoconstriction, with an increase in MAP; a decrease in cardiac output; coronary, pulmonary, and mesenteric blood flow and heart rate; and arrhythmias.[189] A variety of vascular effects in the renal and hepatic arterial beds have been reported. Nitroprusside and nitroglycerin administration may minimize the undesirable cardiovascular and renal side effects of vasopressin but may also result in a deterioration in gas exchange from an increase in the intrapulmonary physiologic shunt.[190] Desmopressin (a synthetic analogue of AVP) may be the preferred agent due to its enhanced antidiuretic potency, virtual absence of vasopressor and oxytocic activity, and a prolonged half-life and duration of action compared with AVP.[191] Schneider and associates reported that kidneys obtained from donors supported with dopamine or vasopressin injection (Pitressin) demonstrated a higher incidence of ATN and a lower rate of graft survival.[192] The use of vasopressin as an antidiuretic and adjunctive pressor agent is preferred by Scheinkestel's group and supported in experimental studies by the work of Blaine and associates.[60, 193] For pressor support in pediatric donors, they recommend adding vasopressin routinely to norepinephrine infusions exceeding 0.5 μg/kg per minute and consider it second-line therapy when refractory hypotension is a problem in adults.[61] In a brain-dead porcine model, Blaine reported physiologic levels of vasopressin, with normal plasma osmolarity and serum sodium; a decrease in urine output, potassium, and fluid requirements; and no effect on the peripheral vascular resistance or microscopic evidence of organ ischemia.[193] Some reports indicate that serum

vasopressin levels in polyuric donors are consistently within or above the normal range, suggesting that these findings may result from a loss of sensitivity of the renal collecting duct to the action of ADH (nephrogenic diabetes insipidus) rather than from central diabetes insipidus.[194]

With currently available information, the benefits of early treatment of the polyuria of diabetes insipidus with a titratable infusion of vasopressin or desmopressin appear to outweigh the potential for ischemic end-organ injury. This would minimize electrolyte abnormalities, fluid shifts, and a reduction in core temperature, which, if left untreated, could contribute to the subsequent development of interstitial edema and myocardial dysfunction. Vasopressin causes increased excretion of urinary phosphate, so inorganic phosphate levels should be monitored and corrected to prevent hypophosphatemia, which could result in a depression of myocardial contractility.[3]

Oliguria suggests hypovolemia, hypoperfusion, disease of the kidney or urinary collecting system, or excessive administration of vasopressin. In the absence of diabetes insipidus, renal management should be based on optimizing filling pressures while monitoring the CVP. If the urine output is inadequate after volume expansion, at a systolic pressure of 90–120 mm Hg, the use of mannitol, furosemide, and renal-dose dopamine[51] or dopexamine may enhance renal function as well as provide protection from preservation injury. If all the above measures fail, placement of a PAC may assist in assessing ventricular function and volume status, facilitating the titration of fluids and inotropic agents to achieve a cardiac index greater than 2.1 liter per minute per sq m.[195]

The infusion of large volumes of glucose-containing solutions, in combination with peripheral insulin resistance resulting from the hormonal stress response, glucocorticoid administration, and inotropic infusions, may significantly exacerbate already increased levels of glucose. The major consequences of hyperglycemia include an increase in the plasma osmolality, metabolic acidosis, ketosis, and osmotic diuresis with a loss of free water and electrolytes, leading to hypovolemia and cardiac instability. Serum glucose, potassium, and ketones must be monitored, and a continuous infusion of insulin (bolus 0.1 U/kg regular insulin, followed by 0.5–2.0 U/hour) should be used to maintain the serum glucose level between 150 and 250 mg/dl. Although supporting experimental and clinical data are limited, nutritional supplementation of the organ donor with 200–400 g glucose and 5–10 units of insulin per 100 g dextrose given over a 24- to 48-hour period before procurement may promote repletion of liver glycogen stores, with a reduction in the risk of injury and posttransplant failure of liver allografts.[196]

Care of the donor can be time consuming and emotionally draining on the resources of a critical care unit. It should be undertaken, however, with the same vigilance and dedication that one would exercise for any patient in an intensive care setting. In 1992, failure to recover organs despite consent occurred in 42% of cases for heart, 20% for liver, and 84% for lungs. The most frequent cause for nonrecovery after consent was poor organ function.[197] Once the process of brain-death certification has been completed, any delays in proceeding immediately to organ recovery may result in hemodynamic collapse of the donor and subsequent loss of organs.[53] The length of donor hospitalization and duration of brain death before procurement also represent a significant donor risk factor for lung, liver, and pancreas graft failure in the recipient.

Respiratory Complications

Pulmonary care is aimed at maintenance of adequate alveolar ventilation and arterial oxygenation, protection of the airways from aspiration and prevention of atelectasis, edema, retention of secretions, and infection. Heart-lung donors must be free of overt pulmonary disease, although 65% demonstrate tracheal aspirates that are culture-positive for bacteria.[198] Treatment of lung donors with intravenous and aerosolized antibiotics has been shown to decrease the incidence of early bacterial pneumonia in the recipient of lung allografts.[199] Currently, only approximately 15–20% of multiple organ donors have lungs suitable for transplantation.[200]

By definition, mechanical ventilation is required in brain-dead patients to ensure adequate systemic oxygenation and acid-base balance. The fraction of inspired oxygen (FIO_2) and minute ventilation should be sufficient to maintain the PaO_2 at 100–150 mm Hg, the arterial blood oxygen saturation (SaO_2) at

95% or greater, $PaCO_2$ at 35–45 mm Hg, and pH, uncorrected for temperature, at 7.40 or greater. Pulmonary edema, whether related to increased endothelial permeability or the result of imbalances in oncotic and hydrostatic pressures and extravasation of fluid into the intraalveolar space, responds to diuresis combined with the application of positive end-expiratory pressure (PEEP). Levels of PEEP in excess of 7.5 cm H_2O are best avoided because of the detrimental effects on thoracic venous return, cardiac output, regional blood flow, and possible barotrauma with lung injury.[201] Adverse humoral effects, including the release of ADH and activation of the renin-angiotensin-aldosterone system, have also been described.[202] If high levels of PEEP are required to maintain adequate oxygenation, the insertion of a PAC may be useful to confirm the diagnosis and monitor therapeutic interventions. Frequent arterial blood gas measurements with appropriate ventilatory adjustments and good pulmonary toilet using aseptic technique are essential.

The FIO_2 should be increased to 100% for transport to the operating room. The important exception is during heart-lung retrieval, when an FIO_2 set as low as possible (less than 40%) to maintain PaO_2 greater than 100 mm Hg, at a normal tidal volume setting of 10–15 cc/kg, and a peak inspiratory pressure less than 30 cm H_2O, is desirable to minimize the possible effects of oxygen toxicity, atelectasis, and pressure injury to the lungs.

Intraoperative Management of the Donor

Declaration of brain death is made by a physician not associated with the transplant team before transporting the donor patient to the operating room. The anesthesiologist should verify the appropriate medical and legal documentation of family consent for organ donation and certification of death. The same fundamentals of donor management apply in the operating room as in the ICU, with an emphasis on optimum organ perfusion and oxygenation together with fluid, electrolyte, temperature, and acid-base balances. Because multiple-organ retrieval is a major thoracoabdominal procedure, which can be associated with considerable blood loss and physiologic derangements, the operating room should be prepared accordingly (Table 4-8).

The management problems are complex and the therapy challenging, yet the therapeutic goals for optimum perioperative therapy are simple. To facilitate rapid recall, they can be summarized as the "rule of 100s": systolic blood pressure (100 mm Hg), CVP (less than 10 mm Hg), pulmonary capillary wedge pressure (PCWP) (less than 10 mm Hg), SVR (less than 1,000 dynes per second^{-5}), heart rate (less than 100 beats per minute), urine output (100 ml/hour), PaO_2 (greater than 100 mm Hg), hemoglobin (100 g/liter), and temperature (100°F).[203]

Monitoring

Cardiovascular instability and hemodynamic changes in the brain-dead organ donor due to autonomous reflexes have been described.[204] There is considerable variability in donors' hemodynamic response to surgical stimulation.[205] Monitoring of the electrocardiogram, CVP, urine output, core temperature, breath sounds, SaO_2, and end-tidal CO_2 is essential, as is placement of an arterial catheter in an upper extremity to facilitate sampling and monitoring of the arterial blood pressure during sequential organ removal. If not already in place, left-sided arterial and right-sided central venous catheters are ideal. The right subclavian artery and left brachiocephalic vein are divided early in the donor operation, with subsequent loss of monitoring and access from right-sided arterial and left-sided venous cannulas.[206] If the donor has a PAC in situ, this should be used, but routine insertion for intraoperative use is currently not a standardized practice. Clinical indications for a PAC include assessment of volume status, measurement of cardiac output, and mixed venous oxygen and calculation of hemodynamic parameters. Patients who may benefit from pulmonary artery monitoring include those with evidence of persistent hypotension despite aggressive resuscitation (CVP greater than 15 mm Hg), when an objective assessment of cardiac function is thought to be crucial to optimizing donor management,[207] for complex fluid management (if one anticipates large fluid volume shifts or in the presence of acute renal failure), and in those requiring increasing levels of PEEP for oxygenation, with or without pulmonary edema. Consideration should be given to the possibility of catheter-induced arrhythmias, trauma to the heart or lungs, and infection, all

Table 4-8. Preoperative Anesthesia Checklist for Organ Recovery

Review
  Declaration of brain death
  Consent for organ donation
  Laboratory data (arterial blood gases, electrolytes, hematocrit, glucose)
  Vital signs, ventilator settings, core temperature, drug infusion dosages
Monitoring equipment and apparatus
  Pressure transducers and display for intra-arterial BP, CVP, PAP, PCWP, CO, mixed venous O_2 saturation
  Urinary catheter
  Esophageal and core temperature probes
  Electrocardiograph
  Pulse oximeter (SaO_2)
  Capnograph (end-tidal CO_2)
  Noninvasive BP monitor
  Mechanical ventilator
  Warming blanket and warmed-air heater ± Heater/humidifier for inspiratory gases
  Nasogastric tube
  Sterile endotracheal suction catheters
  Intravenous fluid warmers
  PEEP valves (2.5- and 5-cm H_2O)
  Calibrated drug-infusion pumps
  Venous and arterial blood sampling syringes and tubes
  Cardiac resuscitation cart (advanced cardiac life support antiarrhythmic drugs and defibrillator)
Drugs
  Vasoactive: dopamine, epinephrine, isoproterenol, vasopressin
  Norepinephrine
  Nitroprusside
  Inhalational agents
  O_2 or air
  Crystalloid, colloid, availability of CMV-compatible donor matched packed RBC (adults 4 units, children 2 units)
  Pancuronium
  Heparin (300 U/kg)
  Diuretics (mannitol 1 g/kg and furosemide 40–100 mg)
  Antibiotics
  Insulin
  Potassium
  Protocol drugs requested by transplant coordinator
      Chlorpromazine 100 mg
      T_3 or T_4
      PGE_1
      Betadine-amphotericin solution for nasogastric instillation in pancreas donors
  Antiarrhythmics: lidocaine, esmolol, sodium bicarbonate, bretylium, epinephrine, calcium, adenosine
Goals of intraoperative management: "rule of 100s"
  Systolic BP >100 mm Hg
  CVP <10 mm Hg
  PCWP <10 mm Hg
  SVR <1,000 dynes/sec^{-5}
  Heart rate <100 beats/min
  PaO_2 >100 mm Hg
  Urine output >100 ml/hr
  Hemoglobin 100 g/liter
  Temperature 100°F

BP = blood pressure; CVP = central venous pressure; PAP = peak airway pressure; PCWP = pulmonary capillary wedge pressure; PEEP = positive end-expiratory pressure; CMV = cytomegalovirus; RBCs = red blood cells; T_3 = triiodothyronine; T_4 = thyroxine; PGE_1 = prostaglandin E_1; SVR = systemic vascular resistance.

of which are detrimental to the donor. Arterial blood gas tensions, acid-base status, hematocrit, electrolytes, and blood glucose should be measured every hour. Aggressive intervention with the use of a warming blanket, warmed air mattress, and intravenous fluid warmers should help to maintain the donor's temperature above 35°C.

Ventilator Settings

Ventilatory requirements include maintaining adequate oxygenation; avoiding atelectasis, barotrauma, and oxygen toxicity; and minimizing disruption of the surgical field and heat loss. Ventilatory settings include an FIO_2 of 1.0 (lungs or heart-lung transplant, FIO_2 of 0.4) while maintaining Pao_2 at 100–150 mm Hg (Sao_2 of at least 95%), PEEP less than 7.5 cm H_2O, tidal volume at 10–15 cc/kg, and a rate adjusted to maintain $Paco_2$ at 35–45 mm Hg. An arterial pH (uncorrected for temperature) kept slightly alkalemic at 7.4 helps to maintain better end-organ function under hypothermic conditions.[134, 208, 209] Correction of a base deficit greater than –5 reduces minute ventilatory requirements and minimizes possible increases in the intrathoracic pressure, which may have a negative impact on the cardiac output. Clearly, with a decrease in oxygen consumption and low CO_2 production (in the absence of cerebral blood flow, central sympathetic drive, and muscle tone), the normal calculated ventilatory settings and gas flow rates based on weight result in hypocapnia. Theoretically, avoiding extensive vascular manipulation and dissection may optimize organ perfusion by avoiding iatrogenic arterial vasospasm. Maintaining $Paco_2$ at greater than or equal to 45 mm Hg may offset vasospasm by a direct vasodilatory effect of hypercapnia resulting in a decreased SVR and an increase in cardiac output from stimulation of the sympathetic nervous system. Mild hypercapnia ($Paco_2$ of 59 mm Hg) increases portal venous blood flow and total hepatic blood flow but also causes a concomitant reduction in liver function. The question of whether hemodynamic responses to alterations of $Paco_2$ parallel changes in end-organ function has been raised.[210, 211] Plasma noradrenaline concentrations increase during apnea,[212] suggesting a sympathoadrenal response at the spinal level in response to acute hypercapnia.

Spinal Reflexes

The declaration of brain death requires the loss of cerebral and brain stem reflexes, leaving responses of spinal origin intact. Clinical observations compatible with the diagnosis of brain death that should not be misinterpreted as evidence for brain stem function include[213]

1. Spontaneous movements of the limbs other than pathologic flexion or extension responses
2. Respiratory-like movements (shoulder elevation and adduction, back arching, intercostal expansion without significant tidal volumes)
3. Muscle stretch reflexes and superficial abdominal reflexes
4. Babinski's reflex
5. Profuse sweating and blushing
6. Tachycardia and sudden increases in blood pressure

Spinal cord responses are observed in approximately 30–70% of brain-dead patients[214, 215] and may occur spontaneously or be elicited by nociceptive stimulation, respiratory acidosis, hypoxia, or brisk neck flexion.[216]

Neuromuscular Reflexes

Reflex muscular contractions, including raising of all limbs off the bed, grasping movements, jerking of one leg, and walking-like movements, have been described. The Lazarus sign includes gooseflesh on arms and trunk, shivering extensor movements, flexion of the arms at the elbow, and bringing the hands to the midsternum as if grasping for the endotracheal tube.[217, 218] For the unsuspecting in the operating room, this can generate tremendous anxiety, and staff may require frequent reassurance that the donor is indeed brain dead. To avoid this reflex neuromuscular activity and to facilitate surgical exposure, the administration of a long-acting nondepolarizing muscle relaxant at the onset of the procedure is important.

Cardiovascular Reflexes

Current definitions of brain death require the absence of medullary respiratory reflexes but not those of cardiovascular control. Explanations for increases in MAP and heart rate have included residual brain stem vasomotor activity, a spinal vasoconstrictor reflex arc between pain and sympathetically mediated efferents, or adrenal medullary stimulation by a spinoadrenal reflex arc.[219–221] Others have found complete cessation of normal variations of the autonomic cardiovascular system, with no evidence of hemodynamic response to noxious stimuli.[222] If left untreated, hypertension and tachycardia may lead to excessive operative blood loss and histopathologic damage to the kidneys, lungs, and heart. Therapy includes adjusting the dosage of inotropic agent and administering a vasodilator, such as nitroglycerin or nitroprusside, although isoflurane is usually more readily available. Some experienced anesthesiologists recommend the use of narcotic analgesics to depress the hemodynamic response elicited on surgical incision.[56, 72, 223] Others question the validity of such a choice.[48, 224]

Hemodynamic Management

Retrieval surgery results in significant hemodynamic effects.[205, 224–226] Pennefather et al. described a biphasic hemodynamic response, with an increase in MAP and SVR after skin incision and sternotomy, followed by a decrease in MAP and PCWP attributed to changes in peripheral vascular resistance.[226]

The first step in resuscitation involves fluid administration with crystalloids, colloids, or blood products, using the hematocrit, electrolytes, filling pressures, heart rate, and possibly cardiac output and mixed venous oxygen saturation as therapeutic endpoints. The specific organs to be donated determine fluid management and the choice of pressor agents. Maintaining a minimum systolic pressure of 90–100 mm Hg, a CVP less than 10 mm Hg, a heart rate less than 100 beats per minute, and hematocrit greater than 24% are the aims to ensure adequate perfusion and oxygen delivery to all vital organs. Remember that the absolute blood pressure measurement in a maximally vasodilated patient may be low, despite adequate end-organ perfusion. In addition to those already mentioned, causes of intraoperative hypotension include rapid infusion of cold preservatives into the portal system, with precipitous hypothermia and cardiovascular instability, and the cardiorespiratory changes inherent in the surgical technique, including

sternotomy, lung retraction, manipulation of the heart, and intraperitoneal dissection of the inferior vena cava (IVC). Intraoperative blood transfusions may be required as a result of losses due to poor surgical technique in conjunction with uncontrolled hypertensive responses to surgical stimulation, continuing resuscitation of the trauma victim, attempted correction of a bleeding diathesis, and excessive blood sampling for tissue typing. Generally, a donor from whom the heart, liver, and kidneys are being removed requires the infusion of 2 units of pRBC during the dissection phases.

The choice of inotropes in order of preference includes dopamine (at a maximum of 10 µg/kg/minute), dobutamine (at a maximum of 15 µg/kg/minute), epinephrine (at less than 0.1 µg/kg/minute), and, when the need is critical, norepinephrine with dopamine for renal protection.

Even with the most rigorous efforts, the inevitable deterioration of the brain-dead patient leads to cardiovascular collapse. Because ventricular arrhythmias and bradycardia are frequent, bretylium, lidocaine, epinephrine, and isoproterenol should be immediately available. Bradycardia in the brain-dead patient is resistant to atropine. In the event of cardiac arrest, cardiopulmonary resuscitation should be initiated, and procurement should proceed rapidly with cross-clamping of the aorta at the diaphragm and infusion of cold preservation solution into the distal aorta and portal vein. Although the heart may not then be usable, maintaining an adequate cardiac output with manual compressions and drug therapy may support the other perfusable organs until core cooling begins.

Pharmacologic intervention has frequently been used to improve the viability of the kidneys before transplantation. Commonly used agents are dopamine, mannitol (1 g/kg), furosemide (40–100 mg), and chlorpromazine (100 mg) given just before division of the renal vascular pedicle. After aortic cannulation and before occlusion of the proximal aorta, heparin (300 U/kg) is administered to prevent intravascular thrombosis.

Anesthetic support of the organ donor is necessary until surgical occlusion of the proximal aorta and start of in situ flushing of organs, after which all monitoring and supportive measures must be discontinued. This limits the amount of emotional distress for operating room personnel involved in witnessing the slow anoxic cardiac death of a donor if only the kidneys and liver are being retrieved. A record should be kept of the time of cross-clamping of the proximal aorta and infusion of cardioplegic solution because it represents the start time of cold ischemia for the transplantable organs.

Multiple Cadaveric Organ Recovery

Surgical techniques for organ recovery have gradually evolved from traditional, extensive in vivo dissection and skeletonization of individual vessels and the removal of warm organs to a coordinated sequence of inspection, mobilization, exsanguination, and preservation with in situ core cooling, followed by surgical removal. If the donor is hemodynamically unstable, an alternate approach has been used of inducing circulatory arrest followed by rapid in situ flushing and "no-touch" en bloc removal of organs. These procurement techniques minimize the possibility of surgically induced warm ischemic injury to perfusable organs from iatrogenic arterial vasospasm, direct trauma, or hypotension from blood loss.

Multiple organ recovery from a heart-beating donor is a sterile procedure usually completed in 6 hours or less, depending on the surgical team's experience, the number of organs intended for retrieval, the presence of accessory vessels, and the donor's hemodynamic stability. When recovery includes the whole pancreas graft with an attached duodenal segment, an additional 45 minutes is required for mobilization. The retrieval team usually consists of one or more visiting surgical groups and transplant coordinators, who work in concert with the operating team of surgeons, nurses, and anesthesiologists from the donor institution. Anesthetic support of the donor is necessary until surgical occlusion of the proximal aorta and the start of in situ flushing of organs with preservation solution, after which the ventilation, monitoring, and intravenous infusions are discontinued.

General Surgical Preparation

The donor should be positioned supine on the operating table with the arms placed in extreme abduction. After surgical preparation and draping, with the thoracic and abdominal teams working simultaneously, a long midline incision is made from the suprasternal notch to the symphysis pubis, and with deflation of the lungs, the sternum is split. Surgically exposing the abdominal and thoracic cavities, even when the heart and lungs are not intended for removal, provides maximum exposure of the abdominal viscera and facilitates resuscitation of the unstable donor in the event of cardiac arrest.

Once the abdomen is opened and exploration of the peritoneal cavity excludes the presence of intra-abdominal sepsis, malignancy, or bowel ischemia, the supporting ligaments of the liver are divided, and the proximal aorta is encircled above the celiac axis (isolating the renal circulation) for future cross-clamping. The liver is inspected for color, consistency, fat content, laceration, hematoma, capillary perfusion, and the presence of arterial anomalies. The splenic or inferior mesenteric vein is cannulated to allow flushing of the liver through the portal system, and a second ligature is placed around the distal abdominal aorta to allow cannulation and retrograde aortic perfusion. During procurement of the heart, the pericardium is opened, and the heart and great vessels are inspected for normal anatomy, contractility, patency of the coronary arteries, and the presence of injury. The aorta and caval vessels are dissected free, and a purse-string suture is placed in the midportion of the ascending aorta to secure the cardioplegia catheter. Hypotension is inherent in this procedure secondary to IVC compression, manipulation of the heart and lungs, hypovolemia, and hypothermia.

Preservation Techniques

Anticoagulation of the donor is necessary to prevent the formation of microvascular thrombi, thereby facilitating uniform distribution of the cooling preservation solution during flushing and optimum reperfusion with revascularization of organs in the recipient. Before insertion of the cardioplegia and lung-perfusion cannulas, heparin is given (3 mg/kg or 300 U/kg) through a central venous catheter, after verification of the ability to freely aspirate blood from this line, or directly into the right atrial appendage. In addition, the transplant coordinator may request the administration of protocol therapy, before cross-clamping the aorta, aimed at improving donor organ preservation. This usually consists of chlorpromazine, phentolamine, prostaglandin E_1 (PGE_1), allopurinol, dextran 40, thyroid hormones, renal-dose dopamine, furosemide, and/or mannitol. Experimental attempts to improve tissue perfusion and limit the cold ischemic injury and reperfusion damage of transplanted organs have been directed almost exclusively toward renal donation, and the question remains whether conclusions drawn from these studies can be extrapolated to multiorgan donation. This includes the use of lidocaine, naloxone, aprotinin, glutathione, albumin flush, dextrose-loading, calcium channel blockers, and atrial natriuretic factor before and during the procurement operation. Methylprednisolone (30 mg/kg) is routinely administered at least 2 hours before organ recovery in an attempt to minimize ischemic injury to the heart and kidneys by membrane stabilization and to eliminate donor lymphocytes from the microcirculation, thereby decreasing antigenicity of the organ graft.[227–229]

After 5 minutes of circulation time, an aortic flush catheter is placed in the distal abdominal aorta above the bifurcation (a portal flush through the inferior mesenteric vein may also be desirable), the central venous catheter is withdrawn, and venous inflow is occluded by first clamping and then dividing the inferior and superior vena cavae at their caval-atrial junctions. The heart is allowed to beat through five or six cardiac cycles until empty, and the aortic cross-clamp is applied. Infusions of cardioplegic solution for cardiac perfusion, lung preservation solution for pulmonary flushing, and cold lactated Ringer's, modified Euro-Collins, or Belzer solution for portal flushing are started simultaneously. Outflow for the perfusate and blood to allow for complete venous decompression of the intra-abdominal viscera is achieved by venting into the pericardium through the divided suprahepatic portion of the IVC or into the abdominal cavity (or the cannula-directed catheter drainage system) through the transected infrarenal vena cava and portal vein. During the flushing phase, the abdomen and chest are filled with cold sterile slush solution to achieve rapid topical cooling while the solid organs are observed for uniform blanching. Palpation of the heart confirms diastolic arrest without ventricular distention. The sequential en bloc removal of organs proceeds according to their anatomic location and susceptibility to ischemia.

Therefore, the heart or heart-lungs are usually secured first, then the liver, and finally the kidneys, with the pancreatectomy performed after the liver or kidneys are removed. The spleen and lymph nodes are removed for tissue typing and immunologic studies, and the aorta, IVC, and iliac vessels are removed for use as vascular grafts. After hypothermic perfusion with a preservation solution, sterile bench dissection (i.e., cholecystectomy, division of the lung bloc, and so on) and biopsies, the donor organs are preserved, without perfusion, by cold storage in sterile bags filled with iced preservation solution and placed in plastic coolers filled with crushed ice.

Heart-Lungs and Lung Procurement

Positioning of the endotracheal tube should be confirmed by the surgeons who will procure the heart-lungs to minimize mucosal injury to the trachea where the suture line will occur. Division of the mediastinal pleura, dissection of the trachea from attachments to the aorta and esophagus, manipulation of the heart and each lung separately out of the mediastinum, and atrial dissection all result in significant mechanical hypotension and difficulties with ventilation and oxygenation. Once adequate fluid volume is restored to a CVP of 8–10 mm Hg, dopamine at less than 10 µg/kg per minute may be required for cardiovascular support, with an acceptable minimum MAP of 60 mm Hg during this interval of manipulation. With cross-clamping of the aorta and administration of cardioplegic solution into the aortic root, cardiac arrest ensues, and pulmonary artery perfusion is begun through a catheter inserted into the main pulmonary artery. The tip of the left atrial appendage of the heart is then excised to prevent distention of the heart by the return of pulmonary perfusate through the pulmonary veins. In this interval, monitoring of the inspiratory O_2 concentration should be continued, with the donor manually ventilated on a maximum FIO_2 of 0.40, at half the normal tidal volumes for four breaths per minute, to aid in even distribution of the preservation solution. Pulmonary artery distention or infusion of solutions of high potassium content or low temperature cause reflex pulmonary vasoconstriction, which impedes complete and uniform distribution of the cooling solution within the pulmonary vasculature.[230] Based on experimental evidence of improvement of gas exchange in the monkey model, the use of PGE_1 to dilate the pulmonary vasculature has become a standardized technique for lung preservation.[231] PGE_1 is either contained in the preservation solution, given as a bolus injection into the pulmonary artery before excision of the heart-lungs bloc, or given 15 minutes before the anticipated clamping of the aorta infused via central venous access at a rate of 15 ng/kg per minute and gradually increased, as long as the MAP is maintained at 55 mm Hg or greater.[230] More recently, prostaglandin I_2 (PGI_2) has also been used as an intravenous infusion or a large bolus just before placement of the aortic cross-clamp.[232] When ventilatory support is discontinued, the airway is suctioned and the endotracheal tube removed. The trachea is divided between clamps, and the lungs, maintained in an inflated state, are removed from the chest. Some centers prefer to remove these organs while the donor is on cardiopulmonary bypass.

Specific Medical and Surgical Considerations

Specific medical and surgical considerations for optimal procurement and subsequent function of each donor include

Heart

1. The requirement for insertion or removal of a PAC
2. The need for withdrawal of the CVP catheter before occlusion of venous inflow to the heart
3. Determination of the optimum drug choice and maximum allowable dose for pressor support:
   Beta agonist: dopamine or dobutamine less than 10 µg/kg per minute
   Alpha agonist: phenylephrine, metaraminol bitartrate, vasopressin
   Hemodynamic goals: "rule of 100s" (see Table 4-8)
4. Avoidance of right- or left-sided myocardial distention
5. Possible use of full hypothermic cardiopulmonary bypass
6. Current standardized method for cardiac graft preservation, including in situ perfusion with venous inflow occlusion and bench perfusion

Future trends in surgical removal of donor hearts for transplant include new cardioplegic solutions containing free radical scavengers (allopurinol), high glucose and ATP content, substrate enhancement with selected amino acids, freezing methods allowing true metabolic arrest, HLA matching, and xenografts. Studies predictive of successful graft outcome include the biochemical evaluation of donor heart damage by measurement of cardiac troponin-I.[233]

Lungs

1. The tip of the endotracheal tube should be positioned at least five cartilaginous rings above the tracheal carina to ensure that the inflated cuff does not contribute to mucosal injury at the site of the anticipated suture line.
2. Insertion of a CVP catheter, with a resultant pneumothorax or hemothorax, may preclude subsequent use of the lung.
3. During the period of infusion of the lung preservation fluid, the transplant team may request manual ventilation of the lungs with FIO_2 at 0.21–0.40, at four breaths per minute with half the normal tidal volume.
4. The lungs may be removed and inflated to two-thirds vital capacity.
5. The use of colloid for intraoperative fluid management and limiting central venous filling pressures to less than 8–10 mm Hg (ideally, CVP less than 6 mm Hg and PCWP less than 10 mm Hg[226]) may help reduce interstitial and intra-alveolar extravasation of fluid in the setting of increased capillary permeability, resulting in subsequent pulmonary insufficiency.
6. Ventilatory settings are chosen to limit toxic exposures to the lung, including
   FIO_2 less than 0.40
   PaO_2 greater than 100 mm Hg, SaO_2 greater than 95%
   Tidal volume 15 cc/kg, PEEP = 5 cm H_2O, peak inflation pressure less than 25–30 cm H_2O
   Areas of atelectasis and collapsed segments should be reinflated by periodic manual ventilation.
7. Susceptibility to infection should be minimized with the use of sterile suction catheters and

endotracheal tubes, frequent suctioning, manual recruitment of lung volume, and prophylactic antibiotics.[185]

8. The use of PGE_1 for pulmonary artery vasodilation has the inherent predictable risk of inducing systemic hypotension.
9. Monitoring of F_{IO_2} until the end is desirable.
10. Fiberoptic bronchoscopy should be available intraoperatively.
11. Cardiopulmonary bypass technique has adverse effects on platelets and alveolar capillary membrane permeability.
12. The sequence for lung procurement and preservation techniques includes
    Pulmonary artery vasodilation
    Flush perfusion cooling
    Simple crystalloid cardioplegia
    En bloc excision of the heart and lungs, followed by "pumpers" (normothermic continuous perfusion) or "freezers" (flush perfusion cooling: hypothermia and metabolic inhibition)

Strategies to enhance lung preservation include magnesium sulfate added to modified Euro-Collins solution, platelet-activating factor antagonist (e.g., TCV-309), oxygen-derived free radical scavengers, PGE_1 or PGI_2, infusion of pulmonary flush solution at less than 10–15 mm Hg, and minimal manipulation of the lungs.

Kidneys

1. Various simple therapeutic interventions are available to maintain an adequate urine output. A urine output greater than 100 ml per hour just before donor nephrectomy is one of the most important factors for posttransplant renal graft function.[234]
2. Desmopressin and vasopressin infusions are discontinued 1 hour before the anticipated cross-clamp of the aorta.
3. Maintaining a systolic blood pressure less than 140–150 mm Hg has been documented as efficacious for renal graft function. Albumin-containing solutions are preferable to artificial plasma expanders for volume replacement because the latter may jeopardize kidney function.[235]

Strategies to enhance renal function include administration of chlorpromazine, naloxone, allopurinol, catalase, superoxide dismutase, prostacyclin, verapamil, and lidocaine.

Donor criteria for the kidney are the broadest of any donated organ due to its ability to recover from ischemic insults and because renal function is not required for recipient survival immediately after transplantation.

Pancreas

1. During procurement, amphotericin irrigation solution and povidone-iodine (Betadine) solution are sequentially instilled through a nasogastric tube whose tip is positioned in the first portion of the duodenum.
2. Hyperglycemia in brain-dead donors is not a sign of endocrine insufficiency in the pancreas but rather represents a state of peripheral insulin resistance.[171, 236, 237] It should be avoided. Major consequences include an increase in plasma osmolality, metabolic acidosis, and osmotic diuresis with loss of free water and electrolytes, which may lead to cardiac instability.

Liver

1. Minimize central venous filling pressures to avoid parenchymal edema and centrilobular ischemia, as evidenced by congestion or solid consistency of the liver and blunting of its edges.
2. Limit the infusion of dopamine to less than 15 μg/kg per minute.[238] Avoid pressor combinations.[239]
3. Control the temperature of the final preservation solution.
4. The nutritional status of the liver is a factor in its sensitivity to ischemia-reperfusion damage: glucose supplementation in an attempt to replenish exhausted liver glycogen stores required for ATP production by anaerobic glycolysis during cold preservation[240, 241] and adenosine flushing of the donor liver to reduce leukocyte adherence, which may contribute to posttransplant reperfusion injury.[242]
5. Minimize preservation time for donors with these factors: advanced age, fatty infiltration, pro-

longed hospitalization, and cardiovascular instability. Traditional donor assessment parameters have not been shown to be reliable predictors of outcome in clinical liver transplantation.[243]

6. Techniques for testing the functional integrity of the donor liver and predicting ultimate graft and patient survival include[244]

- The conversion of lidocaine to its metabolite monoethylglycinexylidide
- Adenine nucleotide content in liver biopsy
- Arterial ketone body ratio as a measure of hepatic mitochondrial redox potential
- Plasma lecithin-cholesterol acyltransferase activity (enzyme that catalyzes the esterification of cholesterol)
- Platelet adhesion to sinusoidal endothelium
- Clearance of indocyanine green

7. Factors contributing to primary graft dysfunction include

Donor factors

- Moderate fatty infiltration (greater than 30% of volume of hepatocyte)
- Age older than 50 years
- Serum sodium greater than 155 mmol/liter (exclusion criteria include serum sodium greater than 170 mmol/liter and hospitalized more than 7 days)[245]

Organ preservation in University of Wisconsin (UW) solution at 4°C

- Cold ischemic time greater than 12–16 hours

Surgical factors

- Prolonged warm ischemic time
- Ischemic-reperfusion injury

Recipient factors

- Retransplantation
- High medical status
- Renal failure

Small Intestine and Abdominal Organ Cluster Recovery

Procurement of small bowel is usually performed simultaneously with that of other visceral organs after institution-specific donor-directed therapy designed to maximize mesenteric perfusion, limit edema formation in the bowel wall, and modulate the immunoreactivity of the gut. Nasogastric instillation of hyperosmolar cathartic solutions and unab-sorbable antibiotics in the ICU is followed by intravenous administration of ampicillin and cefotaxime at the time of operation.

Successful procurement depends on optimum donor management, the technical expertise of the surgical teams, and adherence to the allowable cold ischemia times for optimal organ preservation. Kidneys may be preserved in UW solution with simple cold storage for up to 80 hours, but the rate of ATN increases after 24 hours. Alternatively, preservation time may be further extended for up to 7 days by the use of normothermic "maintenance" machine perfusion.[246] The heart and lungs should be transplanted within 4–6 hours, but ischemic times of up to 8 hours (6 hours for single-lung transplant for primary pulmonary hypertension) are routinely tolerated for the lungs.[247] In the infant donor population, ischemia times for the cardiac graft may range up to 8 hours with normal postoperative function. The primary difficulty in successfully preserving the heart for 24 hours or more is related to its high content of contractile proteins. Normally, ATP is gradually lost in most organs during cold storage and is rapidly regenerated after transplantation, with little impact on immediate organ function or viability. In hearts, as the ATP concentration drops below a critical threshold, contraction-band necrosis and permanent ischemic injury occurs within the actin-myosin complex on reperfusion. Flushing with UW preservation solution has increased the safe cold ischemia time for parenchymal integrity of the liver from 8–24 hours and up to 29 hours for the pancreas. Further investigation is needed to determine whether the incidence of intrahepatic bile duct strictures is increased when the cold storage time exceeds 12–15 hours. Primary nonfunction (6%) or poor initial graft function (16%) in the liver recipient is life threatening. It also significantly drains professional and hospital resources and escalates the hospital charges for the procedure.[246] Retransplantation further depletes the donor pool. Therefore, optimal perioperative care of both the organ donor and transplant recipient is crucial for fostering a favorable outcome after transplantation.

Conclusions

As the scientific basis and clinical practice of organ transplantation continue to evolve, we are faced with many challenging limitations. In this scheme, a relatively underappreciated component has been the identification and perioperative management of the multiorgan donor. Because the demand for vital organs significantly exceeds the potential supply, we must commit energies to maximizing the use of existing resources. The objective is to provide life-saving therapy for patients with end-stage organ failure.

References

1. Potter CD, Wheeldon DR, Wallwork J. Functional assessment and management of heart donors: a rationale for characterization and guide to therapy. J Heart Lung Transplant 1995;14:59–65.
2. United Network for Organ Sharing. Annual Report of the U.S. Scientific Registry of Transplant Recipients and the Organ Procurement and Transplantation Network. Transplant Data: 1988–1998. Richmond, VA: UNOS; and Rockville, MD: the Division of Transplantation, Bureau of Health Resources Development, Health Resources and Services Administration, U.S. Department of Health and Human Services.
3. Soifer BE, Gelb AW. The multiple organ donor: identification and management. Ann Intern Med 1989;110:814–823.
4. Tolle SW, Bennett W, Hickman DH, Benson JA. Responsibilities of primary physicians in organ donation. Ann Intern Med 1987;106:740–744.
5. Evans RW, Orians CE, Ascher NL. The potential supply of organ donors. An assessment of the efficacy of organ procurement efforts in the United States. JAMA 1992;267:239–246.
6. First RM. Transplantation in the nineties. Transplantation 1992;53:1–11.
7. Gabel H. Editorial comment: organ procurement and renal transplants in Spain. The impact of transplant coordination. Nephrol Dial Transplant 1994;9:479–481.
8. Bia MJ, Ramos EL, Danovitch GM, et al. Evaluation of living renal donors. The current practice of US transplant centers. Transplantation 1995;60:322–327.
9. Kasiske BL, Bia MJ. The evaluation and selection of living kidney donors. Am J Kidney Dis 1995;26:387–398.
10. Sutherland DE, Gruessner R, Dunn D, et al. Pancreas transplants from living-related donors. Transplant Proc 1994;26:443–445.
11. Bhatnager V, Rela M, Heaton ND, Tan KC. Liver transplantation from living related donors: review of world experience and its implications for India. Indian J Pediatr 1994;61:387–393.
12. Jurim O, Shackleton CR, McDiarmid SV, et al. Living-donor liver transplantation at UCLA. Am J Surg 1995;169:529–532.
13. Starnes VA, Barr ML, Cohen RG. Lobar transplantation. Indications, technique and outcome. J Thorac Cardiovasc Surg 1994;108:403–410.
14. Nathan HM, Jarrell BE, Broznik B, et al. Estimation and characterization of the potential renal organ donor pool in Pennsylvania. Report of the Pennsylvania Statewide Donor Study. Transplantation 1991;51:142–149.
15. Casavilla A, Ramirez C, Shapiro R, et al. Experience with liver and kidney allografts from non–heart-beating donors. Transplantation 1995;59:197–203.
16. Chang RW. Transplantation of non-heart-beating donor kidneys [letter]. Lancet 1995;346(8970):322.
17. D'Alessandro AM, Hoffman RM, Knechtle SJ, et al. Controlled non-heart-beating donors: a potential source of extrarenal organs. Transplant Proc 1995;27:707–709.
18. Yandza T, Goulao J, Gauthier F, et al. The use of pediatric transplantation of livers from donors who died from anoxia. Transplant Proc 1991;23:2617.
19. Sloand EM, Pitt E, Klein HG. Safety of the blood supply. JAMA 1995;274:1368–1379.
20. Schrieber GB, Busch MP, Kleinman SH, Korelitz JJ. The risk of transfusion—transmitted viral infections. N Engl J Med 1996;334:1685–1690.
21. Bull DA, Stahl RD, McMahan DL, et al. The high risk heart donor: potential pitfalls. J Heart Lung Transplant 1995;14:424–428.
22. Kibbler CC. Infections in liver transplantation: risk factors and strategies for prevention. J Hosp Infect 1995;30:209–217.
23. Gottesdiener KM. Transplanted infections: donor-to-host transmission with the allograft. Ann Intern Med 1989;110:1001–1016.
24. Evans RW. The actual and potential supply of organ donors in the U.S. Clin Transpl 1990:329–341.
25. Brayman KL, Vianello A, Morel P, Payne WD, Sutherland DE. The organ donor. Crit Care Clin 1990;6:821–839.
26. Winton TL, Miller JD, Scavuzzo M, Maurer JR, Patterson GA. Donor selection for pulmonary transplantation. The Toronto Lung Transplant Group. Transplant Proc 1991;23:2472–2474.
27. Bennett LE, First MR, McGaw LJ, et al. Preliminary report of the UNOS Ad Hoc Donation Committee Retrospective Study of Expanded Donors. Abstracts of the 13th Annual Meeting of the American Society of Transplant Physicians, 1994;99.
28. Friedman AL, Nathan HM, Smolinski SE. Remarkable accuracy of a new cadaveric donor evaluation tool. Transplant Proc 1995;27:797–799.
29. Robertson KM, Cook DR. Perioperative management of the multiorgan donor. Anesth Analg 1990;70:546–556.
30. Gelb AW, Robertson KM. Anaesthetic management of the brain dead for organ donation. Can J Anaesth 1990;37:806–812.
31. Levinson MM, Copeland JG. The Organ Donor: Physiology, Maintenance and Procurement Consideration. In BR Brown Jr (ed), Anesthesia and Transplantation

Surgery; Contemporary Anesthesia Practice. Philadelphia: Davis, 1987;31–35.

32. Prager MC. Care of organ donors. Int Anesthesiol Clin 1991;29:1–16.

33. Darby JM, Stein K, Grenvik A, Stuart SA. Approach to management of the heartbeating "brain dead" organ donor. JAMA 1989;261:2222–2228.

34. Grebenik CR, Hinds CJ. Management of the multiple organ donor. Br J Hosp Med 1987;38:62–65.

35. Kozlowski LM. Case study in identification and maintenance of an organ donor. Heart Lung 1988;17:360–371.

36. Trinkle JK, Banowsky LH. Identification and management of organ donors. Tex Med 1988;4:38–43.

37. Powner DJ, Lagler RG, Jastremski M. Medical management of the brain dead patient in preparation for organ donation. Indiana Med 1986;79:966–968.

38. Brown ME. Clinical management of the organ donor. Dimens Crit Care Nurs 1989;8:134–142.

39. Goldsmith J, Montefusco CM. Nursing care of the potential organ donor. Crit Care Nurse 1985;5:22–29.

40. Linde-Zwirble ME, Bishop BS, Menker JB. Management of the organ donor: a first step in transplantation journal. Crit Care Nurs Q 1991;13:19–24.

41. Hill SA, Park GR. Management of multiple organ donors. Clin Anaesthesiol 1990;4:587–605.

42. Turcotte JG. Conventional management of the brain-dead potential multi-organ donor. Transplant Proc 1988;20(Suppl 7):7–8.

43. Freeman JW. Donor Selection and Maintenance Prior to Multi-organ Retrieval. In JL Vincent (ed), Yearbook of Intensive Care and Emergency Medicine. New York: Springer-Verlag, 1993;671–683.

44. Ballew AB, Haid S. Identification and Medical Management of the Pediatric Organ Donor. In DL Levin, FC Morriss (eds), Essentials of Pediatric Intensive Care. St. Louis: Quality Medical Publishing, 1990;212–218.

45. Brayman KL, Vianello A, Morel P, et al. The organ donor. Crit Care Clin 1990;6:821–839.

46. Griepp RB, Stinson EB, Clark DA, et al. The cardiac donor. Surg Gynecol Obstet 1971;133:792–798.

47. Klintmalm GB. The liver donor: special considerations. Transplant Proc 1988;20(Suppl 7):9–11.

48. Bodenham A, Park GR. Care of the multiple organ donor. Intensive Care Med 1989;15:340–348.

49. Jordan CA, Snyder JV. Intensive care and intraoperative management of the brain-dead organ donor. Transplant Proc 1987;19(Suppl 3):21–25.

50. Squifflet JP, Carlier M, Gribomont B, et al. The preoperative management in multiple organ donors; a crucial phase in organ transplantation. Acta Anaesthesiol Belg 1986;37:71–76.

51. Nygaard CE, Townsend RN, Diamond DL. Organ donor management and organ outcome: review from a level 1 trauma center. Trauma 1990;30:728–732.

52. McArthur C, Streat S. Management of the potential organ donor. Anaesth Intens Care 1993;21:712.

53. Ihle BU. Management of the multi-organ donor. Anaesth Intens Care 1993;21:710.

54. Pickett JA, Wheeldon DR, Oduro A. Multi-organ transplantation: donor management. Curr Opin Anaesth 1994;7:80–83.

55. Power BM, Van Heerden PV. The physiological changes associated with brain death—current concepts and implications for treatment of the brain dead organ donor. Anaesth Intensive Care 1995;23:26–36.

56. Odom NJ. Organ donation. I–Management of the multiorgan donor. BMJ 1990;300:1571–1573.

57. Black PM. Brain death. N Engl J Med 1978;299: 338–344.

58. Shivalkar B, Van Loon J, Wieland W, et al. Variable effects of explosive or gradual increase of intracranial pressure on myocardial structure and function. Circulation 1993;87:230–239.

59. Rosner MJ, Newsome HH, Becker BP. Mechanical brain injury: the sympathoadrenal response. J Neurosurg 1984;61:76–86.

60. Scheinkestel CD, Tuxen DV, Cooper DJ, Butt W. Medical management of the (potential) organ donor. Anaesth Intensive Care 1995;23:51–59.

61. Galinanes M, Hearse DJ. Brain-death–induced cardiac contractile dysfunction: studies of possible neurohormonal and blood-borne mediators. J Mol Cell Cardiol 1994;26:481–498.

62. Brink LW, Ballew A. Care of the pediatric organ donor. Am J Dis Child 1992;146:1045–1050.

63. Van Trigt P, Bittner HB, Kendall SW, Milano CA. Mechanisms of transplant right ventricular dysfunction. Ann Surg 1995;221:666–676.

64. Bittner HB, Kendall SW, Chen EP, et al. Myocardial performance after graft preservation and subsequent cardiac transplantation from brain-dead donors. Ann Thorac Surg 1995;60:47–54.

65. Kolin A, Norris JW. Myocardial damage from acute cerebral lesions. Stroke 1984;15:990–993.

66. Novitzky D, Cooper DK, Wicomb WM, Reichart B. Hemodynamic changes, myocardial injury, and pulmonary edema induced by sympathetic activity during the development of brain death in the baboon. Transplant Proc 1986;13:609–612.

67. Rona G. Catecholamine cardiotoxicity. J Mol Cell Cardiol 1985;17:291–306.

68. Sakagoshi N, Shirakura R, Nakano S, et al. Serial changes in myocardial beta-adrenergic receptor after experimental brain death in dogs. J Heart Lung Transplant 1992;11:1054–1058.

69. Randell T, Orko R, Hockerstedt K. Perioperative fluid management of the brain-dead multiorgan donor. Acta Anaesthesiol Scand 1990;34:592–595.

70. Wijnen RMH, van der Linden CJ. Donor treatment after pronouncement of brain death—a neglected intensive care problem. Transpl Int 1991;4:186–190.

71. Ghosh S, Bethune DW, Hardy I, et al. Management of donors for heart and heart-lung transplantation. Anaesthesia 1990;45:672–675.

72. Lindop MJ. Basic principles of donor management for multiorgan removal. Transplant Proc 1991;23:2463–2464.

73. Dawidson I, Berglin E, Brynger H. Perioperative fluid regimen, blood and plasma volumes, and colloid changes in liver related donors. Transplant Proc 1984;16:18–19.

74. Dawidson I, Berglin E, Brynger H, Reisch J. Intravascular volumes and colloid dynamics in relation to fluid management in living related kidney donors and recipients. Crit Care Med 1987;15:631–636.

75. Zikria BA, Subbarao C, Oz MC, et al. Hydroxyethyl starch macromolecules reduce myocardial reperfusion injury. Arch Surg 1990;125:930–934.

76. Legendre CH, Thervet E, Page B, et al. Hydroxyethyl starch and osmotic-nephrosis–like lesions in kidney transplantation [letter]. Lancet 1993;342:248–249.

77. Kormos RL, Donato W, Hardesty RL, et al. The influence of donor organ stability and ischemia time on subsequent cardiac recipient survival. Transplant Proc 1988;20(Suppl 1):980–983.

78. Ali MJ, Gelb AW. Effect of brain death on organ blood flow [abstract]. Anesthesiology 1991;75:A210.

79. Schaer GL, Fink MP, Parrillo JE. Norepinephrine alone versus norepinephrine plus low-dose dopamine; enhanced renal blood flow with combination pressor therapy. Crit Care Med 1985;13:492–496.

80. Goldberg LI. Cardiovascular and renal actions of dopamine: potential clinical applications. Pharmacol Rev 1972;24:1–29.

81. Kelly KJ, Outwater KM, Crone RK. Vasoactive amines in infants and children. Clin Anaesthesiol 1984;2:427–442.

82. Outwater KM, Treves S, Lang P, et al. Renal and hemodynamic effects of dopamine in infants following corrective cardiac surgery [abstract]. Anesthesiology 1984; 61:A130.

83. Whelchel JD, Diethelm AG, Phillips MG, et al. The effect of high-dose dopamine in cadaver donor management on delayed graft function and graft survival following renal transplanation. Transplant Proc 1986;18:523–527.

84. Sanfilippo F, Vaugh W, Spees E, Lucas BA. The effects of delayed graft function on renal transplantation. Transplant Proc 1985;17:13–15.

85. Schneider A, Toledo-Pereyra LH, Zeichner WD, et al. Effect of dopamine and pitressin on kidneys procured and harvested for transplantation. Transplantation 1983;36:110–111.

86. Quesada A, Teja JL, Cotorruelo JG, et al. Inotropic support in 50 brain-dead organ donors: repercussion on renal graft function. Transplant Proc 1991;23:2479–2480.

87. Pienaar H, Schwartz I, Roncone A, et al. Function of kidney grafts from brain-dead donor pigs. The influence of dopamine and triiodothyronine. Transplantation 1990;50:580–582.

88. Nakatani T, Ishikawa Y, Kobayashi K, Ozawa K. Hepatic mitochondrial redox state in hypotensive brain-dead patients and an effect of dopamine administration. Intensive Care Med 1991;17:103–107.

89. Okamoto R, Yamamoto Y, Lin H, et al. Influence of dopamine on the liver assessed by changes in arterial ketone body ratio in brain-dead dogs. Surgery 1990; 107:36–42.

90. Ohkohchi N, Satake M, Yokoi H, et al. A study of donor procurement in 180 liver transplantations-analysis of the pretransplant general condition, liver function test and type of the harvest of donors in the liver transplantation. Jpn J Transplant 1987;22:89.

91. Novitzky D, Wicomb WN, Cooper DK, et al. Prevention of myocardial injury during brain death by total cardiac sympathectomy in the Chacma baboon. Ann Thorac Surg 1986;41:520–524.

92. Goldberg LI. Dopamine—clinical uses of an endogenous catecholamine. N Engl J Med 1974;291:707–710.

93. Walpoth B, Schweizer A, Barbalat-Rey F, Faidutti B. Preischemic conditions affecting myocardial ischemic tolerance. A nuclear magnetic resonance study (31P NMR) Life Support Syst 1985;3(Suppl 1):206–210.

94. Vincent F, Raynal A, Duboust A, et al. Influence of epinephrine treatment of the organ donor on acute tubular necrosis following renal transplantation. Transplant Proc 1995;27:1649.

95. Robie NW, Goldberg LI. Comparative systemic and regional hemodynamic effects of dopamine and dobutamine. Am Heart J 1975;90:340–345.

96. Novitzky D, Wicomb WN, Cooper DK, et al. Electrocardiographic, hemodynamic, and endocrine changes during experimental brain death in the Chacma baboon. J Heart Transplant 1984;4:63–69.

97. Stoelting RK (ed). Sympathomimetics. In Pharmacology and Physiology in Anesthetic Practice (2nd ed). Philadelphia: Lippincott, 1991;264–284.

98. Nagareda T, Kinoshita Y, Tanaka A, et al. Clinicopathology of kidneys from brain-dead patients treated with vasopressin and epinephrine. Kidney Int 1993;43: 1363–1370.

99. Nishimura N, Sugi T. Circulatory support with sympathetic amines in brain death. Resuscitation 1984;12: 25–30.

100. Kinoshita Y, Yahata K, Yoshioka T, et al. Long-term renal preservation after brain death maintained with vasopressin and epinephrine. Transplant Int 1990;3:15–18.

101. Iwai A, Sakano T, Venichi M, et al. Effects of vasopressin and catecholamines on the maintenance of circulatory stability in brain-dead patients. Transplantation 1989;48:613–617.

102. Manaka D, Okamoto R, Yokoyama T, et al. Maintenance of liver graft viability in the state of brain death. Transplantation 1992;53:545–550.

103. Cowley AW Jr, Monos E, Guyton AC. Interaction of vasopressin and the baroreceptor reflex system in the regulation of arterial blood pressure in the dog. Circ Res 1974;34:505–514.

104. Bartelstone HJ, Nasmyth PA. Vasopressin potentiation of catecholamine actions in dog, rat, cat, and aortic strip. Am J Physiol 1965;208:754.

105. Manaka D, Okamoto R, Yokoyama T, et al. Maintenance of liver graft viability in the state of brain death. Transplantation 1992;53:545–550.

106. Van Thiel DH, Schade RR, Hakala TR, et al. Liver procurement for orthotopic transplantation: an analysis of

the Pittsburgh experience. Hepatology 1984;4(Suppl 1): 66S–71S.

107. Mokken FC, Henny CP, Kendaria H, Gelb AW. Hemorrheological changes associated with brain death and their implications for potential organ donors. Transpl Int 1995;8:147–151.

108. Gravlee GP. Blood transfusion and component therapy. ASA Refresher Course Lecture Series 1990;215:1–7.

109. Busson M, Benoit G, N'Doye P, Hors J. Analysis of cadaver donor criteria on the kidney transplant survival rate in 5,129 transplantations. Urol 1995;154:356–360.

110. Cheng SS, Pinson CW, Lopez RR, et al. Effect of donor-disseminated intravascular coagulation in liver transplantation. Arch Surg 1991;126:1292–1296.

111. Kaufman HH, Hui KS, Mattson JC, et al. Clinicopathologic correlations of disseminated intravascular coagulation in patients with severe head injury. Neurosurgery 1984;15:34–42.

112. Deykin D. The clinical challenge of disseminated intravascular coagulation. N Engl J Med 1970;283: 636–644.

113. Miner ME, Kaufman HH, Graham SH, et al. Disseminated intravascular coagulation fibrinolytic syndrome following head injury in children: frequency and prognostic implications. J Pediatr 1982;100:687–691.

114. Shamash FS, Oh HK, Lee MW, Dienst SG. Kidney retrieval from cadaver donors with disseminated intravascular coagulopathy. Curr Surg 1989;46:6–9.

115. Nghiem DD, Palumbi MA, Paul C. The cardiac transplant recipient with disseminated intravascular coagulation—an unusual kidney donor. Transplantation 1993;55:679–680.

116. Hefty TR, Cotterell LW, Fraser SC, Goodnight SH, Hatch TR. Disseminated intravascular coagulation in cadaveric organ donors. Incidence and effect on renal transplantation. Transplantation 1993;55:442–443.

117. Douzdjian V, Gugliuzza KG, Fish JC. Multivariate analysis of donor risk factors for pancreas allograft failure after simultaneous pancreas-kidney transplantation. Surgery 1995;118:73–81.

118. Puig JM, Lloveras J, Oliveras A, et al. Usefulness of diltiazem in reducing the incidence of acute tubular necrosis in Euro-Collins–preserved cadaveric renal grafts. Transplant Proc 1991;23:2368–2369.

119. Logigian EL, Ropper AH. Terminal electrocardiographic changes in brain-dead patients. Neurology 1985;35:915–918.

120. Vaghadia H. Atropine resistance in brain dead organ donors [letter]. Anesthesiology 1986;65:711–712.

121. Walsh CK, Krongraad E. Terminal cardiac electrical activity in pediatric patients. Am J Cardiol 1983;51:557–561.

122. Casavilla A, Famirez C, Shapiro R, et al. Experience with liver and kidney allografts form non–heart-beating donors. Transplantation 1995;59:197–203.

123. Emery RW, Cork RC, Levinson MM, et al. The cardiac donor: a six-year experience. Ann Thorac Surg 1986; 41:356–362.

124. Boucek MM, Kanakriyeh MS, Mathis CM, Trimm RD 3rd, Bailey LL. Cardiac transplantation in infancy: donors and recipients. J Pediatr 1990;116:171–176.

125. Peterseim DS, Chesnut LC, Meyers CH, et al. Stability of the beta-adrenergic receptor/adenylyl cyclase pathway of pediatric myocardium after brain death. J Heart Lung Transplant 1994;13:635–640.

126. Doroshow RW, Ashwal S, Saukel GW. Availability and selection of donors for pediatric heart transplantation. J Heart Lung Transplant 1995;14:52–58.

127. Boucek MM, Mathis CM, Kanakriyeh MS, et al. Donor shortage: use of the dysfunctional donor heart. J Heart Lung Transplant 1993;12(6 pt 2):S186–S190.

128. Reuler JB. Hypothermia: pathophysiology, clinical settings and management. Ann Intern Med 1978;89: 519–527.

129. Takino M, Okada Y. Hyperthermia following cardiopulmonary resuscitation. Intensive Care Med 1991;17:419–420.

130. Schneider SM. Hypothermia: from recognition to rewarming. Emerg Med Rep 1992;13:1–20.

131. American Heart Association. Special Resuscitation Situations: Hypothermia. In RO Cummins (ed), Textbook of Advanced Cardiac Life Support. Dallas, American Heart Association, 1994;10–12.

132. Elenbaas RM, Mattson K, Cole H, et al. Bretylium in hypothermia-induced ventricular fibrillation in dogs. Ann Emerg Med 1984;13:994–999.

133. Buckley JJ, Bosch OK, Bacaner MB. Prevention of ventricular fibrillation during hypothermia with bretylium tosylate. Anesth Analg 1971;50:587–593.

134. Kroncke GM, Nichols RD, Mendenhall JT, et al. Ectothermic philosophy of acid-base balance to prevent fibrillation during hypothermia. Arch Surg 1986;121: 303–304.

135. Swain JA. Hypothermia and blood pH: a review. Arch Intern Med 1988;148:1643–1646.

136. White FN. A comparative physiological approach to hypothermia. J Thorac Cardiovasc Surg 1981;82:821–831.

137. Schrader H, Krogness K, Aakvaag A, et al. Changes of pituitary hormones in brain death. Acta Neurochir (Wien) 1980;52:239–248.

138. Howlett TA, Keogh AM, Perry L, et al. Anterior and posterior pituitary function in brain-stem–dead donors. A possible role for hormonal replacement therapy. Transplantation 1989;47:828–834.

139. Robertson KM, Hramiak IM, Gelb AW. Thyroid function and haemodynamic stability after brain death [abstract]. Can J Anaesth 1988;35:S102.

140. Gifford RR, Weaver AS, Burg JE, et al. Thyroid hormone levels heart and kidney cadaver donors. J Heart Transplant 1986;5:249–253.

141. Theilen EO, Wilson WR. Hemodynamic effects of peripheral vasoconstriction in normal and thyrotoxic subjects. J Appl Physiol 1967;22:207–210.

142. Howitt G, Rowlands DJ. The heart in hyperthyroidism. Am Heart J 1967;73:282–283.

143. Buccino RA, Spann JF, Pool PE, et al. Influence of the thyroid state on the intrinsic contractile properties and energy stores of the myocardium. J Clin Invest 1967; 10:1669–1682.

144. Novitzky D, Cooper DK, Reichart B. Hemodynamic and metabolic responses to hormonal therapy in brain-dead potential organ donors. Transplantation 1987; 43:852–854.

145. Novitzky D, Cooper DK, Chaffin JS, et al. Improved cardiac function following triiodothyronine therapy to both donor and recipient. Transplantation 1990;49: 311–316.

146. Novitzky D, Cooper DK, Morell D, Isaacs S. Change from aerobic to anaerobic metabolism after brain death and reversal following triiodothyronine therapy. Transplantation 1988;45:32–36.

147. Orlowski JP, Spees EK. Improved cardiac transplant survival with thyroxine treatment of hemodynamically unstable donors: 95.2% graft survival at 6 and 30 months. Transplant Proc 1993;25:1535.

148. Wheeldon D, Potter CDO, Dunning J, et al. Haemodynamic correction in multiorgan donation. Lancet 1992;339:1175.

149. Novitzky D, Cooper DK, Chaffin JS, et al. Improved cardiac allograft function following triiodothyronine therapy to both donor and recipient. Transplantation 1990;49:311–316.

150. Novitzky D. Heart transplantation, euthyroid sick syndrome and triiodothyronine replacement. J Heart Lung Transplant 1992;11:196–198.

151. Montero JA, Mallol J, Alvarez F, et al. Biochemical hypothyroidism and myocardial damage in organ donors: are they related? Transplant Proc 1988;20: 746–748.

152. Taniguchi S, Kitamura S, Kawachi K, et al. Effects of hormonal supplements on the maintenance of cardiac function in potential donor patients after cerebral death. Eur J Cardiothorac Surg 1992;6:96–102.

153. Wicomb WN, Cooper DK, Novitzky D. Impairment of renal slice function following brain death, with reversibility of injury by hormonal therapy. Transplantation 1985;41:29–33.

154. Garcia-Fages LC, Antolin M, Cabrer C, et al. Effects of substitutive therapy on intracellular nucleotide levels in donor organs. Transplant Proc 1991;23:2495–2496.

155. Wahlers T, Cremer J, Fieguth HG, et al. Donor heart-related variables and early mortality after heart transplantation. J Heart Lung Transplant 1991;10:22–27.

156. Cooper DKC, Novitzky D, Wicomb WN. The pathophysiological effects of brain death on potential donor organs, with particular reference to the heart. Ann R Coll Surg Engl 1989;71:261–266.

157. Novitzky D. Triiodothyronine replacement, the euthyroid sick syndrome and organ transplantation. Transplant Proc 1991;23:2460–2462.

158. Wheeldon DR, Potter CD, Oduro A, et al. Transforming the "unacceptable" donor: outcomes from the adoption of a standardized donor management technique. J Heart Lung Transplant 1995;14:734–742.

159. Orlowski JP. Evidence that thyroxine (T-4) is effective as a hemodynamic rescue agent in management of organ donors. Transplantation 1993;55:959–960.

160. Bittner HB, Kendall SW, Chen EP, Van Trigt P. Endocrine changes and metabolic responses in a validated canine brain death model. J Crit Care 1995;10:56–63.

161. Masson F, Thicoipe M, Latapie MJ, Maurette P. Thyroid function in brain-dead donors. Transplant Int 1990;3:226–233.

162. Harms J, Isemer FE, Kolenda H. Hormonal alteration and pituitary function during course of brain-stem death in potential organ donors. Transplant Proc 1991;23: 2614–2616.

163. Sazontseva IE, Kozlov IA, Moisuc YG, et al. Hormonal responses to brain death. Transplant Proc 1991;23: 2467.

164. Robertson KM, Hramiak IM, Gelb AW. Endocrine changes and haemodynamic stability after brain death. Transplant Proc 1989;21:1197–1198.

165. Powner DJ, Hendrich A, Lagler RG, et al. Hormonal changes in brain dead patients. Crit Care Med 1990; 18:702–708.

166. Kozlov IA, Jigareva EU, Chestuhin VV, et al. Hormonal therapy and metabolic support efficiency as a criterion in donor heart preoperative evaluation. Transplant Proc 1991;23:2477–2478.

167. Macoviack JA, McDougall IR, Bayer MF, et al. Significance of thyroid dysfunction in human cardiac allograft procurement. Transplantation 1987;43: 1824–1826.

168. Koller J, Wieser C, Gottardis M, et al. Thyroid hormones and their impact on the hemodynamic and metabolic stability of organ donors and on kidney graft function after transplantation. Transplant Proc 1990; 22:355–357.

169. Mariot J, Sadoune LO, Dousset B, et al. Hormone levels, hemodynamics, and metabolism in brain dead organ donors. Transplant Proc 1995;27:793–794.

170. Gifford RR, Weaver AS, Burg JE, et al. Thyroid hormone levels in heart and kidney cadaver donors. J Heart Transplant 1986;5:249–253.

171. Huber TS, Nachreiner R, D'Alecy LG. Hormonal profiles in a canine model of the brain-dead organ donor. J Crit Care 1994;9:7–17.

172. Dyke CM, Yeh TJ, Lehman JD, et al. Triiodothyronine-enhanced left ventricular function after ischemic injury. Ann Thorac Surgery 1991;52:14–19.

173. Wechsler AS, Kadletz M, Ding M, et al. Effects of triiodothyronine on stunned myocardium. J Card Surg 1993;8(Suppl 2):338–341.

174. Meyers CH, D'Amico TA, Peterseim DS, et al. Effects of triiodothyronine and vasopressin on cardiac function and myocardial flow after brain death. J Heart Lung Transplant 1993;12:68–79.

175. Klemperer JD, Zelano J, Helm RE, et al. Triiodothyro-

nine improves left ventricular function without oxygen wasting effects after global hypothermic ischemia. J Thorac Cardiovasc Surg 1995;109:457–465.

176. Bennett-Guerrero E, Jimenez JL, D'Amico EB, et al. Effects of triiodothyronine on hemodynamics and postoperative support in patients undergoing CABG: preliminary results from the Duke T_3 CABG trial. Anesth Analg 1995;80:SCA11.

177. Bennett-Guerrero E, Jimenez JL, White WD, et al. Cardiovascular effects of intravenous triiodothyronine in patients undergoing coronary artery bypass graft surgery. A randomized, double-blind, placebo-controlled trial. Duke T_3 study group. JAMA 1996;275:687–692.

178. Klemperer JD, Klein I, Gomez M, et al. Thyroid hormone treatment after coronary-artery bypass surgery. N Engl J Med 1995;333:1522–1527.

179. Gramm HJ, Meinhold H, Bickel U, et al. Acute endocrine failure after brain death? Transplantation 1992;54:851–857.

180. Wicomb WN, Novitzky D, Cooper DK, et al. Early extranuclear effect of triiodothyronine (T_3) on tissue slices: relevance to organ donor viability. Transplant Proc 1989;21(1 pt 2):1263–1264.

181. Salter DR, Dyke CM, Wechsler AS. Triiodothyronine (T_3) and cardiovascular therapeutics: A review. J Card Surg 1992;7:363–374.

182. Chang MY, Kinos G. Short term effects of triiodothyronine on rat heart adrenoceptors. Biochem Biophys Res Commun 1981;100:313.

183. Jeevanandam V, Todd B, Regillo T, et al. Reversal of donor myocardial dysfunction by triiodothyronine replacement therapy. J Heart Lung Transplant 1994;13;681–687.

184. Fiser DH, Jimenez JF, Wrape V, Woody R. Diabetes insipidus in children with brain death. Crit Care Med 1987;15:551–553.

185. Newsome HH Jr. Vasopressin: deficiency, excess and the syndrome of inappropriate antidiuretic hormone section. Nephron 1979;2:125–129.

186. Staworn D, Lewison L, Marks J, et al. Brain death in pediatric intensive care unit patients: incidence, primary diagnosis and the clinical occurrence of Turner's triad. Crit Care Med 1994;22:1301–1305.

187. Riou B, Kalfon P, Arock M, et al. Cardiovascular consequences of severe hypophosphataemia in brain-dead patients. Br J Anaesth 1995;74:424–429.

188. Ralston C, Butt W. Continuous vasopressin replacement in diabetes insipidus. Arch Dis Child 1990;65:896–897.

189. Hofbauer KG, Studer W, Mah SC, et al. The significance of vasopressin as a pressor agent. J Cardiovasc Pharmacol 1984;6(Suppl 2):S429–438.

190. Mols P, Hallemans R, Van Kuyk M, et al. Hemodynamic effects of vasopressin, alone and in combination with nitroprusside, in patients with liver cirrhosis and portal hypertension. Ann Surg 1984;199:176–181.

191. Debelak L, Pollak R, Reckard C. Arginine vasopressin versus desmopressin for the treatment of diabetes insipidus in the brain dead organ donor. Transplant Proc 1990;22:351–352.

192. Schneider A, Toledo-Pereyra LH, Zeichner WD, et al. Effect of dopamine and pitressin on kidneys procured and harvested for transplantation. Transplantation 1983;36:110–111.

193. Blaine EM, Tallman RD Jr, Frolicher D, et al. Vasopressin supplementation in a porcine model of brain-dead potential organ donors. Transplantation 1984;38:459–464.

194. Hohenegger M, Vermes M, Mauritz W, et al. Serum vasopressin (AVP) levels in polyuric brain-dead organ donors. Eur Arch Psychiatry Neurol Sci 1990;239:267–269.

195. Pagano D, Bonser RS, Graham TR. Optimal management of the heart-lung donor. Br J Hosp Med 1995;53:522–525.

196. Driscoll DF, Palombo JD, Bistrian BR. Nutritional and metabolic considerations of the adult liver transplant candidate and organ donor. Nutrition 1995;11:255–263.

197. Bennett LE, Glascock RF, Breen TJ, et al. Organ donation in the United States: 1988 through 1992. Clin Transpl 1993:85–93.

198. Harjula A, Baldwin JC, Starnes VA, et al. Proper donor selection for heart-lung transplantation. J Thorac Cardiovasc Surg 1987;94:874–880.

199. Dowling RD, Zenati M, Yousem SA, et al. Donor transmitted pneumonia in experimental allografts: successful prevention with donor antibiotic therapy. J Thorac Cardiovasc Surg 1992;103:767–772.

200. Trulock EP. Introduction: infectious complications of organ transplantation. Semin Respir Infect 1993;8:149–151.

201. Dorinsky PM, Whitcomb ME. The effect of PEEP on cardiac output. Chest 1983;84:210–216.

202. Koller J, Wieser C, Kornberger R, et al. Influence of the renin-angiotensin system of the organ donor on kidney function after transplantation. Transplant Proc 1990;22:349–350.

203. Graybar GB, Tarpey M. Kidney Transplantation. In S Gelman (ed), Anesthesia and Organ Transplantation. Philadelphia: Saunders, 1987;80.

204. Conci F, Procaccio F, Arosio M, Boselli L. Viscerosomatic and viscero-visceral reflexes in brain death. J Neurol Neurosurg Psychiatry 1986;49:695–698.

205. Duke PK, Ramsay MA, Paulsen AW, et al. Intraoperative hemodynamic heterogeneity of brain dead organ donors. Transplant Proc 1991;23:2485–2486.

206. Ghosh S, Bethune DW, Hardy I, et al. Management of donors for heart and heart-lung transplantation. Anaesthesia 1990;45:672–675.

207. Wheeldon DR, Potter CD, Jonas M, et al. Using "unsuitable" hearts for transplantation. Eur J Cardiothorac Surg 1994;8:7–10.

208. Swain JA. Hypothermia and blood pH: a review. Arch Intern Med 1988;148:1643–1646.

209. White FN. A comparative physiological approach to hypothermia. J Thorac Cardiovasc Surg 1981;82:821–831.

210. Gelman S. Carbon dioxide and hepatic circulation. Anesth Analg 1989;69:149–151.

211. Fujita Y, Sakai T, Ohsumi A, Takaori M. Effects of hypocapnia and hypercapnia on splanchnic circulation and hepatic function in the beagle. Anesth Analg 1989;69:152–157.

212. Ebata T, Watanabe Y, Amaha K, et al. Haemodynamic changes during the apnoea test for diagnosis of brain death. Can J Anaesth 1991;38:436–440.

213. Report of the Quality Standards Subcommittee of the American Academy of Neurology. Practice parameters for determining brain death in adults [summary statement]. Neurology 1995;45:1012–1014.

214. Ivan LP. Spinal reflexes in cerebral death. Neurology 1973;23:650–652.

215. Jorgensen EO. Spinal man after brain death. The unilateral extension-pronation reflex of the upper limb as an indication of brain death. Acta Neurochir 1973;28:259–273.

216. Wijdicks EF. Determining brain death in adults. Neurology 1995;45:1003–1011.

217. Ropper AH. Unusual spontaneous movements in brain-dead patients. Neurology 1984;34:1089–1092.

218. Jastremski MS, Powner D, Snyder J, et al. Spontaneous decerebrate movement after declaration of brain death. Neurosurg 1991;29:479–480.

219. Gramm HJ, Zimmermann J, Meinhold H, et al. Hemodynamic responses to noxious stimuli in brain-dead organ donors. Intensive Care Med 1992;18:493–495.

220. Wetzel RC, Setzer N, Stiff JL, Rogers MC. Hemodynamic responses in brain dead organ donor patients. Anesth Analg 1985;64:125–128.

221. Aibiki M, Shirakawa Y, Ogura S, et al. Thyrotropin-releasing hormone produces different hemodynamic effects in vegetative and brain-dead patients. Clin Neuropharmacol 1993;16:428–437.

222. Goldstein B, DeKing D, DeLong DJ, et al. Autonomic cardiovascular state after severe brain injury and brain death in children. Crit Care Med 1993;21:228–233.

223. Hill DJ, Munglani R, Sapsford D. Haemodynamic responses to surgery in brain-dead organ donors [correspondence]. Anaesthesia 1994;49:835–836.

224. Chen CL, Chen TL, Sun WZ, et al. Hemodynamic responses to surgical stimuli in brain-death organ donors. Ma Tsui Hsueh Tsa Chi 1993;31:135–138.

225. Fitzgerald RD, Dechtyar I, Templ E, et al. Cardiovascular and catecholamine response to surgery in brain-dead organ donors. Anaesthesia 1995;50:388–392.

226. Pennefather SH, Dark JH, Bullock RE. Haemodynamic responses to surgery in brain-dead organ donors. Anaesthesia 1993;48:1034–1038.

227. Slapak M. The immediate care of potential donors for cadaveric organ transplantation. Anaesthesia 1978;33:700–709.

228. Miller HC, Alexander JW. Protective effect of methyl-prednisolone against ischemic injury to the kidney. Transplantation 1973;16:57–60.

229. Toledo-Pereyra LH, Jara FM. Myocardial protection with methylprednisolone. Evaluation of viability of hearts subjected to warm ischemia before transplantation. J Thorac Cardiovasc Surg 1979;77:619–621.

230. Baldwin JC. Heart-lung and Lung Graft Preservation. In SJ Shumway, NE Shumway (eds), Thoracic Transplantation. Cambridge, MA: Blackwell Science, 1989;71–83.

231. Starkey TD, Sakakibara N, Hagberg RC, et al. Successful six-hour cardiopulmonary preservation with simple hypothermic crystalloid flush. J Heart Transplant 1986;5:291–297.

232. Christie NA, Waddell TK. Lung Preservation. In GA Patterson, JD Cooper (eds), Lung Transplantation. Chest Surg Clin N Am. Philadelphia: Saunders, 1993;29–47.

233. Grant JW, Canter CE, Spray TL, et al. Elevated donor cardiac troponin I. A marker of acute graft failure in infant heart recipients. Circulation 1994;90:2618–2621.

234. Lucas BA, Vaughn WK, Spees EK, Sanfilippo F. Identification of donor factors predisposing to high discard rates of cadaver kidneys and increased graft loss within one year posttransplantation--SEOPF 1977–1982. South-Eastern Organ Procurement Foundation. Transplantation 1987;43:253–258.

235. Pagano D, Bonser RS, Graham TR. Optimal management of the heart-lung donor. Br J Hosp Med 1995;53:522–525.

236. Masson F, Thicoipe M, Gin H, et al. The endocrine pancreas in brain-dead donors. Transplantation 1993;56:363–367.

237. Shaffer D, Madras PN, Sahyoun AI, et al. Cadaver donor hyperglycemia does not impair long-term pancreas allograft survival or function. Transplant Proc 1994;26:439–440.

238. Mor E, Klintmalm GB, Gonwa TA, et al. The use of marginal donors for liver transplantation. Transplant Proc 1992;52:383–386.

239. Mimeault R, Grant D, Ghent C, et al. Analysis of donor and recipient variables and early graft function after orthotopic liver transplantation. Transplant Proc 1989;21:33–55.

240. Adam R, Reynes M, Bao YM, et al. Impact of glycogen content of the donor liver in clinical liver transplantation. Transplant Proc 1993;25:1536–1537.

241. Driscoll DF, Palombo JD, Bistrian BR. Nutritional and metabolic considerations of the adult liver transplant candidate and organ donor. Nutrition 1995;11:255–263.

242. Clavien PA, Harvey PR, Sanabria JR, et al. Lymphocyte adherence in the reperfused rat liver: mechanisms and effects. Hepatology 1993;17:131–142.

243. Makowka L, Gordon RD, Todo S, et al. Analysis of donor criteria for the prediction of outcome in clinical liver transplantation. Transplant Proc 1987;19:2378–2382.

244. Strasberg SM, Howard TK, Molmenti EP, Hertl M.

Selecting the donor liver: risk factors for poor function after orthotopic liver transplantation. Hepatology 1994;20:829–838.

245. Gubernatis G, Tusch G, Oldhafer K, Pichlmayr R. Subjective assessment of donor liver quality. Transplant Proc 1995;27:2191–2194.

246. Southard JH, Belzer FO. Organ preservation. Annu Rev Med 1995;46;235–247.

247. Sundaresan S, Semenkovich J, Ochoa L, et al. Successful outcome of lung transplantation is not compromised by the use of marginal lung donors. J Thorac Cardiovasc Surg 1995;109:1075–1079.

Chapter 5
Mechanical Devices:
A Bridge to Transplantation

John Schweiss and Marc T. Swartz

Chapter Plan

Historic Aspects

Since the early 1950s, physicians have had the clinical capability to support the circulation with mechanical devices. The work of Gibbon led to the first successful clinical use of cardiopulmonary bypass in 1952.[1] This cardiopulmonary bypass system could temporarily support part or all of the circulation during cardiac operations. Soon, other indications were conceived, and attempts were made to support patients with cardiogenic shock after acute myocardial infarction with cardiopulmonary bypass.[2] Temporary use of cardiopulmonary bypass required total heparinization and, in the late 1950s, an operating room environment. Because decompression of the distended heart could not be accomplished using closed-chest cannulation techniques, cardiopulmonary bypass was therefore thought to be ineffective in treating cardiogenic shock. In addition, most patients in cardiogenic shock did not require pulmonary support with an in-line oxygenator, which further complicated coagulopathies and anticoagulation. For these reasons, cardiopulmonary bypass was abandoned as a mechanism to treat cardiogenic shock. It soon became apparent that a temporary mechanical circulatory support device was needed to maintain patients long enough to allow myocardial recovery. It was believed that recovery should occur within 7–10 days. Clinicians then concentrated on the development of integrated systems that would provide isolated ventricular support. Dennis and colleagues introduced the method of left-heart bypass in 1962,[3] a concept that was later modified and used successfully by DeBakey in 1964.[4]

In 1962, the theory of counterpulsation was introduced,[5] and by 1968, diastolic counterpulsation with an intra-aortic balloon pump (IABP) had become a clinical reality.[6] The development of the IABP diminished the need for a more advanced mechanical circulatory support device. Because IABP cannot completely support the circulation, however, its use was limited in critically ill patients with very low cardiac outputs.

In the 1950s, several laboratories began to work on developing an artificial heart. During the 1960s, the National Heart, Lung and Blood Institute began a formal program for the development of mechanical circulatory support. In July 1964, the U.S. Congress approved the first allocation for support of artificial heart research. Initially, the plan was to develop a family of devices for emergency use, for temporary support until the heart recovered, for short- and long-term ventricular assistance, and for cardiac replacement.[7]

During the 1970s, researchers developed elaborate, innovative devices to assist a failing ventricle for longer periods with less blood component damage. These systems included external and internal pneumatic ventricular assist devices (VADs).[8–11] In this interval, the IABP remained the primary method of mechanical circulatory support, and VADs were used only if IABP failed.[12, 13] During the 1980s, technology developed and improvements in clinical management were made. Pneumatic total artificial hearts (TAHs), electrical left VADs, percutaneous cardiopulmonary bypass, and other innovative devices found their way into clinical use.[14–17] Since the late 1980s, improved technology and clinical results have led to a widespread growth of mechanical circulatory support. Survival rates have increased, and morbidity rates are on the decline, especially in patients for whom the device is used as a bridge to transplantation.[18] Several patients have been successfully supported for longer than 1 year with different devices, and successful perfusions of longer than 1 month are now commonplace. Patients are now being discharged from the hospital with the devices in place, to await cardiac transplantation or, in some centers outside the United States, to live the rest of their lives supported by the mechanical VAD.[19, 20] The indications for mechanical circulatory support are varied, and several devices are now available either commercially or with special exemption from the U.S. Food and Drug Administration (FDA) for investigational use. Some devices have been designed for particular circumstances, whereas others are capable of multiple applications.

Intra-Aortic Balloon Counterpulsation

Diastolic augmentation or counterpulsation has been the most commonly used method of mechanical circulatory support since the mid-1970s. Since the first successful application of IABP counterpulsation in 1968, the technique has not changed substantially.[6] Although there have been improvements in the devices and the methods of insertion, the basic theory still applies.[21, 22] This technique involves placing a balloon within the thoracic aorta distal to the left subclavian artery and proximal to the renal arteries (Figure 5-1). The IABP is synchronized with left ventricular contraction by means of the electrocardiogram (ECG) or a systemic arterial blood pressure tracing. A predetermined volume of helium (20–40 cc) is pumped into the balloon during cardiac diastole. This displaces an equivalent amount of blood in the descending aorta, forcing it down the coronary arteries during cardiac diastole when intramyocardial pressures are at their lowest. Just before cardiac systole, the helium is emptied out of the intra-aortic balloon, thereby reducing the pressure inside the ascending aorta so that the left ventricle beats against less resistance. These actions result in a dual response: a reduction in systolic aortic pressure and an increase in diastolic blood pressure. Although the cardiac output may increase 10–40%, the average increase is usually only 10–20%, depending on the condition of the left ventricle and the extent of myocardial infarction or ischemia. The significant effect of IABP assist, other than increasing overall cardiac output, is to improve the myocardial oxygen supply-demand ratio. Often, there is evidence of increased myocardial blood flow, depending on the extent of collateral circulation. Left ventricular wall tension also decreases, and this is sometimes accompanied by a decrease in heart rate. If the IABP improves the patient's condition significantly, it may be possible to reduce the dosages of some of the inotropic drugs, thereby reducing myocardial oxygen consumption.

Clinically, the IABP has been used in nonsurgical patients with low cardiac output and acute myocardial infarctions and in surgical patients who

Figure 5-1. Intra-aortic balloon pump. The balloon is positioned in the descending aorta from placement in the femoral artery. The tip of the balloon is approximately 2 cm distal to the left subclavian

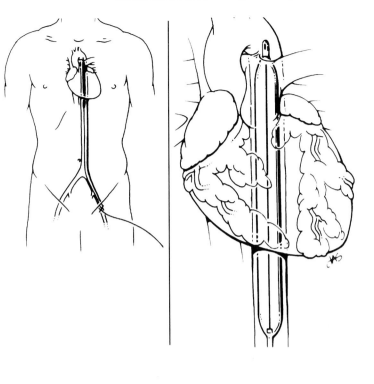

cannot be weaned from cardiopulmonary bypass.[23–25] It also has been used in end-stage cardiac disease patients awaiting cardiac transplantation who deteriorate hemodynamically. Some centers have reported success in supporting patients with IABPs for several weeks before cardiac transplantation.[26–28] Many of these IABP patients, however, are initially stabilized and then again deteriorate and require placement of a more sophisticated mechanical circulatory-support device.[26] VADs and TAHs appear to be a better option than IABP in the bridge-to-transplant patient population because they can provide 100% of circulation needs. This can be accomplished without the use of inotropic drugs; therefore, patients can be free of central intravascular monitoring catheters and therefore managed noninvasively.[29–31] Balloon pumps, on the other hand, require patients to be bed-bound, for the most part. There is often a need for inotropic support in addition to IABP therapy to maintain a cardiac index above 2 liters per minute per m^2. Thus, the need for central venous catheters adds to the risk of infection and immobility. The balloon placed in the femoral artery virtually precludes ambulation. Attempts have been made to place IABPs in the subclavian artery, thereby allowing patient ambula-

tion and greater mobility. These attempts have met with limited success owing to technical design problems of the balloon.[28] After 1–2 weeks, the balloon catheters often crack and leak because they were not designed to stand such stress. Other surgical sites of insertion have included the iliac artery and abdominal aorta.

Contraindications to IABP use include aortic valvular insufficiency and aortic aneurysms of the thoracic or abdominal aorta.

The IABP is associated with many potential complications. Table 5-1 lists these complications in order of seriousness and of when they are recognized.

Five IABPs are commercially available in the United States: Kontron KAAT II (Arrow Kontron International, Everett, MA), Datascope System 97 (Datascope Corporation, Montvale, NJ), St. Jude Model 700 (Cardiac Assist Division, St. Jude Medical, Inc., Chelmsford, MA), TransAct H8000 (C.R. Bard, Inc., Bard Cardiopulmonary Division, Haverhill, MA), and Smeck IABP (Boston Scientific Corporation, Cardiac Assist Division, Mansfield, MA).

For most of the bridge-to-transplant patient population, an IABP is a realistic option that must be considered before VAD placement. Some patients may have an IABP placed and maintained for sev-

Table 5-1. Complications of Intra-Aortic Balloon (IAB) Counterpulsation

Complication	Early	Late
Perforation and dissection of the aorta, femoral, or iliac arteries	✔	✔
Femoral artery damage necessitating open surgical repair	✔	✔
Hematoma at site of entry	✔	✔
Hemorrhage from entry site	✔	✔
Extremity ischemia distal to entry site	✔	✔
Inability to advance IAB due to atheromatous obstruction or stenosis	✔	—
Improper position in thoracic aorta	✔	✔
Thrombosis of femoral artery	✔	✔
Clot formation on catheter or balloon	✔	✔
Embolization of clot on catheter	✔	✔
Aortic wall injury (balloon too large)	✔	✔
Mechanical (e.g., balloon rupture, pump failure, improper timing)	✔	✔
Inadequate support (balloon too small)	✔	—
Infection (local, septicemia)	—	✔
False aneurysm	—	✔
Thrombocytopenia	✔	✔

eral days. This interval of stabilization is often enough to reverse a downward trend. After a brief period of IABP support, the IABP may then be discontinued and the patient maintained on pharmacologic therapy alone. Many patients, however, continue to deteriorate after placement of an IABP or do not show significant improvement after several days of IABP support.[26, 32] At Saint Louis University, it has been our practice to switch these patients over to a VAD in the hope that they can be better rehabilitated. Because the average wait for a suitable donor organ for a status I patient at our university is currently 83 days, we feel much more confident that we can successfully support the transplant candidates with VADs rather than IABPs.

Ventricular Assist Devices and Total Artificial Hearts

The following description derives from a variety of sources, including the Registry for the Clinical Use of Mechanical Ventricular Assist Pumps and Total Artificial Hearts sponsored by the American Society of Artificial Internal Organs (ASAIO) and the International Society of Heart and Lung Transplantation (ISHLT). Some information was obtained from the device manufacturers and a literature review. It must be kept in mind that not all cases are reported to either the registry or the manufacturer and that there are no uniform definitions of complications. For this reason, the information in this chapter must be kept in perspective.

Between 1985 and 1994, more than 2,000 implanted devices have been reported to the combined ASAIO-ISHLT Registry, with 584 of these being placed as a bridge-to-heart transplantation.[18] Figure 5-2 shows the distribution of devices inserted as a bridge to transplantation over 10 years. It can be seen that the most productive years were 1987–1989, with a sharp drop in implants by 1993. Of the 584 patients, 470 were men (84%). The mean age of the men receiving a device was 44 years and 34.3 years for women, which suggests that the population receiving mechanical circulatory support is quite young.

Table 5-2 shows the number of days of mechanical circulatory support according to device type in the bridge-to-transplant population. The shortest duration of support was in patients receiving centrifugal left ventricular assistance (8.1 ± 1.7 days). This short duration of support is related to technical problems with supporting patients for long periods with centrifugal pumps. These problems include anticoagulation, lack of mobility, pump failure, hemolysis, nonpulsatile flow, and higher rates of infection due to the design of the cannulas and position of cannula exit sites. The second shortest duration of support was in the biventricular assistance group. The short duration of support was not a result of early

Figure 5-2. Bridge-to-transplant experience, 1983–1993. Ventricular assist device (VAD) and total artificial heart (TAH) experience. U.S. Food and Drug Administration approval was withdrawn from TAH in 1991.

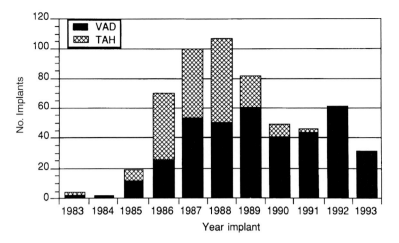

Table 5-2. Days of Support According to Device Type for Bridge-to-Transplant Population

Device Type	Mean ± SEM	Range
LVA	43.7 ± 4.7	0–370
RVA	20.3 ± 17.3	0–72
BVA	17.3 ± 1.9	0–162
TAH	23.4 ± 3.9	0–438

LVA = left ventricular assist; RVA = right ventricular assist; BVA = biventricular assist; TAH = total artificial heart. Source: Adapted from SM Mehta, TX Aufiero, WE Pae, et al. Combined registry for the clinical use of mechanical ventricular assist pumps and the total artificial heart in conjunction with heart transplantation: Sixth Official Report—1994. J Heart Lung Transplant 1995;14:585–593.

transplantation but rather of significant early mortality in a sicker group of patients with biventricular failure and multiorgan dysfunction. Table 5-3 lists the complications of the bridge-to-transplant patient population according to clinical outcome. The most common complication by far was bleeding, with infection and renal failure also being common.

The incidence of technical problems was 6.1% in all patient cohorts, which suggests that the devices' reliability was adequate in these critically ill patients. Table 5-4 shows the rates of transplantation and discharge of the bridge-to-transplant patients based on the type of support received. The best results occurred in patients receiving isolated left ventricular assistance with either pneumatic or electrical VADs. Posttransplant survival was worse in the centrifugal biventricular assistance group and,

surprisingly, in the TAH group. Overall, 68.5% of the patients were transplanted, with 68.5% of the patients transplanted being discharged. This translates to an overall discharge rate of 47%.

Table 5-5 lists posttransplant causes of death. The most common cause of early (<30 days) mortality was ventricular failure due to ischemic injury or rejection, with infection, renal failure, bleeding, and respiratory insufficiency occurring in a significant percentage of the deaths. The most common cause of late (>30 days) mortality was infection (40%), as would be expected in this immunosuppressed population. The 18.9% incidence of late ventricular failure was probably related to graft dysfunction because of rejection.

Figure 5-3 shows the actuarial survival from the time of transplantation in three groups: routine heart transplant recipients (ASAIO-ISHLT Registry data), patients supported with VADs, and all bridge-to-transplant patients, including VAD and TAH patients. The 5-year survival rate in the VAD bridge group is virtually identical to the routine transplant group, which supports the efficacy of VADs. It is not known why patients receiving a TAH fare worse.

Since 1985, 59 patients at Saint Louis University have been placed on advanced mechanical circulatory support devices as a bridge to cardiac transplantation. Thirty-nine were supported with the Thoratec paracorporeal external pneumatic VAD (Thoratec Laboratories, Inc., Berkeley, CA; Figure 5-4). Eighteen patients received an implantable Novacor left ventricular assist system (LVAS) (Novacor Division, Baxter Healthcare Corp.; Figure 5-5), and the remaining two patients received a Jarvik 7-70 TAH (Symbion, Inc.,

Table 5-3. Complications of Bridge-to-Transplant Population According to Clinical Course

Complication	All Patients ($n = 574$) (%)	Not Transplanted ($n = 184$) (%)	Transplanted but Not Discharged ($n = 126$) (%)	Transplanted and Discharged ($n = 274$) (%)
Bleeding/DIC	42.5	59.1	50.0	29.4
Infection	28.5	38.3	30.6	22.0
Renal failure	22.9	46.3	24.5	8.6
Thrombus/emboli	16.6	24.8	10.2	14.5
Hemolysis	10.1	14.1	15.3	5.9
Neurologic	9.1	16.8	10.2	3.9
Technical problems	6.1	8.7	6.1	5.6

DIC = disseminated intravascular coagulopathy.
Source: Adapted from SM Mehta, TX Aufiero, WE Pae, et al. Combined registry for the clinical use of mechanical ventricular assist pumps and the total artificial heart in conjunction with heart transplantation: Sixth Official Report—1994. J Heart Lung Transplant 1995;14:585–593.

Table 5-4. Transplantation and Discharge Rates of Bridge-to-Transplant Population

Device Type	No. of Patients	No. Transplanted (%)	No. Discharged (%)
LVA	187	138 (73.8%)	125 (90.6%)
RVA	5	2 (40.0%)	0 (0%)
BVA	164	113 (68.9%)	77 (68.1%)
Hybrid BVA*	37	12 (32.4%)	6 (50.0%)
TAH	191	135 (70.7%)	66 (48.9%)
Total	**584**	**400 (68.5%)**	**274 (68.5%)**

LVA = left ventricular assist; RVA = right ventricular assist; BVA = biventricular assist; TAH = total artificial heart.
*The hybrid BVA uses two types of devices.
Source: Adapted from SM Mehta, TX Aufiero, WE Pae, et al. Combined registry for the clinical use of mechanical ventricular assist pumps and the total artificial heart in conjunction with heart transplantation: Sixth Official Report—1994. J Heart Lung Transplant 1995;14:585–593.

Table 5-5. Attributable Causes of Death for Transplant Recipients from Bridge-to-Transplant Population

Cause of Death	<30-Day Mortality (%) ($n = 198$)	>30-Day Mortality (%) ($n = 90$)
Ventricular failure	35.7	18.9
Renal failure	28.1	13.3
Respiratory failure	25.3	8.9
Infection	23.2	40.0
Bleeding	21.2	13.3
Transplant problems	10	6.0
Emboli	8.1	6.7

Source: Adapted from SM Mehta, TX Aufiero, WE Pae, et al. Combined registry for the clinical use of mechanical ventricular assist pumps and the total artificial heart in conjunction with heart transplantation: Sixth Official Report—1994. J Heart Lung Transplant 1995;14:585–593.

Tempe, AZ; Figure 5-6). The mean duration of support was 42.4 ± 77 days. Two patients were supported for longer than 1 year. One Novacor patient was supported for 370 days, followed by successful cardiac transplantation. Another patient was supported for 440 days with a Jarvik TAH. The TAH patient died of multiorgan failure approximately 3 months post transplantation, after rejection and infection.

Thirty-six patients (62%) were eventually transplanted, and there were four late deaths at 3, 6, 14, and 68 months. Two more patients (one postpartum cardiomyopathy, one ischemic cardiomyopathy) were weaned from the devices after myocardial recovery at approximately 50 days each. The overall survival rate in the last 20 patients was 83%. There have been no intraoperative deaths for 5 years. Currently, all survivors are New York Heart Association class I.

Figure 5-3. Actuarial survival after primary transplantation compared with bridge-to-transplant recipients. Survival is comparable. (HTX = routine heart transplants; VAD = ventricular assist device; TAH = total artificial heart.)

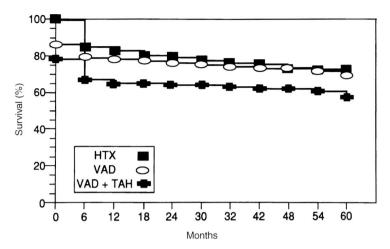

Description of Devices

Various devices for long-term support of the circulation are available both clinically and experimentally. They encompass many designs, which for the most part operate pneumatically or by an electrical power source. The devices can be classified in many ways, ranging from pulsatile or nonpulsatile flow to whether they are positioned externally or internally. Table 5-6 lists and describes the devices currently used clinically for bridging to transplantation in the United States. Some of these devices are considered investigational by the FDA, but two, the ThermoCardioSystems pneumatic HeartMate (ThermoCardioSystems, Inc. [TCI], Woburn, MA; Figure 5-7) and Thoratec (see Figure 5-4), have received FDA approval, and several are very near approval. Some devices were designed using integrated systems specifically for chronic support of the circulation. Others were designed for shorter-term usage and have been modified and used in bridging to transplantation.

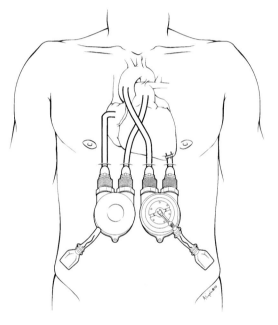

Figure 5-4. Thoratec paracorporeal pneumatic biventricular assist devices. (Thoratec Laboratories Corporation, Pleasanton, CA.)

Centrifugal Pumps

Centrifugal pumps (Figure 5-8) are used widely for short-term support throughout the United States primarily because they are readily available and inexpensive.[33–37] Many perfusionists have been trained in the use of these pumps, and they are commonly used in procedures such as aortic aneurysm repair, liver transplantation, and extracorporeal membrane oxygenation (ECMO). Another typical use is to support the circulation in patients who cannot be weaned from cardiopulmonary bypass after cardiac reparative procedures.[33, 34] They were initially designed to be used during cardiopulmonary bypass for durations of less than 4 hours; therefore, their usage is usually limited from several days to 2 weeks. In most cases, they are used in patients in whom recovery of the natural heart is expected. Some centers do use centrifugal pumps for bridg-

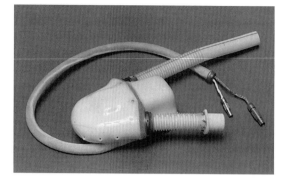

Figure 5-5. Novacor left ventricular assist system (12-V electric). (Courtesy of Baxter Healthcare Corporation, Oakland, CA.)

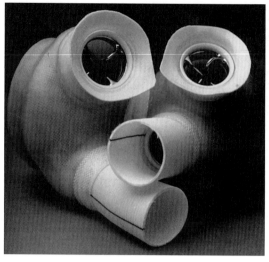

Figure 5-6. Jarvik 7-70 total artificial heart. (Courtesy of Cardiowest, Tucson, AZ.)

Table 5-6. Mechanical Circulatory Support Devices Currently Used in the United States for Bridging to Transplantation

Device (Manufacturer)	Type	Position	Support	Flow Capacity	Requirement for Anticoagulation	Duration of Support
Centrimed (Sarns, Ann Arbor, MI)	Impeller	Extracorporeal	R, L, B	5 liters/min	Moderate continuous heparin	Short (days)
Biomedicus (Medtronic, Minneapolis, MN)	Restrained vortex	Extracorporeal	R, L, B	5 liters/min	Moderate continuous heparin	Short (days)
Thoratec (Thoratec Laboratories, Inc., Berkeley, CA)	Pneumatic sac	Paracorporeal	R, L, B	7 liters/min	Low	Long (mos)
Novacor (Novacor Division, Baxter Healthcare Corp.)	Electrical	Internal	L	10 liters/min	Low	Long (indefinite)
ThermoCardio-Systems Heart-Mate (Thermo CardioSystems, Inc. [TCI], Woburn, MA)	Pneumatic piston or electrical	Internal	L	10 liters/min	Low	Long (indefinite)
Cardiowest TAH (formerly Jarvik) (Symbion, Inc., Tempe, AZ)	Pneumatic sac	Internal	Total	10 liters/min	Low-moderate	Long (indefinite)

R = right heart; L = left heart, B = both right and left heart; TAH = total artificial heart.

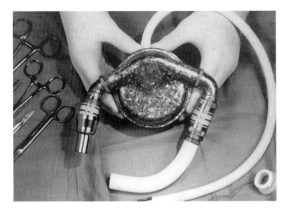

Figure 5-7. HeartMate pneumatic model. (Courtesy of ThermoCardioSystems, Inc., Woburn, MA.)

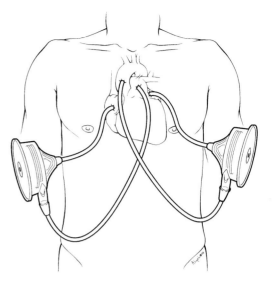

Figure 5-8. Centrifugal ventricular assist device, biventricular configuration. (Courtesy of Medtronics Biomedicus, Minneapolis, MN.)

ing to transplantation, but this is changing rapidly due to the wider availability of more sophisticated pulsatile devices.[35–37] Surgical placement of centrifugal pumps is less complicated than it is for the pulsatile systems. It involves placing standard cardiopulmonary bypass catheters in either atria or the left ventricle for blood removal and standard cardiopulmonary bypass inflow cannulas into the pulmonary artery or aorta, or both. They can be placed with or without full cardiopulmonary bypass support. These devices have impellers or rotating cones coupled electromagnetically to produce energy that generates pressure and flow work.[38]

There are several disadvantages to using centrifugal devices in bridge-to-transplant candidates. The greatest concern is that the average time necessary to locate a donor heart in the United States now exceeds 6 months. Status I (urgent need) categorization of bridge-to-transplant candidates gives them priority over nonurgent candidates, but the wait is often 1–3 months. Centrifugal pumps, with their limited duration of support, are therefore of questionable value in most bridge candidates. The second factor is that the extracorporeal nature of the devices requires a large control console, which limits patient mobility. Centrifugal pump devices are not designed for and cannot be rigged for extended support. The cannula design and the connectors' propensity to cause hemolysis and thromboembolism make them far from ideal. Commercially available centrifugal pumps include the Biomedicus (Medtronic, Minneapolis, MN), Centrimed (Sarns, Ann Arbor, MI), and the St. Jude (Chelmsford, MA).

Centrifugal pumps are sometimes used to bridge children to cardiac transplantation because the more sophisticated devices used in adults are not available for children. The same inherent problems with the centrifugal design that are present in adults also pertain to children.[39]

Pneumatic Ventricular Assist Devices

Several pneumatic external VADs can be used for bridging to cardiac transplantation. For example, the Abiomed BVS (BVS 5000, Danvers, MA; Figure 5-9), is an extracorporeal pneumatic VAD that can provide biventricular support. It has FDA approval for postcardiotomy support in the United States, but it is not approved for bridging to transplantation. There has been some experience in Europe using the Abiomed BVS to bridge patients to transplantation.[40] A second example is the Thoratec VAD (see Figure 5-4), which was designed by a group at Pennsylvania State University in Hershey, Pennsylvania. The Thoratec VAD can support both the right and left heart and can be inserted without cardiopulmonary bypass. Several hundred patients have been bridged to cardiac transplantation with the Thoratec device in the United States, and many more in Europe. The device has proved

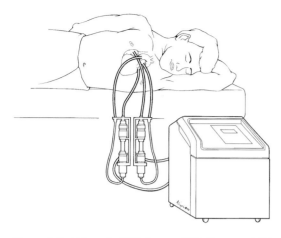

Figure 5-9. Abiomed's BVS System 5000 (Danvers, MA) with console.

to be reliable and effective for durations of up to 6 months, and the FDA approved it for bridge-to-transplant use in December of 1995.

The Thoratec VAD consists of a polyurethane blood sac attached to inlet and outlet conduits that can be placed in either the left atrium, right atrium, or left ventricle (inlet), with the outlet conduits being sutured to the aorta or pulmonary artery, or both (Figure 5-10). The Thoratec device uses Björk-Shiley monostrut valves to provide unidirectional flow. It can operate in three modes: an ECG-synchronous mode, a fixed-rate mode, and a fill-to-empty mode, which uses a sensor that detects blood-sac filling. The stroke volume of the device is 65 ml, and it can pump 6.5–7.0 liters per minute.

The paracorporeal nature of the device permits ambulation and exercise for physical conditioning. Left ventricular apex cannulation is usually used in bridge-to-transplant candidates because it maximizes pump washing and output. If the left ventricle is small and of a normal configuration (e.g., in acute myocardial infarction patients), however, left atrial cannulation is used. The Thoratec VAD can also support the right ventricle, and biventricular assist devices (BVADs) are usually necessary in approximately 20–25% of bridge-to-transplant patients.

Implantable Blood Pumps

Two implantable blood pumps are available, and both have had extensive testing. They have been used in the United States and Europe for bridging to transplantation and have successfully supported patients for longer than 1 year. They are the pneumatic and electrical HeartMate 1000 IP LVAS and the electrical Novacor LVAS. Both were designed for chronic support of the left heart.

The HeartMate 1000 IP LVAS (see Figure 5-7) is a pneumatically driven blood pump that is implanted in the abdomen with a percutaneous driveline attached to a portable external drive console.[30] The blood pump is formed by a rigid titanium housing enclosing a flexible polyurethane diaphragm that divides the pump into an air chamber and a blood chamber. The drive console operates in one of two modes: rate responsive or set rate. Blood inflow is from the left ventricular apex, and

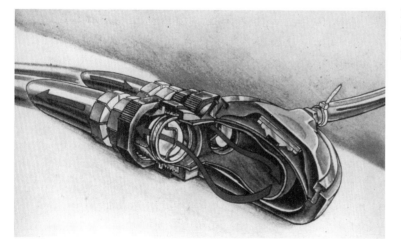

Figure 5-10. Thoratec ventricular assist device. (Courtesy of Thoratec Medical Laboratories, Pleasanton, CA.)

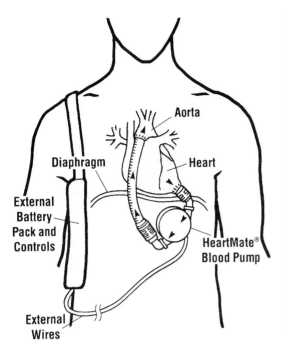

Figure 5-11. ThermoCardioSystems (Woburn, MA) Electric Left Ventricular Assist Device (VE-LVAD) System with battery pack, controls, and external vent line.

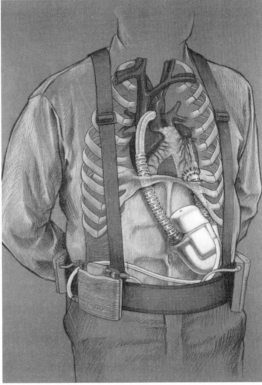

Figure 5-12. Novacor Left Ventricular Assist System. (Courtesy of Novacor Division, Baxter Healthcare Corporation, Oakland, CA.)

pump filling is passive. The device uses bioprosthetic porcine valves. Blood is ejected through the outflow conduit, which is anastomosed to the ascending aorta.

The textured surface of titanium microspheres on the rigid metallic blood-contacting surface promotes the formation of an intimal fiber and cellular component that evolves into a blood-compatible biological lining. For this reason, it is generally believed that the HeartMate requires less anticoagulation than do some of the devices that use ultrasmooth polyurethane sacs. Several reports have documented the effectiveness of this device and have shown the results with its use to be comparable to those achieved by both Thoratec and Novacor.[30, 41, 42]

An electrically driven, externally vented left ventricular assist device (LVAD) is made by Thermo-CardioSystems, Inc. (Figure 5-11). The HeartMate vented electrical device is identical in design to the pneumatic HeartMate, with the exception that it is electrically actuated. A portable, wearable 12-volt system has been developed for use in conjunction with the electrical HeartMate VE-LVAD. This allows patients to be ambulatory and untethered. It

has also allowed several patients to be discharged from the hospital to await location of a donor heart in an outpatient environment.[20]

The Novacor LVAS (Figure 5-12) is an electrically powered ventricular assist system that uses spring-loaded, solenoid-activated compression of a sac chamber by a dual pusher plate hinged mechanism.[41] A microprocessor controls the solenoid. Current designs require a percutaneous electrical cable and a vent tube. The device is connected by a Dacron conduit to the left ventricular apex, and the outflow graft is anastomosed to the ascending aorta. The percutaneous vent tube with its electrical conduit is tunneled subcutaneously to the right lower quadrant. The pump is positioned in the left upper abdominal quadrant preperitoneally. This device is capable of flows of up to 10 liters per minute and permits full ambulation when the wearable controller and battery pack are used. The Novacor LVAS uses bioprosthetic inlet and outlet valves, and

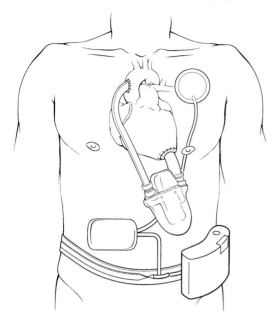

Figure 5-13. Novacor Left Ventricular Assist System. It is totally implantable with volume compensator, belt transformer (primary), implanted secondary, external power and status monitor, electronic controller, and external battery power source. (Courtesy of Novacor Division, Baxter Healthcare Corporation, Oakland, CA.)

Table 5-7. Criteria for Investigational Device Insertion

Cardiac index <2.0 liters/min/m^2
Pulmonary capillary wedge pressure or right atrial pressure >18 mm Hg
Systemic hypotension
Evidence of reversible end-organ damage from low cardiac output (i.e., blood urea nitrogen, creatinine, bilirubin, or hypoxemia secondary to pulmonary edema)
Refractory life-threatening arrhythmias

---

the pump has an ultrasmooth polyurethane sac. Current protocols call for anticoagulation with warfarin and low-dose aspirin.

From experience in the bridge-to-transplant population, it seems that prolonged mechanical circulatory support is a realistic option to pursue. A totally implantable Novacor system is currently being tested and developed (Figure 5-13). Clinical trials with this device could begin within 3–5 years.

Patient Selection

Some devices used for bridging to transplantation described in this chapter are investigational and under strict FDA protocols, but two have been approved for commercial use as a bridge to transplantation. Specific and rigid patient selection criteria were derived for each clinical trial. The selection criteria are similar among studies, however, and are identical in some cases. Patients considered for mechanical circulatory support before cardiac transplantation are transplant candidates without the usual transplant exclusion criteria (e.g., age older than 65

years, pulmonary artery hypertension, diabetes) and should have refractory heart failure (acute or chronic).[43, 44] Usual conventional therapy (i.e., IABP, drugs) should have been tried and determined to be ineffective. For investigational devices, the patient should usually meet the criteria listed in Table 5-7.

Most patients meeting these conditions are considered for emergent placement of a VAD. Other patients, however, have repeated episodes of congestive heart failure and gradual multiorgan deterioration. For these patients, a more elective approach may be chosen, and the device can be inserted during an optimal interval. Because bridge-to-transplant procedures are so costly in terms of labor and resources, once devices are approved by the FDA and commercially available, the criteria for patient selection that were used during the clinical trials generally remain the standard by which patients are selected. Due to the diversity of clinical situations, however, there are definite advantages to not being confined by stringent hemodynamic criteria when choosing patients.

Anesthetic Management

Candidates for bridging to transplantation are often in cardiogenic shock. They always have low cardiac output and are compromised metabolically. They are being pharmacologically supported as well as maximally sympathetically stimulated endogenously and often have an IABP in place. A small percentage of patients may be supported with emergency venoarterial ECMO.[45]

Preoperative Preparation

We have avoided unsupervised preoperative sedation in settings outside the operating room to avoid circulatory depression and the potential reduction in endogenous catecholamines. Often, preoperative medications are administered only after the patient is positioned on the operating table with monitoring established and under the direction of the anesthesiologist. Small doses of opioids, usually fentanyl, are intermittently administered intravenously in 50- to 100-mg doses, frequently combined with benzodiazepines (diazepam or midazolam) in 0.5- to 1.0-mg boluses to facilitate the establishment of invasive monitoring, if it is not already in place. Table 5-8 lists our standard equipment and vasoactive drugs immediately available. Before initiation of surgery, 1 million units of aprotinin are infused followed by an infusion (250,000 IU/hour) throughout the surgery. The perfusionist also adds 1 million units to the pump prime.

The critical period after the patient's arrival in the operating room until the cardiopulmonary bypass begins is particularly challenging. Rapid deterioration may occur spontaneously or be associated with an inadvertent alteration in the flow of inotropes and supportive drugs during transfer to or positioning in the operating room. Emergency drugs, particularly epinephrine and calcium chloride, should be available. Pacing capability via esophageal or intracardiac leads, or provisions for external pacing, should be available. Leads 2 and 5 of the ECG, pulse oximetry, an intra-arterial pressure catheter (radial, femoral, or from the IABP), and a thermodilution catheter with oximetry are placed before induction if time permits, and if they are not already functional. Multigas and agent analyses are standard routine care. Although venous access is always present on arrival, it is frequently not appropriately sized to manage major blood replacement needs, and at a minimum, two large-bore intravenous access sites are established, preferably 14 gauge or larger. Smaller existing catheters (18 or 20 gauge) can be replaced with a 7 French exchange device using the Seldinger technique or with similar central access devices inserted when peripheral access is limited or impossible. Central venous access insertion is facilitated by the use of portable ultrasound visualization.

Our experience with mixed venous oxygen saturation has made us prefer a 7.5 French Svo_2-enhanced thermodilution catheter. We prefer to place it via the right internal jugular vein through a 9.0 French sheath. After entry into the chest via a median sternotomy, a left atrial catheter is usually placed in

Table 5-8. Standard Anesthetic Setup

Monitors
    ECG leads II and V5
    Blood pressure, noninvasive, radial arterial catheter
    Pulse oximeter
    Pulmonary artery catheter (PAC) via internal jugular vein with continuous mixed venous oximetry
    Temperature probe, esophageal and PAC
    Esophageal stethoscope
    Transesophageal echocardiography
    Anesthetic gas and end-tidal CO_2 monitors
    Foley catheter, for urine output
    Two-channel EEG
Equipment
    Anesthetic machine with tidal volume, minute ventilation, and peak inspiratory pressure monitoring and variable PEEP valve
    Red blood cell scavengers
    Intra-aortic balloon pump
    Dual atrial-ventricular demand pacemaker
    Blood gas, electrolyte analyzer
    Pneumatic pressure infusers
    Intravenous fluid infusion pump
    Syringe pumps
    Neuromuscular stimulator
    ECMO
Temperature maintenance
    Heated humidifier
    Thermal mattress
    Fluid or blood warmer
Vasoactive drugs
    Ephedrine (5 mg/ml D_5W)
    Epinephrine (5 mg/250 ml D_5W)
    Dopamine (200 mg/100 ml D_5W)
    Dobutamine (250 mg/125 ml D_5W)
    Isoproterenol (1 mg/250 ml D_5W)
    Norepinephrine (4 mg/250 ml D_5W)
    Milrinone (50 mg/250 ml D_5W)
    Phenylephrine (10 mg/250 ml D_5W)

ECG = electrocardiogram; EEG = electroencephalogram; PEEP = positive end-expiratory pressure; ECMO = extracorporeal membrane oxygenation; D_5W = 5% dextrose in water.

the right pulmonary vein before initiating mechanical circulatory support. The use of a right internal jugular vein for thermodilution catheter placement does not appear to compromise its use for subsequent access for endocardial biopsy. Every effort should be made to ensure sterility in placing invasive devices to avoid subsequent device-related infections.

Emergency ECMO initiation via the femoral arterial and venous access routes may have been required before transfer, and although it indicates deteriorating status, ECMO usually stabilizes the patient. It may be necessary to initiate cardiopulmonary bypass in the operating room emergently on arrival using similar femoral-femoral access. Complicating the problem is the fact that many patients have had a previous cardiac surgical procedure. This lengthens the interval between induction and completion of the surgical exposure of the mediastinal structures.

Induction

Induction of anesthesia may precipitate collapse by depressing cardiac contractility, producing vasodilatation, or depressing endogenous catecholamine production. Therefore, the hemodynamic status of the patient on arrival in the operating room determines the induction technique. We have usually used a high-dose narcotic technique of 50–75 μg/kg of fentanyl with success. It must be administered very slowly, titrating cautiously, or by using a slow, continuous infusion. Incrementally administered amnestic agents (0.5–1.0 mg lorazepam, 0.5–1.0 mg of midazolam, or 1–2 mg of diazepam) are frequently used, but their hypotensive potential when combined with fentanyl should be anticipated.

Although vecuronium (0.1 mg/kg) would appear to be a good choice, its use in the presence of fentanyl may sometimes be a disadvantage, due to vecuronium's minimal effect on heart rate. We have used a combination of pancuronium and metocurine (1–4 mg) for two reasons: cost and a sympathomimetic effect in overcoming the bradyarrhythmias often seen with a high-dose narcotic technique. If a pre-existing bradycardia and hypotension are present, pancuronium is most appropriate (0.1 mg/kg). The muscle relaxants rocuronium and mivacurium may also be considered.

If a rapid-sequence induction is necessary, ketamine, etomidate, or pentothal, with succinylcholine or rocuronium, may be considered. Even their rapid administration, however, may lead to a loss of hemodynamic stability. Reversal of this induced hypotension has almost always followed administration of 500 mg calcium chloride or epinephrine (10–50 μg), or both, as a bolus through the right atrial port of the thermodilution catheter.

A review of our bridge experience revealed that most patients arrive in the operating room unintubated. Although they are hemodynamically compromised, they tolerate a narcotic-based induction with fentanyl and an intubating dose of pancuronium (1.0 mg/kg). After induction, we favor the continued use of fentanyl as an infusion (0.22 μg/kg/minute) throughout the intraoperative period. Because early hospital discharge is not a consideration, a few more hours of intubation before extubation is considered advantageous, particularly because bleeding and the necessity for re-exploration (up to 50%) are common complications of the postoperative course.

The bridge-to-transplant patient is in a delicate balance involving preload, vascular resistance, and ventricular function. Volume loss is poorly tolerated, as is vascular overload. Profound hemodynamic changes can be the result of relatively small variations in volume associated with blood loss or fluid loading. Central venous and pulmonary artery wedge pressure observations are essential to maintain adequate preload by infusion of colloid and crystalloid solutions. Hemodynamic support may need to be increased, or alternate inotropic drugs substituted or added, to restore hemodynamic stability. Dopamine and dobutamine infusions may need to be increased, and epinephrine, isoproterenol, amrinone, or milrinone infusions may have to be initiated.

Intraoperative Management

Once the patient is anesthetized, sternotomy and mediastinal exposure of the heart and great vessels is done. With the heart exposed, the abdominal pocket for the implantable LVAS can be prepared. If a paracorporeal or external device is used, percutaneous cannula exit sites are created to minimize dissection while heparinized and to minimize the time on cardiopulmonary bypass. The patient is then heparinized to achieve an activated clotting time (ACT) of 450–500 seconds. Another method to reduce the time on cardiopulmonary bypass is to anastomose the grafts onto the aorta or pulmonary artery before initiating bypass. Once the VAD outflow cannulas have been placed, attention is turned to VAD inflow.

Many of the patients bridged to transplant have LVAD inflow cannulas placed within the left ventricular apex, and this requires cardiopulmonary bypass. Depending on the preference of the implanting surgeon, cardioplegic arrest may or may not be used for placement of the left ventricular apex cannula. In some patients, it may be preferable to use the left atrium as the source of VAD inflow. Left atrial cannulation can be performed without cardiopulmonary bypass in stable patients, and the cannula can be placed in several sites, including the left atrial appendage, the dome of the left atrium, or the right superior pulmonary vein. If the patient is receiving BVADs, right VAD (RVAD) pump inflow is placed in the right atrium. Cannulation of the right ventricle has proved to be unsuccessful owing to the small size of the chamber. During device implantation, cardiopulmonary bypass may or may not be used, but the patient is maintained at normothermia. Once all the cannulas have been placed, the VADs are connected to the cannulas, and all air is removed from the system.

Once the air has been removed, the VADs are activated at a rate of 15–30 beats per minute while cardiopulmonary bypass flow is reduced. Weaning from cardiopulmonary bypass is usually fairly rapid (less than 5 minutes). During this time, left atrial and right atrial pressure should be continuously monitored. In patients receiving only LVADs, the left atrial pressure should be maintained at 5–10 mm Hg, with VAD pump indices greater than 2.2 liters per minute per m^2. At the same time, the right atrial pressure should be less than 15 mm Hg. In approximately 20–25% of patients receiving LVADs, acute right ventricular failure develops. This is manifested by a high right atrial pressure, a low left atrial pressure, and low LVAD flow indices. Some patients may respond to increasing inotropic support, and our drug of choice is isoproterenol. We have found prostaglandin E_1 ineffective in reversing right ventricular failure. Pulmonary artery pressures decrease, but right ventricular function does not improve. The decision to place an RVAD occurs when, despite moderate inotropic support (combination of isoproterenol and dopamine or dopamine and milrinone), the LVAD flow remains low with a low left atrial pressure and high right atrial pressure. Some clinicians advocate placement of a BVAD from the outset to eliminate some of the more common complications, including right ventricular failure, ventricular arrhythmias, and hypoxia from a patent foramen ovale (PFO). Our approach at Saint Louis University is to place an LVAD device ini-

tially and provide pharmacologic support as indicated. If the patient develops right ventricular failure that is refractory to conventional therapy, an RVAD is placed.

VAD filling is not as efficient as that of the natural heart. Elevated filling pressures are usually required (left atrial pressure and right atrial pressure of 10–15 mm Hg) to maintain VAD flows above 2 liters per minute per m^2. Without adequate preload pressure to the artificial ventricle, adequate pump output cannot be maintained. During and immediately after weaning from cardiopulmonary bypass, volume loading requires coordination between the anesthesiologist and perfusionist.

As for the natural heart, elevated afterload reduces the volume of blood that is ejected from the VAD, resulting in a decrease in the cardiac output. In addition, residual stagnant blood in the pumping chamber increases the risk of clot formation and subsequent thromboembolization. For this reason, intravenous vasodilators are frequently required within a few hours of VAD placement to maintain the mean arterial pressure at 70–80 mm Hg. In some patients, oral vasodilators are needed for the duration of VAD support.

An elevated pulmonary vascular resistance that was present preoperatively, or a transient elevation that may have developed during weaning from cardiopulmonary bypass or because of blood transfusions, further impairs right ventricular performance. Elevated pulmonary vascular resistance may respond to the infusion of sodium nitroprusside or prostaglandin E_1. In most patients, the pulmonary vascular resistance drops dramatically once the LVAD has been activated. The pulmonary capillary wedge pressure sometimes drops from 30–40 mm Hg to 5–10 mm Hg within minutes of LVAD activation.

Once it has been determined that the VAD or BVADs are functioning correctly, heparinization may be reversed with protamine, and the transfusion of fresh frozen plasma and platelets to normalize coagulation factors should begin.

When right atrial pressure exceeds left atrial pressure in the presence of an otherwise insignificant PFO after initiation of LVAD support, shunting from right to left at the atrial level may occur, producing arterial hypoxemia. We routinely check for a PFO by digital palpation of the atrial septum or by transesophageal echocardiographic visualization with agitated saline at the beginning of the procedure.

Although not always detectable, especially while on cardiopulmonary bypass, an otherwise insignificant PFO may produce profound arterial hypoxemia if right atrial pressure is higher than left atrial pressure once bypass is discontinued. Because LVADs significantly decrease left atrial pressure, it is not unusual to see this right-greater-than-left atrial pressure relationship in patients with an LVAD only. For this reason, once bypass is terminated, an arterial blood sample should be obtained to detect any hypoxemia. In patients who receive BVADs, the right and left atrial pressures are usually lowered to near normal levels, and even if a PFO is present, there is little, if any, right-to-left shunting.

After VAD placement, bleeding is a frequent complication, requiring re-exploration in 30–50% of VAD patients. A number of factors contribute to this bleeding, including preoperative anticoagulation therapy, cardiogenic shock, previous surgery, cardiopulmonary bypass, and the cannulation or anastomosis of multiple great vessels. Foreign surfaces, multiple homologous transfusions, re-exploration, and hypothermia further complicate the bleeding problem. It is important to anticipate this problem, to establish meticulous surgical hemostasis, and to provide appropriate platelet, fresh frozen plasma, and packed red blood cell (RBC) products to avoid the development of a major coagulopathy. In the group of 24 patients from Saint Louis University who had VADs as a bridge to cardiac transplantation (April 1991–December 1995), eight required re-exploration (33%). On average, each patient received 5 scavenged, packed, washed cell products; 2 units of bank packed RBCs; 3 units of fresh frozen plasma; and 1.5 pheresis products of platelets at the time of implant in the operating room. Despite the high percentage of re-exploration for bleeding, considerable progress has been made in this area.

To reduce the development of circulating antibodies after device insertion (which appears to be associated with homologous transfusion), we routinely use autotransfusion of shed, scavenged, washed blood intraoperatively and leukocyte-poor filters on all homologous RBC transfusions. Only single-donor platelets obtained by pheresis (rather than random donor platelet concentrates) are administered. Postoperatively, we process the chest drainage in the blood bank with a COBE blood cell processor. After these measures were instituted, the incidence and severity of circulating antibody development were reduced. These circulating antibodies can make it extremely difficult to locate a compatible donor organ. If significant amounts of antibodies are present, a pretransplant donor-recipient crossmatch must be obtained. This often reduces the number of potential donor organs. In addition, only cytomegalovirus (CMV)-negative blood products are administered to avoid the potential of CMV sepsis in immunosuppressed posttransplant recipients. This strategy, in which the anesthesiologist corrects the prothrombin time, partial thromboplastin time (PTT), and platelet count to as near normal as possible while the surgeon corrects any surgical bleeding and controls any oozing, may require several hours before chest closure is considered.

The combination of fluid retention before VAD insertion and fluid loading during cardiopulmonary bypass is usually associated with a brisk postoperative diuresis. An increase in urine output usually begins after the initiation of cardiopulmonary bypass. However, we sometimes give a diuretic shortly after the device has been activated and an adequate mean arterial blood pressure and cardiac output have been established. Because many patients have chronic congestive heart failure and arrive in the operating room with expanded intravascular volumes, hemoconcentration is frequently used during cardiopulmonary bypass to reduce excess water and potentially limit the number of RBC transfusions. Blood collected from the operative field is washed using a cell-saver device. Shed blood from the chest tubes is collected and returned to the blood bank, where it is washed and then reinfused. Blood loss is preferably replaced by the administration of leukocyte-filtered homologous (or autologous washed) RBCs, fresh frozen plasma, or platelets rather than by crystalloid.

Immediate Postanesthetic Care

Although early extubation and mobilization are desirable goals, the high incidence of immediate postoperative bleeding and the need to achieve a stable hemodynamic state do not always lend themselves to early extubation. However, 50% of the bridge-to-transplant patients at Saint Louis University were extubated within 24–36 hours. Once the patient was awake and alert, measured parameters of ventilation were obtained and the potential for extubation was analyzed. The high-dose narcotic technique has not delayed the goal of early extubation in these patients, which at this point is rarely expected to occur within 12 hours. One of the major limiting factors for early extubation has been pulmonary congestion, which is often present preoperatively in the form of diffuse infiltrates or pulmonary edema, or both. Ventilation-perfusion problems are sometimes present postoperatively for at least 1–2 days. Low levels of positive end-expiratory pressure (2.5–5 cm H_2O) are routinely used for these patients to hasten fluid displacement out of the lung parenchyma and to promote alveolar aeration. The combination of a lowered left atrial pressure and diuresis also results in clearing of the interstitial lung edema. These patients, who are often severely volume overloaded, require diuresis once to twice daily for up to 2 weeks after device insertion before all evidence of pulmonary congestion and peripheral edema is gone. Other, rather common complications, which include bleeding, right ventricular failure, and renal insufficiency, also prolong the need for ventilatory assistance.

Another potential problem is embolization in the form of air or thrombus. Many in this patient group have a moderate amount of clot in the native heart, and manipulation of the heart during device implantation could break loose a thrombus. In addition, when the devices are de-aired, it is possible that a bolus of air could be delivered into either the pulmonary artery or aorta. Although the therapeutic benefit of electroencephalographic (EEG) monitoring is questionable, it is reassuring to observe the return of EEG activity. It also documents the time of adverse events, such as air or particulate emboli, hypoxemia, inadequate perfusion, misdirected aortic-input cannulas, and superior canal obstruction.

Arrhythmias are rare in this group, but if they develop, they are often clinically insignificant. Whether an LVAD or BVAD is present, arrhythmias usually cause little problem, especially in the early postoperative period.

Renal failure is an exclusion criterion for VAD implantation. Therefore, most patients come to the operating room with near-normal renal function. Some do not begin to spontaneously diurese, and they require diuretics. The perfusion staff at Saint Louis University routinely place a hemoconcentrator in the line of the cardiopulmonary bypass circuit

and remove a minimum of 2–3 liters of fluid from each patient. Although this technique may aggravate early hypovolemia in a bleeding patient, it helps with pulmonary congestion, reduces edema, and decreases the need for later diuretics.

The immediate postoperative management of these patients is not very complicated. If their volume status can be stabilized and maintained at the appropriate levels, and if proper support has been placed (biventricular support for biventricular failure), the first 24 hours are usually spent allowing the patient some period of stabilization. For this reason, inotropic and vasodilator drugs are minimally manipulated. In the nonbleeding patient, minimal blood transfusions are required. Device function (device flows) is optimized and maintained at a constant level for at least 24 hours to minimize ischemic damage to the major organs. Patients may be extubated within 12–24 hours, but there is generally no rush, as long as extubation can be accomplished within 2 days.

After a 24-hour period of stabilization, weaning from pharmacologic support begins. In addition, some of the invasive monitoring catheters (left atrial pressure, pulmonary artery catheter) and drainage tubes (chest tubes or pump pocket drain) can be discontinued as appropriate. Physical therapy can be started within the first 24 hours and continued throughout the period of hospitalization. Nutritional status is evaluated on an individual basis. Some patients, especially those who deteriorated acutely or are extubated early, begin to take adequate oral nutrition on their own. Other, more chronically ill patients may require total parenteral nutrition, and this would be initiated within the first 48 hours and continued until they were able to take approximately 2,000 calories a day.

Long-Term Postanesthetic Care

The first priority of mechanical circulatory support is to establish high systemic flows as soon as possible to reverse any prior ischemic injury to the vital organs. Because there is usually systemic acidosis from low perfusion, a minimal total flow (natural heart output plus device flow) of 2 liters per minute per m^2 is crucial for a successful outcome. Higher perfusion levels, usually in the range of 2.5–3.0 liters per minute per m^2, are probably optimal.

Device regulation depends on the type of device used. Centrifugal pumps are driven at rates (revolutions per minute) that produce optimal flow without regard to the patient's natural heart rate. Pneumatic pulsatile devices, such as the Pierce-Donachy Thoratec VAD, can function in several modes, including an asynchronous mode, a fill-to-empty volume mode, and an ECG-synchronous mode. Much of the experience with these pneumatic-type devices has been with the fill-to-empty mode because it provides the highest output and optimal blood sac washing to reduce the incidence of thrombus formation and subsequent thromboembolism. Electrical LVASs also have several control parameters, including asynchronous, ECG-synchronous, and volume modes. Because the electrical devices do not have to compensate for the transit time of compressed air, they are much easier to synchronize to the natural heart's ECG. For this reason, most electrical devices are run at rates equal to the patient's native heart rate.

When using the Thoratec VAD for biventricular support, the left and right pumps are usually both run in a fill-to-empty volume mode. Although other combinations of control parameters have been used, this appears to be the most practical and physiologic. The technique provides an excellent response to increased demands of pump output due to patient mobilization and exercise. When both devices are run in a fill-to-empty mode, little regulation is required because the devices compensate for any increased flow (VAD preload) by automatically increasing VAD rate. Both pumps are also always filling and emptying, which reduces the likelihood of thrombus formation in the device. BVADs running in the fill-to-empty mode rarely run at the same rate. LVADs and RVADs are not synchronized to the natural heart or to each other. This technique, in which stroke volume stays constant and the rate varies, may be the best mode to operate univentricular or biventricular devices. Several studies have demonstrated that ECG synchronization of the VADs to the natural heart is not beneficial. TAHs do not have to contend with the problem of working in synchrony with the natural heart because the native ventricles are removed at the time of TAH implantation.

Once the patient's volume status has been stabilized (right atrial and left atrial pressures of 10–15 mm Hg) and postoperative bleeding, if any, is under control, attempts are made to reduce the amount of inotropic drug support. Inotropes should

be weaned slowly and, if necessary, vasodilating drugs added to the pharmacologic regimen. Ideally, within 48–72 hours, the patient is weaned to very low doses of drugs (renal-dose dopamine or low-dose isoproterenol).

As shown in Table 5-3, bleeding is one of the most common postoperative complications, occurring in as many as 50% of mechanical circulatory support patients. Clinical studies done to date have not identified a particular coagulopathy associated with assist-device patients. The derangement of the coagulation parameters is very similar to that of patients who have undergone prolonged cardiopulmonary bypass runs. We have found it most effective to deal with this coagulopathy by infusing large amounts of fresh frozen plasma and platelets. With most of the more sophisticated devices, such as the Novacor, ThermoCardioSystems HeartMate, Thoratec, and Cardiowest TAH (formerly Jarvik), intraoperative heparin required for cardiopulmonary bypass can be completely reversed with protamine. The coagulation factors can be normalized using blood component transfusions. There is usually no need to begin anticoagulating the patient until at least 24–48 hours postoperatively.

Our protocol at Saint Louis University calls for the initiation of low molecular weight dextran at 25 ml per hour once the bleeding has reached less than 100 ml per hour from the chest tubes for 3 consecutive hours. Patients are usually maintained for approximately 48 hours on dextran and then switched to intravenous heparin to keep the PTT at 1.5 times control. The contraindications to dextran are active bleeding, platelet consumption, or a platelet count less than 75,000/µl. Once patients are extubated and able to take oral nutrition and medications, they are switched to an oral regimen of warfarin. Low-dose aspirin (80 mg/day) may be added.

Late bleeding and cardiac tamponade are also common problems in these patients due to the requirement to begin early anticoagulation with either heparin or warfarin. It is not unusual to see late tamponade 1–2 weeks after device insertion. However, the location of bleeding is usually limited to the surgical exposure areas of the mediastinum. Other late bleeding complications are also frequently encountered because of placement of vascular access lines. Because these patients have frequent bleeding and infection complications and often require parenteral nutrition for an extended period, we have become more aggressive in placing Hickman catheters for

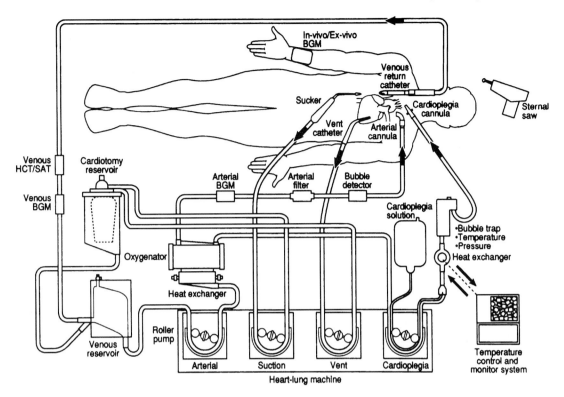

Figure 5-14. Cardiopulmonary bypass, typical membrane oxygenator setup. (HCT/SAT = hematocrit and oxygen saturation; BGM = blood gas measurement.)

long-term access in patients approximately 1 week postoperatively. We begin total parenteral nutrition on the second postoperative day and continue it until the patient is able to take approximately 2,000–2,500 calories per day by mouth. If the patient is intubated or has neurologic problems that preclude oral feeding for a prolonged period, then total parenteral nutrition is changed to enteral feedings.

Late infection, which is often related to the device cannula sites or power cable exit sites, occurs in approximately 30% of patients on mechanical circulatory support. For this reason, these patients undergo frequent courses of intravenous antibiotics and are often on antibiotics at the time of transplantation. The development of bacteremia in patients with a VAD in place is a significant but not insurmountable problem. Several of our patients developed positive blood cultures during the interval of support. In each case, we were able to sterilize the blood, and in seven of eight cases, we proceeded with successful transplantation. The eighth patient was successfully weaned from the device and discharged.

Considerable progress has been made in the field of mechanical circulatory support over the last decade. Patients are now routinely supported for longer than 1 month, and a growing number of institutions are gaining experience with supporting patients outside the hospital. At Saint Louis University, we have now had two patients discharged from the hospital while being supported with the Novacor LVAS to unsponsored outpatient facilities to await location of a donor heart. These patients were fully ambulatory and able to move throughout the city freely. Both were successfully transplanted and had no infectious, thromboembolic, or mechanical complications.

Cardiopulmonary Bypass

Venoarterial or cardiopulmonary bypass is the method by which the work of the heart and the gas-exchange roles of the lung are temporarily substituted by a mechanical pump-oxygenator system[46] (Figure 5-14). A variety of cannulation techniques can be used to connect the patient to the bypass system. One or more cannulas are placed in the right atrium, inferior vena cava, superior vena cava, or one of the large peripheral veins to drain blood into the venous side of the system. Blood is then pumped into the oxygenator, where carbon dioxide is removed and oxygen is added. The oxygenated blood is returned to the patient through the ascending aorta or one of the large peripheral arteries. Since the early 1950s, cardiopulmonary bypass technology has undergone countless modifications. Many different types of circuits are currently in use, but some components are common to most systems. A venous reservoir is usually used and is positioned to provide adequate gravity drainage. This reservoir allows air to escape from the venous return lines, and it can be used to store excess volume. Bubble oxygenators act as their own venous reservoir, whereas hollow-fiber and membrane oxygenators have a separate reservoir.

Several types of oxygenators are commercially available, including bubble, membrane, and hollow fiber. Each has a unique system of gas exchange. Although there are some minor differences in terms of cost and blood-handling capabilities, no distinct advantage has been documented for one type of oxygenator over another in routine cardiac surgical procedures. A heat exchanger is necessary and is an integral component of the oxygenator.

In a large percentage of cases, a roller pump is used and, to a lesser extent, a centrifugal pump. Although there are clear differences between these types of pumps, one design has not been demonstrated to be superior to another for cardiopulmonary bypass runs of less than 3 hours. Other secondary components include an arterial line pressure monitor, arterial line bubble trap, arterial filter, and cardiotomy suction lines.

Pulsatile versus Nonpulsatile Flow

When the ability to support the circulation with cardiopulmonary bypass was introduced, it was recognized that normal physiology was keyed to pulsatile flow, and methods of combining pulsatile flow with perfusion techniques were introduced. The recognition that short periods of support were tolerated without a pulsatile component and the complexity associated with pulsatile techniques led to abandoning attempts to provide a pulsatile component during cardiopulmonary bypass.

There was evidence that nonpulsatile flow may be deleterious. Activation of the renin-angiotensin system led to hypertension during bypass as well as the development of progressive systemic arterial vasoconstriction, which persisted into the early post-bypass period. If pulsatile bypass is provided, the systemic vasoconstriction is attenuated. This results in a lessened work requirement for the ventricle when bypass is terminated, and the incidence of low cardiac output syndrome is reduced. This vasoconstrictor response has been linked to catecholamine release, activation of the renin-angiotensin system, an increase in antidiuretic hormone secretion, and the production of vasoactive substances locally. Thromboxane release is thought to be associated with nonpulsatile perfusion and platelet activation. The effect of mean flow and pressure on renal arteries is associated with an increase in renin secretion and angiotensin II levels.[47–54]

Providing a pulsatile component for routine bypass is hampered by arterial cannula size, the use of membrane oxygenators in the arterial side of the roller pump, the nature of the pumping mechanism (roller or centrifugal), the lengthy lines from the pump head to the patient cannula, and arterial filters, all of which dampen the pulsatile nature of the flow. The simplest solution is a "stepped" roller pump. This is accomplished by varying the pump speed cyclically in each rotation of the roller pump. Another solution is the insertion of an IABP and the fixed-rate activation of the balloon during bypass.

Experience with continuous-flow devices for long periods of support indicates that nonpulsatile flow devices (e.g., centrifugal VADs, ECMO) can provide support for longer intervals in animals. Normal sheep and calves have been supported for up to 5 months, and investigation into this area is ongoing.[55] There is evidence that higher flows (100 ml/kg/minute) overcome some of the adverse effects of nonpulsatile flow. Another option is partial support, with a component of ventricular output retained through the aortic valve. This may provide both support and pulsatile flow.

For most procedures involving cardiopulmonary bypass, the ascending aorta is the most frequently used site of arterial cannulation. Femoral artery input is occasionally used. There appears to be no hemodynamic difference between arterial inflow in the ascending aorta or the femoral artery. The more centrally positioned and larger the venous cannula, the better the venous return. The venous return is augmented by intracardiac vents and cardiotomy suction lines used to remove blood from the surgical field. The perfusion flow rate can be manipulated by regulating venous return or pump speed. The optimal pump flow index is usually 2.0–2.5 liters/m^2 per minute, but it varies with body size and temperature. Perfusion flow rates and venous return are usually maintained at levels that keep the atrial pressures as low as possible. At normothermia, pump flow indices less than 1.6 liters per m^2 per minute commonly result in systemic acidosis; higher flow indices often result in increased blood trauma from higher shear rates.

Temperature Regulation

Temperature is easily regulated with the use of heat exchangers. Mild (28–32°C) to profound hypothermia (18–20°C) is used for virtually all cardiac operations, depending on the type of repair and degree of myocardial protection needed. For routine cardiac surgical procedures, there is a trend toward normothermic perfusion without "active cooling."

Priming

The priming solution for the cardiopulmonary bypass circuit is also an important consideration. Hematocrits of 20–25% provide adequate oxygen-carrying capacity and lower the blood viscosity, thereby providing lower shear rates and better perfusion of the microcirculation compared to blood with higher hematocrits (>30%). Albumin is often used to offset the reduction in colloidal osmotic pressure and reduce the volume of fluid transfer from the intravascular space to interstitial spaces. Mannitol, antibiotics, and buffers are also added to promote diuresis, reduce infection, and normalize the pH, respectively. Blood gases are maintained at a pH of 7.35–7.45, a PaO_2 of 200–300 mm Hg, and a $PaCO_2$ of 30–40 mm Hg measured at 37°C (alpha stat).

Effects on Blood Components

Despite the improvements in technology and techniques, cardiopulmonary bypass is known to have rather dramatic detrimental effects on all blood components. Blood is an intricate mix of RBCs and white blood cells (WBCs), platelets, and plasma proteins. During cardiopulmonary bypass, blood is subjected to increased shear rates, nonendothelialized surfaces, and accumulation of altered or foreign substances, such as fibrin particles, platelet aggregates, and bubbles.[56] The damage that occurs when blood contacts a foreign surface is related to the amount of blood surface interaction. Blood surface interaction can involve both the prosthetic surface area and the duration of time the blood is in contact with the prosthetic material. Blood in the boundary area of the circuit is most likely to be affected. There is a large boundary area in oxygenators and heat exchangers; the amount of blood surface interaction is less in the tubing and cannula.

All artificial surfaces have a deleterious effect on platelets.[57, 58] Platelets clump, their numbers are reduced, and their adhesion and aggregating properties are decreased. Platelet counts are significantly reduced after cardiopulmonary bypass, which is a major factor affecting postoperative bleeding. Exposure to artificial surfaces also has undesirable effects on the erythrocytes and leukocytes, which experience damage that can result in cell disruption. In addition, cardiopulmonary bypass results in the activation of several other systems, including the coagulation cascade, humoral amplification, fibrinolytic cascade, complement, and kallikrein-bradykinin. Activation of these systems often results in pulmonary dysfunction and the development of anaphylatoxins (C3a, C5a).[59, 60] Production of C3a and C5a reduce the available supply of complement and may lessen the normal immune response.

Anticoagulation

The ability to bind heparin to plastic surfaces has been available since 1963, when Gott introduced the heparin-coated Gott shunt.[61] Coated cardiopulmonary bypass components using the Carmeda (Medtronic, Inc., Minneapolis, MN) and Duraflo II (Baxter-Bently, Irvine, CA) processes are available. The ability to use these coated-device components with low heparinization and without systemic heparinization is being investigated. This technology has been reported to reduce complement activation and thrombus formation in the presence of less-than-full systemic heparinization.[62] In a study of 104 randomized patients undergoing bypass, the low-heparin group had decreased blood loss (postoperative drainage), decreased packed homologous RBC transfusion requirements (300 ± 354 ml versus 957 ± 596 ml [full-heparin group]), and a decrease in fresh frozen plasma and platelet use. They attributed this reduction to reduced platelet depletion, better preservation of platelet function, and an improved function of the coagulation system in the low-heparin group. No visible clots were noted on any component of the extracorporeal circuitry.[63]

Although encouraging results are evident from coating the extracorporeal circuitry, the majority of patients undergoing bypass will remain fully heparinized until the safety and efficacy of low or no heparin is clarified. We know of no plan to use heparin bonding on the blood-contacting components of any pulsatile long-term VAD or TAH. For cardiopulmonary bypass and for insertion of VADs, patients are fully heparinized with a dose of 3 mg/kg; aprotinin is also administered. The ACT is maintained at more than 500 seconds throughout the procedure. After the device is in place and functioning with adequate flows, protamine is given to completely reverse the heparin and normalize the ACT. No anticoagulation is given for at least the first 16–24 hours, until chest tube drainage decreases to below 100 ml per hour for 3 consecutive hours and coagulation parameters (international normalized ratio [INR], PTT, platelet count) have begun to normalize. Dextran is initiated at 25 mg per hour or heparin at 10 μg/kg per hour at a constant rate for the next several days. Once the patient is capable of receiving oral medications, warfarin is started to maintain the INR at 2.5–3.0. The heparin dose is increased to maintain the PTT at 1.5–2.0 times control while waiting for the warfarin to take effect.

Cardiopulmonary bypass has the capability to provide more than adequate flow, perfusion pressure, and gas exchange in a resting individual. A number of potentially hazardous factors are not easily controlled, which creates an abnormal physiologic state that should be kept as short as possible. Patients on cardiopulmonary bypass should always be considered at risk for a number of complications, including blood coagulation disorders, hemolysis, complement activation, and gas or particulate emboli.

Scavenging

Cardiopulmonary bypass patients are estimated to require up to 20% of the nation's blood supply annually. At one time, this was of national concern, and the Red Cross's ability to meet these needs was questioned.[64] The risks associated with blood transfusions (e.g., hepatitis, human immunodeficiency virus, mismatch, immune response) have emphasized the need for blood conservation to reduce the number of homologous transfusions.

Centrifugal scavenging devices designed for retrieval of shed blood from surgical wounds have been available for general use since 1974, when the Haemonetics Cell Saver (Haemonetics, Inc., Braintree, MA) was introduced.[65] Several manufacturers now produce instruments that enable shed scavenged blood to be collected, anticoagulated, filtered, packed by centrifugation, washed with saline in the operating suite, and made immediately available for reinfusion as a packed, washed RBC product.

The surgical suction wand is connected to a regulated source of vacuum (vacuum of less than 120 cm H_2O is recommended) to minimize the trauma that can result in the hemolysis of RBCs. The aspirate (shed blood) is mixed with an anticoagulant of either heparinized saline or citrate (acid citrate dextrose or citrate phosphate dextrose) as the blood is drawn into the cardiotomy collection reservoir, where initial 40-μm filtration occurs. The filtered product is then transferred by a roller pump to a centrifuge bowl and concentrated to a hematocrit of approximately 60%. This is associated with plasma removal (waste). The collected packed RBC mass is then washed with 1,000–1,500 ml of 0.9% saline to remove residual plasma, particulate matter, activated coagulation factors, debris smaller than 40 μm, activated complement (C3a and C5a), and the anticoagulant. The washed, packed product is then transferred to a reinfusion bag for return to the patient. Forty-μm filtration at the time of infusion is recommended. We use an in-line blood pump set to facilitate the reinfusion of packed RBCs. We have averaged 3.5 units of the washed cell product per open-heart patient and 5 units in our bridge-to-transplant device insertions.

Figure 5-15 shows the circuitry of the collection process. Although the potential for contamination is present, washing appears to minimize infection. In

Figure 5-15. Intraoperative Red Blood Cell Scavenger Centrifugal System. (AAL = anticoagulant aspiration line; BRB = blood reinfusion bag; BSWB = blood separation wash bowl; CYA = cardiotomy Y-adapter; OEL = oxygenator extension line; VEL = vacuum extension line; WCB = waste collection bag.)

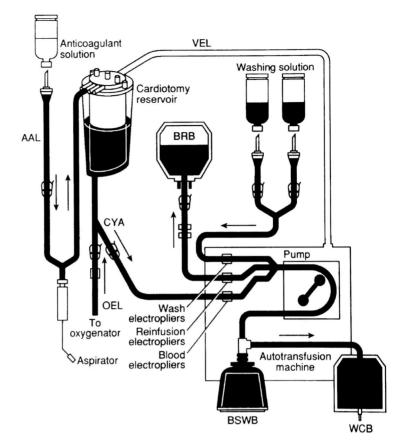

addition, the same blood is suctioned into the heartlung machine during bypass. The equipment is simple to operate, microprocessor based, and designed to eliminate the possibility of air embolism.

In addition to conserving blood, scavenging has a second advantage when the patient is being bridged to transplantation. The use of autologous scavenged RBCs, combined with the removal of WBCs by leukocyte-poor filters on banked homologous RBCs, has virtually eliminated the allogenic reactions that were seen when unfiltered blood was used during VAD insertions. In the past, some patients required several months to allow the antibody titers to fall so that a suitable match of donor and recipient was possible. This is no longer a major problem in our bridge-to-transplant candidates.[29]

Four scavenging units are available in this country: the BRAT (COBE Laboratories, Inc., Lakewood, CO), the Dideco (Sorin Biomedical, Inc., Irvine, CA), Electromedics (Medtronic, Inc., Parker, CO)

and the Haemonetics (Braintree, MA). Several of the cell-saver devices can also be configured and used in the operating theater for platelet pheresis before bypass.

Also available are devices that collect and anticoagulate the shed blood for transfer to transfusion services for washing and subsequent reinfusion (Sorenson, ATS-120S, Abbott Laboratories, Salt Lake City, UT). They are useful in situations of controlled small blood losses (less than 1,000 ml) in which immediate reinfusion can be delayed by volume replacement with fluids or colloid-containing fluids. Postoperative blood loss from chest tube drains can also be retrieved by this processing technique. Removal of the scavenged blood from the surgical theater requires accurate identification and reverification by retyping of the product to prevent a wrong product infusion, a problem that does not exist with intraoperative processing in the operating suite. Intraoperative cell-washing scavenging techniques are almost always used in cardiac and liver transplantation. Intraoperative scavenging techniques are rarely used in renal, pancreas, and lung transplantation.

Because blood banks usually own equipment for cell washing and have personnel to process the collected scavenged blood, the cost of processing (disposable supplies and personnel costs) is often less than $50. This cost compares favorably to the acquisition costs of intraoperative dedicated cell-processing devices ($15,000) for immediate reinfusion in the operating room and to the more expensive disposables ($150). Add to this the cost of a dedicated operator for each site of processing, which usually requires at least 4–6 hours of presence.

Scavenging of fewer than 2 units is generally not considered cost-effective. An institution providing transplantation services is expected to provide scavenged RBC processing in the operating room. Most cardiac and liver transplants are associated with losses exceeding 2 units. In our setting, scavenged losses averaged 5 units in cardiac transplantation (range, 2–8 units) and 10 units in hepatic transplantation (range, 2–30 units).

Because this service is used in situations where perfusionists are unavailable, our anesthesia department is responsible for all intraoperative scavenging. Medicare considers blood scavenging a hospital entity and does not reimburse the physician for services related to collection, processing, and reinfusion. The hospital must render the charge and reimburse the department.

Other Devices

Several other mechanical devices are useful in the setting of transplantation. Two are directly related to the infusion of blood and other fluids at body temperature in situations of massive losses, particularly in liver transplantation and trauma. They are the Rapid Infusion System (RIS) (Haemonetics, Inc., Braintree, MA) and the Level I Blood Warmer (Level I Technologies, Rockland, MA). Both units permit the rapid infusion of bank blood products at near body temperature under conditions of very rapid administration (500 ml/minute or more).

A schematic representation of an RIS is shown in Figure 5-16. The RIS is a recirculating system with a cardiotomy reservoir that has an integral heat exchanger designed for the rapid infusion of blood and blood products by a roller pump at approximately body temperature. It is programmable, and it has safety controls to prevent mishaps. It is frequently used in conjunction with the autotransfusion scavenging systems in liver transplantation, when massive losses are anticipated or occurring. The 3-liter reservoir is augmented by 4 additional liters of infusables, which can be added to the reservoir during the infusion of the reservoir contents to maintain a level of blood in the reservoir. Up to 1,500 ml per minute can be rapidly infused with a DeBakey roller pump. The infusate is 40-μm filtered with an in-line filter of high capacity. Fluid level detectors, pressure sensors, two air detectors, and temperature sensors are monitored by a visual display control panel (see Figure 5-16). Rate of infusion, temperature, and pressure are displayed, and the rate of infusion is operator adjustable. Flow rate varies from 25 ml per minute to 1,500 ml per minute.

Washed, packed RBCs processed by a cell saver (autologous scavenged) are also returned to the RIS cardiotomy reservoir for reinfusion. A mix of 2 units of fresh frozen plasma to each unit of packed, scavenged RBCs or packed RBCs (bank) is added to the cardiotomy reservoir. Platelets should not be added to the reservoir of the RIS; they should be infused directly to the patient via venous access to avoid recirculating damage and removal of platelets from the micropore filter and their adherence onto foreign surfaces.

Conclusions

The clinical results of bridging to cardiac transplantation continue to improve as experience grows. Nonetheless, only a limited number of transplants can be performed per year due to the limited supply of donor hearts. It is currently estimated that 30,000–60,000 patients per year in the United States are candidates for heart transplantation or permanent mechanical circulatory support. If the bridge-to-transplant results continue to improve and the technology is refined, permanent mechanical circulatory support will become a reality. Without the bridge-to-transplant experience, this hoped-for accomplishment would be impossible.

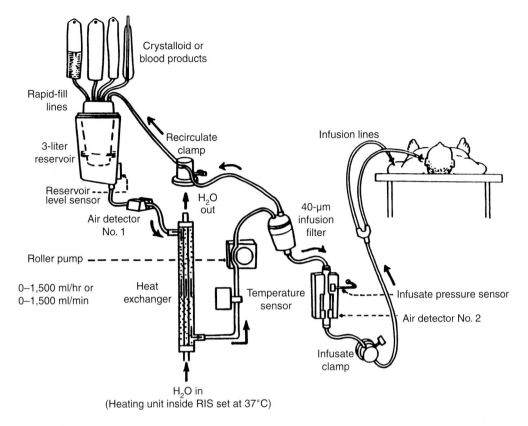

Figure 5-16. Schematic representation of a rapid infusion system (RIS).

Suggested Reading

Grablee GP, Davis RF, Utley JR (eds). Cardiopulmonary Bypass, Principles and Practice. Baltimore: Williams & Wilkins, 1993.

Lewis T, Graham TR (eds). Mechanical Circulatory Support. London: Edward Arnold, 1995.

Ott RA, Gutfinger DE, Gazzaniga AB (eds). Cardiac Surgery: State of the Art Reviews, Mechanical Cardiac Assist (Vol 7, No. 2). Philadelphia: Hanley and Belfus, 1993.

References

1. Gibbon JH Jr. Application of a mechanical heart and lung apparatus to cardiac surgery. Minn Med 1954;37: 171–173.
2. Stuckey JH, Newman MM, Dennis C, et al. The use of the heart-lung machine in selected cases of acute myocardial infarction. Surg Forum 1957;8:342–344.
3. Dennis C, Carlens E, Senning A, et al. Clinical use of a cannula for left heart bypass without thoracotomy. Ann Surg 1962;156:623–626.
4. DeBakey ME. Left ventricular bypass pump for cardiac assistance. Clinical experience. Am J Cardiol 1971;27: 3–11.
5. Moulopoulos SD, Topaz S, Kolff WJ. Diastolic balloon pumping (with carbon dioxide) in the aorta. Mechanical assistance of the failing circulation. Am Heart J 1962;63:669–675.
6. Kantrowitz A, Tjonneland S, Freed PS, et al. Initial clinical experience with intra-aortic balloon pumping in cardiogenic shock. JAMA 1968;203:135–140.
7. The Working Group on Mechanical Circulatory Support of the National Heart, Lung and Blood Institute. Artificial Heart and Assist Devices: Directions, Needs, Costs, Societal, and Ethical Issues. NIH publication No. 85-2723. Washington, DC: U.S. Department of Health and Human Services. Public Health Service, National Institutes of Health, 1985;9.
8. Bernhard WF, Poirier V, LaFarge CG, et al. A new method for temporary left ventricular bypass: preclinical appraisal. J Thorac Cardiovasc Surg 1975;70:880–895.
9. Pierce WS, Brighton JA, O'Bannon W, et al. Complete

left ventricular bypass with paracorporeal pump: design and evaluation. Ann Surg 1974;180:418–426.

10. Norman JC. Intracorporeal partial artificial hearts: initial results in ten patients. Artif Organs 1977;1:41–52.

11. Boretos JW, Pierce WS. Segmented polyurethane: a new elastomer for biomedical applications. Science 1967;158:1481–1482.

12. McEnany MT, Kay HR, Buckley MJ, et al. Clinical experience with intra-aortic balloon pump support in 728 patients. Circulation 1978;58(Suppl 1):24–32.

13. Norman JC, Cooley DA, Igo SR, et al. Prognostic indices for survival during postcardiotomy intra-aortic balloon pumping. J Thorac Cardiovasc Surg 1977;74:709–720.

14. DeVries, WC, Anderson JL, Joyce LD, et al. Clinical use of the total artificial heart. N Engl J Med 1984;310:5–12.

15. Portner PM, Oyer PE, Pennington DG, et al. Implantable electrical ventricular assist system: bridge-to-transplantation and the future. Ann Thorac Surg 1989;47:142–150.

16. Phillips SJ, Zeff RH, Kongtahworn C, et al. Percutaneous cardiopulmonary bypass: application and indication for use. Ann Thorac Surg 1989;47:121–123.

17. Frazier OH, Nakatani T, Duncan JM, et al. Clinical experience with the hemopump. Trans Am Soc Artif Intern Organs 1989;35:604–606.

18. Mehta SM, Aufiero TX, Pae WE, et al. Combined registry for the clinical use of mechanical ventricular assist pumps and the total artificial heart in conjunction with heart transplantation: sixth official report—1994. J Heart Lung Transplant 1995;14:585–593.

19. Dew MA, Kormos RL, Roth LH, et al. Life quality in the era of bridging to cardiac transplantation. Bridge patients in an outpatient setting. ASAIO J 1994;39:145–152.

20. Frazier OH. Outpatient LVAD: its time has arrived. Ann Thorac Surg 1994;58:1309–1310.

21. Bergman D, Nicholas AB, Weiss MB, et al. Percutaneous intra-aortic balloon insertion. Am J Cardiol 1980;46:261–264.

22. Bolooki H. Physiology of Balloon-Pumping. In H Bolooki (ed), Clinical Application of Intra-aortic Balloon Pump. Mount Kisko, NY: Futura, 1984;57–126.

23. Pennington DG, Swartz MT, Codd JE, et al. Intra-aortic balloon pumping in cardiac surgical patients: a nine-year experience. Ann Thorac Surg 1983;36:125–131.

24. DiLello F, Mullen DC, Flemmon RJ, et al. Results of intra-aortic balloon pumping after cardiac surgery: experience with the Percor balloon catheter. Ann Thorac Surg 1988;46:442–444.

25. Downing TP, Miller DC, Stofer R, Shumway NE. Use of the intra-aortic balloon pump after valve replacement. J Thorac Cardiovasc Surg 1986;92:210–217.

26. Reedy JE, Pennington DG, Miller LW, et al. Status I heart transplant patients. Conventional vs ventricular assist device (VAD) support. J Heart Lung Transplant 1992;11(2):246–252.

27. Hardesty RL, Griffith BP, Trento A, et al. Mortally ill patients and excellent survival following cardiac transplantation. Ann Thorac Surg 1986;41:126–129.

28. McBride LR, Miller LW, Naunheim KS, Pennington DG. Axillary artery insertion of an intra-aortic balloon pump. Ann Thorac Surg 1989;48:874–875.

29. Pennington DG, McBride LR, Peigh PS, et al. Eight years experience with bridging to cardiac transplantation. J Thorac Cardiovasc Surg 1994;107(2):472–481.

30. McGee MC, Parnis SM, Nakatani T, et al. Extended clinical support with an implantable left ventricular assist device. Trans Am Soc Artif Intern Organs 1989;35:614–616.

31. Joyce LD, Johnson KE, Toninato CJ, et al. Results of the first 100 patients who received Symbion total artificial hearts as a bridge-to-cardiac transplantation. Circulation 1989;80(Suppl 3):192–201.

32. Naunheim KS, Swartz MT, Pennington DG, et al. Intra-aortic balloon pumping in cardiac surgical patients: risk analysis and long-term follow-up. J Thorac Cardiovasc Surg 1992;104:1654–1661.

33. Magovern GJ, Park SB, Maher TD. Use of a centrifugal pump without anticoagulants for postoperative left ventricular assist. World J Surg 1985;9:25–36.

34. Golding LR, Groves LK, Peter M, et al. Initial clinical experience with a new temporary left ventricular assist device. Ann Thorac Surg 1980;29:66–69.

35. Bolman RM, Spray TL, Cox JL, et al. Heart transplantation in patients requiring preoperative mechanical support. J Heart Transplant 1987;6:273–280.

36. Joyce LD, Emery RW, Eales F, et al. Mechanical circulatory support as a bridge-to-cardiac transplantation. J Thorac Cardiovasc Surg 1989;98:935–941.

37. Golding LAR, Stewart RW, Sinkewich M, et al. Nonpulsatile ventricular assist bridging to transplantation. Trans Am Soc Artif Intern Organs 1988;3:476–479.

38. Pennington DG, Swartz MT. Selection of circulatory support devices. Heart Failure 1988;4(1):5–12.

39. Pennington DG, Swartz MT. Circulatory support in infants and children. Ann Thorac Surg 1993;55:233–237.

40. Champsaur G, Ninet J, Vigneron M, et al. Use of the Abiomed BVS 5000 System as a bridge to cardiac transplantation. J Thorac Cardiovasc Surg 1990;100:122–128.

41. Portner PM, Oyer PE, Pennington DG, et al. Implantable electrical ventricular assist system: bridge-to-transplantation and the future. Ann Thorac Surg 1989;47:142–150.

42. Farrar DJ, Lawson JH, Litwak P, Cederwall G. Thoratec VAD system as a bridge to heart transplantation. J Heart Transplant 1990;9:415–423.

43. Pennington DG, Swartz MT. Patient Selection for Mechanical Circulatory Support. In R Ott (ed), Cardiac Surgery: State of the Art Reviews (Vol 7, No. 2). Philadelphia: Hanley and Belfus, 1993:2;229–239.

44. Reedy JE, Swartz MT, Pennington DG, et al. Bridge-to-cardiac transplantation—importance of patient selection. J Heart Transplant 1990;9:473–481.

45. Raithel SC, Swartz MT, Braun PR, et al. Experience

with an emergency resuscitation system. Trans Am Soc Artif Intern Organs 1989;35:475–477.

46. Casthely PA. The Anatomy of Cardiopulmonary Bypass. In PA Casthely, D Bregman (eds), Cardiopulmonary Bypass: Physiology, Related Complications and Pharmacology. Mount Kisko, NY: Futura, 1991.

47. Geha AS, Salaymeh MT, Tomio A, et al. Effect of pulsatile cardiopulmonary bypass on cerebral metabolism. J Surg Res 1972;12:381.

48. Landymore RW, Murphy DA, Kinley CE, et al. Does pulsatile flow influence the incidence of postoperative hypertension? Ann Thorac Surg 1979;28:26.

49. Watkins L Jr, Lucas SK, Gardner TJ, et al. Angiotensin II levels during cardiopulmonary bypass: a comparison of pulsatile and non-pulsatile flow. Surg Forum 1978;29:229.

50. Philbin DM, Levine FH, Emerson CW, et al. Plasma vasopressin levels and urinary sodium excretion during cardiopulmonary bypass in patients with valvular disease: effect of pulsatile flow. J Thorac Cardiovasc Surg 1979;78:779.

51. Philbin DM, Levine FH, Kono K, et al. Alteration of the stress response to cardiopulmonary bypass by the addition of pulsatile flow. Circulation 1981;64:808.

52. Taylor KM, Wright GS, Reid JM, et al. Comparative studies of pulsatile and nonpulsatile flow during cardiopulmonary bypass II: the effects of renal secretion of cortisol. J Thorac Cardiovasc Surg 1978;75:574.

53. Angell James JE, de Burgh Daly M. Effects of graded pulsatile pressures on the reflex vasomotor responses elicited by changes of mean pressure in the perfused carotid sinus-aortic arch regions of the dog. J Physiol (Lond) 1971;214:51.

54. Frater RWM, Wakagama S, Oka Y, et al. Pulsatile cardiopulmonary bypass: failure to influence hemodynamics or hormones. Circulation 1980;62(Suppl 1):19.

55. Macris MP, Myers TJ, Jarvik R, et al. In vivo evaluation of an intraventricular electric axial flow pump for left ventricular assistance. ASAIO J 1994;40:M719-M722.

56. Salzman EW, Merrill EW. Interaction of Blood with Artificial Surfaces. In RW Coleman, J Hirsh, VJ Marder, EW Salzman (eds), Hemostasis and Thrombosis. Philadelphia: Lippincott, 1987;1335–1337.

57. Turitto T, Baumgartner HR. Platelet-Surface Interactions. In RW Coleman, J Hirsh, VJ Marder, EW Salzman (eds), Hemostasis and Thrombosis. Philadelphia: Lippincott, 1987;555–571.

58. Joist JH, Pennington DG. Platelet reactions with artificial surfaces. Trans Am Soc Artif Intern Organs 1987; 33:341–344.

59. Boralessa H, Shifferli JA, Zame F, et al. Perioperative changes in complement associated with cardiopulmonary bypass. Br J Anaesth 1982;54:1047–1052.

60. Craddock PR, Fehr J, Brigham KL, et al. Complement and leukocyte-mediated pulmonary dysfunction in hemodialysis. N Engl J Med 1982;196:769–774.

61. Gott VL, Whiffen JD, Dutton RC. Heparin bonding on colloidal graphite surfaces. Science 1963;142: 1297–1298.

62. Von Segesser LK, Weiss BM, Garcia E, et al. Reduction and elimination of systemic heparinization during cardiopulmonary bypass. Thorac Cardiovasc Surg 1992;103:790–799.

63. Von Segesser LK, Weiss BM, Pasic M, et al. Risk and benefit of low systemic heparinization during open heart operations. Ann Thorac Surg 1994;58:391–397.

64. Roch JK, Stengle JM. Open heart surgery and the demand for blood. JAMA 1973;225(12):1516–1521.

65. Watson-Williams EJ. Use of the Haemonetics centrifuge to conserve blood during open heart surgery. Presented at the Haemonetics Advanced Pheresis Seminar. Haemonetic Research Institute, 1974.

Chapter 6
Heart and Heart-Lung Transplantation

Rajiv Jhaveri, R. Duane Davis, Barbara Tardiff,
and Bruce Leone

Chapter Plan

Heart Transplantation

Although the first clinical heart transplantation was performed in 1967 by Christiaan Barnard,[1] the initial poor results[2] led to the discontinuation of several heart transplant programs in the early years. A better understanding of the problems of organ preservation, infection, rejection, physiology of the transplanted heart, and the development of superior immunosuppressants (such as cyclosporine) contributed to a more consistent and successful outcome. This led to a resurgence of heart transplant programs all over the world in the early 1980s. Thus, the annual number of heart transplant procedures rose from 62 in 1981 to 2,127 in 1991 in the United States alone.[3]

Since 1981, more than 40,137 heart transplants have been reported from 297 centers worldwide to the Registry of the International Society for Heart and Lung Transplantation (ISHLT).[4] The number of heart transplants has plateaued since 1988, with 3,800–3,900 transplants being performed annually, 2.7% of those being retransplants. The actuarial survival rate of heart transplant recipients is 80% at 1 year after transplant, although there is a steep decline over the ensuing years, with 62% surviving at 5 years and less than 40% surviving at 12 years (Figure 6-1). Although actuarial survival showed a substantial improvement after 1982, the rate of improvement has been much slower in the second

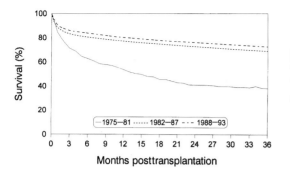

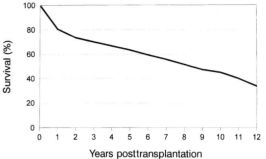

Figure 6-1. Actuarial survival after heart transplantation. (Reprinted with permission from JD Hosenpud, RJ Novick, TJ Breen, OP Daily. The Registry of the International Society of Heart and Lung Transplantation: eleventh official report—1994. J Heart Lung Transplant 1994;13:562.)

Figure 6-2. Heart transplantation actuarial survival by era. (Reprinted with permission from JD Hosenpud, RJ Novick, TJ Breen, OP Daily. The Registry of the International Society of Heart and Lung Transplantation: eleventh official report—1994. J Heart Lung Transplant 1994;13:562.)

half of the decade (Figure 6-2). Recipients older than age 65 years have a significantly higher mortality, and actuarial survival is lower in retransplant recipients (48% vs. 78% at 1 year).[4–6] Those retransplanted within 6 months have a worse outcome than those retransplanted after 6 months (1-year actuarial survival 36% vs. 61%).[4,5]

The quality of life after heart transplantation is an important measure of the effectiveness and benefits of this form of therapy. The National Cooperative Transplantation Study has explored this issue in detail.[7] In this study, more than 80% of the surviving heart transplant recipients were reported to be physically active based on global measures of activity. Activity level was equivalent to that experienced by kidney, liver, or pancreas transplant recipients. Thirty-two to 50% of the surviving recipients were employed, and overall satisfaction with life was high.

Pathophysiology of Heart Failure

Optimal medical management of chronic heart failure requires an understanding of the pathophysiologic mechanisms involved. The failure of the heart as a pump may be due to a systolic or diastolic dysfunction.[8] The resultant low cardiac output state initiates a number of major adaptive changes in the heart, lungs, peripheral circulation, and skeletal muscles in an attempt to maintain function.[8–10] In chronic heart failure, the myocardium undergoes

structural remodeling with myocyte loss, segmental and interstitial fibrosis, myocyte slippage, abnormal fiber orientation, and myocyte hypertrophy.[8,11,12] These structural changes eventually lead to severe ventricular dysfunction and clinical end-stage heart failure. The sympathetic and renin-angiotensin systems are activated early in heart failure. The degree of rise in plasma norepinephrine level has a prognostic value in patients with chronic heart failure.[13] The chronically elevated catecholamine levels cause downregulation (decreased receptor density) of beta$_1$ receptors as well as subsensitivity of beta$_2$ receptors.[14,15] Beta$_2$ receptors are also downregulated in heart failure due to mitral valve disease or ischemic cardiomyopathy.[16] The mechanisms of increased peripheral vascular resistance in chronic heart failure are poorly understood, but it may result from an abnormal vascular endothelial function[17] or structural abnormalities of resistance vessels.[18] Atrial natriuretic peptide, important in hemodynamic and fluid homeostasis in normal patients, appears to play a minor role in patients with severe cardiac failure in the immediate perioperative period.[19–21]

Easy fatigability and shortness of breath are the most debilitating symptoms of heart failure. Diminished cardiac output and increased left ventricular end-diastolic pressure only partly contribute to these symptoms. Pulmonary compliance is reduced due to venous congestion and lymphatic distention. A number of studies have demonstrated diaphragmatic weakness. In addition, skeletal muscle atrophy and deconditioning occur in congestive heart failure, which leads to fatigue before attainment of maximal oxygen consumption.[22] Activation of ergoreceptors in the skeletal muscle may also play a role in the sensation of breathlessness.[8]

Medical Management of Patients Awaiting Heart Transplant

The advances in pharmacotherapy for chronic heart failure since the early 1990s has considerably improved the outlook for these patients. A detailed discussion of the treatment of chronic heart failure is beyond the scope of this chapter, but we do discuss management options available to patients with persistent heart failure who are awaiting a heart transplant.

A potential candidate with relatively stable symptoms may be managed with conventional therapy for heart failure. This includes a low-sodium diet, avoidance of drugs that are known to adversely affect cardiac function (e.g., disopyramide, flecainide, nonsteroidal anti-inflammatory agents, first-generation calcium channel blockers), and pharmacologic treatment of heart failure and of arrhythmias, if they develop. The drug therapy usually consists of a combination of diuretics, angiotensin-converting enzyme (ACE) inhibitors, vasodilators, and inotropic agents.

Many patients with heart failure develop fluid and sodium retention because of activation of the renin-angiotensin system. Persistent heart failure frequently requires high doses of diuretics and/or a combination of loop, thiazide, and potassium-sparing diuretics. Electrolyte imbalance often occurs, especially hypokalemia, hypomagnesemia, and metabolic alkalosis, and requires close scrutiny. Electrolyte imbalance has been held responsible for sudden cardiac death in these patients by some investigators.

A number of major studies have documented a small but significant decrease in mortality with ACE inhibitors,[23–26] and these have become the cornerstone of treatment of congestive heart failure. ACE inhibitors not only reduce mortality, even in New York Heart Association (NYHA) class IV patients,[27] but they also produce functional improvement[25] and a reduction in the number of hospital admissions.[23] The putative mechanisms of the beneficial effects of ACE inhibitors include vasodilatation as well as prevention of myocardial

remodeling, possibly through their action on the cardiac renin-angiotensin system.[28, 29]

Vasodilating drugs, such as hydralazine and nitrates, exert short-term beneficial effects by reducing left ventricular filling pressure (nitrates) or afterload (hydralazine), although tachyphylaxis can develop rapidly.[30, 31] The addition of hydralazine and isosorbide dinitrate to digoxin and diuretics has been shown to reduce mortality in chronic heart failure patients, but their role in patients already treated with ACE inhibitors is unclear.[32] In addition, hydralazine activates the renin-angiotensin system, leading to further fluid and sodium retention and attenuation of clinical response.[33] The calcium channel–blocking drugs, such as diltiazem and nifedipine, are effective in the presence of diastolic dysfunction, although cardiac function may deteriorate in a patient with systolic dysfunction,[34, 35] and caution is advocated in their use.

Digitalis has been in clinical use for treatment of heart failure for more than 200 years. Its continuing popularity was demonstrated in the Studies of Left Ventricular Dysfunction report, which stated that digitalis was taken by 45% of patients.[36] Its usage in heart failure was second only to diuretics, which were prescribed for 62% of patients. Despite widespread use, its role in the treatment of mild or severe heart failure has been questioned. It is superior to placebo in patients with a moderate degree of heart failure; however, the improvement in systolic function is similar to that seen with ACE inhibitors. Improved survival with long-term digoxin has not been demonstrated. Implication of digoxin as an independent risk factor for mortality and its association with a higher incidence of cardiac events in survivors of myocardial infarction has brought this drug into further disrepute.[37]

Demonstration of downregulation and subsensitivity of beta-adrenergic receptors in the presence of chronically elevated catecholamine levels has revived interest in beta blockers in the treatment of severe heart failure. Metoprolol[38–41] and bucindolol[42, 43] are the two agents most extensively studied and shown to reduce morbidity, improve exercise tolerance, reduce hospital admissions, increase ejection fraction, and reduce the need for transplantation. However, metoprolol does not appear to significantly reduce mortality[38] or produce a decrease in plasma norepinephrine levels,[44] which is a prognostic marker in congestive heart failure.[13] Domanski and Eichhorn[45] argued for the need for a definitive trial to study the role of beta blockers in congestive heart failure.

Asymptomatic venous thromboses have been reported in up to 60% of patients with chronic heart failure[46]; these thromboses subject patients to a high risk of pulmonary and systemic embolism. Insertion of central venous catheters for long-term administration of inotropic agents further increases this risk. Therefore, anticoagulation with low-dose warfarin (Coumadin) (international normalized ratio 1.3–1.5) has been recommended even in patients in sinus rhythm.[47, 48] Anticoagulant therapy should be carefully monitored if liver function is impaired due to hepatic congestion.

Some patients deteriorate while awaiting heart transplantation despite optimal medical therapy. Failure of orally administered vasodilators and diuretics necessitates intravenous treatment with vasodilators and inotropic agents. Sodium nitroprusside is commonly used because it reduces afterload and increases stroke volume while reducing left ventricular end-diastolic pressure and volume and mitral regurgitation. Nitroprusside, however, is a short-term measure due to its potential for cyanide and thiocyanate toxicity. Intravenous nitroglycerin may be used as an alternative to nitroprusside. It acts mainly as a venodilator and therefore reduces preload. It is not as effective in increasing cardiac output as nitroprusside, however, and tolerance frequently develops, thereby limiting its usefulness.

Prostacyclin has been used for short-term treatment of refractory heart failure. Beneficial acute hemodynamic effects are produced due to pulmonary and systemic vasodilation. Its inhibition of platelet adhesion and prevention of thrombus formation may add to its value. Tolerance develops less commonly than with intravenous nitrates. However, long-term benefit or improvement in survival has not been demonstrated.[49]

Inotropic agents commonly used for rapidly deteriorating heart failure are dopamine, dobutamine, and phosphodiesterase III inhibitors. Although these agents do not alter the long-term prognosis in heart failure, they buy time to locate a cardiac donor. Waiting cardiac recipients who require inotropic support in the intensive care unit are placed in status I category by the United Network for Organ Sharing (UNOS) and receive the donor organ on a priority basis.

Dopamine stimulates alpha$_1$- and beta$_1$-adrenergic receptors as well as dopaminergic receptors. At doses under 5 μg/kg per minute, it mainly acts on the dopaminergic receptors, increasing the renal blood flow. At higher doses, beta$_1$ receptors are stimulated, thus increasing myocardial contractility. At even higher doses, peripheral vasoconstriction and tachycardia are observed, and the benefit derived from increased inotropy may be mostly negated. Dobutamine acts on beta$_1$ adrenoreceptors, increasing contractility without significantly altering the systemic vascular resistance. Tachycardia, however, can be troublesome, limiting dobutamine's use in some patients. Development of tolerance due to desensitization of beta receptors remains a major problem with both of these drugs. Chronic intermittent dobutamine therapy, although it prevents desensitization and increases dobutamine's effect on myocardial performance,[50, 51] has been associated with a higher mortality when compared with placebo.[52] In addition, such therapy requires central venous access, which introduces the risk of infection and catheter-tip thrombus formation.

The phosphodiesterase III–inhibiting drugs, amrinone, milrinone, and enoximone, increase intracellular calcium availability by increasing the cyclic adenosine monophosphate (AMP) levels. These agents increase myocardial contractility, reduce afterload, and improve diastolic compliance of the left ventricle. The myocardial efficiency is improved more with dobutamine and amrinone than with dobutamine alone in patients with severe cardiomyopathy.[53] Clear hemodynamic benefits can be shown in the treatment of acute heart failure. When used to supplement conventional therapy in chronic heart failure, however, milrinone was associated with a 28% increase in mortality from all causes, a 37% increase in mortality from cardiovascular causes, and a significant increase in morbidity compared with placebo.[54] The increased mortality observed in these patients has been attributed to increased intracellular cyclic AMP and calcium-dependent arrhythmias.[55] Nevertheless, a number of reports have demonstrated effectiveness of phosphodiesterase III–inhibiting agents as a bridge to transplantation in moribund cardiac recipients on the waiting list.[56–58]

Mechanical Support of the Pretransplant Patient

Failure of maximal pharmacotherapy leads to severe debility and deterioration of other organ systems. The need for a transplant is urgent in such patients if they are to survive. With the aggressive use of mechanical support devices, many patients can be maintained and stabilized while awaiting cardiac transplantation. At present, intra-aortic balloon pump counterpulsation (IABP) and left ventricular assist devices (LVADs) are the mainstays of mechanical cardiovascular support for bridging these patients to cardiac transplantation.

Intra-Aortic Balloon Pump Counterpulsation

IABP has been used since the 1970s to provide mechanical support for patients with ischemic heart disease. Expansion of a helium-filled balloon during the diastolic phase of the cardiac cycle increases the diastolic blood pressure and improves cardiac perfusion. The deflation of the balloon immediately before the onset of ventricular contraction serves to unload the left ventricle, decreasing the impedance to ejection and thus augmenting forward blood flow to the periphery.[59, 60]

IABP has had limited applicability as a mechanical support to the pretransplant patient with failing ventricular function. Several authors have documented successful support of patients with IABP for prolonged periods while awaiting a donor organ. Due to the necessity of intra-arterial placement, however, patient mobility may be limited, thus contributing to morbidity of patients awaiting transplantation. Device failure, limb ischemia, and platelet destruction are all recognized complications of IABP use. Some patients have been maintained on IABP with alternative arterial approaches to balloon placement. Axillary artery access has been used with some success.[61]

Left Ventricular Assist Devices

Many attempts have been made to obviate orthotopic heart transplantation by the development of an effective "artificial heart." This technology, although not successful, fostered research into techniques of mechanical circulatory support. Several devices were developed for temporary circulatory support as a bridge to cardiac transplantation.

LVADs generally involve extraperitoneal placement with exteriorization of the portion of the device that imparts energy for forward flow. These devices do not provide support for the right ventricle; thus, adequate right ventricular function must be maintained to enable the patient to be supported. Inflow to the device is via the left atrium or ventricle, and outflow is into the proximal aortic root.[62, 63]

LVADs have been used with great success as bridges to cardiac transplantation. In many patients, establishment of LVAD mechanical support allows recovery of organ function by optimizing cardiovascular performance.[64] LVADs have provided prolonged support for patients awaiting donor organs. Some patients have used a portable device to enable discharge from the hospital and resumption of daily activities.[65] At present, although not approved for mechanical cardiac replacement, LVADs provide a significant degree of support to patients with end-stage cardiac function and allow increased survival in the pretransplant period.[66–70] See Chapter 5 for a more detailed discussion of devices used for mechanical support of the pretransplant patient.

Indications for Heart Transplantation

All patients with end-stage heart failure with NYHA class III or IV symptoms who have failed to respond to maximal medical or surgical therapy are considered potential candidates for heart transplantation. Annually, more than 40,000 patients younger than age 65 years may benefit from heart transplantation,[71] but the pool of potential donors is less than 10,000, of which only 26–44% are being used.[72] This imbalance of supply and demand necessitates application of more restricted criteria for candidate selection.

Ischemic heart disease (47.2%) and idiopathic dilated cardiomyopathy (43.5%) are the primary underlying causes of congestive heart failure in adult recipients of heart transplants[4] (Figure 6-3). Other indications are retransplantation (2.3%), valvular heart disease (4.2%), congenital heart disease (1.3%), and miscellaneous causes (1.5%). Patients with restrictive cardiomyopathies secondary to infiltrative processes, such as sarcoidosis or amyloidosis, have been successfully transplanted. Progression of sarcoidosis and amyloidosis has been shown to occur in the transplanted heart, however, leading to reduced long-term survival.[73] Some centers also consider transplantation a therapeutic alternative in symptomatic patients who have undergone repeated coronary revascularization procedures and in selected patients with valvular disease, in whom conventional surgical treatment

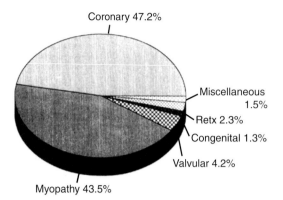

Coronary 47.2%

Miscellaneous 1.5%

Retx 2.3%

Congenital 1.3%

Valvular 4.2%

Myopathy 43.5%

Figure 6-3. Indications for adult heart transplantation. (Retx = retreatment.) (Reprinted with permission from JD Hosenpud, RJ Novick, TJ Breen, OP Daily. The Registry of the International Society of Heart and Lung Transplantation: eleventh official report—1994. J Heart Lung Transplant 1994;13:561.)

Table 6-1. Suggested Guidelines for Selection of a Cardiac Recipient

Indications for transplantation
$\dot{V}o_2$max <10 cc/kg/min or $\dot{V}o_2$max, 10–14 cc/kg/min with severely limited daily activity
Severe or recurrent unstable ischemia not amenable to angioplasty or coronary artery bypass graft
Recurrent symptomatic ventricular arrhythmias refractory to therapy
Insufficient indications for transplantation (unless other criteria are present)
Ejection fraction <20%
History of functional class III or IV symptoms of heart failure
Previous ventricular arrhythmias
$\dot{V}o_2$max >15 cc/kg/min without other indications

$\dot{V}o_2$max = maximum oxygen consumption.
Source: Adapted from GH Mudge, S Goldstein, LJ Addonizio, et al. Task Force 3: recipient guidelines/prioritization. J Am Coll Cardiol 1993;22:21–30.

with valve replacement is deemed to be associated with a high risk.[74]

Recipient Selection

Objective criteria for selecting potential candidates from a large pool of patients with end-stage heart disease should describe the degree of disability as well as assessing the survival of these patients with and without transplantation. The risk of the procedure should be assessed after maximal medical therapy has been instituted. Guidelines for selection of recipients are presented in Table 6-1.

Patients with severe or recurrent unstable angina that is not amenable to angioplasty or coronary bypass surgery are suitable candidates for cardiac transplantation. Recurrent refractory ventricular arrhythmias pose a constant threat of sudden cardiac death and warrant consideration for transplantation, although a previous history of arrhythmia in isolation is not an indication for transplantation.[74] Patients with NYHA class IV symptoms (symptomatic despite optimal medical therapy) have less than 50% annual survival rates.[27, 75] Although 1-year survival in patients with NYHA class III symptoms has been previously reported as 40–70%,[27, 76] progress in medical management of these patients appears to have improved their prognosis.[23–25] Thus, only selected

patients with NYHA class III symptoms are considered for cardiac transplantation.

NYHA classification of functional status has been criticized for its subjective nature and because the assessment is influenced by patient deconditioning and pulmonary disease. As such, measurement of oxygen consumption at peak exercise ($\dot{V}o_2$max) provides a more objective determination of a patient's functional capacity. $\dot{V}o_2$max has been shown to be a univariate predictor of survival in patients with chronic heart failure.[77–79] Cardiac transplantation can be safely deferred in patients with $\dot{V}o_2$max greater than 14 ml/kg per minute, unless confounding factors, such as recurrent ventricular arrhythmias, fluid retention, or unstable angina, alter the prognosis.[74, 78] Cardiac transplantation is indicated in patients with $\dot{V}o_2$max less than 14 ml/kg per minute, with $\dot{V}o_2$max less than 10 ml/kg per minute being a strong indication.[74, 78]

Ejection fraction has been shown to be a prognostic indicator in patients with congestive heart failure in a number of studies.[26, 80, 81] Although its usefulness as an indication for cardiac transplantation has been questioned,[74] many transplant centers consider ejection fraction less than 20% in association with other criteria as an indication for transplantation.

Candidates with certain comorbid conditions are excluded from consideration for heart transplantation, although traditional beliefs are challenged as experience with "high-risk" patients accumulates

Table 6-2. Exclusion Criteria for Heart Transplantation

Age >65 years
Severe, irreversible pulmonary hypertension: pulmonary
　　vascular resistance >6 Wood units, transpulmonary gra-
　　dient >15 mm Hg (despite maximal medical therapy)
Severe hepatic or renal dysfunction
Severe peripheral or cerebral vascular disease
Contraindications to immunosuppression (e.g., human
　　immunodeficiency virus infection, malignancy)
Brittle diabetic control or complications of diabetes
Major psychiatric disorder
Noncompliance with medical therapy
Continued tobacco or substance abuse

(Table 6-2). Earlier transplants were limited to patients younger than age 55 years. Although experience indicates a successful outcome in elderly patients,[82] the mortality in recipients older than 65 years remains significantly higher than in those younger than age 65.[4] One report from France also indicates that the mortality at 1 and 5 years in heart transplant recipients older than age 60 years is significantly higher compared to heart transplant recipients ages 20–50 years.[83]

Severe pulmonary hypertension with irreversible, high pulmonary vascular resistance (PVR) entails a high risk of acute right ventricular failure in the immediate postoperative period due to the normal donor heart's inability to adapt rapidly to the increased workload. One study suggested that a preoperative transpulmonary gradient may be more useful in predicting mortality at 6 and 12 months after heart transplantation than the more conventional measures of pulmonary hypertension (pulmonary arterial systolic pressure, PVR, and PVR index).[84] Patients with PVR greater than 6 Wood units or a transpulmonary gradient greater than 15 mm Hg, despite appropriate maximal medical therapy, are excluded from consideration for heart transplantation, although they may be candidates for heart-lung transplantation (HLT). The evaluation of potential candidates with pulmonary hypertension should include a pharmacologic trial with a pulmonary vasodilator. We commonly use prostaglandin E_1 (PGE_1) in such patients to assess the reversibility of PVR. Alternatives to PGE_1 include prostacyclin, phosphodiesterase III inhibitors, sodium nitroprusside, dobutamine, and nitric oxide. Patients in whom

a reduction in PVR below 6 Wood units or in transpulmonary gradient below 15 mm Hg can be achieved are deemed suitable for heart transplantation. However, use of vasodilators is often associated with systemic hypotension, alterations in cardiac output, and hypoxemia due to increased intrapulmonary shunting. Nitric oxide, because of its short half-life and its selective action on the pulmonary vasculature without systemic effects, may be more suitable in this setting. In a report by Adatia et al.,[85] heart transplantation was successfully performed in two patients with pulmonary hypertension reversible with 80 parts per million inhaled nitric oxide. Both of these patients had normal or moderately elevated pulmonary artery pressure postoperatively. Nitric oxide is similarly used to test pulmonary vasodilator capacity in children with pulmonary hypertension and congenital heart disease.[86]

Patients in whom immunosuppressant therapy would be contraindicated due to coexistent malignancy or human immunodeficiency virus (HIV) infection are not candidates for transplantation. Severe renal or hepatic dysfunction is also generally regarded as a contraindication for heart transplantation, although successful combined heart and renal transplantation[87] and heart and liver transplantation[88] have been described. Severe peripheral vascular and cerebrovascular diseases are likely to limit rehabilitation before and after transplantation and preclude insertion of IABP; therefore, they are considered relative contraindications for transplantation. Patients with recent pulmonary embolism or infarction are also excluded from consideration for transplantation because they are at increased risk of pulmonary infection. Several centers now accept insulin-dependent diabetic patients for transplantation if diabetic control is good and there is no evidence of diabetic nephropathy or neuropathy.

A psychosocial evaluation is valuable in identifying patients who may not be able to cope with the stress of transplantation and in whom noncompliance with medical regimen may endanger graft survival. Patients with a history of ongoing substance abuse are deemed unsuitable for heart transplantation. Patients with major psychiatric disorders and those with a history of noncompliance are also excluded from consideration. However, some degree of depression from a chronic debilitating disease is manifest in a number of patients and is not necessarily an indicator of posttransplantation psychiatric problems.[89] Identification of a support person is essential for a successful outcome. In one international survey,[90] the percentage of patients rejected for heart transplantation on psychosocial grounds ranged from 0 to 37%, with an average of 5.6% being rejected in the United States.

Patients requiring intravenous inotropic or mechanical support were once considered too sick for transplantation. Several centers have now reported successful outcomes in such patients.[91–95] In a retrospective analysis of cardiac transplantations performed at three centers in a 2-year period, however, O'Connell et al.[91] reported that although the mortality in patients requiring mechanical assistance was higher at 1 month posttransplant than in patients on either oral medical therapy or on intravenous inotropic support, mortality figures were similar at 3 months and 1 year. Griffith et al.[95] retrospectively studied 162 recipients of LVADs who had the device for 60 days or more. Of the 125 patients who subsequently received heart transplantation, 115 (93%) survived the procedure. The analysis also revealed that the incidence of complications was substantially higher in patients who were supported by the device for more than 100 days.

Evaluation of the Recipient

Careful screening of a potential transplant candidate requires a multidisciplinary approach. The heart transplant team at our institution consists of the cardiac surgeon; cardiologist; anesthesiologist; transplant coordinator; specialists from infectious diseases, pathology, immunology, and psychiatry; medical social worker; and physical therapist. Although most of the preoperative screening can be done on an outpatient basis, hospitalization facilitates evaluation while allowing time for the transplant team members to interact with the patient and his or her family. The team can address many of their questions and fears in an unhurried manner.

Table 6-3 presents a protocol for evaluation of the cardiac recipient. The value of many of these tests is self-evident. They are intended to assess the extent of the disease and its effects on various body systems and to determine the presence of comorbid conditions that may have a bearing on the patient's acceptance for heart transplantation.

Table 6-3. A Suggested Protocol for Evaluation of a Potential Cardiac Recipient

General assessment
  Complete blood count, including differential count
  Serum electrolytes
  Serum creatinine, blood urea nitrogen, urinalysis, creatinine clearance, and 24-hour total protein
  Liver function tests, including total protein and albumin levels
  Coagulation profile
  Stool for guaiac examination (three times); colonoscopy in men >50 years old
  Thyroid function tests
  Pulmonary function tests, including arterial blood gas analysis
  Lung ventilation-perfusion scanning*
  Mammography*
  Papanicolaou smear*
  Carotid Doppler ultrasound examination*
  Ultrasound examination of the gallbladder
  Lipoprotein profile
  Consultation: psychology, social services, physical therapy,* dental,* psychiatry*
  Nutritional status and diet history
Cardiovascular system assessment
  Electrocardiogram
  Chest radiograph
  Exercise test with oxygen consumption (peak $\dot{V}_{O_2}$)
  Hemodynamic measurements with right heart cardiac catheterization
  Echocardiogram
  Radionuclide ventriculogram*
  Left heart catheterization*
  Endomyocardial biopsy*
Immunologic assessment
  Blood type and antibody screen
  HLA typing
  Panel of reactive antibody screen
  Prostate-specific antigen assay in men >45 years old
  Carcinoembryonic antigen assay
Infectious disease assessment
  Hepatitis B surface antigen and hepatitis C serology screen
  Herpes simplex antibody assay
  Human immunodeficiency virus antibody assay
  CMV immunoglobulin M (IgM) and IgG antibody assay
  Toxoplasma antibody screen
  Varicella-zoster and rubella viral titers
  Epstein-Barr viral capsid IgG, IgM antibodies
  VDRL test
  Urine for viral cultures (CMV, adenovirus)
  Urine culture and sensitivity
  Standard battery of eight skin tests, including purified protein derivative, mumps, histoplasmosis, and coccidioidomycosis

CMV = cytomegalovirus; $\dot{V}_{O_2}$ = oxygen consumption per unit time.
*If clinically indicated.

Myocardial biopsy provides histopathologic confirmation of the diagnosis of cardiomyopathy and identifies the occasional patient with ongoing acute myocarditis, infiltrative disease, or unsuspected systemic disease that may benefit from medical therapy, thus obviating heart transplantation.[96] Preformed immunoglobulin G (IgG) antibodies in recipient serum against the donor HLA can lead to hyperacute rejection and fulminant graft failure. Therefore, potential recipients are screened for the presence of antibodies by testing their sera against an HLA panel (panel of reactive antibody [PRA]). The PRA level appears to be related to previous blood transfusions or pregnancies, which may have exposed the patient to nonhomologous HLAs. When the PRA level exceeds 10%, most centers require a negative prospective cross-match between donor cells and recipient serum before transplantation.[97] The requirement of a negative prospective cross-match, however, limits the donor pool for a given recipient, thereby increasing the waiting time on the transplant list and attendant mortality. The presence or absence of cytomegalovirus (CMV) antibodies in the recipient is important because the CMV-negative recipient transplanted with a CMV-positive organ has a higher risk of developing a severe form of CMV disease. *Toxoplasma* infection is more likely to manifest in cases in which a mismatch has occurred; such recipients may require prophylactic treatment with co-trimoxazole or pyrimethamine.

The psychosocial assessment of the candidate includes identification of stressors, supportive friends or family members, presence or absence of personality disorder, and history of drug or alcohol abuse. It also assesses the quality of family relationships, the level of the patient's and spouse's education, occupation, the need for vocational rehabilitation, and the need for relocation. A formal psychiatric assessment is performed only if indicated.

Donor Selection

The need for donor organs outweighs the availability of organs by a considerable margin. In addition, by one estimate, only 10–20% of suitable cardiac donors become actual donors.[98] The mortality in patients with NYHA class IV congestive heart failure remains high (30–40%) despite maximal medical therapy. Therefore, transplant centers are faced with increasing pressure to broaden the donor selection criteria to expand the donor pool. Efforts are also made to increase donor awareness and to educate both the medical and nonmedical community about transplantation.

Initial screening of a potential donor is usually performed at the donor hospital (Table 6-4). Screening includes the details of the present illness, such as the etiology of brain death, duration of pulselessness, severity and duration of hypotension or hypoxemia, length of cardiopulmonary resuscitation (CPR), life-threatening arrhythmias, extent of thoracic trauma (if present), hemodynamic status, and the nature and quantity of inotropic support. Other relevant information includes age; height; weight; history of tobacco, alcohol, or drug use; history indicative of ischemic or valvular heart disease; prior medications; previous cardiac or thoracic surgery; and ABO blood group. Risk factors for atherosclerosis are noted.

Although ST segment changes or T-wave abnormalities on electrocardiogram (ECG) may be com-

Table 6-4. Selection Criteria for Heart Donors

Preliminary evaluation
  Age <55 years
  ABO blood group compatibility
  Hemodynamically stable (mean arterial pressure >80 mm Hg) with minimum inotropic support (dopamine or dobutamine <10 µg/kg/min)
  No history of prolonged hypotension (systolic blood pressure <60 mm Hg for 6 hours) or prolonged or repeated cardiopulmonary resuscitation
  Absence of risk factors for coronary atherosclerosis or presence of normal coronary arteries
  No major thoracic trauma (blunt, penetrating)
  No previous cardiac or major thoracic surgery
  Normal electrocardiogram (see text for changes in ST segments)
  Normal echocardiography
  Smoking <20 pack-years
  Adequate size match
  Negative serology for hepatitis B or human immunodeficiency virus infection
Final evaluation (at time of harvest)
  No cardiac contusion
  Normal coronary arteries
  Normal size and contractility
  No evidence of valvular disease

mon secondary to brain death, Q waves or evidence of significant ischemia should be viewed with suspicion. Coronary arteriography should be performed when possible in donors at high risk for coronary atherosclerosis such as older donors, those with a strong family history of coronary artery disease, long-standing history of tobacco abuse, severe hypertension, diabetes mellitus, or marked abnormalities of lipid metabolism. Although most centers require normal cardiac function, as evaluated by echocardiography and ventriculography, hearts with regional wall motion abnormalities or those requiring high inotropic support have been used successfully, though with an increased risk of posttransplantation mortality. Notably, the University of California at Los Angeles group has used donor hearts with normal ventricular function but documented coronary artery atherosclerosis.[99] Saphenous vein bypass grafting was performed before implantation.

Past medical history of malignancy, infectious diseases, diabetes mellitus, or other significant systemic disease is obtained. A baseline 12-lead ECG, chest x-ray, arterial blood gases, routine blood chemistry, and echocardiography are obtained. Blood samples are also drawn for HLA type and serology for CMV; HIV; hepatitis A, B, and C; *Toxoplasma gondii*; and herpes simplex. Many centers use positive serology for CMV to alter their perioperative prophylaxis against the CMV virus. Hepatitis B or HIV infection would preclude tissue donation; however, some centers would use hepatitis C-positive donors for hepatitis C-positive recipients, in some circumstances.

Many centers consider age 40 years the upper limit for an acceptable cardiac donor. The number of hearts harvested from donors up to age 65 has steadily increased. Although some centers have reported no increase in early mortality in recipients of such hearts,[100, 101] the ISHLT Registry considers a donor older than 40 years an increased risk.[4] Donor age older than 50 is associated with an increased risk of posttransplant death,[102] earlier development of posttransplant coronary artery disease,[103] and a greater incidence of chronotropic incompetence.[104] If an older donor is accepted, coronary arteriogram is indicated in men older than 40 years and women older than 50. It is also recommended that the recipient not receive an organ from a donor who is substantially older than him- or herself.[105] For example, a 60-year-old donor heart should not be used in a 20-year-old recipient but may be acceptable for a 55-year-old recipient.

A chest radiograph is useful in assessing the size of the cardiac silhouette and examining the lung fields for pulmonary edema, effusions, or other evidence of significant thoracic trauma. Cardiac echocardiography is an invaluable bedside aid in assessing global cardiac function, wall motion abnormalities, estimated ejection fraction, and valvular morphology. If transthoracic echocardiography is unable to provide an acceptable image, a transesophageal approach may be necessary. Patients who continue to require more than 10 µg/kg per minute of dopamine or dobutamine to maintain a mean blood pressure above 80 mm Hg after adequate volume resuscitation (central venous pressure of 8–12 mm Hg) are not suitable candidates. Patients who have had extensive thoracic trauma or cardiac contusion are unsuitable donors. Patients who had prolonged hypotension (systolic blood pressure less than 60 mm Hg for more than 6 hours) or who required prolonged or repeated CPR are also not considered.

The donor must have an intact cardiovascular system (beating-heart donor). Although liver, kidneys, and lungs have been retrieved from non–beating-heart donors, such donors have not been used for heart transplantation. However, a number of groups continue to investigate cardiac resuscitation in non–beating-heart donors. The cause of brain death does not appear to have a predictable effect on posttransplant survival in adult donors, but in pediatric donors, death from causes other than head trauma appear to have a negative impact on posttransplant survival. The injury leading to brain death is often associated with hemodynamic compromise or respiratory insufficiency. Cardiac arrest may be primary, may accompany the brain injury, or be secondary to a respiratory arrest. The interval without circulation, the interval with circulation through CPR, and the interval of marked hypotension are related to posttransplantation cardiac dysfunction.

The final decision to use the heart is made at the time of the harvest procedure. At this time, the right and left ventricular contractility is visually assessed. The coronary arteries are examined digitally for evidence of atherosclerotic disease, and the heart chambers are palpated for thrills indicative of significant valvular abnormalities. Pulmonary artery, left atrial, and central venous pressures are estimated. The pulmonary artery or left atrial pressures may be formally measured by placing in the chamber a needle catheter connected to a pressure transducer. Elevation of these pressures correlates with an increased risk to the recipient.

Recipient-Donor Matching

UNOS allocates the donor heart based on the geographic location of the donor, severity of the recipient's illness (status), ABO blood type, and the time on the waiting list.[106] The recipients are classified as status I if they require cardiac support with total artificial heart, left or right ventricular assist device, or IABP; inotropic agents to maintain adequate cardiac output in the intensive care unit; or mechanical ventilation of their lungs. Such patients receive a higher priority than the more stable patients (status II). A detailed protocol has been devised for allocation of the hearts based on the geographic location of the donor. The allocation takes place in the following sequence: local status I heart recipient, local heart-lung recipient, local status II heart recipient, and national allocation based on geographic zones. In each location, recipients who have been on a waiting list the longest receive the donor organ. Recipients with ABO blood type identical to that of the donor take priority over those with a compatible blood group.[106]

The prospective recipient is matched to the donor based on comparison of the body surface area and weight. An acceptable donor has a body surface area equal to or up to 20% greater than the recipient. Compatibility in exposure to CMV and a prospective PRA cross-matching (if the recipient PRA level is greater than 10%) are also taken into consideration.

Ischemic time less than 3 hours is desirable. Although little difference in survival can be demonstrated with ischemic times less than 4 hours, the risk of posttransplant death increases markedly when ischemic time surpasses 4 hours.[102] Shorter ischemic times usually correlate with less need for posttransplant inotropic support and mortality. A combination of adverse risk factors, such as older donor age plus prolonged ischemic time, dramatically increase the risk of patient mortality, whereas otherwise ideal characteristics mitigate the risk associated with one adverse risk factor. For example, a 55-year-old male donor who is larger than the recipient, has normal ventricular function on no inotropic therapy, and has an ischemic time of 6 hours would place the recipient at a significantly greater risk than an ideal donor would.

Heart-Lung Transplantation

Encouraged by the success of Reitz et al. in obtaining long-term survival in monkeys after HLT,[107] Stanford University embarked on a clinical HLT program in 1981. First report of a successful clinical HLT[108] was followed by establishment of similar programs at other centers. The early indications for HLT included Eisenmenger's syndrome as well as a number of primarily pulmonary diseases. In these early years, HLT was the preferred operation in some patients with primary pulmonary pathology due to several considerations. HLT was considered a technically easier procedure than double-lung transplantation.[109] The incidence of tracheal anastomotic dehiscence (a major early complication of double-lung transplantation) was lower in the recipients of HLT due to preservation of tracheobronchial circulation and development of collaterals from the coronaries.[110] Ventilation-perfusion imbalance was not encountered, and cross-contamination of the transplanted lung from the remaining lung was avoided. In addition, a major advantage was thought to be the ease of monitoring rejection of cardiac and pulmonary allografts by serial endomyocardial biopsies. This stemmed from the initial hypothesis that rejection occurred simultaneously in the two organs.[111] The error of such reasoning became evident when several centers reported independent or asynchronous rejection of lungs[112–115] and, therefore, the necessity of simultaneous surveillance of both organs for rejection.

The number of HLT procedures reported annually to the ISHLT Registry peaked at 214 in 1989, but it has declined every year since then.[4] Overall, primary pulmonary hypertension (PPH) (31.5% of total) and congenital heart disease (27% of total) comprise the most common indications for HLT, although the indications are being redefined due to the success of single and bilateral sequential lung transplantations in patients with primary pulmonary disease, including those with PPH or secondary pulmonary hypertension. Comparison of PPH patients undergoing single or bilateral lung transplantation to those undergoing HLT shows a trend toward a poorer survival rate after HLT.[4] Even among patients with Eisenmenger's syndrome, some may benefit from the surgical correction of a cardiac defect in conjunction with single or bilateral lung transplantation. Thus, increasingly, HLT is indicated only in patients with Eisenmenger's syndrome and an uncorrectable cardiac defect or left ventricular dysfunction.

The actuarial survival of HLT recipients has remained unchanged over the years,[4] with 1-year and 3-year survival rates being 59% and 49%, respectively. Early mortality is often due to primary graft failure, infection, or bleeding.

Recipient Selection and Evaluation

HLT is considered in patients with end-stage cardiopulmonary disease when the patient has rapidly worsening functional disability despite maximal medical therapy and when his or her expected survival without transplantation is 6–12 months. Most transplant centers currently limit HLT to patients younger than age 50 years because of increased surgical and postoperative risks in older patients. This age limit, however, like the age limits for other solid organ transplantations, is arbitrary, and physiologic age is often considered more important than actual age. As with heart transplantation, patients with comorbid conditions are excluded from consideration for HLT. These conditions include severe hepatic or renal dysfunction, HIV infection, hepatitis B or C infection, complicated diabetes mellitus, malignancy, substance abuse, active extrapulmonary infection, or severe peripheral or cerebral vascular disease. Previous major thoracic surgery is no longer considered a contraindication because of the effectiveness of aprotinin in substantially reducing blood loss during repeated thoracic procedures. Psychosocial considerations described for heart transplantation candidates also apply to potential HLT recipients. Earlier fears of poor tracheobronchial healing and anastomotic breakdown in patients on steroids preoperatively have been refuted.[116] Low-dose steroids (less than 20 mg prednisolone per day) are no longer considered a contraindication to lung transplant or HLT.

Evaluation of the recipient is similar to that of a potential cardiac recipient. It is designed to assess the extent of the primary disease and the degree of involvement of other organ systems. Another aim is to avoid risk factors that may adversely affect their survival after the transplantation.

Donor Selection

Availability of suitable donors with both heart and lungs in optimal condition for transplantation is very low. Lungs in many donors are rendered unusable because of neurogenic pulmonary edema, aspiration pneumonia, chest infection, fat embolism, or contusion due to chest trauma. Egan et al.[117] estimated that only 25% of cardiac donors have acceptable lungs for transplantation. Moreover, because status I patients on heart transplant lists receive the highest priority, most suitable heart-lung blocks are used for heart recipients and lung recipients. The use of a suitable heart-lung block is especially unusual for a heart-lung recipient with blood type O. Donor criteria have been successfully liberalized to include older donors and those with smoking history, gram-negative rods in sputum, and small pulmonary infiltrate on radiography.[118] Due to the severe shortage, marginal donors are more likely to be used. Heart-lung blocks from donors who test serologically positive for the hepatitis C virus are more likely to be used because of the severe shortage, particularly for recipients who are blood group O.

In addition to the acceptance criteria for a suitable heart, pulmonary suitability is assessed as outlined in Table 6-5.[119] Details of thoracic trauma and duration of ventilatory support are sought. Previous history of major thoracic surgery, smoking, asthma, and pulmonary infections, such as tuberculosis, is obtained. Evidence of pulmonary edema, aspiration, and infection is sought by means of a chest radiograph, fiberoptic bronchoscopy, and microbiological examination of the tracheobronchial secretions. During bronchoscopy, secretions that clear easily should not be a contraindication to lung donation. Poorly compliant lungs are not suitable for transplantation. Arterial Po_2 greater than 300 mm Hg, with inspired oxygen concentration of 100% and 5 cm H_2O of positive end-expiratory pressure, provides evidence of overall adequacy of gas exchange. Presence of a mass, especially in a donor with a history of smoking, should be viewed with suspicion. The final decision to accept the heart-lung block is not made until the time of harvest. Provided the chest radiograph or

Table 6-5. Selection Criteria for Heart-Lung Donors

Preliminary evaluation (in addition to criteria for heart donors)
    No evidence of pulmonary infection, aspiration, or
        edema on chest radiograph and bronchoscopy
    Negative Gram's stain and culture if prolonged intubation
    Arterial oxygen tension >300 mm Hg on F_{IO_2} = 1.0 and
        PEEP 5 cm H_2O
    Adequate size match
    No evidence of pulmonary mass
Final evaluation
    Chest radiograph shows no unfavorable changes (as
        listed above)
    Oxygenation has not deteriorated
    Bronchoscopy shows no aspiration or mass
    Visual and manual assessment during organ harvest
    Parenchyma satisfactory
    No adhesions or masses

F_{IO_2} = fraction of inspired oxygen; PEEP = positive end-expiratory pressure.
Source: Adapted from S Sundaresan, GD Trachiotis, M Aoe, et al. Donor lung procurement: assessment and operative technique. Ann Thorac Surg 1993;56:1409–1413.

oxygenation has not deteriorated by this time, the thoracic cavity and the lungs are examined for adhesions, masses, and areas of contusion or consolidation. On palpation, the lung should not feel boggy or edematous. Obvious evidence of emphysema is a contraindication to donation. In practice, the drastic shortage of available heart-lung donor blocks often necessitates the use of marginal lungs. Bilateral lung blocks with a small area of contusion or infiltrate have been successfully used. Similarly, many groups have used lungs in which bronchoscopy demonstrated a moderate amount of purulent secretions but the mucosa appeared to be normal after aspirating the purulent secretions. Areas of apical blebs have been excised using stapling techniques. Providing the remaining lung was of normal quality, good results have been obtained.

The donor and recipient are matched for size, ABO blood group compatibility, and CMV status. Size matching is based more on donor and recipient height than weight. A range 20% larger or smaller than the recipient is considered appropriate. In patients with restrictive lung disease associated with heart failure, such as sarcoidosis, the pleural space may be considerably smaller than that of a similarly sized (by height) donor. In such cases, a comparison of the chest cavities may be estimated from the recipient and donor chest films by measuring the vertical dimension at the midclavicular line and the horizontal measurement at the level of the domes of the diaphragm. Alternatively, the lungs may be surgically reduced in size at the time of implantation. This is usually performed by staple resection of the middle lobe, lingular, or upper lobe apices.

Ischemic time of 4–6 hours is considered acceptable. The histocompatibility complex matching is not obtained before transplantation because of the relatively long time required for such testing.

Donor Operative Procedures

Procurement of the Donor Heart

The initial experiences with heart transplant and HLT involved donors who either were present in the implanting institution or were transported to the implanting institution. With the increase in numbers of transplants performed and with most donors providing multiple organs, often involving multiple procurement teams, this practice is no longer feasible. Because multiple organs may be procured and multiple teams may be involved, an understanding of each implanting team's needs is imperative to optimize results for all the recipients.

The donor's anterior torso, from chin to midthigh, is prepared and draped. A midline incision is performed from the donor's sternal notch to the level of the pubis. The thymic tissue may be excised or divided in the midline. A pericardial cradle is created. Once the donor's heart has been examined and deemed suitable for transplantation, the implanting surgical team is informed. The aorta is dissected free from the main pulmonary artery and the right pulmonary artery. The IVC and the superior vena cava (SVC) are mobilized, and either umbilical tapes or O-silk sutures are placed around the SVC.

When all procurement teams are ready to proceed with organ flushing, heparin is administered (200–300 U.S. Pharmacopeia units/kg) through a central vein. If the central access is not available, the surgeon may administer heparin directly through the SVC. A purse-string suture using 4-0 prolene is placed in the ascending aorta, and the cardioplegia needle (24 French right-angle arterial cannula) is inserted and secured using this suture. In smaller donors, the size of the cannula must be adjusted appropriately. All central venous cannulas are withdrawn. The SVC is occluded using either the previously placed suture or tape or the vascular staple load. The right side of the donor's heart is vented by dividing the anterior surface of the IVC above the pericardial reflection. The left side of the heart is vented by dividing the left atrial appendage. When lungs are not to be harvested, division of the right or left superior pulmonary vein is acceptable. A vascular clamp is placed across the aorta immediately below the innominate artery. To arrest the donor's heart, most centers use a cold (less than 4°C), high-potassium, crystalloid cardioplegia (15–20 ml/kg) delivered into the ascending aortic cannula. The cardioplegia is delivered using an intravenous pressure bag. Alternatively, University of Wisconsin solution has been used with excellent results. During cardioplegia delivery, the surgeon should assess that adequate perfusion pressure is present by palpating the aortic root and that cardiac distention is not occurring by palpating the heart chambers.

After administration of the cardioplegia preservation solution, excision of the donor's heart is begun. The left side of the left atrium is incised midway between the coronary sinus and the anterior portion of the orifices of the left superior and inferior pulmonary veins. The incision is then carried rightward. The anterior aspect of the right pulmonary veins is visualized from within the left atrium. The incision is continued superiorly, leaving a 5-mm to 10-mm cuff of left atrium with the pulmonary veins. The incision between the left and right sides is connected by dividing the roof of the left atrium. The IVC incision is completed. The SVC is then divided, taking care to preserve the right pulmonary artery, which traverses posterior to the SVC. When additional caval length is needed, a vascular clamp may be used to occlude the SVC instead of ligating the cava. The left innominate vein and jugular vein are mobilized, allowing the entire SVC to be preserved. The aorta is then divided at the level of the arch. Similarly, if more length is needed, dissection can be carried out onto the arch, and transection can be performed distally. The pulmonary artery is then divided at the level of the bifurcation. If the lungs are not to be used, additional pulmonary artery may be used. The donor's heart is then removed from the field and transported to the back table, where it is packaged and stored on ice for immediate delivery to the implanting hospital.

Procurement of the Donor Heart-Lung Block

The heart-lung harvest procedure is similar to that described for the heart donor. The additional steps are described here. Before heparinization, the donor's trachea is mobilized in the space between the ascending aorta and the SVC, and an umbilical tape is placed around it. A purse-string suture is placed in the main pulmonary artery immediately below the bifurcation. Once the pulmonary artery cannula is inserted and secured with the purse-string suture, 500 g PGE_1 is administered directly into the pulmonary artery or the SVC. The pulmonary preservation solution is administered via the pulmonary artery cannula simultaneously with the cardioplegia solution. The most common pulmonary preservation solutions are modified Euro-Collins or University of Wisconsin solution (2–5 liters). The pulmonary solution is infused with the bag elevated no more than 30 cm above the pulmonary artery to prevent pulmonary edema. During delivery of the pulmonary preservation solution, the donor's lungs should be ventilated using normal tidal volumes (12–15 cc/kg). After the cardioplegia and pulmonary preservation solution have been administered, the frequency of ventilation and the tidal volume may be decreased during organ removal to facilitate surgery.

The donor's heart and lungs may be excised using a variety of techniques. The simplest technique involves removing the heart and lung with the posterior mediastinal block. In this technique, the IVC is completely divided. The gastric tube is removed from the donor and his or her esophagus is freed using blunt dissection at the level of the pericardium, where it is divided using a gastrointestinal anastomosis (GIA) stapler. Using a scalpel, the remaining mediastinal tissue is divided above the diaphragm to the spine. The incision is carried superiorly along the spine immediately posterior to the thoracic aorta on the left and posterior to the hemiazygos vein on the right, to a level above the aortic arch. If the donor's trachea was previously dissected free, the umbilical tape is drawn and pulled upward. The anesthesiologist is asked to inflate the donor's lungs to approximately two-thirds of maximal distention. The trachea is ligated using a surgical stapler. After the tracheal tube is removed, a second row of staples is applied more proximally, and the trachea is divided between the staple lines. The donor's esophagus is freed from

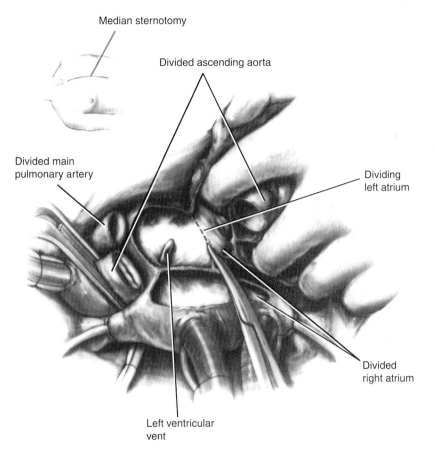

Median sternotomy

Divided ascending aorta

Divided main
pulmonary artery

Dividing
left atrium

Divided
right atrium

Left ventricular
vent

Figure 6-4. Bicaval cannulation through the lateral aspect of the right atrium, with snares placed around each caval cannula. A left ventricular vent via the superior pulmonary vein is also shown. The arterial cannula is placed through the ascending aorta. The recipient's heart is excised at the level of the atrioventricular groove and across the great vessels just above the two valves. (Reprinted with permission from P Van Trigt III. Cardiac Transplantation. In DC Sabiston Jr [ed], Atlas of Cardiothoracic Surgery. Philadelphia: Saunders 1995;509.)

surrounding structures and divided using a GIA stapler. The remaining mediastinal structures are sharply divided to the donor's spine, and the entire heart, lung, and mediastinal block is removed from the chest and transported to a separate sterile table, where the remaining dissection is performed. During this back-table dissection, topical hypothermia is maintained by placing the heart-lung block in a basin containing ice slush. The donor's esophagus and aorta are excised using sharp dissection immediately adjacent to the respective wall. Pericardium is excised. The heart-lung block is then packaged for transport in cold lung-preservation solution. The entire package is placed in a cooler surrounded by ice and transported to the implanting hospital as quickly as possible.

Recipient Surgical Procedures

Heart Transplantation Procedure

In the heart transplantation recipient, the venous cannulas may be placed through the lateral wall of the right atrium into the vena cava (Figure 6-4). Alternatively, direct caval cannulation may be used and is required when bicaval anastomoses are planned. In patients who have undergone multiple cardiac procedures and in whom either cardiac chambers or conduits are likely to adhere to the posterior table of the sternum, femoral artery and venous cannulation is performed. Tapes are placed around the SVC and IVC to enable total cardiopulmonary bypass (CPB). A left ventricular vent is routinely placed via the

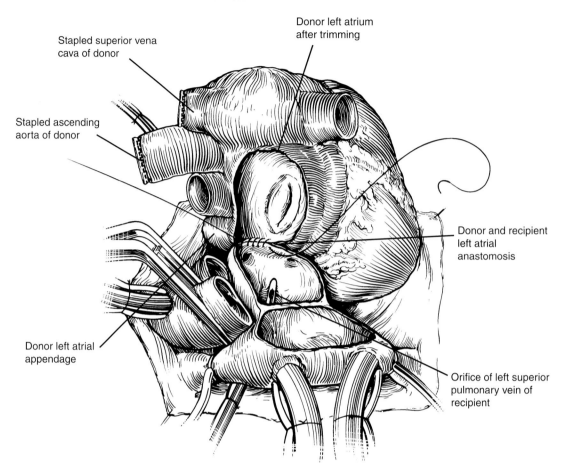

Donor left atrium
after trimming

Stapled superior vena
cava of donor

Stapled ascending
aorta of donor

Donor and recipient
left atrial
anastomosis

Donor left atrial
appendage

Orifice of left superior
pulmonary vein of
recipient

Figure 6-5. The left atrial anastomosis is begun at the area of the left atrial appendage, progressing down the lateral free wall to the interatrial septum. Cardioplegia can then be delivered to the donor heart via the ascending aorta. (Reprinted with permission from P Van Trigt III. Cardiac Transplantation. In DC Sabiston Jr [ed], Atlas of Cardiothoracic Surgery. Philadelphia: Saunders 1995;510.)

right superior pulmonary vein. When the donor heart arrives in the operating room, the ascending aorta is occluded with a vascular clamp and the patient is placed on total CPB.

The native heart is excised at the level of atrioventricular junction and immediately above the semilunar valves. The left atrial cuff is trimmed to the appropriate size to match the donor left atrial cuff, usually excising the native left atrial appendage. The donor atrial septum is inspected for a patent foramen ovale or a septal defect. If present, these should be closed before the anastomosis is begun. Similarly, the valves are visualized and repaired if necessary. The left atrial anastomosis is performed first. The suture line is begun by approximating the donor left atrial appendage to the corresponding area

on the recipient left atrium (Figure 6-5). The anastomosis is performed with a running suture, extending the suture line along the lateral free wall to the interatrial septum. The septal portion is completed with the same suture line. Before the left atrial anastomosis is completed, the left ventricular vent should be positioned through the mitral valve into the donor left ventricle. Cardioplegia is administered via the ascending aorta, taking care to vent any existing air.

The systemic venous connections may be made using either the cuff technique of Shumway and Lower, in which the right atria are anastomosed, or by direct bicaval anastomoses. When using the right atrial cuff technique, the donor right atrium is incised from the anterior vena cava toward the right atrial appendage. The anastomosis is begun along the medial side of the donor right atrial cuff at the level of the IVC–right atrial juncture, which is anastomosed to the septal portion of the recipient atrium. After this portion is complete, the lateral wall of the donor atrium is anastomosed to the lateral wall of the right atrium.

When performing caval anastomoses, the surgeon fully develops the interatrial groove on the recipient heart. After the Swan-Ganz catheter is withdrawn, the SVC is transected immediately above the juncture between the cava and the right atrium. The inferior aspect of the right atrium is divided above the level where the right inferior pulmonary vein enters the left atrium. The residual areas of right atrial free wall are excised. Several vessels traversing the septum and the mediastinum require control using either cautery or suture ligation. The caval anastomoses are performed using a 5-0 prolene suture in a running fashion. The IVC anastomosis is usually performed first. The pulmonary artery catheter should be advanced through the donor heart before the SVC anastomosis is completed. This may save considerable time because placement of the pulmonary artery catheter after completion of the anastomosis may be difficult. When the ischemic time has been prolonged (more than 210 minutes), these anastomoses may be performed after the aortic anastomosis.

The aortic anastomosis is performed using a 4-0 prolene suture in a running fashion. It is important to de-air the donor heart chambers and aorta as much as possible before release of the cross-clamp. This may require adding a large volume to the perfusion circuit. During this period, the patient's lungs are ventilated to evacuate air trapped in the pulmonary veins. Rewarming the patient is initiated before the aortic anastomosis is completed.

The pulmonary artery anastomosis is performed using a 4-0 polypropylene suture as a running stitch. Again, this may be performed after the aortic anastomosis. If the ischemic time is not prolonged, however, completing the posterior row of the anastomoses before releasing the aortic cross-clamp makes this anastomosis easier.

After completing the anastomoses and defibrillating the heart, and while the heart is being reperfused, the anastomoses are inspected and bleeding sites corrected. During this period, the aorta should be vented for any residual air. When the patient's temperature reaches 34°C, inotropic support (discussed in further detail under Anesthesia for Heart and Heart-Lung Transplantation) is initiated. If adequate contractility is present, the vent from the left ventricle is removed. After an appropriate reperfusion period, and when the patient has been rewarmed, the patient is weaned from CPB. The most common difficulty encountered while weaning the patient from CPB is right ventricular dysfunction, usually secondary to pulmonary vascular hypertension. Techniques to mitigate this difficulty include delivery of inhaled nitric oxide and administration of PGE_2 via the pulmonary artery catheter, with left atrial administration of norepinephrine or phenylephrine to maintain systemic vascular resistance. Right ventricular assist devices (e.g., the Abiomed BVS, Danvers, MA) have been used in cases refractory to pharmacologic treatment with reasonable results.

Heart-Lung Transplantation Procedure

Once the donor heart-lung block has been accepted by the retrieving surgeon, the recipient is brought to the operating room and anesthetized. In recipients who are likely to tolerate single-lung ventilation, a double-lumen tracheal tube may be used to improve surgical exposure when mobilizing the pulmonary structures. The operation may be performed through a median sternotomy or a bilateral anterotranssternal (clamshell) thoracotomy. In patients who have significant adhesions between their lungs and chest wall, in whom significant bronchial collateral or systemic artery-to-pulmonary connections exist, or in whom previous thoracic surgical procedures have been performed, the clamshell incision offers greater visualization and decreases the technical complexity. The ascending aorta, IVC, and SVC are mobilized. The trachea is mobilized between the SVC and the aorta, and umbilical tape is placed around its distal end above the carina. The patient is placed on CPB using the ascending aorta for the arterial cannulation site and bicaval cannulation for venous return. Both pleural cavities are opened. Any adhesions between the patient's lung and chest wall are divided using electrocautery. Initial dissection and mobilization of the hilar structures is performed when possible. Because most patients undergoing HLT have pulmonary artery hypertension, dissection and mobilization of the hilar structures are often not possible before initiating CPB.

After dissection and mobilization are complete, and after the donor organs have arrived at the recipient hospital, the patient can be placed on CPB. Cessation of mechanical ventilation improves exposure and the technical ease of removing the patient's lungs. The patient is systemically cooled, usually to 28–32°C. The pericardium is excised around the level of the hilar structures. The pulmonary arteries and veins are mobilized in the intrapericardial space. After ligating these structures proximally and distally, they are divided between the ligatures. Similarly, the bronchi are mobilized and ligated proximally using a surgical stapler. The bronchi are divided distal to the staple line, allowing removal of the patient's lungs. It is important to identify and preserve the phrenic nerve at all times. After the patient's lungs are removed, the opening in the pericardium is extended inferiorly and superiorly to enable positioning of the donor lungs into the appropriate pleural cavities.

A vascular occlusion clamp is placed across the ascending aorta below the aortic cannula. Tapes are placed and used to occlude the cava around the cannula to place the patient on complete bypass. The right atrium is excised adjacent to the atrioventricular groove anteriorly. This incision is extended circumferentially along the atrial septum. The aorta is divided above the aortic valve and retracted superiorly. The remaining pulmonary arteries, left atrium, and ventricular structures are dissected free from the surrounding mediastinal tissue, and the patient's heart is removed. By retracting the umbilical tape surrounding the trachea, the bronchi and carinal structures may be mobilized more easily from the mediastinal tissue. Often, many enlarged bronchial and systemic arteries in this region must be ligated. Obtaining hemostasis before performing the anastomoses is critical. Exposure to these regions after implantation of the donor heart-lung block is difficult. The patient's trachea is divided immediately above the carina using a fresh scalpel blade, and hemostasis is carefully achieved (Figure 6-6). It is useful to place a 2-0 silk suture through the anterior aspect of the tracheal wall to serve as a traction stitch.

The donor heart-lung block is brought into the field, maintaining topical hypothermia throughout. The donor lungs are passed through the opening in the pericardium posterior to the phrenic nerve into the patient's pleural cavities. The tracheal anastomosis is performed first. The donor trachea is divided one to two rings above the carina. Keeping this distance short minimizes the risk of ischemia in the donor airway. The anastomosis is performed using a running stitch. Surrounding peritracheal tissue may be approximated over the suture line.

The systemic venous anastomosis may use either direct caval anastomoses or a right atrial cuff technique (see previous section) (Figure 6-7). Before completing this anastomosis, it is important to advance the pulmonary artery catheter into the pulmonary artery. This anastomosis can be performed after the aortic anastomosis if the ischemic time is prolonged. The aortic anastomosis is performed using a running stitch of 4-0 prolene. Before tying this anastomosis, the heart-lung block is carefully de-aired.

Systemic rewarming is initiated. A vent is placed via the right superior pulmonary vein into the left ventricular vein. When the patient's temperature reaches 34°C and adequate ventricular function is present, the left ventricular vent may be removed. Attention to de-airing the cardiac chambers is imperative. Transesophageal echocardiography is extremely useful in assessing the amount of residual air. The level of inotropic support required to separate the HLT recipient from CPB is often less than that required for patients with moderate pulmonary hypertension undergoing cardiac transplantation. In patients whose lung allografts develop moderate to severe reperfusion injury, pharmacotherapy, including inhaled nitric oxide and PGE_2, may be used to lower the pulmonary artery pressure. Mechanical assistance with extracorporeal membrane oxygenation may be necessary in patients who do not respond to pharmacologic intervention.

Anesthesia for Heart and Heart-Lung Transplantation

Preoperative Considerations

Although heart and heart-lung recipients undergo extensive evaluation before they are placed on the waiting list, their end-stage disease and the often long waiting times cause significant deterioration by the time they arrive for transplant. Therefore, careful assessment of their current physical status is necessary before induction of anesthesia. Routine preanesthetic considerations, including examination of the patient's airway, determination of the time of last meal, and notation of allergies and ongoing medical therapy, also apply to transplant patients. Availability of blood products should be ascertained before surgery. Blood chemistry, automated blood count, coagulation profile, recent ECG, and chest radiograph should be reviewed.

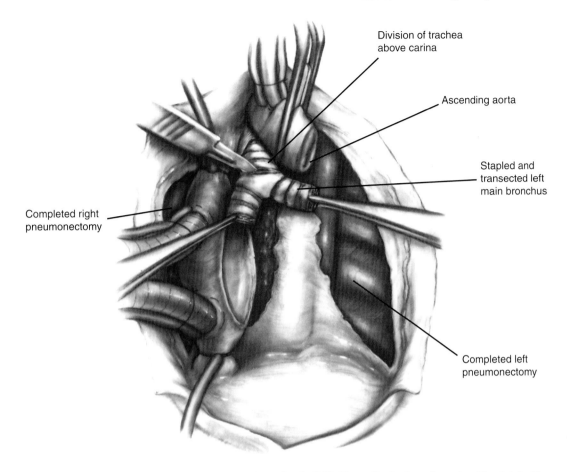

Figure 6-6. Aorta is retracted to expose the trachea. The trachea is divided immediately above the carina. (Reprinted with permission from P Van Trigt III. Cardiac Transplantation. In DC Sabiston Jr [ed], Atlas of Cardiothoracic Surgery. Philadelphia: Saunders 1995;523.)

Preoperatively, H_2 antagonists or nonparticulate antacids may be administered because many patients may have delayed gastric emptying. Ongoing medical therapy should be maintained until the time of transplant. In some patients, failure of medical therapy may have necessitated the use of mechanical devices as a bridge to transplantation. Arrangements may have to be made to coordinate transport of these critically ill patients from the intensive care unit to the operating room along with multiple intravenous infusions and perfusion-support devices. Heparin infusion in patients with unstable angina should be discontinued on arrival in the operating room.

A 5-lead ECG, peripheral oxygen saturation, nasal and urinary bladder temperatures, urine output, and capnography are routinely monitored.

Systemic arterial and pulmonary arterial catheters, with continuous oximetric monitoring of mixed venous oxygen saturation, are placed before induction of anesthesia. Intravenous hypnotics and narcotics may be judiciously titrated to allay anxiety during placement of invasive monitoring devices. Some centers favor routine placement of a femoral arterial catheter, which provides more reliable arterial pressure monitoring postbypass as well as offering ready access for placement of an IABP if necessary. Catheters capable of measuring right ventricular ejection fraction have also been used in this setting.[120] The benefit of pulmonary artery catheters in the transplant patient has been debated because insertion introduces a potential infection risk and measured pressures may not accurately reflect ventricular volumes in the presence of pul-

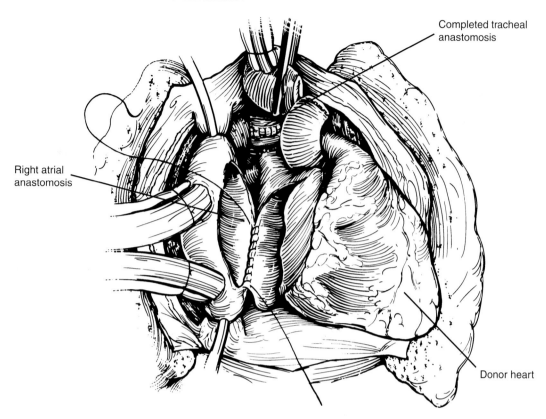

Figure 6-7. Right atrial anastomosis. Injury to the sinus node should be carefully avoided when opening the donor atrium. Direct vena caval anastomoses may also be performed instead of the atrial anastomosis. (Reprinted with permission from P Van Trigt III. Cardiac Transplantation. In DC Sabiston Jr [ed], Atlas of Cardiothoracic Surgery. Philadelphia: Saunders 1995;524.)

monary hypertension.[121] However, the information provided by a pulmonary artery catheter is useful for following trends in the indices of cardiac function and in measuring responses to interventions in these critically ill patients. Moreover, monitoring of right ventricular function and pulmonary impedance may be needed to optimize ventricular performance. Because it is difficult to predict the degree of posttransplantation right ventricular dysfunction in most cases, a prudent course is the insertion of a pulmonary artery catheter as part of routine monitoring. During the cardiectomy, the pulmonary artery catheter is either coiled in the operative field or withdrawn into the protective sleeve. It can be reinserted under visual guidance by the surgeon through the grafted heart or flow-directed after circulation is restored. Intraoperative transesophageal echocardiography is useful in assessing ventricular filling and function as well as inspecting the atrial anastomotic site and pul-

monary venous blood flow and is routinely used at many centers.[122]

Strict aseptic precautions during invasive procedures are essential because of the risk of infection in the immunosuppressed patient. Some institutions use a sterile laryngoscope, but, with widespread availability of prepackaged, factory-sterilized tracheal tubes, this usage appears to have little impact on infection control.[123] Vascular catheter sites should be covered with sterile dressings. Stopcocks and access ports should be capped when not being used for sampling blood or infusing drugs. Patients with congenital heart disease presenting for HLT may have an intracardiac shunt, and the risk of paradoxical air embolism should be recognized. Some centers prefer to use the left internal jugular approach for placement of the pulmonary artery catheter, preserving the right internal jugular vein for future use for serial endomyocardial biopsies. However, right-sided cannulation has been routinely performed at our institution (and many others) intraoperatively without jeopardizing subsequent access for biopsies.[124, 125]

HLT candidates may have severe pulmonary hypertension, often to near systemic levels, in addition to right or biventricular failure. Preoperative hypoxemia is often seen in these patients due to pulmonary congestion, pulmonary hypertension, and reduced pulmonary compliance. Exacerbation of hypoxemia and hypercarbia due to a combination of sedative administration and supine or Trendelenburg position during invasive line insertion before induction of anesthesia can produce further increase in PVR and deterioration in right ventricular function. Thus, due care should be exercised when administering sedative drugs. The patient should be supine for the least possible time.

Induction and Maintenance of Anesthesia

A variety of regimens is used for the induction and maintenance of anesthesia in cardiac transplant patients with satisfactory results.[126–128] No clear outcome data favor any one technique. A combination of narcotic and muscle relaxant with hypnotics as an adjunct is commonly used.[129] Ketamine is relatively contraindicated in patients with pulmonary hypertension because of its effect on PVR.[130] Inhalational agents may also be used as part of a balanced anesthetic technique with acceptable results.[131, 132] An anesthetic regimen commonly used before initiation of bypass at our institution is given in Table 6-6. Because of the relatively short notice with which these procedures are usually performed and because of the possibility of reduced gastric motility due to gut hypoperfusion, we routinely perform rapid-sequence induction in these patients. Although we do not routinely use inhalational agents to maintain anesthesia, the occasional patient may require volatile anesthetic (usually isoflurane) due to hemodynamic response to surgery to supplement the infusions of narcotic and sedative agents.

Drug dosages should be adjusted for a prolonged circulation time and the reduced volume of distribution associated with low cardiac output. Although the required tissue concentrations of the anesthetic agents are normal and the total cumulative dose is only modestly decreased at most, slow administration of the induction agent allows for better ongoing assessment of the patient's pharmacodynamic

Table 6-6. A Sample Anesthetic Regimen in the Prebypass Period during Heart and Heart-Lung Transplantation

	Agents
Induction	Midazolam, 0.02–0.05 mg/kg
	Fentanyl, 5–10 µg/kg
Muscle relaxant	Succinylcholine, 1.0–1.5 mg/kg
	Pancuronium, 0.1 mg/kg
Maintenance	Midazolam, 0.02–0.04 mg/kg/hr
	Fentanyl, 0.03–0.05 µg/kg/min
	Isoflurane, 0–0.5% if necessary

response. Comparison of the pressure-volume loops from a normal heart and a severely myopathic heart in Figure 6-8 shows the increases in chamber volumes and a severe reduction in stroke volume and stroke work in dilated cardiomyopathy.[126] The ventricular performance is critically affected by small changes in the preload and afterload.

Exogenous catecholamine administration can be associated with an unpredictable and diminished response in the patient on chronic beta-agonist inotropes secondary to downregulation of beta-receptors and receptor subsensitivity, thereby further complicating acute management.[55–57] Mannitol or furosemide may be necessary to maintain urine output in many patients due to a markedly expanded blood volume and chronic diuretic therapy. Transesophageal echocardiography may be useful in assessing left ventricular contractility and filling.

Vasoactive drugs initiated in the pretransplant patient are normally continued until bypass. Infusion rates may need to be adjusted in response to anesthetic induction and surgical manipulation to maintain adequate cardiac output and coronary and cerebral perfusion pressures. In patients with pulmonary hypertension undergoing HLT, pharmacologic manipulations of PVR may be necessary. Nitroglycerin (0.1–7.0 µg/kg/minute), PGE_1 (0.05–0.50 µg/kg/minute), and a phosphodiesterase III inhibitor, such as milrinone (0.375–0.750 µg/kg/minute), are commonly used to this end. However, intravenous pulmonary vasodilators also produce systemic vasodilation and hypotension as well as worsening of gas exchange due to inhibition of hypoxic pulmonary vasoconstriction. For these reasons, the most beneficial dose to reduce pulmonary hypertension is often not attained. Accordingly,

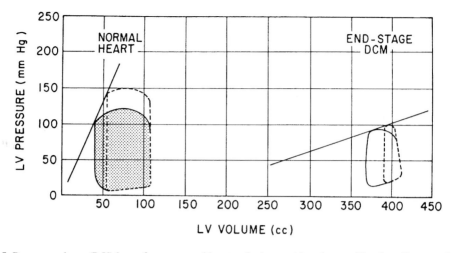

Figure 6-8. Pressure-volume (P-V) loops from a normal heart and a heart with end-stage dilated cardiomyopathy (DCM). The P-V loop at an elevated peak systolic pressure (*dotted line*) is superimposed on the resting P-V loop (*solid line*). The tangents depict the slopes of the end-systolic P-V relationships. Note the marked decrease in stroke volume in cardiomyopathy when the systolic pressure is mildly elevated. (LV = left ventricular.) (Reprinted with permission from NJ Clark, RD Martin. Anesthetic considerations for patients undergoing cardiac transplantation. J Cardiothorac Anesth 1988;2:523.)

nitric oxide may be more useful for selective pulmonary vasodilation, although it seems to have a less prominent effect in patients with long-standing pulmonary hypertension, and no definitive outcome studies have been done.

Antifibrinolytic agents, such as aprotinin, epsilon-aminocaproic acid, and tranexamic acid, have been demonstrated to reduce postoperative blood loss and blood requirement in patients who have had previous cardiac or thoracic surgery, although only aprotinin has been studied specifically in heart transplant recipients.[133-135] In one prospective study, blood and blood product requirements were not altered by administration of aprotinin in patients undergoing primary sternotomy for heart transplantation.[135] In patients undergoing a repeat sternotomy for heart transplantation, however, aprotinin significantly reduced blood and blood product requirements compared to patients who did not receive aprotinin. Aprotinin was administered in a 1-ml test dose, followed by a 200-ml loading dose intravenously and an additional 200 ml in the CPB circuit. This was followed by a continuous infusion of 50 ml per hour until the end of surgery. These patients showed no evidence of increased occurrence of renal dysfunction. The authors recommend use of aprotinin only in patients undergoing reoperative heart transplantation.

Hypothermic CPB is instituted and managed in the usual manner. Hemodynamic instability at induction or at the beginning of the procedure may require urgent establishment of CPB. Hypokalemia due to chronic and vigorous diuretic therapy and metabolic acidosis from chronic low cardiac output are often seen in recipients. These electrolyte and acid-base derangements should be corrected intraoperatively. In patients with evidence of significant preoperative fluid retention or renal insufficiency, hemofiltration during bypass may be beneficial.[136, 137]

Weaning from Cardiopulmonary Bypass

After rewarming the patient to 34°C, infusion of inotropes is begun in preparation for weaning from the cardiopulmonary bypass. The level of inotropic support depends on the quality of the donor heart, the ischemic time, and the degree of the recipient's pulmonary vascular hypertension. Dopamine in renal dose is administered routinely. At our institution, epinephrine in a low dose (0.1–0.5 µg/kg/minute) is the inotrope of choice. A phosphodiesterase III antagonist, such as milrinone (0.375–0.750 µg/kg/minute) may be added in patients with pre-existing pulmonary hypertension or in whom right ventricular dysfunction in the immediate post-bypass period is anticipated. Epinephrine infusion may subsequently be adjusted to clinical response. Some centers prefer to use isoproterenol (0.01–0.10 mg/kg/minute) as the primary inotropic agent because of its direct effect on the denervated transplanted heart and its pulmonary vasodilator effect.[138] The usual criteria that guide separation from the bypass include cardiac index greater than 2 liters per minute per m², mixed venous oxygen saturation greater than 60%, pulmonary artery occlusion pressure (PAOP) less than 20 mm Hg, and central venous pressure less than PAOP. Failure to meet weaning criteria, despite optimization of preload and afterload, the use of two inotropic agents, and echocardiographic evidence of hypocontractile left ventricle, indicate the need for insertion of an IABP.

The values of cardiac filling pressures to achieve optimal cardiac performance depend on cardiac compliance and contractility. Preload should be carefully and gradually increased to obtain maximal cardiac output, indicating optimal position on the Frank-Starling curve. In our experience, fluid loading to a PAOP value of 15–17 mm Hg is usually necessary to attain this goal. A mild reduction in afterload may be useful in reducing ventricular wall stress and increasing the cardiac index.

Cardiac output may depend on an adequate heart rate and a sinus rhythm in the presence of a relatively fixed stroke volume. Bradyarrhythmias, usually slow junctional rhythms secondary to varying degrees of sinoatrial or atrioventricular nodal dysfunction, are relatively common.[139] The transplant recipient may have two anatomic sinoatrial nodes. Both atria are often electrically evident initially, but electrical activity originating from the native atria may be variable and tends to disappear over time. Some authorities recommend the routine use of isoproterenol in weaning from CPB and throughout the immediate postoperative period.[125] Epicardial pacing may be necessary to ensure a satisfactory rate and rhythm (usual target range 70–100 beats per minute) in the acute posttransplant period.

Acute right ventricular failure is the most common problem after heart transplantation. Increased PVR associated with refractory chronic heart failure may be exacerbated in the perioperative period and may place a significant right ventricular afterload burden on the fresh transplant.[140–143] Pharmacologic agents used to reduce PVR and improve right ventricular function include phosphodiesterase III inhibitors, such as amrinone and milrinone; PGE_1; prostacyclin; vasodilators, such as sodium nitroprusside and nitroglycerin; and more recently, selective pulmonary vasodilator nitric oxide. Kieler-Jensen et al.[144] compared the effects of nitric oxide with those of intravenous prostacyclin, PGE_1, and sodium nitroprusside after heart transplantation and found prostacyclin the most effective agent. The effects of intravenous agents on pulmonary circulation are accompanied by a decrease in systemic vascular resistance, however, which may lead to significant hypotension. Inhaled nitric oxide acts selectively on pulmonary vasculature and has been shown to be effective in treating acute pulmonary hypertension after heart transplantation,[145–147] although its use in a large series and subsequent outcome data are not yet available. Mechanical assistance, including the use of right ventricular assist devices, may be necessary when pharmacologic therapy fails. Temporary placement of a venoarterial right-to-left shunt has been used successfully to treat severe right ventricular failure after transplant.[148] Pulmonary vascular dynamics commonly improve in the early postoperative period.

Prolonged total ischemic time and time on CPB are the most important predictors of need for inotropic support and poor outcome.[122, 149] Serum levels of myosin light chain I, a biochemical marker of myocardial cell damage, correlates with ischemic time and need for inotropic support, which emphasizes the importance of good graft preservation and operative techniques.[150]

After extracorporeal support has been terminated, monitoring and maintenance of hemodynamic values are similar to those required for other patients after CPB. Hemorrhage is a common early complication, as in other thoracic cases. Neutralization of heparin with protamine is done according to usual practice after CPB. The use of blood products should be tailored to the laboratory coagulation profile and clinical setting. Packed red cells are transfused to keep the hematocrit at the desired level. A hematocrit of 35% may be appropriate in patients receiving HLT, to compensate for impaired gas exchange in the postischemic lung and to preserve oxygen delivery to tissues while maintaining a low fraction of inspired oxygen to minimize oxygen toxicity.

Anesthetic Considerations during Heart-Lung Transplantation

HLT recipients present with severe pulmonary hypertension and a low, fixed cardiac output due to right or biventricular failure. In addition, intracardiac shunting is present in patients with Eisenmenger's syndrome. These patients have severely limited cardiorespiratory reserves, may be hypoxic despite supplemental oxygen therapy, and may be orthopneic. Deterioration in their oxygenation can be rapid and difficult to reverse. Hypoxia can further increase the PVR and worsen right-sided heart failure. Thus, pre- and intraoperative management of these patients requires meticulous attention to avoid hypoxia and preserve myocardial function.

HLT recipients are monitored similarly to cardiac recipients. Lung isolation improves surgical exposure when mobilizing the pulmonary structures; therefore, a double-lumen tube should be inserted if the patient can tolerate single-lung ventilation. The risk of paradoxical air embolism should be recognized in patients with right-to-left shunt.

The choice of specific anesthetic agents is not critical. The objectives should be to minimize cardiac depression and prevent exacerbation of pulmonary hypertension. (Anesthetic agents commonly used at our institution are given in Table 6-6.) Ketamine may be avoided because of its detrimental effect on PVR. Inhalational agents, used judiciously, lower the PVR without significantly altering myocardial contractility. Many recipients may need preoperative inotropic support. Inotropes should be continued intraoperatively until CPB can be established. Their dose may need to be adjusted after induction of anesthesia because of changes in preload, afterload, systemic vascular resistance, and PVR. The pulmonary artery catheter may be either withdrawn into the sterile sheath or coiled and left in the surgical field. It is repositioned, with guidance by the surgeon, at the end of the implantation procedure.

The management during CPB follows the principles outlined under Heart Transplantation Procedure. The time spent on bypass is likely to be more prolonged than for heart transplant due to the additional surgical time necessary for bilateral pneumonectomy and for implantation of the donor lungs. The newly transplanted lungs are prone to pulmonary edema due to ischemic injury, reperfusion injury, damage to the lymphatics, and physical trauma due to manipulation during surgery.[151] Therefore, careful avoidance of fluid overload is essential. We usually aim to keep the central venous pressure between 8 and 10 mm Hg and the PAOP between 12 and 15 mm Hg (lower than in heart transplant recipients). Marginal quality of the cardiac allograft, prolonged bypass time, and long ischemic period may result in poor cardiac function initially, however, requiring higher filling pressures for adequate cardiac index (2.0 liter/minute/m²). Hemofiltration may be useful in patients with chronically expanded blood volume. After reperfusion, ventilation with a positive end-expiratory pressure of 5–10 cm H_2O and intravenous diuretics may also help to reduce lung water and expand atelectatic areas. Inspired oxygen concentration should be adjusted to the lowest level necessary to obtain an arterial PO_2 of approximately 100 mm Hg to minimize the risk of oxygen toxicity.

Separation from the CPB is frequently easier than during cardiac transplantation. Right ventricular dysfunction is less commonly a problem because of a normal or moderately elevated PVR. Cardiac function as well as arterial anastomoses should be assessed with transesophageal echocardiography.

Conclusions

Both heart transplantation and HLT have become established modes of treatment for end-stage cardiopulmonary disease. Surgical techniques have improved immeasurably since the early 1980s. Criteria for recipient and donor selection have become more established, but they continue to evolve. Greater understanding of physiology and immunology has improved long-term results of these procedures. The functional outcome is comparable to that after solid-organ transplantations. The greatest barriers to greater applicability of heart transplants and HLT are the development of chronic rejection, manifest as graft coronary artery disease and obliterative bronchiolitis, and the shortage of organs. With the addition of new immunosuppressants, and with a greater understanding of the mechanisms that cause chronic graft failure, the long-term results continue to improve.

References

1. Barnard CN. A human cardiac transplant: an interim report of a successful operation performed at Groote Schuur Hospital, Cape Town. S Afr Med J 1967;41:1271.

2. Thompson T. The tragic record of heart transplants. The year they changed hearts. Life Magazine 1971;Sept 17:56–70.

3. Evans RW, Manninen DL, Dong FB. The National Cooperative Transplantation Study: Final Report. Seattle: Battelle-Seattle Research Center, 1991.

4. Hosenspud JD, Bennett LE, Keck BM, et al. The Registry of the International Society for Heart and Lung Transplantation: fourteenth official report–1997. J Heart Lung Transplant 1997;16:691–712.

5. Karwande SV, Ensley RD, Renlund DG, et al. Cardiac retransplantation: a viable option? Registry of the International Society for Heart and Lung Transplantation. Ann Thorac Surg 1992;54:840–845.

6. Ensley RD, Hunt S, Taylor DO, et al. Predictors of survival after repeat heart transplantation. Registry of the International Society for Heart and Lung Transplantation. J Heart Lung Transplant 1992;11:S142–158.

7. Evans RW. Executive summary: The National Cooperative Transplantation Study: BHARC-100-91-020. Seattle: Battelle-Seattle Research Center, June 1991.

8. Poole-Wilson PA. Relation of pathophysiologic mechanisms to outcome in heart failure. J Am Coll Cardiol 1993;22:22A–29A.

9. Poole-Wilson PA. Future perspectives in the management of congestive heart failure. Am J Cardiol 1990;66:462–467.

10. Poole-Wilson PA, Buller NP, Lindsay DC. Blood flow and skeletal muscle in patients with heart failure. Chest 1992;101:330S–332S.

11. Francis GS, McDonald K, Chu C, Cohn JN. Pathophysiologic aspects of end-stage heart failure. Am J Cardiol 1995;75:11A–16A.

12. Schaper J, Schaper W. Ultrastructural correlates of reduced cardiac function in human heart disease. Eur Heart J 1993;4(Suppl A):35–42.

13. Cohn JN, Levine TB, Olivari MT, et al. Plasma norepinephrine as a guide to prognosis in patients with congestive heart failure. N Engl J Med 1984;311:819–823.

14. Bristow MR, Ginsburg R, Minobe W, et al. Decreased catecholamine sensitivity and β-adrenergic receptor density in failing human hearts. N Engl J Med 1982;307:205–211.

15. Bristow MR, Ginsburg R, Umans V, et al. β_1- and β_2-adrenergic receptor subpopulations in nonfailing and failing human ventricular myocardium: coupling of both receptor subtypes to muscle contraction and selective β_1 receptor down-regulation in heart failure. Circ Res 1986;59:297–309.

16. Brodde OE, Zerkowski HR, Doetsch N, et al. Myocardial beta-adrenoreceptor changes in heart failure: concomitant reduction in beta$_1$- and beta$_2$-adrenoreceptor

17. function related to the degree of heart failure in patients with mitral valve disease. J Am Coll Cardiol 1989;14:323–331.

17. Katz SD. The role of endothelium-derived vasoactive substances in the pathophysiology of exercise intolerance in patients with congestive heart failure. Prog Cardiovasc Dis 1995;38(1):23–50.

18. Wroblewski H, Kastrup J, Norgaard T, et al. Evidence of increased microvascular resistance and arteriolar hyalinosis in skin in congestive heart failure secondary to idiopathic dilated cardiomyopathy. Am J Cardiol 1992;69:769–774.

19. Sakai T, Latson TW, Whiten CW, et al. Perioperative measurement of interleukin-6 and alpha-melanocyte stimulating hormone in cardiac transplant patients. J Cardiothorac Vasc Anesth 1993;7:17–22.

20. Glisson SN, Gutzke GE, Pifarre R, et al. Atrial natriuretic peptide responses during anaesthesia in patients with refractory cardiomyopathies. Can J Anaesth 1991;38:572–577.

21. Hare JM, Baughman KL, Kass DA, et al. Influence of dilated cardiomyopathy, myocarditis and cardiac transplantation on the relation between plasma atrial natriuretic factor and atrial pressures. Am J Cardiol 1991;67:391–397.

22. Wilson JR, Martin JL, Schwartz D, Ferraro N. Exercise intolerance in patients with chronic heart failure: role of impaired nutritive flow to skeletal muscle. Circulation 1984;69:1079–1087.

23. SOLVD Investigators. Effect of enalapril on survival in patients with reduced left ventricular ejection fractions and congestive heart failure. N Engl J Med 1991;325:293–302.

24. Cohn JN, Archibald DG, Ziesch S, et al. Effect of vasodilator therapy on mortality in chronic congestive heart failure. Results of a Veterans Administration Cooperative Study. N Engl J Med 1986;314:1547–1552.

25. Cohn JN, Johnson G, Ziesch S, et al. A comparison of enalapril with hydralazine-isosorbide dinitrate in the treatment of chronic congestive heart failure. N Engl J Med 1991;325:303–310.

26. Cohn JN, Archibald JG, Francis GS, et al. Veterans Administration Cooperative Study on vasodilator therapy of heart failure: influence of prerandomization variables on the reduction of mortality by treatment with hydralazine and isosorbide dinitrate. Circulation 1987;75(5 pt 2):IV49–54.

27. The CONSENSUS Trial Study Group. Effects of enalapril on mortality in severe congestive heart failure. Results of the Cooperative North Scandinavian Enalapril Survival Study (CONSENSUS). N Engl J Med 1987;316:1429–1435.

28. Johnston CI, Fabris B, Yoshida K. The cardiac renin-angiotensin system in heart failure. Am Heart J 1993;126:756–760.

29. Dzau VJ. Tissue renin-angiotensin system in myocardial hypertrophy and failure. Arch Intern Med 1993;153:937–942.

30. Packer M, Meller J, Medina N, et al. Hemodynamic characterisation of tolerance to long-term hydralazine therapy in severe chronic heart failure. N Engl J Med 1982;306:57–62.

31. Reifart N, Kaltenbach M, Bussmann WD. Loss of effectiveness of dihydralazine in the long-term treatment of chronic heart failure. Eur Heart J 1984;5:568–580.

32. Cohn JN. Mechanisms of action and efficacy of nitrates in heart failure. Am J Cardiol 1992;70:88B–92B.

33. Armario P, Hernandez del Rey R, Pardell H. Adverse effects of direct-acting vasodilators [review]. Drug Saf 1994;11(2):80–85.

34. Lang R. Medical management of chronic heart failure: Inotropic, vasodilator or inodilator drugs? Am Heart J 1990;6:1558–1564.

35. Olivari MT, Levine TB, Cohn JB. Acute hemodynamic effects of nitrendipine in chronic congestive heart failure. J Cardiovasc Pharmacol 1984;6:S1002–1005.

36. Young JB, Weiner DH, Yusuf S, et al. Patterns of medication use in patients with heart failure: a report from the Registry of Studies of Left Ventricular Dysfunction (SOLVD). South Med J 1995;88:514–523.

37. Kober L, Torp-Pedersen C, Gadsboll N, et al. Is digoxin an independent risk factor for long-term mortality after acute myocardial infarction? Eur Heart J 1994;15:382–388.

38. The MDC trial study group. Metoprolol in dilated cardiomyopathy, multicenter randomized placebo-controlled trial (abstract). Circulation 1992;86(Suppl I):1–118.

39. Engelmeier RS, O'Connell JB, Walsh R, et al. Improvement in symptoms and exercise tolerance by metoprolol in patients with dilated cardiomyopathy: a double-blind, randomized, placebo-controlled trial. Circulation 1985;72:536–546.

40. Heilbrunn S, Shah P, Bristow M, et al. Increased β-receptor density and improved response to catecholamine stimulation during long term metoprolol therapy in heart failure from dilated cardiomyopathy. Circulation 1989;79:484–490.

41. Eichhorn EJ, Heesch CM, Barnett JH, et al. Effect of metoprolol on contractility in dilated cardiomyopathy: a double-blind, placebo-controlled trial [abstract]. Circulation 1993;88:1–105.

42. Eichhorn EJ, Bedotto JB, Malloy CR, et al. Effect of beta-adrenergic blockade on myocardial function and energetics in congestive heart failure: improvements in hemodynamic, contractile, and diastolic performance with bucindolol. Circulation 1990;82:473–483.

43. Woodley SL, Gilbert EM, Anderson JL, et al. β-blockade with bucindolol in heart failure due to ischemic vs idiopathic dilated cardiomyopathy. Circulation 1991;84:2426–2441.

44. Lijnen PJ, Amery AK, Fagard RH, et al. The effects of beta-adrenoceptor blockade on renin, angiotensin, aldosterone and catecholamines at rest and during exercise. Br J Pharmacol 1979;7:175–181.

45. Domanski MJ, Eichhorn EJ. Beta blockade in congestive heart failure—the need for a definitive study. Am J Cardiol 1994;73:597–599.

46. Roberts WC, Siegel RJ, McManus BM. Idiopathic dilated cardiomyopathy: Analysis of 152 necropsy patients. Am J Cardiol 1987;60:1340–1355.

47. Stratton JR, Nemanich JW, Johannessen K, Resnick AD. Fate of left ventricular thrombi in patients with remote myocardial infarction or idiopathic cardiomyopathy. Circulation 1988;78:1388–1393.

48. Keogh AM, Freund J, Baron DW, Hickie JB. Timing of cardiac transplantation in idiopathic dilated cardiomyopathy. Am J Cardiol 1988;61:418–422.

49. Haywood GA, Adams KF Jr, Gheorghiade M, et al. Is there a role for epoprostenol in the management of heart failure? Am J Cardiol 1995;75:44A–50A.

50. Unverferth DV, Magorien RD, Altschuld R, et al. The hemodynamic and metabolic advantages gained by a three-day infusion of dobutamine in patients with congestive cardiomyopathy. Am Heart J 1983;106:29–34.

51. Applefeld MM, Newman KA, Grove WR, et al. Intermittent continuous outpatient dobutamine infusion in the management of congestive heart failure. Am J Cardiol 1983;51:455–458.

52. Dies F, Krell MJ, Whitlow P, et al. Intermittent dobutamine in ambulatory outpatients with chronic cardiac failure. Circulation 1986;74(Suppl):38A.

53. Sundram P, Reddy HK, McElroy PA, et al. Myocardial energetics and efficiency in patients with idiopathic cardiomyopathy: response to dobutamine and amrinone. Am Heart J 1990;119:891–898.

54. Packer M, Carver JR, Rodeheffer RJ, et al. Effect of oral milrinone on mortality in severe chronic heart failure. The PROMISE study research group. N Engl J Med 1991;325:1468–1475.

55. Lubbe WF, Podzuweit T, Opie LH. Potential arrhythmogenic role of cyclic adenosine monophosphate (AMP) and cytosolic calcium overload: implications for prophylactic effects of beta-blockers in myocardial infarction and proarrhythmic effects of phosphodiesterase inhibitors. J Am Coll Cardiol 1992;19:1622–1633.

56. O'Connell JB, Gilbert EM, Renlund DG, Bristow MR. Enoximone as a bridge to heart transplantation: the Utah experience. J Heart Lung Transplant 1991;10:477–481.

57. Skoyles JR, Sherry KM, Price C. Intravenous milrinone in patients with severe congestive cardiac failure awaiting heart transplantation. J Cardiothorac Vasc Anesth 1992;6:222–225.

58. Uretsky BF, Hua J. Combined intravenous pharmacotherapy in the treatment of patients with decompensated congestive heart failure. Am Heart J 1991;121:1879–1886.

59. Kern MJ. Intra-aortic balloon counterpulsation. Coron Artery Dis 1991;2:649–660.

60. Bhayana JM, Scott SM, Sethi GK, Takaro T. Effects of intraaortic balloon pumping on organ perfusion in cardiogenic shock. J Surg Res 1979;26:108–113.

61. Kormos RL. The role of the intra-aortic balloon as a bridge to cardiac transplantation. Cardiac Assists 1987; 3:1–4.

62. Wiebalck AC, Wouters PF, Waldenberger FR, et al. Left ventricular assist with an axial flow pump (Hemopump): clinical application. Ann Thorac Surg 1993;55: 1141–1146.

63. Farrar DJ, Hill JD. Univentricular and biventricular Thoratec VAD support as a bridge to transplantation. Ann Thorac Surg 1993;55:276–282.

64. Farrar DJ, Hill JD. Recovery of major organ function in patients awaiting heart transplantation with Thoratec ventricular assist devices. Thoratec ventricular assist device principal investigators. J Heart Lung Transplant 1994;13:1125–1132.

65. Korfer R, el-Banayosy A, Posival H, et al. Mechanical circulatory support: the Bad Oeynhausen experience. Ann Thorac Surg 1995;59(Suppl 2):S56–62.

66. Frazier OH, Macris MP, Myers TJ, et al. Improved survival after extended bridge to cardiac transplantation. Ann Thorac Surg 1994;57:1416–1422.

67. Frazier OH, Rose EA, McCarthy P, et al. Improved mortality and rehabilitation of transplant candidates treated with a long-term implantable left ventricular assist system. Ann Surg 1995;222:327–336.

68. Lewandowski AV. The bridge to cardiac transplantation: ventricular assist devices. Dimens Crit Care Nurs 1995;14(1):17–26.

69. Loisance D, Benvenuti C, Lebrun T, et al. Cost and cost effectiveness of the mechanical and pharmacologic bridge to transplantation. ASAIO Trans 1991;37(3): M125–127.

70. McCarthy PM. HeartMate implantable left ventricular assist device: bridge to transplantation and future applications. Ann Thorac Surg 1995;59:46–51.

71. O'Connell JB, Gunnar RM, Evans RW, et al. Task force 1: organization of heart transplantation in the U.S. J Am Coll Cardiol 1993;22:8–14.

72. Orians CE, Evans RW, Ascher NL. Evidence of organ specific availability for the United States. Transplant Proc 1993;25:1541–1542.

73. Hosenspud J, DeMarco T, Frazier H, et al. Progression of systemic disease and reduced long term survival in patients with cardiac amyloidosis undergoing heart transplantation: follow-up results of a multicenter survey. Circulation 1991;84(Suppl III):338–343.

74. Mudge GH, Goldstein S, Addonizio LJ, et al. Task Force 3: recipient Guidelines/Prioritization. J Am Coll Cardiol 1993;22:21–30.

75. Wilson JR, Schwartz JS, Sutton MS, et al. Prognosis in severe heart failure: relation to hemodynamic measurements and ventricular ectopic activity. J Am Coll Cardiol 1983;2:403–410.

76. Franciosa JA, Wilen M, Ziesche S, Cohen JN. Survival in men with severe chronic left ventricular failure due to either coronary heart disease or idiopathic dilated cardiomyopathy. Am J Cardiol 1983;51:831–836.

77. Szlachcic J, Massie BM, Kramer BI, et al. Correlates and prognostic implications of exercise capacity in chronic congestive heart failure. Am J Cardiol 1985;55:1037–1042.

78. Mancini DM, Eisen H, Kussmal W, et al. Value of peak oxygen consumption for optimal timing of cardiac transplantation in ambulatory patients with heart failure. Circulation 1991;83:778–786.

79. Cohn JN, Rector TS. Prognosis of congestive heart failure and predictors of mortality. Am J Cardiol 1988; 62:1636–1641.

80. Califf RM, Bounous P, Harrell FE, et al. The Prognosis in the Presence of Coronary Artery Disease. In E Braunwald, MB Mock, JT Watson (eds), Congestive Heart Failure: Current Research and Clinical Applications. New York: Grune & Stratton, 1982;31–40.

81. Keogh AM, Baron DW, Hickie JB. Prognostic guides in patients with idiopathic or ischemic dilated cardiomyopathy assessed for cardiac transplantation. Am J Cardiol 1990;65:903–908.

82. Olivari MT, Antolick A, Kaye MP, et al. Heart transplantation in elderly patients. J Heart Transplant 1988; 7:258–264.

83. Robin J, Ninet J, Tronc F, et al. Long term results of heart transplantation deteriorate more rapidly in patients over 60 years of age. Eur J Cardiothorac Surg 1996;10:259–263.

84. Erickson KW, Costanzo-Nordin MR, O'Sullivan EJ, et al. Influence of preoperative transpulmonary gradient on late mortality after orthotopic heart transplantation. J Heart Transplant 1990;9:526–537.

85. Adatia I, Perry S, Lanzberg M, et al. Inhaled nitric oxide and hemodynamic evaluation of patients with pulmonary hypertension before transplantation. J Am Coll Cardiol 1995;25:1656–1664.

86. Berner M, Beghetti M, Spahr-Schopfer I, et al. Inhaled nitric oxide to test the vasodilator capacity of the pulmonary vascular bed in children with long-standing pulmonary hypertension and congenital heart disease. Am J Cardiol 1996;77:532–535.

87. Gonwa TA, Husberg BS, Klintmalin GB, et al. Simultaneous heart-kidney transplantation: a report of three cases and review of the literature. J Heart Lung Transplant 1992;11:152–155.

88. Olivieri NF, Liu PP, Sher GD, et al. Brief report: combined liver and heart transplantation for end-stage iron-induced organ failure in an adult with homozygous beta-thalassemia. N Engl J Med 1994;330:1125–1127.

89. Kuhn WF, Myers B, Brennan AF, et al. Psychopathology in heart transplant candidates. J Heart Transplant 1988;7:223–226.

90. Olbrisch ME, Lebenson JL. Psychosocial evaluation of heart transplant candidates: an international survey of process, criteria and outcomes. J Heart Lung Transplant 1991;10:948–955.

91. O'Connell JB, Renlund DG, Robinson JA, et al. Effect of preoperative hemodynamic support on survival after

cardiac transplantation. Circulation 1988;78(Suppl III):78–82.

92. Bolman RM, Spray TL, Cox JL, et al. Heart transplantation in patients requiring preoperative mechanical support. J Heart Transplant 1987;6:273–280.

93. Reedy JE, Pennington G, Miller LW, et al. Status I heart transplant patients: conventional versus ventricular assist device support. J Heart Lung Transplant 1992; 11:246–252.

94. McCarthy PM. HeartMate implantable left ventricular assist device: bridge to transplantation and future applications. Ann Thorac Surg 1995;59:S46–51.

95. Griffith BP, Kormos RL, Nastala CJ, et al. Results of extended bridge to transplantation—window into the future of permanent ventricular assist devices. Ann Thorac Surg 1996;61:396–398.

96. Levine AB, Levine TB. Patient evaluation for cardiac transplantation. Prog Cardiovasc Dis 1991;33:219–228.

97. O'Connell JB, Bourge RC, Costanzo-Nordin MR, et al. Cardiac transplantation: recipient selection, donor procurement, and medical follow-up. A statement for health professionals from the Committee on Cardiac Transplantation of the Council on Clinical Cardiology, American Health Association. Circulation 1992;86: 1061–1079.

98. Fragomeni LS, Rogers G, Kaye MP. Donor Identification and Organ Procurement for Cardiac Transplantation. In R Thompson (ed), Cardiovascular Clinics: Cardiac Transplantation. Philadelphia: Saunders, 1990.

99. Laks H, Gates RN, Ardehali A, et al. Orthotopic heart transplantation and concurrent coronary bypass. J Heart Lung Transplant 1993;12:810–815.

100. Sweeny SM, Lammermeier DE, Frazier OH, et al. Extension of donor criteria in cardiac transplantation: surgical risk versus supply-side economics. Ann Thorac Surg 1990;50:7–11.

101. Pflugfelder PW, Singh NR, McKenzie FN, et al. Extending cardiac allograft ischemic time and donor age: effect on survival and long-term cardiac function. J Heart Lung Transplant 1991;10:394–400.

102. Young JB, Nafter DC, Bourge RC, et al. Matching the heart donor and heart transplant recipient—clues for successful expansion of the donor pool: a multivariate, multiinstitutional report. J Heart Lung Transplant 1994;13:353–365.

103. Gao SZ, Hunt SA, Alderman EL, et al. Relationship of donor age and pre-existing coronary disease by angiography and intracoronary ultrasound to later development of cardiac allograft coronary artery disease. J Heart Lung Transplant 1995;14:S40.

104. Chau EMC, McGregor CGA, Rodeheffer RJ, et al. Increased incidence of chronotropic incompetence in older donor hearts. J Heart Lung Transplant 1995;14:743–748.

105. Baldwin JC, Anderson JL, Boucek MM, et al. 24th Bethesda Conference—Cardiac Transplantation. Task force 2: donor guidelines. J Am Coll Cardiol 1993;22: 15–22.

106. Organ Distribution Policy Document. United Network for Organ Sharing, Richmond, VA. March 1996. 3.1–3.31.

107. Reitz BA, Burton NA, Jamieson SW, Pennock JL, Stinson EB, Shumway NE. Heart and lung transplantation—autotransplantation and allotransplantation in primates with extended survival. J Thorac Cardiovasc Surg 1980;80:360–372.

108. Reitz BA, Wallwork JL, Hunt SA, et al. Heart-lung transplantation: successful therapy for patients with pulmonary vascular disease. N Engl J Med 1982;306:557–564.

109. Merz B. New techniques enable "heartless" lung transplants. JAMA 1987;257:728.

110. Starnes VA. Heart-lung transplantation: an overview. Cardiol Clin 1990;8:159.

111. Reitz BA, Gaudiani VA, Hunt SA, et al. Diagnosis and treatment of allograft rejection in heart-lung transplant recipients. J Thorac Cardiovasc Surg 1983;85:354.

112. Cooper DK, Novitzky D, Rose AG, et al. Acute pulmonary rejection precedes cardiac rejection following heart-lung transplantation in a primate model. J Heart Transplant 1986;5:29.

113. McGregor CGA, Baldwin JC, Jamieson SW, et al. Isolated pulmonary rejection after combined heart-lung transplantation. J Thorac Cardiovasc Surg 1985;90:623.

114. Novitzky D, Cooper DKC, Rose AG, et al. Acute isolated pulmonary rejection following transplantation of the heart and both lungs: experimental and clinical observations. Ann Thorac Surg 1986;42:180.

115. Scott WC, Haverich A, Billingham ME, et al. Lethal rejection of the lung without significant cardiac rejection in primate heart-lung allotransplants. J Heart Transplant 1984;4:33.

116. Bryan CL, Anzueto A, Levine SM, et al. Corticosteroid therapy does not potentiate bronchial anastomotic complications in single lung transplantation (SLT). Am Rev Respir Dis 1991;143(Part 2):A461.

117. Egan TM, Boychuk JE, Rosato K, et al. Whence the lungs? A study to assess suitability of donor organs for transplantation. Transplantation 1992;53:420.

118. Shumway SJ, Hertz MI, Petty MG, et al. Liberalization of donor criteria in lung and heart-lung transplantation. Ann Thorac Surg 1994;57:92–95.

119. Sundaresan S, Trachiotis GD, Aoe M, et al. Donor lung procurement: assessment and operative technique. Ann Thorac Surg 1993;56:1409–1413.

120. Gasior T, Armitage J, Stein K, et al. Right ventricular performance in the transplanted heart. Anesthesiology 1989;71:A86.

121. Berberich J. Anesthesia for Heart and Heart-Lung Transplantation. In JA Fabian (ed), Anesthesia for Organ Transplantation. Philadelphia: Lippincott, 1992;1–19.

122. Kaye DM, Bergin P, Buckland M, Esmore D. Value of postoperative assessment of cardiac allograft function by transesophageal echocardiography. J Heart Lung Transplant 1994;13:165–172.

123. Haverich A, Dammenhayn L, Albes J, et al. Heart transplantation: intraoperative management, postoperative

therapy and complications. Thorac Cardiovasc Surg 1990;38:280.

124. Baum VC. Anesthesia for heart transplantation recipients. Semin Anesth 1990;4:298.

125. Firestone L. Heart transplantation. Int Anesthesiol Clin 1991;29:41–58.

126. Clark NJ, Martin RD. Anesthetic considerations for patients undergoing cardiac transplantation. J Cardiothorac Anesth 1988;2:519–542.

127. Gutzke GE, Shah KB, Glisson SN, et al. Cardiac transplantation: a prospective comparison of ketamine and sufentanil for anesthetic induction. J Cardiothorac Anesth 1989;3:389–395.

128. Baum VC. Anesthesia for heart transplantation recipients. Semin Anesth 1990;4:298–304.

129. Hensley FA Jr., Martin DE, Larach DR, Romanoff ME. Anesthetic management for cardiac transplantation in North America—1986 survey. J Cardiothorac Anesth 1987;1:429–437.

130. White PF, Way WL, Trevor AJ. Ketamine: its pharmacology and therapeutic uses. Anesthesiology 1982;65:119.

131. Demas K, Wyner J, Mihm FG, et al. Anaesthesia for heart transplantation: a retrospective study and review. Br J Anaesth 1986;58:1357–1364.

132. Zickmann B, Boldt J, Hempelmann G. Anesthesia in pediatric heart transplantation. J Heart Lung Transplant 1992;11:S272–S276.

133. Havel M, Owen AN, Simon P, et al. Decreasing use of donated blood and reduction of bleeding after orthotopic heart transplantation by use of aprotinin. J Heart Lung Transplant 1992;11:348–349.

134. Propst JW, Siegel LC, Feeley TW. Effect of aprotinin on transfusion requirements during repeat sternotomy for cardiac transplantation surgery. Transplant Proc 1994;26:3719–3721.

135. Prendergast TW, Furukawa S, Beyer AJ III. Defining the role of the aprotinin in heart transplantation. Ann Thorac Surg 1996;62:670–674.

136. Hakim M, Wheeldon D, Bethune DW, et al. Haemodialysis and haemofiltration on cardiopulmonary bypass. Thorax 1985;40:101–106.

137. Wheeldon DW, Bethune DW, Gill RD. Perfusion for cardiac transplantation. Perfusion 1986;1:57–61.

138. Cabrol C, Gandjbakhch I, Pavie A, et al. Surgical Procedure. In J Wallwork (ed), Heart and Heart-Lung Transplantation. Philadelphia: Saunders, 1989;119–144.

139. DiBiase A, Tse T-K, Schnittger I, et al. Frequency and mechanism of bradycardia in cardiac transplant recipients and need for pacemakers. Am J Cardiol 1991;67:1385–1389.

140. Bourge RC, Kirklin JK, Naftel DC, et al. Analysis and predictors of pulmonary vascular resistance after cardiac transplantation. J Thorac Cardiovasc Surg 1991;101:432–445.

141. Kawaguchi A, Gandjbakhch I, Pavie A, et al. Cardiac transplantation recipients with preoperative pulmonary hypertension: evolution of pulmonary hemodynamics and surgical options. Circulation 1989;80(Suppl III):90–96.

142. Bhatia SJ, Kirshenbaum JM, Shemion RJ, et al. Time course of resolution of pulmonary hypertension and right ventricular remodeling after orthotopic cardiac transplantation. Circulation 1987;76:819–826.

143. Hosenspud JD, Norman DJ, Cobanaglu A, et al. Serial echocardiographic findings early after heart transplantation: evidence for reversible right ventricular dysfunction and myocardial edema. J Heart Transplant 1987;6:343–347.

144. Kieler-Jensen N, Lundin S, Rickstein SE. Vasodilator therapy after heart transplantation: effects of inhaled nitric oxide and intravenous prostacyclin, prostaglandin E_1 and sodium nitroprusside. J Heart Lung Transplant 1995;14:436–443.

145. Williams TJ, Salamonsen RF, Snell G, et al. Preliminary experience with inhaled nitric oxide for acute pulmonary hypertension after heart transplantation. J Heart Lung Transplant 1995;14:419–423.

146. Semigran MJ, Cockrill BA, Kacmarek R, et al. Hemodynamic effects of inhaled nitric oxide in heart failure. J Am Coll Cardiol 1994;24:982–988.

147. Girard C, Durand PG, Pannetier JC, et al. Inhaled nitric oxide for right ventricular failure after heart transplantation. J Cardiothorac Vasc Anesth 1993;7:481–485.

148. Oz MC, Slater JP, Edwards N, Dickstein ML, Beck JR, Spotnitz HM, Levin HR. Desaturated venous-to-arterial shunting reduces right-sided heart failure after cardiopulmonary bypass. J Heart Lung Transplant 1995;14:172–176.

149. Forester A, Abdelnoor M, Geiran O, et al. Risk factors for total and cause-specific mortality in human cardiac transplantation. Eur J Cardiothorac Surg 1991;5:641–647.

150. Uchino T, Belboul A, El-Gatit A, et al. Assessment of myocardial damage by circulating cardiac myosin light chain I after heart transplantation. J Heart Lung Transplant 1994;13:418–423.

151. Bonser RS, Jamieson SW. Heart-lung transplantation. Clin Chest Med 1990;11:235–246.

Chapter 7
Lung Transplantation

Peter E. Krucylak and Lawrence J. Baudendistel

Chapter Plan

Historic Aspects

Early Attempts

Early investigational work with surgical techniques in lung transplantation used a canine model. The pioneering work was performed in the 1950s by Metras, Demikhov, and Hardin. The work of Henri Metras is of particular interest because he described most of the basic surgical techniques in use today, particularly the use of a left atrial cuff to simplify the anastomosis of the pulmonary veins.[1] Metras also was the first investigator to perform bronchial artery revascularization; Hardin and Kittle used the canine model to evaluate survival of grafts after transplantation.[2] Their report emphasized the importance of rejection in limiting survival after lung transplant. Various methods of immunosuppression were used, including corticosteroids, splenectomy, and total body irradiation. Demikhov's work (the first successful canine heart-lung transplant before coronary artery bypass) was not appreciated until relatively recently because of the late translation of his works from Russian.[3]

The first human lung transplant was reported by Hardy et al. in 1963.[4] The recipient was a man with squamous cell carcinoma involving the left mainstem bronchus. He had preoperative symptoms of weight loss, hemoptysis, and dyspnea. It was thought that, after a left pneumonectomy, his remaining right lung would have insufficient reserve to support respiratory function. He therefore underwent left pneumonectomy followed by single-lung transplantation (SLT). The lung was harvested from a donor who died after a fatal myocardial infarction. Immunosuppression consisted of azathioprine, corticosteroids, and thymic irradiation. Although the single-lung graft was successful and supported his respiratory function in the immediate postoperative period, the recipient died of postoperative renal failure and malnutrition on the eighteenth postoperative day. No evidence of rejection was seen on postmortem examination.

A total of 20 lung transplants were reported in the late 1960s to early 1970s.[5] There was only one case of survival to discharge: a 23-year-old man with pulmonary fibrosis, who survived for 10 months before dying with evidence of chronic rejection.[6] Early postoperative problems included infection (*Pseudomonas* and *Klebsiella* sepsis treated with gentamicin), airway complications (stenosis at the site of bronchial anastomosis), and rejection (treated with increased doses of corticosteroids). The recipient eventually died from *Pseudomonas* pneumonia with attendant septic shock.

By 1978, 38 lung transplants were reported, with a mean survival time of 8.5 days.[7] Patients died of graft dysfunction, rejection, or bronchial dehiscence. The longest survivals noted at that time were 6 and 10 months. The available immunosuppressive drugs did not allow for adequate selective immunosuppression after lung transplant.

The Modern Era

Reitz et al. introduced heart-lung transplantation (HLT) in 1981 as a treatment for pulmonary hypertension.[8] Use of cyclosporine-based immunosuppression allowed for reduced corticosteroid use and improved patient survival. Replacement of the heart and both lungs offered technical simplicity and the elimination of all diseased lung tissue. The clinical success of HLT proved that implanted lungs would function in a human recipient. Also, the ability of the heart-lung graft to provide adequate blood flow to the tracheal anastomosis allowed patients to survive without significant airway complications.

When HLT was introduced into clinical practice, research was being performed to deal with the problems of rejection, infection, and airway complications. The discovery and subsequent use of cyclosporine led to reduced rejection rates as well as lower rates of opportunistic infections. Cyclosporine also allowed the avoidance of corticosteroids in the routine immunosuppressant regimen. Cooper et al. described the use of a pedicle of omentum to "wrap" the bronchial anastomosis (omentopexy) to protect it and to provide increased vascularity to the area.[9] They also identified the use of high-dose corticosteroids as a reason for poor bronchial healing. The Lung Transplantation Program at the University of Toronto reported the successful use of SLT for patients with idiopathic pulmonary fibrosis (IPF).[10] Patients with pulmonary fibrosis were considered the ideal model for the development of SLT techniques because the ventilation and perfusion after SLT would preferentially be directed to the grafted lung, thus eliminating the theoretical concern of ventilation-perfusion mismatch. Gradually, the indications for SLT broadened to other disease states, such as emphysema and pulmonary hypertension. This allowed for wider use of donor organs because one donor could donate intrathoracic organs to three recipients. The same group at the University of Toronto developed double-lung transplantation (DLT) with an en bloc implantation technique for use in recipients with bilateral infectious lung disease, such as cystic fibrosis.[11] However, DLT has since fallen out of use as a result of high rates of airway complications.[12] A more recent approach to the replacement of both lungs is bilateral single-lung transplantations (BLTs), in which consecutive single-lung grafts are placed.[13]

Pathology of Recipients

Most lung transplant recipients have pulmonary disease that falls into one of four categories: obstructive pulmonary disease, restrictive pulmonary disease, septic lung disease, and pulmonary vascular disease. The preoperative diagnosis defines the patient's condition at time of transplantation as well as the patient's transplant strategy. Table 7-1 lists the distribution of lung transplants by diagnosis.

Obstructive lung disease, particularly emphysema, is the most common cause of terminal lung dysfunction. Standard medical treatment for emphysema includes inhaled beta-agonists, theophylline

Table 7-1. Distribution of Lung Transplantations by Diagnosis

	Single-Lung Transplantation (%)	BLT/DLT (%)
Emphysema	44.3	17.2
alpha$_1$-Antitrypsin deficiency	11.9	10.9
Pulmonary fibrosis	20.1	6.9
Primary pulmonary hypertension	5.9	10.4
Cystic fibrosis	1.6	33.8
Retransplant	3.4	2.8
Miscellaneous	12.8	18.1

BLT = bilateral single-lung transplantation; DLT = double-lung transplantation.
Source: Adapted from JD Hosenpud, LE Bennett, MK Berkeley, et al. The Registry of the International Society for Heart and Lung Transplantation: fourteenth official report—1997. J Heart Lung Transplant 1997;16:691–712.

preparations, and corticosteroids. New developments in surgical treatment of emphysema are discussed at the end of this chapter.

Restrictive lung disease is usually in the form of IPF. Once patients with pulmonary fibrosis become oxygen dependent and develop oxygen desaturation with minimal exertion, life expectancy is less than 1 year.[14] Current therapy for pulmonary fibrosis consists of corticosteroids with a second cytotoxic agent, such as cyclophosphamide or methotrexate.[15] Although these agents possess broad anti-inflammatory actions, their specific mechanisms of action in IPF are unknown.

Septic lung disease occurs most commonly in the form of cystic fibrosis or bronchiectasis. Patients with cystic fibrosis have adhesions in their pleural spaces secondary to repeated infections.[16, 17] Cystic fibrosis is an autosomal recessive genetic disorder, with 1 in 25 whites being carriers of the gene.[18] There are approximately 30,000 people with cystic fibrosis in the United States with a median survival of 29 years.[19, 20] Patients born in 1990 with cystic fibrosis have an estimated life span of 40 years.[20] Respiratory pathology in this population includes bronchitis, which develops into bronchiectasis. The pathophysiology is that of obstructive disease progressing to fibrosis.[18] Colonization of the distal air-ways occurs with *Haemophilus influenzae, Staphylococcus aureus, Pseudomonas aeruginosa*, and occasionally *Pseudomonas cepacia*.

Current treatment for respiratory compromise with cystic fibrosis consists of chest physical therapy and antibiotics. Sputum in these patients is especially thick because of increased protein glycoprotein sulfation and because of the presence of DNA from dead leukocytes.[18] Dornase alfa (Pulmozyme) is a human recombinant DNase that is administered by inhalation of an aerosol mist. Dornase alfa hydrolyzes the DNA in the sputum and reduces sputum viscosity.

Pulmonary vascular disease is either primary pulmonary hypertension (PPH) or secondary to congenital heart disease with resultant Eisenmenger's syndrome. PPH is defined as a mean pulmonary artery pressure greater than 25 mm Hg at rest or greater than 30 mm Hg during exercise in the setting of a normal pulmonary artery wedge pressure and absence of secondary causes.[21] Syncopal episodes in patients with pulmonary hypertension are related to effort and are thought to occur as a result of limitation in cardiac output. Several predictive factors of shortened survival are identifiable: mean pulmonary artery pressure exceeding 85 mm Hg, absence of response to vasodilators, New York Heart Association class III or IV, right atrial pressure exceeding 20 mm Hg, and cardiac index less than 2.0 liters per minute per m^2.[21] Estimated mean survival of patients with PPH from time of diagnosis is 2.8 years.[22]

Several new approaches have been used to treat patients with PPH. These strategies are also used as a bridge to transplantation. Prostacyclin has been used as a test to determine vascular reactivity and also as a long-term intravenous infusion.[23, 24] Patients treated with long-term prostacyclin infusion demonstrate greater exercise tolerance, improved cardiac index, lower pulmonary artery pressure, and improved survival.[23] Calcium channel antagonists, particularly nifedipine and diltiazem, are used in cases of PPH. The goal of vasodilator therapy is reduction of pulmonary artery pressure, increased cardiac output, and maintenance of systemic blood pressure.[21] Nifedipine and diltiazem are the calcium channel antagonists of choice in this population.

Anticoagulant therapy is recommended for patients with PPH.[25] They are at risk for throm-

Table 7-2. Selection Criteria for Lung Transplant Recipients

End-stage lung disease with life expectancy of 12–18 months
No other systemic disease
History of compliance with medical advice
No contraindications to immunosuppression
Psychological stability
Ambulatory status or potential for physical rehabilitation
Abstinence from tobacco for >6 months
No extrapulmonary sites of infection
No marked obesity
Age: SLT <65; BLT <60

SLT = single-lung transplantation; BLT = bilateral single-lung transplantation.

Table 7-3. Selection Criteria for Lung Transplantation by Diagnosis

Obstructive airway disease (emphysema, alpha$_1$-antitrypsin deficiency)
   Postbronchodilator FEV_1 <500 ml (<20% predicted)
   Rapid FEV_1 decline
   Hypoxia (PaO_2 <55 mm Hg), hypercapnia
   Secondary pulmonary hypertension
Pulmonary vascular disease (primary pulmonary hypertension)
   Mean PA pressure >55 mm Hg
   Mean RA pressure >10 mm Hg
   Cardiac index <2.5 liters/min/m^2
   Nonresponder to vasodilator drugs
Septic lung disease (cystic fibrosis)
   Postbronchodilator FEV_1 <30% of predicted
   Rapid decline in FEV_1
   Hypoxia, hypercapnia
   Increased frequency and severity of lung infections
   Hemoptysis, pneumothorax
Restrictive lung disease (idiopathic pulmonary fibrosis)
   VC or TLC <65% of predicted
   Hypoxia with exercise
   Secondary pulmonary hypertension
   DLCO <30% of predicted

FEV_1 = forced expiratory volume in 1 second; PA = pulmonary artery; RA = right atrial; VC = vital capacity; TLC = total lung capacity; DLCO = carbon monoxide diffusing capacity of the lungs.

boemboli due to their decreased physical exertion, venous insufficiency, and dilated right atrium and ventricle.[21] Even a small pulmonary embolus can be life threatening. Use of warfarin is particularly recommended in patients who do not respond to pulmonary vasodilators.[26]

Indications for Lung Transplantation

The general criterion for lung transplantation is irreversible, progressive, terminal pulmonary disease in which the life expectancy is 12–18 months despite maximal medical and surgical therapy (Table 7-2). Table 7-3 sets out the selection criteria by diagnosis. Contraindications to lung transplantation are categorized as either relative or absolute (Table 7-4).

Low doses of prednisone (up to 0.3 mg/kg/day) are acceptable before lung transplantation.[27] Patients who are mechanically ventilated are not normally candidates for lung transplant unless they have already been evaluated for transplant and have spent enough time on a transplant list to have a reasonable chance of obtaining an organ.[28] Patients who have been ventilated more than a few days and who are still considered candidates for transplantation probably need BLT because of colonization of the airway. There is no absolute cutoff in evaluating left ventricular ejection fraction in this population, but patients with severe left ventricular dysfunction or coronary artery disease are probably best treated with HLT.[29]

Choice of Procedure

Lung transplantation encompasses a number of different surgical procedures. In general, patients will have better pulmonary function when both lungs are replaced. The limited number of available donor lungs has led investigators to identify situations in which replacement of a single lung will be sufficient to meet clinical goals. In addition to these considerations, operations that replace both lungs, such as BLT, are associated with more postoperative morbidity than SLT, particularly in older patients. These factors often dictate the choice of a particular type of lung transplant procedure. Trulock summarized the choice of procedure in this way: "the *best* transplant procedure is the one that can be done when the patient needs it."[30] Table 7-5 summarizes the number of transplants performed in 1996 by surgical procedure.

SLTs are performed for indications of emphysema and pulmonary fibrosis and in selected

Table 7-4. Contraindications to Lung Transplantation

Absolute
  Systemic disease with nonpulmonary organ involvement
  Significant hepatic or renal disease
  Malignancy
  Active infection (pulmonary or extrapulmonary)
  Current tobacco use
  History of medical noncompliance
Relative
  Previous thoracic surgery
  Heavy steroid use (>0.3 mg/kg/day)
  Left ventricular dysfunction or coronary artery disease
  Long-term ventilator dependence

Table 7-5. Total Number of Lung Transplantations Classed by Type of Procedure (1996)

Procedure	Number of Recipients
Single-lung transplantation	500
Bilateral single-lung transplantation	498
Heart-lung transplantation	76

Source: Adapted from JD Hosenpud, LE Bennett, MK Berkeley, et al. The Registry of the International Society for Heart and Lung Transplantation: fourteenth official report—1997. J Heart Lung Transplant 1997;16:691–712.

patients with pulmonary hypertension. SLT allows maximal use of a donor's organs and offers the practical advantage of possibly avoiding cardiopulmonary bypass (CPB) if the recipient tolerates intraoperative one-lung ventilation (OLV). Postoperatively, the carina remains innervated, allowing for a more normal cough. Patients with emphysema have large thoracic cavities, which makes SLT a technically straightforward procedure. SLT is particularly suited to patients with pulmonary fibrosis and older patients with emphysema, who may not be able to tolerate replacement of both lungs.

The nomenclature describing the procedure to replace both lungs is confusing. DLT refers to the procedure originally described by Patterson, in which both lungs are implanted en bloc while the recipient is supported with CPB.[11] DLT has been associated with a high incidence of catastrophic airway complications and so has been largely abandoned.[12] The preferred current procedure is BLT, in which each lung is replaced separately, with separate bronchial anastomoses.[13] This is performed either through a bilateral transverse anterolateral thoracotomy (clamshell approach) or bilateral posterolateral thoracotomies. The indications for DLT and BLT are roughly the same. Patients receiving BLT appear to tolerate the development of obliterative bronchiolitis (OB) better than do patients receiving SLT because they have better pulmonary reserve. BLT is frequently performed for patients with cystic fibrosis, in whom both lungs must be removed to prevent infection spreading from a diseased native lung. Risk factors for poor outcome after BLT include age older than 50 years, congen-

ital heart disease as the indication for transplant, and admission to the intensive care unit (ICU) before transplantation.[31]

HLT refers to the procedure in which the heart and both lungs are transplanted as one block. It is reserved for situations in which both the heart and the lungs need replacement, as with a patient with congenital heart disease who develops Eisenmenger's syndrome. Waiting time for HLT is three to six times longer than that for lung transplantation.[32] HLT was initially the only available surgical option for patients with Eisenmenger's syndrome. Several case reports have described SLT in association with intracardiac repair of the congenital defect. In some cases, this approach maximizes the benefit of donor availability.

Donor Lung

Donor lung availability is a severe limitation for most lung transplantation programs. According to the United Network for Organ Sharing (UNOS), as of August 31, 1998, 3,027 patients had registered for lung transplant and 240 had registered for HLT.[33] As of April 30, 1998, 5,540 patients had received lung transplants (both single and bilateral) and 608 patients had received a heart-lung transplant.[33]

The number of organ donors in the United States has remained stable since the early 1990s while the number of potential recipients has increased.[33] All potential HLT and lung transplant recipients are grouped into one priority category. The waiting time for an organ, which begins when the patient is listed with UNOS for transplant, is the primary criterion for selection. Patients with the diagnosis of pulmonary fibrosis have a higher mortality rate during the waiting period and are awarded 90 days of waiting time when they are listed for lung transplant.[34] When an organ becomes available, it is offered to patients with the most seniority within 500 miles of the donor hospital (zone A). If no suitable recipients are found, the search is extended to 500–1,000 miles away (zone B) and then to more than 1,000 miles away (zone C).

Problems with donor availability mean that a certain percentage of patients die while awaiting a donor lung. Six-month survival has been defined for subjects awaiting lung transplantation: It is highest in cases of Eisenmenger's syndrome (89%) compared to emphysema (81%), cystic fibrosis (74%), PPH (60%), and interstitial lung disease (38%).[35] Mean survival after diagnosis of PPH is 42 months.[36] Demise occurs as a sudden event or as a result of progressive right ventricular failure. Syncope is a predictor of early mortality in patients with PPH.[37] The presence of elevated right atrial pressure in PPH correlated with worsened survival.[35] IPF has a 40–80% mortality rate within 5 years of diagnosis.[38]

The vast majority (98%) of patients with cystic fibrosis die because of pulmonary complications.[38] Markers of early mortality in cystic fibrosis include a forced expiratory volume in 1 second (FEV_1) less than 30% of predicted, carbon dioxide retention, required use of supplemental oxygen, frequent pulmonary infection, and failure to maintain weight.[39] One-third of patients with cystic fibrosis die while awaiting transplantation.[40]

Assessment of Donor Lung

Assessment of donor lung suitability typically involves a preliminary phase and a final phase. The preliminary phase is performed at the institution where the donor receives care. The donor should be younger than 55 years old. Chest x-ray is used to rule out parenchymal disease and to allow for size matching. Relevant history to be obtained includes smoking history, lack of significant trauma, exclusion of aspiration, and exclusion of previous cardiac or pulmonary operation. Donors who have a smoking history longer than 10 pack-years are usually unacceptable.[41] Oxygenation is assessed by measuring serial blood gases on a fraction of inspired

Table 7-6. Donor Selection Criteria

Age <55 years
No parenchymal disease seen on chest x-ray
Exclusion of aspiration
Exclusion of previous thoracic or cardiac surgery
Adequate oxygenation
Negative hepatitis B and human immunodeficiency virus serology
Negative examination by fiberoptic bronchoscopy

oxygen (FIO_2) of 1.0. Adequate gas exchange is defined as a PaO_2 of 300 mm Hg or greater on FIO_2 of 1.0. Fiberoptic bronchoscopy is performed to exclude the possibility of aspirated masses. Hepatitis B and human immunodeficiency virus serologies are performed to verify negative results. ABO crossmatch is performed. The retrieval team makes the final assessment with a review of a recent chest x-ray, bronchoscopy, review of recent blood gases, and direct visual inspection of the lungs to be harvested. The donor selection criteria are summarized in Table 7-6.

Donor lungs are obtained from donors that meet criteria for brain death. Few lungs are suitable for transplantation. Only 5–10% of acceptable heart donors have usable lungs.[42] Acceptability factors include the length of mechanical ventilation and the possibility of bacterial colonization of the tracheobronchial tree. Resuscitation maneuvers for these patients, such as infusion of large amounts of intravenous fluid, may predispose their lungs to pulmonary edema. Irreversible brain death may cause neurogenic pulmonary edema and may also reduce pulmonary vascular resistance.[43] As the pulmonary vascular resistance decreases, the lungs are subject to a hyperdynamic state that makes them prone to edema from noncardiogenic causes. Chest trauma may result in an unacceptable amount of pulmonary contusion. Lungs with small contusions may be acceptable. BLT in the setting of marginal donor lungs probably provides a greater degree of safety. It may be possible to perform single-lung harvests from donors with unilateral pathology, such as trauma or contralateral aspiration.[44]

Initial size matching is done using vertical and transverse measurements obtained from chest x-ray. Patients with obstructive lung disease should receive lungs 10–20% smaller than the removed lung, whereas patients with pulmonary fibrosis should receive lungs 10–20% larger than the removed lung.[45]

General guidelines for the management of lung donors include maintenance of mean blood pressure above 70 mm Hg and a pulmonary capillary wedge pressure below 12 mm Hg. Fluid replacement should be targeted to maintain a urine output of 1–2 ml/kg per hour. Desmopressin (DDAVP) should be used for documented cases of diabetes insipidus. Pressors should be used in place of large volumes of intravenous fluid to support blood pressure. Dopamine in doses below 10 μg/kg per minute is recommended. The lowest FIO_2 compatible with a Pao_2 greater than 100 mm Hg is used. Arterial blood gases should be obtained every 2 hours to detect deterioration in oxygenation.

The acceptable degree of graft dysfunction depends on the indication for SLT. Patients with pulmonary hypertension should receive single-lung grafts of the highest quality because that lung will receive 90% of the cardiac output. In the event of graft dysfunction, the remaining lung will be unable to support respiratory gas exchange while the grafted lung recovers. Patients with emphysema tolerate some degree of graft dysfunction because the remaining lung usually produces adequate oxygenation. Using lungs from marginal donors who do not meet one or two criteria does not worsen posttransplant survival.[46] Liberalization of donor criteria should help increase the number of available donor organs.

Organ Harvest

Lung transplantation is unique in that it is the only solid-organ transplant in which the arterial supply to the graft is not routinely re-established. Blood flow to the bronchial anastomosis occurs through collateral blood vessels from the pulmonary artery.[47] In addition, the bronchial anastomosis is continuously subjected to a nonsterile environment. In light of these circumstances, it is not surprising that airway and infectious complications are common.

Initial methods of lung preservation centered around topical cooling of the donor lung. This approach was used during the initial phases of the lung transplant program at the University of Toronto.[48] Topical cooling limited the tolerable duration of ischemia to 4–6 hours.[48] Current preservation strategies involve single-flush perfusion of the donor lung with maintenance in a cold medium for transport. Prostaglandin or prostacyclin is used as an adjunct to this method to prevent reflex pulmonary vasoconstriction from cold flush solutions.[48]

Harvesting of both lungs is possible without affecting cardiac procurement.[49] Systemic heparin (250–300 units/kg) is administered before placement of vascular clamps. Prostaglandin E_1 (PGE_1) (500 mg) is given directly into the pulmonary artery. Modified Euro-Collins solution is delivered at 4°C into the main pulmonary artery. The lungs are ventilated with 100% oxygen and are partially inflated before removal.[50] This maintains the lung in a state consistent with normal end-tidal inspiration and improves the preservation process.[48]

Cold ischemia is well tolerated for 6 hours. Ischemia times of up to 10 hours result in functioning lungs. Factors associated with improved graft function include partial lung inflation, use of PGE_1, ventilation of the donor lung with 100% oxygen, and transport at 10°C. Maintenance of hypothermia below this temperature worsened subsequent gas exchange in a rabbit lung model.[51] Trials using University of Wisconsin solution demonstrated improved organ preservation.[52, 53] Improvements in this field may allow more distant procurement or even harvesting organs from non–beating-heart cadavers.

Transplant Procedure

SLT is performed via a lateral thoracotomy. The anastomoses are typically done in the order of left atrium (pulmonary veins), bronchus, and pulmonary artery. The pulmonary artery is initially clamped for 5 minutes to determine whether CPB is necessary. During performance of the bronchial anastomosis, the donor bronchus is excised to within two bronchial rings of the takeoff of the upper-lobe bronchus to keep it as short as possible. This anastomosis is done in either an end-to-end fashion or by using a telescoping anastomosis with overlap of short sections of the donor and recipient bronchus. The pulmonary venous anastomosis is done by anastomosing a cuff of the donor left atrium to the cuff of the recipient left atrium. The pulmonary artery is typically anastomosed with a single running suture.[54] SLT is used with obstructive lung disease, fibrosing lung disease, and selectively for pulmonary hypertension. Suggested guidelines for use of SLT for pulmonary hypertension include a right ventricular ejection fraction (RVEF) greater than 20% and an echocardiogram demonstrating lack of severe disease in the right ventricle.[55]

In the case of SLT, the choice of which side to transplant depends on three factors: (1) prior surgery, (2) ventilation-perfusion mismatch, and (3) donor factors.[38] It is preferable to transplant the previously unoperated side. The side of worse function is preferentially replaced, and the best donor lung is grafted. Transplantation of the left lung may increase the incidence of CPB because of the increased traction on the heart during pneumonectomy.

The effect of leaving a diseased native lung must be evaluated before SLT. SLT is usually not recommended for recipients with cystic fibrosis due to the risk of transmitted infection from the remaining native lung.[56] The use of SLT along with simultaneous removal of the remaining native lung has been reported in this population.[57, 58] Patients having chronic obstructive pulmonary disease with a component of infectious bronchitis are not suitable candidates for SLT because of concerns about infecting the newly transplanted organ. Patients with severe bullous emphysema may require BLT or bullectomy of the native lung to prevent overexpansion of the native lung.[59] Native lung pathology contributed significant morbidity in 27% of cases from St. Vincent's Hospital.[60]

SLT is an option in cases of Eisenmenger's syndrome if it is done simultaneously with repair of the cardiac anomaly. Atrial septal defects and ventricular septal defects may be corrected through a right thoracotomy followed by replacement of the right lung.[61] Patients with a patent ductus arteriosus may have it ligated through a left-sided thoracotomy followed by replacement of the left lung.[62]

Initial attempts to protect the bronchial anastomosis involved the use of an omental wrap (omentopexy) around the bronchus. The highly vascular omentum quickly provided collateral circulation to the anastomosis. Use of omentopexy complicated the transplant procedure by requiring a laparotomy. Kjaghani evaluated the survival advantage of using an omentopexy and concluded that it did not improve success rates.[63] Calhoon described a telescoping bronchial anastomosis, which has become the preferred method of bronchial anastomosis.[54]

BLT is typically performed via a clamshell incision (bilateral transverse anterolateral thoracotomy), which allows for better access and hemostasis. Approximately 25% of patients transplanted via median sternotomy required re-exploration for bleeding, with none requiring re-exploration after transplantation using the clamshell approach.[11] Access to the lower lobes through a median sternotomy is restricted.[64] The lung with less perfusion, as detected by preoperative perfusion scan, is transplanted first.[65] The anastomoses are performed similarly to those done during SLT.

During the implantation of the second lung, there is often progressive pulmonary hypertension, pulmonary edema, and worsened gas exchange in one-third of patients with cystic fibrosis undergoing BLT.[11] Use of partial CPB may be necessary to allow implantation of the second lung.

BLT offers several advantages over DLT. First, it often avoids use of CPB. Second, the absence of mediastinal dissection reduces the risk of hemorrhage and injury to the vagus and phrenic nerves. Third, there are fewer complications at the site of the bronchial anastomoses than at the tracheal anastomoses.

DLT and HLT are becoming increasingly rare. With DLT, ischemic complications at the site of the tracheal anastomosis resulted in a 25% mortality rate.[14] HLT is declining in frequency, representing only 10% of thoracic transplants in some centers.[66] Reasons for this decline include the difficulty in obtaining the block of organs and the decreased incidence of Eisenmenger's syndrome because of the early repair of congenital cardiac defects.

Lobar transplantation is a new option in the pediatric population. Indications for lobar transplants do not differ from the indications for whole-lung transplants. Acute deterioration without expectation of receiving a cadaver organ is the indication for the cases reported to date.[67] The mean age of donors is 45 years (range, 38–55).[68] The right lower lobe and left lower lobe are preferred for harvest.[69] The right middle lobe is the easiest to harvest but behaves more like a segment than a lobe.[69] Living-related transplant has been described for cystic fibrosis with use of bilateral lobar grafts (one lobe from each biological parent).[70] Perioperative survival for bilateral lobar transplant is reported as 83%.[67] Unilateral grafts receive the majority of blood flow. This procedure may be most beneficial in recipients that weigh 20–50 kg.[67] Canine studies indicate that transplanted lobes from larger animals physiologically behave as a single lung from the standpoint of segmental blood flow and vascular resistance.[71] Prolonged air leak is the frequent complication of the donor lobectomy, occurring in three of eight donors in one series.[69] Living-related donors exhibit a 15–20% decrease in FEV_1 and forced vital capacity (FVC) at the time of postoperative spirometry 3 months after surgery.[69]

Anesthetic Management

Preoperative Testing

Theodore described who should be considered for transplant: "Anyone with lung disease who is sick enough to need the operation, well enough to survive the waiting period of several months for a donor organ, fit enough to survive the surgery, and courageous enough to deal with the complex postoperative care."[72] The proper goal of preoperative testing is the identification of transplant recipients who can make a full recovery despite life-threatening pulmonary disease. Preoperative testing should also identify patients who will die of their pulmonary disease within 12–18 months. This involves evaluation of other organ systems to determine underlying physiologic reserve. It also involves investigation to exclude conditions that would jeopardize the survival of the graft and of the recipient. Such conditions would include extrapulmonary sources of infection and current malignancies. Patients with a history of malignancy should demonstrate a 5-year disease-free period.[29]

Exercise testing in lung transplant recipients is generally limited to a 6-minute walk test with oximetry or a modified Bruce protocol treadmill study. Data from the University of Toronto Lung Transplant program indicate 6-minute walk distances of 200–500 meters.[73] The distance covered in a 6-minute walk test correlates with maximal oxygen consumption.[74] More formal testing is used to measure and guide the postoperative course.

Cardiac catheterization is routinely performed in patients with pulmonary hypertension. It is also used to evaluate the presence of coronary artery disease. The screening process involved in selecting recipients removes patients with symptomatic coronary artery disease. The appropriate role for coronary angiography is to exclude coronary artery disease in patients who are asymptomatic but have significant risk factors for coronary artery disease.[75]

Chronic pulmonary parenchymal disease may hinder acquisition of a technically adequate transthoracic echocardiogram.[76] Preoperative transesophageal echocardiography (TEE) is useful in evaluating patients, particularly patients with PPH. Gorscan reported the usefulness of TEE in this population: 25% of patients studied with TEE had findings that altered the surgical approach.[77] These findings included atrial septal defect, ventricular septal defect, and proximal pulmonary artery thrombi. TEE was well tolerated in these patients.

Evaluation of right ventricular function is important in assessing the recipient's ability to withstand lung transplant without the use of CPB. Transthoracic echocardiography is often technically unsatisfactory, especially in patients with emphysema. Assessment of right ventricular function has been studied, comparing preoperative measurement of RVEF by pulmonary artery catheter with a first-pass multiple-gated acquisition radionuclide scan (MUGA). The catheter-derived RVEF better represents the forward ejection fraction in patients with tricuspid regurgitation.[78]

Pretransplant testing of cigarette smokers requires particular attention. There must be evidence of abstinence from tobacco use for 2 years before evaluation for lung transplantation. Additionally, other smoking-related illnesses must be excluded, especially peripheral vascular disease and airway malignancy.[29] Left heart catheterization and coronary angiography may be necessary to exclude significant coronary disease that would prevent lung transplantation. The presence of severe left ventricular dysfunction may cause the patient to be referred for HLT.[29]

Abnormal hepatic function (defined as total bilirubin greater than 2.5 mg/dl despite maximal diuresis) must be excluded before lung transplantation. The risks of hepatic dysfunction in the postoperative period include coagulopathy, hepatic encephalopathy, infection, poor wound healing, reduced clearance of cyclosporine, and increased postoperative mortality.[29]

Induction

Lung transplant recipients have terminal pulmonary dysfunction and limited pulmonary reserve. Conacher summarized the situation in these patients as "a pneumonectomy in a patient who, under normal circumstances, would be adjudged as unfit for such an operation."[79] The anesthetic goals of hemodynamic stability and normal ventilation are often mutually exclusive during lung transplantation; the risks of these two goals must be continuously balanced and re-evaluated intraoperatively.

As with most organ transplants, lung transplants occur on an emergency basis. Despite this urgency, Myles and associates discovered that 60% of their patients had been fasted appropriately before induction of anesthesia, whereas another 19% had received antacid prophylaxis.[80] Singh and associates have recommended a modified rapid-sequence induction.[81] Bracken and colleagues suggested a typical induction regimen of 5–10 μg/kg of fentanyl and half the usual induction dose of thiopental or etomidate, followed by 0.5–1.0 mg/kg of rocuronium.[82] Because postoperative ventilation is common after lung transplantation, the use of a high-dose narcotic anesthetic technique may be a useful alternative in cases that are expected to involve periods of hemodynamic instability, such as transplantation for pulmonary hypertension. The use of such techniques also does not inhibit hypoxic pulmonary vasoconstriction and does not cause myocardial depression.[83]

Myles reported two cases of circulatory arrest after induction of anesthesia in patients with emphysema secondary to alpha$_1$-antitrypsin deficiency.[84] Both cases were attributed to "pulmonary tamponade" during positive-pressure ventilation and air trapping leading to electromechanical dissociation. The treatment in each case consisted of intravenous epinephrine, volume expansion, and disconnection from the ventilator circuit to allow lung deflation. Both cases proceeded using the technique of permissive hypoventilation, in which conventional positive pressure is limited and the arterial P_{CO_2} is allowed to rise.

Maintenance

Hypoxic pulmonary vasoconstriction (HPV) is the major compensatory mechanism involved in reducing blood flow to areas of hypoxic lung.[85] The use of intravenous anesthetics or one minimal alveolar concentration of inhaled anesthetic agents does not inhibit HPV.[86] Intravenous agents are useful in situations in which an ICU-type ventilator is needed or when deliberate hypoventilation is needed. Inhalational agents are familiar to most anesthesiologists, are potent bronchodilators, and offer the advantage of being easily titrated. Nitrous oxide is best avoided to prevent increases in pulmonary vascular resistance and to allow the delivery of high oxygen concentrations.[87]

Intraoperative Monitoring

Patients undergoing lung transplantation experience large changes in cardiac and pulmonary function. In addition to the standard anesthetic monitors (electrocardiography, noninvasive blood pressure, oximetry, temperature, and end-tidal CO_2), other monitoring devices are intended to permit early detection of these changes, instigate treatment, and verify the efficacy of treatment.

The lung transplant group at Washington University has recommended that intra-arterial and pulmonary artery catheters be placed before induction of anesthesia because of the changes in hemodynamic status that occur during induction and when spontaneous ventilation is replaced by controlled ventilation.[88] The placement of catheters before induction provides additional information and confers the added benefit that the anesthesiologist's attention is not diverted after induction by performing an invasive procedure. Patients with restrictive pulmonary disease have difficulty tolerating placement of central venous catheters before induction of anesthesia because they do not tolerate the supine position. Furthermore, due to their accentuated negative intrathoracic pressures during spontaneous ventilation, they are prone to air embolism.[89] Many patients are normally dyspneic, and this is exacerbated while in the Trendelenburg position, making central line placement uncomfortable for the patient. Preinduction placement of a central venous catheter may need to be deferred until anesthesia has been induced.

Conacher has reported the results of using pulmonary artery catheters with the ability to measure mixed venous saturation.[90] Mixed venous oximetry allows for continuous monitoring of oxygen usage as well as providing a printed copy of events that occur intraoperatively. Demajo uses mixed venous oximetry information as one of his criteria for placing recipients on CPB; he requires a mixed venous saturation of less than 65% as evidence of need for CPB.[91]

Right ventricular function is stressed, particularly during SLT. Diminished right ventricular performance is one of the major reasons to use CPB. Baseline studies of right ventricular function are typically performed as a MUGA scan. Determination of thermodilution RVEF allows for immediate measurement of improvement in right ventricular function after SLT for pulmonary hypertension.[92]

There are limitations to the information derived from a pulmonary artery catheter. Despotis reported the pressure gradient across the pulmonary artery anastomosis in 10 patients receiving BLTs.[93] Presence of the catheter proximal to the pulmonary artery anastomosis may represent a falsely elevated pulmonary artery pressure, even if the anastomosis appears to be technically adequate. Measurement of the pulmonary artery pressure distal to the anastomosis is recommended before instituting therapy directed at reducing right ventricular afterload.

Respiratory monitoring during lung transplantation has traditionally been limited to periodic blood gas monitoring, end-tidal CO_2 determination, pulse oximetry, and measurement of volatile agent levels. Advances in technology have resulted in the manufacture of continuous blood-gas monitoring (CBGM) optodes.[94] The technique has been reported to be useful during OLV for lobectomy.[95] Haller reported results with CBGM in patients with severe respiratory failure, noting that the device overestimated $Paco_2$ when the true value was greater than 60 mm Hg.[96] CBGM was still useful in this setting to help determine trends. Groh[97] reported the results of CBGM in three cases of lung transplantation, noting that CBGM allowed earlier detection of changes in blood-gas parameters than did pulse oximetry and intermittent blood-gas analysis. Bardoczky reported the use of side-stream spirometry during SLT as an early means of detecting endotracheal tube malposition and pulmonary edema after reperfusion of the grafted lung.[98] Capnography is not a reliable monitor in estimating Pco_2 in this population. Jellinek reported the use of capnography in seven patients who underwent BLT demonstrating large amounts of dead-space ventilation due to ventilation-perfusion mismatch.[99]

TEE has been used to help monitor and guide therapy of right ventricular dysfunction. TEE also is used to evaluate the left atrial anastomosis and to diagnose pulmonary venous thrombosis. Proponents of using TEE conclude that the device allows for earlier and more accurate diagnosis of right ventricular failure with improved therapy. A preliminary report from Brown and colleagues identifies TEE as the modality that best distinguishes hypovolemia from right ventricular dysfunction.[100] Disadvantages of TEE include the costly nature of the technology and the diversion of attention from patient care while performing the examination.[89] Use of TEE is most valuable in helping to interpret pulmonary artery pressures in the lateral position, to assess right ventricular function after pulmonary artery clamping, to monitor intracardiac air, to visualize suture lines and check blood flow, and to rule out a patent foramen ovale.

Modes of Ventilation

The majority of patients undergoing lung transplantation are sufficiently well ventilated with conventional intermittent positive-pressure ventilation (IPPV). Preoperative need for supplemental oxygen at rest and an elevated $Paco_2$ were suggested as predictive of the inadequacy of IPPV for patients undergoing SLT for chronic obstructive pulmonary disease (COPD).[101] Recommended ventilator settings for patients with COPD are tidal volume of 8–10 ml/kg, increased respiratory rate (15–25 breaths/minute), and a long expiratory time (inspiratory to expiratory [I:E] ratio of 1 to 4-5).[88]

Treatment of hypoxemia during lung transplant is similar to that for other thoracic procedures. Positive end-expiratory pressure (PEEP) applied to the nonoperative lung and continuous positive airway pressure (CPAP) applied to the operative lung may be used to improve oxygenation and decrease venous admixture.[102] Hogue reported the use of two low levels of CPAP (2 and 5 cm H_2O) to be useful in improving oxygenation.[103] Venous admixture is no longer an issue once the pulmonary artery is clamped before removal of the native lung.

High-frequency ventilation (HFV) has not been found to be helpful compared to IPPV modes of ventilation.[89] HFV modes that use passive exhalation may cause air trapping.[104] HFV may be easily accomplished with anesthesia ventilators such as the Ohmeda 7800 (Ohmeda, Madison, WI) and Drager Narkomed AV-E ventilator (North American

Drager, Telford, PA). This technique has been used while anesthetizing a patient with severe emphysema for coronary artery bypass grafting.[105] The flexibility of a readily available ventilator may warrant a trial of HFV, especially if the alternative is using CPB.

Lung transplant recipients with cystic fibrosis may require special modes of ventilation. Robinson reported the use of slow-rate, high-pressure ventilation in two patients with cystic fibrosis.[106] The ventilator settings were 6 breaths per minute, sustained peak inspiratory pressure at 75 cm H_2O, and I:E ratio of 1. This mode of ventilation decreased arterial carbon dioxide levels and allowed surgery to proceed without CPB.

Abnormalities in pulmonary function in lung transplant recipients often preclude normal modes of ventilation designed to keep arterial Pco_2 at 40 mm Hg. Permissive ventilatory techniques are often necessary to reduce the amount of IPPV used. Permissive hypercapnia is a strategy in which alveolar distention is restricted by limitations of pressure or ventilation and the effects of respiratory acidosis are tolerated.[107] This technique is useful in patients with emphysema. Inflation of emphysematous lungs with tidal volumes of 10 ml/kg causes overinflation with possible air trapping and decreased venous return, decreased cardiac output, and arterial hypotension. This has been termed *pulmonary tamponade*[88] or *dynamic hyperinflation*.[108] Generally, our practice is to limit the peak inspiratory pressure to 35–40 cm H_2O to prevent this overdistention and also to reduce the risk of pneumothorax in patients with bullous emphysema.

Permissive hypercapnia has been used in cases of adult respiratory distress syndrome (ARDS) with relative safety. Levels of $Paco_2$ up to 100 mm Hg have been tolerated. The first report of hypercapnia during lung transplantation was from Rolly in 1972.[109] His group reported the anesthetic management of the first long-term survivor of SLT for silicosis. Intraoperative $Paco_2$ values of 120 mm Hg were tolerated with adequate oxygenation. The recipient had pre-existing hypercarbia, exhibited by a $Paco_2$ of 120 mm Hg immediately after induction of anesthesia. Quinlan reported a case of deliberate hypoventilation during bilateral SLT in a 28-year-old woman with cystic fibrosis.[110] Severe hemodynamic instability developed during OLV for removal of the first native lung. Hemodynamic stability was restored by decreasing the minute ventilation and allowing the $Paco_2$ to rise as high as 162 mm Hg.

One-Lung versus Two-Lung Anesthesia

OLV greatly improves the surgical field and is probably mandatory for lung transplantation. There are two basic techniques to accomplish OLV. Double-lumen endotracheal tubes (DLETT) allow for selective ventilation and bronchoscopic access to each lung. The techniques necessary for placement are familiar to most thoracic anesthesiologists. Placement may be confirmed by either auscultation or by using fiberoptic bronchoscopy. Because of the great importance of proper positioning of the DLETT, use of the fiberoptic bronchoscope is strongly recommended. The experience at Saint Louis University with patients undergoing thoracoscopic lung-volume reduction for end-stage emphysema confirms this recommendation because most of these patients do not have audible breath sounds.[111] Usually a left-sided DLETT is placed because it is the simplest to position and does not interfere with surgical exposure.[88, 112] If a left-sided DLETT is used in a BLT for cystic fibrosis, it may be necessary to intubate the patient with a single-lumen tube and use a 5.5-mm bronchoscope to suction the lungs before placing the DLETT.[37]

Bronchial blockade can be accomplished either by a single-lumen endotracheal tube with a Fogarty balloon-tipped catheter placed alongside it, or with a Univent tube (Fuji Systems Corp., Tokyo, Japan), which is a single-lumen endotracheal tube with an enclosed bronchial blocker. Patients with cystic fibrosis may be better served with a Univent tube because its larger internal diameter allows the use of a larger suction catheter or fiberoptic bronchoscope (5.5 mm) to remove tenacious secretions.[83, 113] Use of the Univent tube offers the theoretical advantage of avoiding changing endotracheal tubes at the conclusion of surgery. Bronchial blockers may be subject to a higher incidence of displacement than are DLETTs.

Pulmonary Vasodilators

Right ventricular function is particularly taxed during lung transplantation performed without use of CPB. Appropriate use of pulmonary vasodilators reduces the impedance to flow of the right ventricle during these stressed conditions. Conventional pulmonary vasodilators have been used, including nitroglycerin, sodium nitroprusside, and phosphodiesterase inhibitors (primarily amrinone). All these previously used agents have the complication of producing systemic vasodilation. Some investigations have centered on three new agents that are relatively selective in their ability to produce pulmonary vasodilation: nitric oxide, PGE_1, and prostacyclin.

Nitric oxide mimics the effect of endothelium-derived relaxing factor.[114] Nitric oxide is a labile agent with a biological half-life of approximately 120 milliseconds. It is quickly inactivated by hemoglobin, which prevents systemic effects. Rajek reported the use of nitric oxide after cardiac transplantation, demonstrating improved RVEF and lower pulmonary artery pressures compared to a group receiving PGE_1.[115] Triantafillou reported using nitric oxide postoperatively in patients after SLT with improved oxygenation and lack of systemic vasodilation.[116]

PGE_1 has received the most use as a pulmonary vasodilator. PGE_1 is a vasodilator with a predominant site of action in the pulmonary vasculature.[117] It is almost entirely metabolized within the first pass through the lung. Norepinephrine administered through a left atrial catheter may be necessary to support arterial blood pressure.[118] This approach of combining PGE_1 and norepinephrine has been demonstrated as effective in patients who have undergone mitral valve replacement with associated pulmonary hypertension and right heart failure.[119]

Prostacyclin (prostaglandin I_2) is a potent pulmonary vasodilator that has been used in the treatment of PPH. Administration of intravenous prostacyclin in patients with PPH reduces pulmonary vascular resistance and increases cardiac output.[120] Investigations have evaluated inhaled prostacyclin as a pulmonary vasodilator. Walmrath reported the use of inhaled prostacyclin in three patients with ARDS.[121] In these cases, pulmonary vascular resistance decreased by 30%, with little change in systemic arterial pressure. A comparison of inhaled prostacyclin with nitric oxide in a canine model of HPV demonstrated that both agents decreased right ventricular afterload but that nitric oxide reduced pulmonary vascular resistance 35% more than prostacyclin.[122] Increasing the dose of nebulized prostacyclin is limited by the amount that "spills over" into the systemic circulation with attendant systemic hypotension.

Fluid Management

There are no clear recommendations for administration of intravenous fluids during lung transplantation. Because lymphatic drainage is interrupted as a result of lung transplantation, there may be theoretical reasons to limit the amount of fluids administered because the recipient has a limited ability to eliminate excess fluids. Approximately 70% of alveolar edema is cleared by direct absorption through alveolar epithelial cells; the remainder is cleared by the lymphatic system.[123] Despite this theoretical concern, Karanikolas has reported that there was no correlation between amount of fluid administered and incidence of adverse effects.[124] During BLT, an average of 4 more liters of crystalloid fluid are administered than in SLT.[125] The use of colloids instead of crystalloids may be attractive, but it is of unproved benefit. The temptation to administer intravenous fluids to treat episodes of hypotension should be controlled, and the early use of pressors, such as dopamine, should be considered to maintain acceptable hemodynamic parameters. The use of TEE to estimate left ventricular preload is particularly helpful in deciding the amount of fluids to administer.

Blood Products

Average blood usage for lung transplantation is 5 units of packed red blood cells. There is little use of other blood components. Use of leukoreduction filters or ultraviolet radiation is recommended to reduce the risk of HLA alloimmunization.[126] Red cell salvage devices are useful in cases of nonseptic lung disease in decreasing use of exogenous blood.

The use of aprotinin is a promising method to reduce the need for transfusion during lung transplantation, particularly in cases performed with CPB. Aprotinin is a serine protease inhibitor that inhibits a range of proteases, such as trypsin, plasmin, and kallikrein. It reduces fibrinolysis and protects platelet function.[126] Its blood-conserving properties are best demonstrated in cases that are at high risk for bleeding, such as repeat cardiac surgery. It has been reported in use during HLT in a patient with cystic fibrosis.[16] Aprotinin is recommended in cases of retransplantation.[127] It is also recommended for patients with cystic fibrosis because of pleural adhesions and the unpredictable need for use of CPB.[11] Prior exposure to aprotinin carries a risk of allergic reaction on subsequent administration, which makes administration of a test dose prudent. Rapid injection of aprotinin may cause an anaphylactoid reaction secondary to histamine release.[128] Our intraoperative protocol for use of aprotinin during lung transplantation is the administration of 1,000,000 units before skin incision and an infusion of 250,000 units per hour until completion of the procedure.

Cardiopulmonary Bypass

Increased experience with lung transplantation has decreased the need for CPB. Advances such as BLT, TEE, deliberate hypoventilation, and the use of selective pulmonary vasodilators have allowed more cases to be completed without CPB. Specific indications for the elective use of CPB include HLT, DLT, and SLT for pulmonary hypertension. Lobar transplantation is also performed using CPB to avoid having the entire cardiac output perfuse one pulmonary lobe.[67, 129]

The Lung Transplant Group at Washington University has analyzed its data with regard to the use of CPB. It was rare in cases of SLT but was necessary in 26.5% of bilateral SLT, particularly during implantation of the second lung.[130] There is an increased use of CPB during BLT in cases where marginal donor lungs were implanted.[46] During BLT, the use of CPB did not increase time to extubation, ICU stay, or time required to reach a room air Pao_2 greater than 60 mm Hg. CPB may be more likely necessary during a left-sided transplant because of the compression of the heart that occurs during left pneumonectomy and lung implantation.[131]

De Hoyos reported the experience at the University of Toronto, where the use of CPB was not predictable with preoperative variables.[132] CPB is used in approximately 10% of SLTs and 10% of BLTs.[133] Systemic cooling is usually avoided on bypass, keeping the temperature at 34–35°C.[131] Lee reported the use of partial CPB during bilateral SLT

for the purpose of rewarming a patient whose temperature had decreased to 32.6°C.[134]

CPB is deleterious to the grafted lung. Aeba summarized the experience with CPB in cases of lung transplantation.[135] In cases in which CPB was used, gas exchange was worse, chest x-ray appearance was worse, there was a greater incidence of prolonged intubation (7 days or longer), and more blood was used compared to cases performed without CPB. Canine studies suggest that transplants performed with CPB increase pulmonary vascular resistance.[136] Egan has reported the increased incidence of blood transfusion in cases of lung transplantation for cystic fibrosis in which CPB was used (21.5 vs. 6.05 units of packed red cells).[129] There were also associated increases in the period of postoperative ventilation and hospital stay.

Postoperative Care

The goals of postoperative care are to monitor the hemodynamic and respiratory status of the patient, manage complications, induce immunosuppression, and avoid infections. The goal of ventilatory management is the use of the lowest concentration of oxygen and the lowest peak inspiratory pressures compatible with adequate oxygen delivery. Peak inspiratory pressures should be kept below 50 cm H_2O to prevent barotrauma to the airway anastomosis.[137] FIo_2 is kept at the lowest level that keeps the Po_2 at or above 90 mm Hg. Early extubation after lung transplant for emphysema helps to avoid problems with overdistention of native emphysematous lung.[138] There have been case reports using OLV postoperatively because of hyperinflation of the native lung. Smiley reported a case of SLT for emphysema in which the patient received independent lung ventilation postoperatively for 6 days to prevent hyperinflation of the native lung.[139] Hyperinflation of the native lung was not a problem with spontaneous ventilation. Popple reported the use of a similar strategy in a case in which the patient received SLT for lymphangioleiomyomatosis.[140] The native lung exhibited auto-PEEP postoperatively, which prolonged the process of weaning the patient from mechanical ventilation.

Extubation is accomplished in the setting of good allograft lung function, satisfactory conscious state, adequate analgesia, and stable hemodynamic state. Attempts to wean patients from mechanical ventilation occur as soon as possible, except in cases of pulmonary hypertension. Patients with pulmonary hypertension who receive SLTs have 90–95% of the cardiac output in the grafted lung. Heavy sedation and muscle paralysis helps to limit the frequency and severity of hypertensive crises.

Systemic hypotension is common after lung transplantation, particularly if CPB was used during the procedure. It is typically characterized by decreased systemic vascular resistance, adequate filling pressures, and normal or elevated cardiac output.[141] Given the desirability of maintaining a negative fluid balance postoperatively, it is prudent to use vasopressors to maintain an adequate systemic arterial pressure rather than relying on a strategy of liberal fluid administration.

The reimplantation response (noncardiogenic pulmonary edema in the transplanted lung) is seen in 80% of patients.[142] Clinically, it presents as a combination of poor pulmonary compliance, compromised gas exchange, radiographic infiltrates, and disordered fluid elimination. It represents either reperfusion injury or preservation injury. The increased frequency of this response with prolonged ischemic times supports the argument that it is a result of preservation injury. Diagnoses that should be excluded are hypervolemia, left ventricular failure, rejection, infection, and atelectasis.

Negative fluid balance is produced postoperatively, with inotropes being used to support hemodynamic status instead of additional intravascular volume. Diuretics are administered with a goal of reaching a body weight 2–3 kg below preoperative weight.[143] Attention must be paid to the cyclosporine dose and blood level during this period of diuresis. The dose of furosemide typically must be increased during the first week of therapy.

Postoperative Analgesia

Epidural analgesia has become standard therapy for pain control after thoracic procedures.[144, 145] Triantafillou reported the comparison of lumbar epidural analgesia with continuous morphine infusion to intravenous patient-controlled analgesia in patients who had undergone lung transplantation.[146] Patients receiving epidural morphine were extubated earlier (2.8 vs. 6.2 days) and had shorter stays in the ICU (4.9 vs. 9.66 days). Body reported the experience with thoracic epidural catheters using a mixture of bupivacaine with fentanyl or meperidine.[147] Epidural catheters were in place for an average of 7.6 days. There was a universal elevation of $PaCO_2$, which did not require reintubation of any patient. The elevated postoperative $PaCO_2$ is probably multifactorial in origin, with other possible etiologies (e.g., pre-existing hypercapnia, central action of epidural narcotics, fluid restriction, or use of diuretics).

Technical aspects of epidural catheter placement must be considered. Epidural catheters are preferentially placed with the patient in a sitting position to minimize dyspnea. Timing is an important issue when instituting epidural analgesia. The Lung Transplant Group at Washington University advocates placement of a lumbar epidural catheter before induction of anesthesia in patients in whom they expect to avoid CPB.[148] Their rationale is that many patients have normal coagulation status preoperatively but will develop coagulation disorders postoperatively. Placement of an epidural catheter preoperatively allows sufficient time for a clot to form in the event of a traumatic insertion before CPB being instituted.

The protocol at Saint Louis University Hospital is to place an epidural catheter postoperatively after testing the patient for coagulopathy. Our preference is placement of a thoracic epidural catheter, although lumbar catheters have been used successfully. Prothrombin time, partial thromboplastin time, platelet count, and bleeding time are confirmed to be in the normal range before catheter placement. After successful placement of the epidural catheter, we administer a bolus of preservative-free morphine (Duramorph) followed by an infusion of morphine (with a lumbar epidural catheter) or a mixture of bupivacaine and fentanyl (with a thoracic catheter). This protocol avoids the uncertainty about whether CPB will be used intraoperatively and expedites the start of the surgical procedure. There are few recommendations concerning the use of adjuvant analgesic agents. Nonsteroidal anti-inflammatory agents are avoided because of the possibility of cyclosporine-induced nephrotoxicity.[131]

Immunosuppression

A review of immunosuppressive agents is beyond the scope of this chapter. Interested readers are encouraged to refer to several comprehensive reviews of the subject[149–151] and to Chapter 17. This discussion is limited to the anesthetic effects of commonly used immunosuppressive agents.

Cyclosporine's activity is mediated by its ability to block the secretion of interleukin-2.[152] Three-fourths of patients receiving cyclosporine have hypertension, which is usually treated with diltiazem and an angiotensin-converting enzyme inhibitor.[133] Other adverse effects of cyclosporine include renal dysfunction, hepatic dysfunction, seizures, tremor, paresthesia, gingival hyperplasia, and hirsutism.[153] Trough levels of 100–300 ng/liter are therapeutic, whereas levels greater than 1,000 ng/liter are associated with renal toxicity.[152] Cyclosporine has also been shown to augment the effects of pentobarbital and fentanyl in mice.[154] Muscle relaxation with vecuronium is prolonged in patients receiving cyclosporine.[155]

Tacrolimus (FK506) is a macrolide immunosuppressant produced by *Streptomyces tsukubaensis*. It suppresses some humoral immunity but mostly suppresses cell-mediated reactions. It produces T-lymphocyte activation by an undefined mechanism. Mild-to-moderate hypertension is a common effect of FK506 treatment. It responds to treatment with commonly used antihypertensive drugs. Given FK506's ability to cause hyperkalemia, potassium-sparing diuretics are contraindicated. Thirty to 40% of liver transplant patients treated with FK506 develop nephrotoxicity. Neurotoxicity, as evidenced by tremor, headache, and changes in motor function, were noted in 55% of recipients. These patients respond to dosage adjustment. Seizures associated with high serum levels can develop. Patients receiving FK506 may develop an anaphylactic reaction. Use of FK506 leads to fewer episodes of acute and chronic rejection. There is a lower incidence of bacterial infections compared to cyclosporine but a higher incidence of fungal infections.[156]

Azathioprine acts on the DNA synthetic phase of the cellular cycle.[152] The use of azathioprine requires white blood cell (WBC) monitoring. If the WBC count falls below 4.0×10^9, the drug should be stopped. It may also cause hepatic dysfunction, specifically elevation of aspartate transaminase and alanine aminotransferase. Cyclophosphamide may be substituted for azathioprine in cases of hepatic impairment. Azathioprine may cause leukopenia, thrombocytopenia, macrocytic anemia, hepatitis, pancreatitis, and cholestatic jaundice.[153]

The effects of corticosteroids are well known to most anesthesiologists. Corticosteroids can cause obesity, cushingoid body habitus, hyperlipidemia, sodium retention, hypertension, cataracts, osteoporosis, peptic ulcer disease, diabetes, avascular necrosis, and, in children, growth retardation.[153]

Complications

In the early posttransplant period, mechanical complications of the airway and cardiac complications are the major causes of death. Eighty-three percent of deaths occur in the first 3 months after lung transplant.[142] Late deaths are the result of chronic rejection and its subsequent management. Infection often occurs during periods of supplemented immunosuppression. Hypoxemia after lung transplantation generally occurs because of pulmonary edema, rejection, or infection. Distinguishing between these clinical entities is aided by knowledge of their temporal relationship to the transplant. Bacterial pneumonia usually occurs after the second postoperative day, acute rejection after day 5, and cytomegalovirus (CMV) pneumonia after day 16.[157] These data help to focus clinical and laboratory investigation on the most likely diagnoses.

Donor lung dysfunction (DLD), defined as an increased alveolar-to-arterial oxygen gradient and decreased lung compliance in the presence of a persistent diffuse infiltrate on chest x-ray, has been described as a complication of lung transplantation in 20% of cases.[158] DLD may occur as a result of technical complications during surgery, as a result of a postoperative complication, or without an obvious precipitating event. The hallmark of care in these cases is the continuation of intensive supportive modalities, including ventilatory and nutritional support. DLD is not related to the length of donor ischemic time. Nitric oxide has been used to treat DLD. Adatia et al. have reported their results using nitric oxide in 10 patients with DLD and posttransplant pulmonary hypertension.[159] Nitric oxide results in lower pulmonary artery pressures, improved oxygenation, improved cardiac index, and stable systemic blood pressure.

Reperfusion injury occurs in 20% of recipients and consists of pulmonary edema, reduced lung compliance, and impaired gas exchange.[160] Reperfusion pulmonary edema is probably related to graft ischemia, preservation technique, manipulation of the organ, and the interruption of lymphatic drainage.[161] Pulmonary edema is not cardiogenic in etiology in the majority of cases. Conventional treatment of this syndrome consists of maintaining ventilation with the use of PEEP and, in severe cases, using inverse-ratio ventilation and extracorporeal membrane oxygenation (ECMO). A novel treatment modality in the form of nebulized synthetic surfactant has been reported.[160] Treatment with nebulized surfactant resulted in improved lung compliance and improved oxygenation. The mechanisms of improvement are unknown.

Chronic and acute rejection are frequent complications of lung transplantation. Hyperacute rejection is rare in lung transplantation, however, with an incidence of 1%.[141] Clinical signs of acute rejection include dyspnea, fatigue, dry cough, low-grade fever, hypoxemia, development of a new radiographic infiltrate, and at least a 10% decrease in FEV_1.[161] Differential diagnosis of acute rejection includes infection (viral and pneumocystic pneumonia), reperfusion injury, and lymphoproliferative disorders. Histologic specimens obtained by fiberoptic bronchoscopy and biopsy are needed to confirm the diagnosis. Acute graft rejection is characterized histologically by perivascular mononuclear infiltrates, which may be accompanied by lymphocytic bronchitis or bronchiolitis.[162] The development of acute rejection is one of the most important factors for developing chronic rejection.[161] Most recipients of lung transplants have at least one episode of acute rejection within the first 3 weeks, which is easily treatable with high-dose corticosteroids or OKT3 along with optimization of cyclosporine and azathioprine dosage.[163]

Chronic rejection is histologically described as OB, an obstructive and restrictive condition caused by progressive obstruction of bronchioles in the setting of a chronic inflammatory response in the distal airways. Histologically, OB is characterized by the progressive submucosal scarring of membranous and respiratory bronchioles.[164] It results in a decrease in FEV_1 and increasing dyspnea on exercise. The FEV_1 is thought to most closely correlate with other clinical parameters.[165] Because of the importance of early detection of decreases in FEV_1, patients are asked to maintain a daily log of their medical regimen, respiratory symptoms, and results of daily spirometry, including FEV_1. The incidence of OB is approximately 25% in long-term survivors.[163] The treatment of OB consists of antilymphocyte agents (antithymocyte globulin or OKT3) along with corticosteroids.[166]

Mortality in patients with OB does not usually occur from respiratory failure but from sepsis occurring during periods of intense immunosuppression.[167] Persistent cases of OB are an indication for retransplantation. OB does not recur in an accelerated manner after retransplantation.[168]

Infection is twice as common in the lung transplant population as it is in heart and liver transplant recipients.[141] Infection is the leading cause of death after lung transplantation at the University of Toronto.[169] The lung is susceptible to bacterial infection because of its direct communication to the atmosphere as well as decreased or absent mucociliary function in the grafted organ. Bacterial pneumonia accounts for 66% of infections in data reported by the Toronto Lung Transplant Group.[170] Gram-negative organisms, such as *Klebsiella*, *Pseudomonas,* and *H. influenzae*, are the most common pathogens isolated. One-third of lung transplant recipients acquire pneumonia during the first 2 weeks after transplantation.[167] This early incidence of pneumonia represents the airway colonization that occurs with intubation and mechanical ventilation of the donor. Cultures taken at the time of organ harvest help to guide early antibiotic therapy. In general, bacterial pneumonia typically occurs in the first 6 months after transplantation.[171]

CMV infection is the most common infection after lung transplantation, occurring 1–4 months after transplant.[141] It can be diagnosed by lung biopsy (open or bronchoscopic) or bronchoalveolar lavage. CMV infection is associated with an increased incidence of chronic rejection. Ganciclovir is effective treatment for CMV pneumonia and is occasionally used for prophylaxis. Some published data indicate that CMV mismatch (donor positive, recipient negative), absence of CMV prophylaxis, and development of CMV disease are markers for increased mortality.[172]

Fungal infections occur early and late in the postoperative course. *Candida albicans* is the most common fungus isolated in the postoperative period and is usually associated with colonization of the airway.[171] *Candida* pneumonitis is relatively rare despite its frequent presence. Disseminated or locally invasive *Candida* can be treated with amphotericin B or fluconazole. *Aspergillus* is also seen in as many as 20–40% of cases and is considered a more serious infection than *Candida*. *Aspergillus* may present as bronchitis, pneumonia, or disseminated aspergillosis, with the site of infection being the transplanted lung.[171] Bronchitis is successfully treated with itraconazole or aerosolized amphotericin, whereas pneumonia is treated with intravenous amphotericin. (See Chapter 18 for a more detailed discussion of infections associated with transplantation.)

The high incidence of airway complications has resulted in cessation of performance of en bloc DLT.[12, 173] Approximately 15% of patients develop airway anastomotic complications (stenosis, bronchomalacia, or dehiscence) after SLT and BLT.[174] Airway stents are placed when there is a 50% or greater reduction in lumen size.[170] Placement of endobronchial stents improves results in pulmonary function tests, with FEV_1 improving from 58% of predicted to 77% of predicted.[175]

Abdominal complications have been described as a major source of morbidity and mortality after lung transplantation.[176–178] These complications included ileus, ischemic bowel, colitis, colonic perforation, and cholelithiasis. There was a delay of 6 days between presentation of symptoms and diagnosis and treatment. Patients in this series underwent a variety of diagnostic and therapeutic procedures, including colonoscopy, colectomy, small bowel resection, cholecystectomy, and liver biopsy. Abdominal pathology accounted for 22% of deaths after lung transplantation at the University of Minnesota. Colonic perforation had a 50% mortality rate in one small series.[177] It has been noted that patients who required abdominal surgery had a higher incidence of rejection, higher steroid dosages, and a lower posttransplant FEV_1 compared to patients who did not require such surgical intervention.[178] In addition to these complications, symptomatic gastroparesis is a frequent complication of lung transplantation.[179] The mechanism of gastroparesis is unclear and is only partially responsive to metoclopramide or cisapride.

Pulmonary venous stenosis was found in 29% of patients on postoperative TEE after lung transplantation.[180] The degree of obstruction correlated with short-term outcome. Clinical presentation of pulmonary venous abnormalities may include hypoxemia and interstitial infiltrates, which mimic other postoperative morbidities such as infection, rejection, and reperfusion injury.[181] It is therefore important to consider pulmonary venous obstruction, particularly when other causes of hypoxemia and interstitial infiltrates on chest x-ray have been ruled out. Complete obstruction of a pulmonary vein results in lobar infarction within 4–6 hours.[182] Once

a lobe has infarcted, the treatment options are either lobectomy or retransplantation. A novel approach reported by Schmid is the use of tissue plasminogen activator to lyse the thrombus.[183]

Pulmonary emboli are a unique risk to the transplanted lung because there is no collateral bronchial circulation. Prophylaxis against deep venous thrombosis is necessary postoperatively. Six percent of patients had symptomatic pulmonary emboli in one series from the University of Minnesota.[184] All patients in this series underwent postoperative ventilation-perfusion scans as part of their routine postoperative testing. Follow-up ventilation-perfusion scans were done at 6 months and 1 year after transplantation. Presenting symptoms included pleuritic chest pain, cardiac arrhythmias (atrial fibrillation or supraventricular tachycardia), and hemoptysis. Three of seven patients had resolution of their pulmonary emboli after selective pulmonary artery infusion of urokinase. The mortality rate after developing a pulmonary embolus is high: 42% of those developing pulmonary emboli died. Based on this experience, the authors recommended that these patients be treated as a high-risk group for developing pulmonary emboli, receiving routine ventilation-perfusion scans and lower-extremity duplex scanning. Confirmation of a suspected pulmonary embolus should be obtained by pulmonary angiography if the clinical suspicion is high.

Posttransplantation lymphoproliferative disorder (PTLD) is a complication of immunosuppression.[152] PTLD is defined as a predominantly B-lymphocyte tumor that occurs after transplantation.[185] PTLD may occur in the transplanted organ or in other locations. It may initially appear as an incidental change on chest x-ray, such as nodules or an unexplained infiltrate. Symptoms are vague and include low-grade fever, weight loss, fatigue, and nonspecific gastrointestinal complaints.[186] Physical findings are usually limited to mild adenopathy. Abdominal involvement may present as an acute abdomen. The cornerstone of therapy is reduction of immunosuppression. Chemotherapy, irradiation, or both may be necessary if there is no response to reduction in immunosuppression. Patients with head and neck or abdominal involvement appear to have the best outcomes. Cases of abdominal PTLD can be treated by curative resection. Despite this, data from the St. Louis International Lung Transplant Registry indicate that 7% of deaths in lung transplant recipients are caused by malignancy.[153]

Table 7-7. Actuarial Survival after Lung Transplantation

Center	Type	Number	1-Year Survival (%)	2-Year Survival (%)
University of Toronto[175]	SLT	45	65	58
University of Toronto[175]	DLT	37	69	69
San Antonio[54]	SLT	22	77	73
Washington University[196]	SLT	73	87	87
Washington University[196]	BLT	58	76	73
University of Pittsburgh[197]	SLT	68	70	—
University of Pittsburgh[197]	BLT/DLT	80	65	—
International Registry[198]	SLT	1,943	70	60
International Registry[198]	BLT/DLT	943	70	60

SLT = single-lung transplantation; DLT = double-lung transplantation; BLT = bilateral single-lung transplantation.

Outcome

Overall Function

Improvements in spirometry occur for the first 2 months after transplantation.[167] Improvements are usually seen in total lung capacity, vital capacity, FEV_1, and carbon monoxide diffusing capacity of the lungs.[187] Hypercapnia persists for 2–3 weeks in patients with preoperative hypercapnia. Blunting of the ventilatory response curve in response to carbon dioxide occurs in these patients and resolves at the same time the hypercapnia resolves.[167]

Six-minute walk test results are 500–700 meters after HLT and SLT.[66] Maximum oxygen uptake ($\dot{V}o_2$) is reduced to 44.2% of predicted after SLT and 48.5% of predicted in patients after DLT.[188] This decrease is not due to limitations in ventilatory parameters. Deconditioning appears to play a role in this.

Hemodynamic parameters improve immediately after SLT for pulmonary hypertension as exhibited by decreased pulmonary artery pressures and increases in cardiac output.[189] RVEF increased in patients after both SLT and DLT for a variety of indications.[190] Cardiac index improves significantly only in BLT or HLT.[191]

Survival

Patients receiving SLT rather than BLT for COPD tend to have less physiologic reserve in the setting of illness.[192] Changes in pulmonary function tests in patients receiving SLT are impressive. In a series reported from Papworth Hospital, FEV_1 improved from 17.8% of predicted to 54% of predicted 6

months after transplantation.[193] Actuarial survival in this series is 82% at 1 year and 74% at 3 years.[194] Arterial blood gases improve after SLT with an increase in Pao_2 from 58 mm Hg to 86 mm Hg 3 months after SLT.[194] Results of a 6-minute walk test improve from 99 meters to 587 meters at 6 months.[195]

The reported survival data from large centers are summarized in Table 7-7. The results from Washington University are particularly impressive for SLTs. The inference is that large surgical volume produces superior results.

Survival is best in patients with emphysema and worst in patients with pulmonary hypertension.[167] The results in the pediatric population are not as good as in adults. Survival data from the International Lung Transplant Registry indicate an actuarial survival of 65% at 1 year for pediatric lung transplant.[199] More current results indicate an actuarial survival of 73% at 1 year.[200]

Financial

The cost of a lung transplant is approximately $150,000 (U.S. currency) for the first year and $20,000 annually thereafter.[201] The Lung Transplant Group at the University of Toronto has estimated the cost per year of life gained at $63,000 (Canadian currency).[202] Major commercial insurers started coverage for lung transplants in 1990–1991 as the techniques became an accepted form of therapy for lung failure.[203] By comparison, the average yearly cost of conventional therapy for a patient with cystic fibrosis is $27,500.[204] Patients feel better after lung transplantation, with 80% of them able to return to their former employment.[137]

Future Strategies

Due to the shortage of donor lungs, many patients die before transplantation. This reality has spurred the investigation of other modalities of treating end-stage lung disease. Use of these modalities is intended to support patients until a donor lung can be found or to eliminate the need for transplantation.

Nonsurgical treatments of lung disease are increasing. The use of genetic engineering in treating patients with cystic fibrosis is currently under investigation. One strategy involves the use of recombinant human DNase (rhDNase) to decrease the viscosity of secretions. The use of rhDNase has improved FEV_1 and FVC[205] and decreased the use of parenteral antibiotics.[206] A more direct approach is the use of gene transfer to transfer normal genes for cystic fibrosis transmembrane conductor regulator to replace the defective genes in patients with cystic fibrosis.[207]

Emphysema caused by alpha$_1$-antitrypsin deficiency may be preventable in the future. A commercial form of the enzyme, Prolastin, is currently available. Prolastin (Miles Inc., West Haven, CT) is a lyophilized preparation of alpha$_1$-proteinase inhibitor that is pooled from the serum of normal donors. It is indicated for the chronic replacement therapy of individuals having congenital alpha$_1$-antitrypsin deficiency.

The prevalence of Eisenmenger's syndrome should decrease in the future as congenital heart disease is surgically corrected earlier in life, before pulmonary hypertension develops. The development of catheter-delivered devices to close atrial septal defects and ventricular septal defects may allow more patients to have early cardiac repair.

The use of mechanical support devices has been disappointing to date. There have been case reports of using ECMO to bridge patients to transplant. This has occurred in the setting of acute lung failure (i.e., ARDS) or in the case of early graft dysfunction refractory to more conservative treatment. This is not possible in the United States because a lung cannot be obtained on short notice for such a purpose. Demertizis reported a DLT in a patient who developed ARDS.[208] The patient was supported by ECMO for 4 days before transplant. Jurmann described two patients supported by ECMO after graft failure.[209] The first patient was placed on ECMO once a donor was identified for retransplan-

tation. The total time of ECMO was 8 hours. The second patient required the use of ECMO for 232 hours, until retransplantation was possible. The shortage of donor organs precludes the routine use of ECMO as a bridge to subsequent transplantation.

Lung transplantation is usually not offered to patients supported by mechanical ventilators. The exception to this occurs when a patient has already been fully evaluated for transplantation and has been awaiting an organ for long enough that obtaining one is likely.[28] The concern with patients who are on ventilators is that the trachea will be colonized and that they will become deconditioned while ventilated.

Lung volume reduction is an attractive new surgical option for patients with emphysema. The initial concept was described by Otto Brantigan in 1959.[210] Brantigan proposed that reducing overall lung volume would restore the outward elastic pull on small airways and reduce expiratory airway obstruction. His initial series was not well received because of skepticism and because of the lack of objective outcome data. Cooper has reported the results of his lung volume reduction efforts.[211] The operation consists of a median sternotomy with removal of 20–30% of each lung by using a linear stapling device to perform nonanatomic resections. Results after 1 year reveal an increase in FEV_1 of 68%, an increase in FVC of 32%, and an increase in the distance covered during a 6-minute walk test by 25%. Gaissert reported the results of bilateral lung volume reduction performed via median sternotomy in patients who were otherwise eligible for lung transplantation.[212] The functional results were comparable to those achieved after SLT for emphysema and offered the advantage of avoiding the complications of infection and immunosuppression.

Advances in the techniques of thoracoscopy and linear stapling devices have allowed lung reduction to be performed using this less invasive technique. Naunheim reported the results at Saint Louis University in 50 patients undergoing unilateral thoracoscopic lung reduction.[213] Keller has compared results of this type of surgery to SLT.[214] Although the patients receiving SLT had superior functional results, the patients receiving lung reduction had acceptable improvement in respiratory function. Zenati has reported the use of thoracoscopic lung volume reduction surgery as a bridge to lung transplantation in two patients.[215] Our experience at Saint Louis University includes three patients who underwent SLT after unilateral thoracoscopic lung reduction. In all cases, the patients were able to discontinue use of corticosteroids and improve their exercise performance during a pretransplant rehabilitation protocol that they were unable to tolerate previously.

Diversion of patients into a lung-reduction program may increase the number of available lungs for patients with other diagnoses while avoiding transplant-related complications in these patients. Issues that must be resolved include the duration of benefit after lung reduction, the optimal type of surgery, and the optimal timing for eventual transplantation.

These examples of nontransplant forms of treating terminal lung disease are expanding as the underlying mechanisms of disease are uncovered. This type of approach allows earlier and more effective therapy for all types of diagnoses.

Conclusions

Since the early 1990s, lung transplantation has become an accepted mode of treatment for severe pulmonary disease. Survival rates and recipient's functional capacity continue to improve for all types of lung transplantations. Anesthesiologists have contributed to these developments through their intraoperative care, their expertise in the ICU, and advances in analgesic techniques. Anesthesiologists are involved in the care of these patients during transplantation and afterward, as they present for nonpulmonary surgery. Lessons learned in the care of these patients help practitioners care for patients with respiratory difficulties.

References

1. Metras D. Henri Metras: a pioneer in lung transplantation. J Heart Lung Transplant 1992;11:1213–1216.
2. Hardin CA, Kittle CF. Experiences with transplantation of the lung. Science 1954;119:97–98.
3. Shumacker HB Jr. A surgeon to remember: Vladimir Demikhov. Ann Thorac Surg 1994;58:1196–1198.
4. Hardy JD, Webb WR, Dalton ML Jr, Walker GR Jr. Lung homotransplantation in man: report of the initial case. JAMA 1963;186:1065–1074.
5. Veith FJ, Kamholz SL, Mollenkoff FP, Montefusco CM. Lung transplantation. Transplantation 1983;35:271–278.
6. Derom F, Barbier F, Ringoir S, et al. Ten-month survival after lung homotransplantation in man. J Thorac Cardiovasc Surg 1971;61:835–846.
7. Veith FJ, Montefusco CM. Long-term fate of lung autografts charged with providing total pulmonary function. II. Hemodynamic, functional and angiographic studies. Ann Surg 1979;190:654–656.
8. Reitz BA, Wallwork JL, Hunt SA, et al. Heart-lung transplantation—successful therapy for patients with pulmonary vascular disease. N Engl J Med 1982;306:557–564.
9. Cooper JD, Pearson FG, Patterson GA, et al. Technique of successful lung transplantation in humans. J Thorac Cardiovasc Surg 1987;93:173–181.
10. Grossman RF, Frost A, Zamel N, et al. Results of single-lung transplantation for bilateral pulmonary fibrosis. The Toronto Lung Transplant Group. N Engl J Med 1990;322:727–733.
11. Patterson GA. Bilateral lung transplant: indications and technique. Semin Thorac Cardiovasc Surg 1992;4:95–100.
12. Patterson GA, Todd TR, Cooper JD, et al. Airway complications after double lung transplantation. J Thorac Cardiovasc Surg 1990;99:14–21.
13. Pasque MK, Cooper JD, Kaiser LR, et al. Improved technique for bilateral lung transplantation: rationale and initial clinical experience. Ann Thorac Surg 1990;49:785–791.
14. Cooper JD. Current status of lung transplantation. Transplant Proc 1991;23:2107–2114.
15. Hunninghake GW, Kalica AR. Approaches to the treatment of pulmonary fibrosis. Am J Respir Crit Care Med 1995;151:915–918.
16. Peterson KL, DeCampli WM, Feeley TW, Starnes VA. Blood loss and transfusion requirements in cystic fibrosis patients undergoing heart-lung or lung transplantation. J Cardiothorac Vasc Anesth 1995;9:59–62.
17. Starnes VA, Lewiston N, Theodore J, et al. Cystic fibrosis: target population for lung transplantation in North America in the 1990s. J Thorac Cardiovasc Surg 1992;103:1008–1014.
18. Aitken ML, Fiel SB. Cystic fibrosis. Dis Mon 1993; 39:11–52.
19. Fiel SB, FitzSimmons S, Schidlow D. Evolving demographics of cystic fibrosis. Semin Respir Crit Care Med 1994;15:349–355.
20. Crystal RG. Chairman's summary. Am J Respir Crit Care Med 1955;151:S45–S46.
21. Rubin LJ. Primary pulmonary hypertension. Chest 1993;104:236–250.
22. D'Alonzo GE, Barst RJ, Ayres SM, et al. Survival in patients with primary pulmonary hypertension. Ann Intern Med 1991;115:343–349.
23. Barst RJ, Rubin LJ, McGoon MD, et al. Survival in primary pulmonary hypertension with long-term continuous intravenous prostacyclin. Ann Intern Med 1994; 121:409–415.

24. Rubin LJ, Mendoza J, Hood M, et al. Treatment of primary pulmonary hypertension with continuous intravenous prostacyclin (epoprostenol). Ann Intern Med 1990;112:485–491.

25. Fuster V, Steele PM, Edwards WD, et al. Primary pulmonary hypertension: natural history and the importance of thrombosis. Circulation 1984;70:580–587.

26. Rich S, Kaufmann E, Levy PS. The effect of high doses of calcium-channel blockers on survival in primary pulmonary hypertension. N Engl J Med 1992;327:76–81.

27. Schafers HJ, Wagner TOF, Demertzis S, et al. Preoperative corticosteroids: a contraindication to lung transplantation? Chest 1992;102:1522–1525.

28. Low DE, Trulock EP, Kaiser LR, et al. Lung transplantation of ventilator-dependent patients. Chest 1992;101: 8–11.

29. Marshall SE, Kramer MR, Lewiston NJ, et al. Selection and evaluation of recipients for heart-lung and lung transplantation. Chest 1990;98:1488–1494.

30. Trulock EP. Lung transplantation. Am J Respir Crit Care Med 1997;155:789–818.

31. Shumway SJ. Bilateral Sequential Lung Transplantation. In SJ Shumway, NE Shumway (eds), Thoracic Transplantation. Cambridge, MA: Blackwell, 1995; 415–419.

32. Jenkinson SG, Levine SM. Lung transplantation. Dis Mon 1994;40:5–38.

33. U.S. Scientific Registry for Transplant Recipients and the Organ Procurement and Transplantation Network. www.unos.org

34. Bollinger RR. The Role of UNOS in Thoracic Organ Transplantation. In SJ Shumway, NE Shumway (eds), Thoracic Transplantation. Cambridge, MA: Blackwell, 1995;141–148.

35. Hayden AM, Robert RC, Kriett JM, et al. Primary diagnosis predicts prognosis of lung transplant candidates. Transplantation 1993;55:1048–1050.

36. Glanville AR, Burke CM, Theodore J, Robin ED. Primary pulmonary hypertension—length of survival in patients referred for heart-lung transplantation. Chest 1987;91:675–681.

37. Patterson GA, Cooper JD. Lung Transplantation. In TW Shields (ed), General Thoracic Surgery. Baltimore: Williams & Wilkins, 1994;1064–1091.

38. Egan TM, Kaiser LR, Cooper JD. Lung transplantation. Curr Probl Surg 1989;679–751.

39. Kerem E, Reisman J, Corey M, et al. Prediction of mortality in patients with cystic fibrosis. N Engl J Med 1992;326:1187–1191.

40. Sharples L, Hathaway T, Dennis C, et al. Prognosis of patients with cystic fibrosis awaiting heart and lung transplantation. J Heart Lung Transplant 1993;12:669–674.

41. Kaiser LR, Cooper JD. The current status of lung transplantation. Adv Surg 1992;25:259–307.

42. Griffith BP, Zenati M. The pulmonary donor. Clin Chest Med 1990;11:217–226.

43. Colice GL, Matthay MA, Bass E, Matthay RA. Neurogenic pulmonary edema. Am Rev Respir Dis 1984;130: 941–948.

44. Puskas JD, Winton TL, Miller JD, et al. Unilateral donor lung dysfunction does not preclude successful contralateral single lung transplantation. J Thorac Cardiovasc Surg 1992;103:1015–1018.

45. Davis RD Jr, Pasque MK. Pulmonary transplantation. Ann Surg 1995;221:14–28.

46. Sundaresan S, Semenkovich J, Ochoa L, et al. Successful outcome of lung transplantation is not compromised by the use of marginal donor lungs. J Thorac Cardiovasc Surg 1995;109:1075–1080.

47. Waters PF. Lung transplantation. Trans Assoc Life Insurance Med Dir Am 1992;75:48–54.

48. Kirk AJB, Colquhoun IW, Dark JH. Lung preservation: a review of current practice and future directions. Ann Thorac Surg 1993;56:990–1000.

49. Todd TR, Goldberg M, Koshal A, et al. Separate extraction of cardiac and pulmonary grafts from a single organ donor. Ann Thorac Surg 1988;46:356–359.

50. Sundaresan S, Trachiotis GD, Aoe M, et al. Donor lung procurement: assessment and operative technique. Ann Thorac Surg 1993;56:1409–1413.

51. Egan TM. Lung preservation. Semin Thorac Cardiovasc Surg 1992;4:83–89.

52. Kawahara K, Itoyanagi N, Takahashi T, et al. Transplantation of canine lung allografts preserved in UW solution for 24 hours. Transplantation 1993;55:15–18.

53. Hardesty RL, Aeba R, Armitage JM, et al. A clinical trial of University of Wisconsin solution for pulmonary preservation. J Thorac Cardiovasc Surg 1993;105:660–666.

54. Calhoon JH, Grover FL, Gibbons WJ, et al. Single lung transplantation: alternative indications and technique. J Thorac Cardiovasc Surg 1991;101:816–825.

55. Tanoue LT. Lung transplantation. Lung 1992;170: 187–200.

56. Tsang V, Hodson ME, Yacoub MH. Lung transplantation for cystic fibrosis. Br Med Bull 1992;48:949–971.

57. Shennib H, Massard G, Gauthier R, et al. Single lung transplantation for cystic fibrosis: is it an option? J Heart Lung Transplant 1993;12:288–293.

58. Forty J, Hasan A, Gould FK, et al. Single lung transplantation with simultaneous contralateral pneumonectomy for cystic fibrosis. J Heart Lung Transplant 1994;13:727–730.

59. Egan TM. Single-Lung Transplantation. In SJ Shumway, NE Shumway (eds), Thoracic Transplantation. Cambridge, MA: Blackwell, 1995;395–405.

60. Glanville A, Rowland M, MacDonald P, et al. Native lung pathology after single lung transplantation [abstract]. J Heart Lung Transplant 1994;13:S32.

61. McCarthy PM, Rosenkranz ER, White RD, et al. Single-lung transplantation with atrial septal defect repair for Eisenmenger's syndrome. Ann Thorac Surg 1991; 52:300–303.

62. Fremes SE, Patterson GA, Williams WG, et al. Single lung transplantation and closure of patent ductus arte-

riosus for Eisenmenger's syndrome. J Thorac Cardio-vasc Surg 1990;100:1–5.

63. Khaghani A, Tadjkarimi S, Al-Kattan K, et al. Wrapping the anastomosis with omentum or an internal mammary artery pedicle does not improve bronchial healing after single lung transplantation: results of a randomized clinical trial. J Heart Lung Transplant 1994;13:767–773.

64. Bains MS, Ginsberg RJ, Jones WG II, et al. The clamshell incision: an improved approach to bilateral pulmonary and mediastinal tumor. Ann Thorac Surg 1994;58:30–33.

65. Bisson A, Bonnette P. A new technique for double lung transplantation: "bilateral single lung" transplantation. J Thorac Cardiovasc Surg 1992;103:40–46.

66. Dark JH. Lung transplantation. Transplant Proc 1994; 26:1708–1709.

67. Starnes VA, Barr ML, Cohen RG. Lobar transplantation: indications, technique and outcome. J Thorac Cardiovasc Surg 1994;108:403–411.

68. Schenkel FA, Barr ML, Cohen RG, et al. Living-related pulmonary transplantation: an evolving role for the cardiothoracic transplant program [abstract]. J Heart Lung Transplant 1994;13:S44.

69. Cohen RG, Barr ML, Stares VA. Lobar Pulmonary Transplantation. In SJ Shumway, NE Shumway (eds), Thoracic Transplantation. Cambridge, MA: Blackwell, 1995;406–414.

70. Starnes VA, Barr ML, Cohen RG, et al. Bilateral living-related lobar transplantation for cystic fibrosis: initial experience [abstract]. J Heart Lung Transplant 1994;13: S57.

71. Kitamura M, Stares VA, Tagusari O, et al. Segmental flow-resistance relationship in pulmonary lobar transplantation: possibility for donor lobe evaluation in pediatric lung transplantation. J Heart Lung Transplant 1994;13:319–324.

72. Theodore J, Lewiston N. Lung transplantation comes of age. N Engl J Med 1990;322:772–774.

73. Howard DK, Iademarco EJ, Trulock EP: The role of cardiopulmonary exercise testing in lung and heart-lung transplantation. Clin Chest Med 1994;15:405–420.

74. Cahalin L, Pappagianopoulos P, Prevost S, et al. The relationship of the 6-min walk test to maximal oxygen consumption in transplant candidates with end-stage lung disease. Chest 1995;108:452–459.

75. Thaik CM, Semigram MJ, Ginns L, et al. Evaluation of ischemic heart disease in potential lung transplant recipients. J Heart Lung Transplant 1995;14:257–266.

76. Vigneswaran WT, McDougall JC, Olson LJ, et al. Right ventricular assessment in patients presenting for lung transplantation. Transplantation 1993;55: 1051–1055.

77. Gorcsan JG III, Edwards TD, Ziady GM, et al. Transesophageal echocardiography to evaluate patients with severe pulmonary hypertension for lung transplantation. Ann Thorac Surg 1995;59:717–722.

78. Keller CA, Ohar J, Ruppel G, et al. Right ventricular function in patients with severe COPD evaluated for lung transplantation. Chest 1995;107:1510–1516.

79. Conacher ID. Isolated lung transplantation: a review of problems and guide to anaesthesia. Br J Anaesth 1988;61:468–474.

80. Myles PS, Weeks AM, Buckland MR, et al. Anesthesia for bilateral sequential lung transplantation: experience of 64 cases. J Cardiothorac Vasc Anesth 1997;11:177–183.

81. Singh H, Bossard R. Perioperative anaesthetic considerations for patients undergoing lung transplantation. Can J Anaesth 1997;44:284–299.

82. Bracken CA, Gurkowski MA, Naples JJ. Lung transplantation: historical perspective, current concepts, and anesthetic considerations. J Cardiothorac Vasc Anesth 1997;11:220–241.

83. Soberman MS, Kraenzler EJ, Licina M, et al. Airway management during bilateral sequential lung transplantation for cystic fibrosis. Ann Thorac Surg 1994;58: 892–894.

84. Myles PS, Weeks AM. Alpha 1-antitrypsin deficiency: circulatory arrest following induction of anaesthesia. Anaesth Intensive Care 1992;20:358–362.

85. Siegel LC. Choice of anesthetic agent for thoracic surgery. Probl Anesth 1990;4:249–263.

86. Benumof JL. One-lung ventilation and hypoxic pulmonary vasoconstriction: implications for anesthetic management. Anesth Analg 1985;64:821–833.

87. Schulte-Sasse U, Hess W, Tarnow J. Pulmonary vascular responses to nitrous oxide in patients with normal and high pulmonary vascular resistance. Anesthesiology 1982;57:9–13.

88. Triantafillou AN. Anesthetic Considerations. In GA Patterson, L Couraud (eds), Lung Transplantation. Amsterdam: Elsevier, 1995;171–190.

89. Triantafillou AN, Heerdt PM. Lung transplantation. Int Anesthesiol Clin 1991;29:87–109.

90. Conacher ID, Paes ML. Mixed venous oxygen saturation during lung transplantation. J Cardiothorac Vasc Anesth 1994;8:671–674.

91. Demajo WA. Pulmonary Transplantation. In JA Kaplan (ed), Thoracic Anesthesia. New York: Churchill Livingstone, 1991;555–562.

92. Triantafillou AN, Heerdt PM, Pasque MK, et al. Immediate improvement of pulmonary hemodynamics and right ventricular function after single lung transplantation for primary pulmonary hypertension [abstract]. Circulation 1991;84:1277.

93. Despotis GJ, Karanikolas M, Triantafillou AN, et al. Pressure gradient across the pulmonary artery anastomosis during lung transplantation. Ann Thorac Surg 1995;60:630–634.

94. Wahr JA, Tremper KK. Continuous intravascular blood gas monitoring. J Cardiothorac Vasc Anesth 1994;8: 342–353.

95. Greenblott GB, Tremper KK, Barker SJ, et al. Continuous blood gas monitoring with an intraarterial optode

during one-lung anesthesia. J Cardiothorac Vasc Anesth 1991;5:365–367.

96. Haller M, Kilger E, Briegel J, et al. Continuous intra-arterial blood gas monitoring in patients with severe respiratory failure [abstract]. Anesthesiology 1993;79:A566.

97. Groh J, Haller M, Kilger E, et al. Continuous blood gas monitoring during lung transplantation [abstract]. Anesthesiology 1994;81:A617.

98. Bardoczky GI, deFrancquen P, Engelman E, Capello M. Continuous monitoring of pulmonary mechanics with the sidestream spirometer during lung transplantation. J Cardiothorac Vasc Anesth 1992;6:731–734.

99. Jellinek H, Hiesmayr M, Simon P, et al. Arterial to end-tidal CO_2 tension difference after bilateral lung transplantation. Crit Care Med 1993;21:1035–1040.

100. Brown MJ, Licina MG, Savage RM, et al. Transesophageal echocardiography should be used during anesthesia for lung transplantation [abstract]. Anesthesiol 1994;81:A547.

101. Rogers J, Sharp T, Hantler C, et al. Is conventional ventilation adequate in COPD patients during single lung transplantation (SLT) [abstract]? Anesthesiology 1990;73:A1184.

102. Alfery D, Benumof JL, Trousdale FR. Improving oxygenation during one lung ventilation: the effects of PEEP and blood flow restoration to the non-ventilated lung. Anesthesiology 1981;55:381.

103. Hogue CW. Effectiveness of low levels of nonventilated lung continuous positive airway pressure in improving arterial oxygenation during one-lung ventilation. Anesth Analg 1994;79:364–367.

104. Froese AB, Bryan AC. High frequency ventilation. Am Rev Respir Dis 1987;135:1363–1374.

105. Heres EK, Shulman MS, Krenis LJ, Moon R. High-frequency ventilation with a conventional anesthetic ventilator during cardiac surgery. J Cardiothorac Vasc Anesth 1995;9:63–65.

106. Robinson RJS, Shennib H, Noirclerc M. Slow-rate, high-pressure ventilation: a method of management of difficult transplant recipients during sequential double lung transplantation for cystic fibrosis. J Heart Lung Transplant 1994;13:779–784.

107. Bidani A, Tzouanaki AE, Cardenas VJ Jr, Zwischenberger JB. Permissive hypercapnia in acute respiratory failure. JAMA 1994;272:957–962.

108. Myles PS, Ryder IG, Weeks AM, et al. Diagnosis and management of dynamic hyperinflation during lung transplantation. J Cardiothorac Vasc Anesth 1997;11:100–104.

109. Rolly G, Malcolm-Thomas B, Verschraegen R, et al. Anesthesia during human lung transplantation and early postoperative respiratory treatment. Int Anesthesiol Clin 1972;10:79–92.

110. Quinlan JJ, Buffington CW. Deliberate hypoventilation in a patient with air trapping during lung transplantation. Anesthesiol 1993;78:1177–1181.

111. Krucylak PE, Naunheim KS, Keller CA, Baudendistel LJ. Anesthetic management of patients undergoing unilateral video-assisted lung reduction for treatment of end-stage emphysema. J Cardiothorac Vasc Anesth 1996;10:850–853.

112. Slinger P. The Univent tube is not the best method of providing one-lung ventilation. J Cardiothorac Vasc Anesth 1993;7:108–112.

113. Scheller MS, Kriett JM, Smith CM, Jamieson SW. Airway management during anesthesia for double-lung transplantation using a single-lumen endotracheal tube with an enclosed bronchial blocker. J Cardiothorac Vasc Anesth 1992;6:204–207.

114. Lunn RJ. Inhaled nitric oxide therapy. Mayo Clin Proc 1995;70:247–255.

115. Rajek MA, Hiesmayr M, Heilinger D, et al. Controlled trial on prevention of acute right failure after heart transplantation with nitric oxide inhalation or prostaglandin infusion [abstract]. Anesth Analg 1995;80:SCA101.

116. Triantafillou AN, Pohl MS, Okayabashi K, et al. Effects of inhaled nitric oxide and prostaglandin E_1 on hemodynamics and arterial oxygenation in patients following single lung transplantation [abstract]. Anesth Analg 1995;80:SCA40.

117. Said SI. Pulmonary metabolism of prostaglandin and vasoactive peptides. Ann Rev Physiol 1982;44:257–268.

118. Vincent JL, Carrier E, Pinky MR, et al. Prostaglandin E_1 infusion for right ventricular failure after cardiac transplantation. J Thorac Cardiovasc Surg 1992;103:33–39.

119. D'Ambra MN, LaRaia PJ, Philbin DM, et al. A new therapy for refractory right heart failure and pulmonary hypertension after mitral valve replacement. J Thorac Cardiovasc Surg 1985;89:567–572.

120. Rubin LJ, Groves BM, Reeves JT, et al. Prostacyclin-induced acute pulmonary vasodilation in primary pulmonary hypertension. Circulation 1982;66:334–338.

121. Walmrath D, Schneider T, Pilch J, et al. Aerosolised prostacyclin in adult respiratory distress syndrome. Lancet 1993;342:961–962.

122. Zwissler B, Welte M, Messmer K. Effects of inhaled prostacyclin as compared with inhaled nitric oxide on right ventricular performance in hypoxic pulmonary vasoconstriction. J Cardiothorac Vasc Anesth 1995;9:283–289.

123. Cooper JD, Vreim CE. Biology of lung preservation for transplantation. Am Rev Respir Dis 1992;146:803–807.

124. Karanikolas MS, Triantafillou AN, Pond CG, et al. Outcome of lung transplantation in relation to intraoperative crystalloid fluid administration [abstract]. Anesthesiology 1994;81:A1464.

125. Low DE, Trulock EP, Kaiser LR, et al. Morbidity, mortality, and early results of single versus bilateral lung transplantation for emphysema. J Thorac Cardiovasc Surg 1992;103:1119–1126.

126. Ramsey G, Sherman LA. Transfusion therapy in solid organ transplantation. Hematol Oncol Clin North Am 1994;8:1117–1129.

127. Miller JD, Patterson GA. Retransplantation following isolated lung transplantation. Semin Thorac Cardiovasc Surg 1992;4:122–125.

128. Westaby S. Aprotinin in perspective. Ann Thorac Surg 1993;55:1033–1041.

129. Egan TM, Detterbeck FC, Mill MR, et al. Improved results of lung transplantation for patients with cystic fibrosis. J Thorac Cardiovasc Surg 1995;109:224–235.

130. Triantafillou AN, Pasque MK, Huddleston CB, et al. Predictors, frequency, and indications for cardiopulmonary bypass during lung transplantation in adults. Ann Thorac Surg 1994;57:1248–1251.

131. Esmore DS, Brown R, Buckland M, et al. Techniques and results in bilateral sequential single lung transplantation. J Card Surg 1994;9:1–14.

132. de Hoyos A, Demajo W, Snell G, et al. Preoperative prediction for the use of cardiopulmonary bypass in lung transplantation. J Thorac Cardiovasc Surg 1993; 106:787–796.

133. Boscoe M. Anesthesia for patients with transplanted lungs and heart and lungs. Int Anesthesiol Clin 1995; 33:21–44.

134. Lee BS, Sarnquist FH, Starnes VA. Anesthesia for bilateral single-lung transplantation. J Cardiothorac Vasc Anesth 1992;6:201–203.

135. Aeba R, Griffith BP, Kormos RL, et al. Effect of cardiopulmonary bypass on early graft dysfunction in clinical lung transplantation. Ann Thorac Surg 1994; 57:715–722.

136. Fullerton DA, McIntyre RC Jr, Mitchell MB, et al. Lung transplantation with cardiopulmonary bypass exaggerates pulmonary vasomotor dysfunction in the transplanted lung. J Thorac Cardiovasc Surg 1995;109:212–217.

137. Judson MA. Clinical aspects of lung transplantation. Clin Chest Med 1993;14:335–357.

138. McCarthy PM. Immediate Postoperative Care After Thoracic Organ Transplantation. In SJ Shumway, NE Shumway (eds), Thoracic Transplantation. Cambridge, MA: Blackwell, 1995;205–218.

139. Smiley RM, Navedo AT, Kirby T, Schulman LL. Postoperative independent lung ventilation in a single-lung transplant recipient. Anesthesiology 1991;74:1144–1148.

140. Popple C, Higgins TL, McCarthy B, et al. Unilateral auto-PEEP in the recipient of a single lung transplant. Chest 1993;103:297–299.

141. de Hoyos A, Maurer JR. Complications following lung transplantation. Semin Thorac Cardiovasc Surg 1992;4:132–146.

142. Bierman MI, Stein KL, Stuart RS, Dauber JH. Critical care management of lung transplant recipients. Intensive Care Med 1991;6:135–142.

143. Todd TRJ. Early postoperative management following lung transplantation. Clin Chest Med 1990;11:259–267.

144. Lubenow TR, Faber LP, McCarthy RJ, et al. Postthoracotomy pain management using continuous epidural analgesia in 1,324 patients. Ann Thorac Surg 1994;58:924–930.

145. Kavanaugh BP, Katz J, Sandler AN. Pain control after thoracic surgery: a review of current techniques. Anesthesiology 1994;81:737–759.

146. Triantafillou AN, Heerdt PM, Hogue CW, et al. Epidural vs. intravenous morphine for postoperative pain management after lung transplantation [abstract]. Anesthesiology 1992;77:A858.

147. Body S, Fanciullo G, Ferrante M, et al. Thoracic epidural analgesia after lung transplantation [abstract]. Anesthesiology 1994;81:A1285.

148. Karanikolas MS, Triantafillou AN, Pond CG, et al. Epidural catheter placement in lung transplantation. Before or after the operation [abstract]? Anesth Analg 1995;80:SCA30.

149. Griffith BP, Hardesty RL, Armitage JM, et al. Acute rejection of lung allografts with various immunosuppressive protocols. Ann Thorac Surg 1992;54:846–851.

150. Griffith BP, Bando K, Hardesty RL, et al. A prospective randomized trial of FK506 versus cyclosporine after human pulmonary transplantation. Transplantation 1994;57:848–851.

151. Briggs JD. A critical review of immunosuppressive therapy. Immunol Lett 1991;29:89–94.

152. Payne N. Anesthetic implications of immunosuppressants used for transplantation. Int Anesthesiol Clin 1995;33(2):93–106.

153. Cohen RG, Barr ML, Starnes VA. Pediatric lung transplantation. Semin Pediatr Surg 1993;2:279–288.

154. Cirella VN, Pantuck CB, Lee YJ, Pantuck EJ. Effects of cyclosporine on anesthetic action. Anesth Analg 1987;66:703–706.

155. Sharpe M, Gelb A. Cyclosporin potentiates vecuronium blockade and prolongs recovery time in humans [abstract]. Can J Anesth 1992;39:A126.

156. Keenan RJ, Konishi H, Kawai A, et al. Clinical trial of Tacrolimus versus cyclosporin in lung transplantation. Ann Thorac Surg 1995;60:580–585.

157. Paradis IL, Duncan SR, Duaber JH, et al. Distinguishing between infection, rejection, and the adult respiratory distress syndrome after human lung transplantation. J Heart Lung Transplant 1992;11:S232–S236.

158. Haydock DA, Trulock EP, Kaiser LR, et al. Management of dysfunction in the transplanted lung: experience with 7 clinical cases. Ann Thorac Surg 1992;53: 635–641.

159. Adatia I, Lillehei C, Arnold JH, et al. Inhaled nitric oxide in the treatment of postoperative graft dysfunction after lung transplantation. Ann Thorac Surg 1994; 57:1311–1318.

160. Struber M, Cremer J, Harringer W, et al. Nebulized synthetic surfactant in reperfusion injury after single lung transplantation. J Thorac Cardiovasc Surg 1995; 110:563–564.

161. King-Biggs MB. Acute pulmonary allograft rejection: mechanisms, diagnosis, and management. Clin Chest Med 1997;18:301–310.

162. Berry GJ, Billingham ME. The Pathology of Combined Heart-Lung and Lung Transplantation. In SJ Shumway, NE Shumway (eds), Thoracic Transplantation. Cambridge, MA: Blackwell, 1995;331–347.

163. Trulock EP. Management of lung transplant rejection. Chest 1993;103:1566–1576.

164. Miller-Catchpole R. Diagnostic and therapeutic technology assessment (DATTA): lung transplantation. JAMA 1993;269:931–936.

165. Cooper JD, Billingham M, Egan T, et al. A working formulation for the standardization of nomenclature and for clinical staging of chronic dysfunction in lung allografts. J Heart Lung Transplant 1993;12:713–716.

166. Midthun DE, McDougall JC, Peters SG, Scott JP. Medical management and complications in the lung transplant recipient. Mayo Clin Proc 1997;72:175–184.

167. Ettinger NA, Cooper JD. Lung Transplantation. In GL Baum, E Wolinsky (eds), Textbook of Pulmonary Diseases. Boston: Little, Brown, 1994;1245–1261.

168. Novick RJ, Schafers H, Stitt L, et al. Seventy-two pulmonary retransplantations for obliterative bronchiolitis: predictors of survival. Ann Thorac Surg 1995;60:111–116.

169. Chaparro C, Maurer JR, Chamberlain D, et al. Causes of death in lung transplant recipients. J Heart Lung Transplant 1994;13:758–766.

170. Maurer JR. Therapeutic challenges following lung transplantation. Clin Chest Med 1990;11:279–290.

171. Chaparro C, Kesten S. Infections in lung transplant recipients. Clin Chest Med 1997;18:339–351.

172. Bando K, Paradis IL, Komatsu K, et al. Analysis of time-dependent risks for infection, rejection, and death after pulmonary transplantation. J Thorac Cardiovasc Surg 1995;109:49–59.

173. Griffith BP, Magee MJ, Gonzalez IF, et al. Anastomotic pitfalls in lung transplantation. J Thorac Cardiovasc Surg 1994;107:743–754.

174. Kshettry VR, Kroshus TJ, Hertz MI, et al. Early and late airway complications after lung transplantation: incidence and management. Ann Thorac Surg 1997;63:1576–1583.

175. de Hoyos AL, Patterson GA, Maurer JR, et al. Pulmonary transplantation: early and late results. J Thorac Cardiovasc Surg 1992;103:295–306.

176. Smith PC, Slaughter MS, Petty MG, et al. Abdominal complications after lung transplantation. J Heart Lung Transplant 1995;14:44–51.

177. Beaver TM, Fullerton DA, Zamora MR, et al. Colon perforation after lung transplantation. Ann Thorac Surg 1996;62:839–843.

178. Pollard TR, Schwesinger WH, Sako EY, Sirineck KR. Abdominal operations after lung transplantation: indications and outcome. Arch Surg 1997;132:714–718.

179. Berkowitz N, Schulman LL, McGregor C, Markowitz D. Gastroparesis after lung transplantation: potential role in postoperative respiratory complications. Chest 1995;108:1602–1607.

180. Leibowitz DW, Smith CR, Michler RE, et al. Incidence of pulmonary vein complications after lung transplantation: a prospective transesophageal echocardiographic study. J Am Coll Cardiol 1994;24:671–675.

181. Pham SM, Armitage JM, Katz WE, Griffith BP. Left atrial thrombus after lung transplantation. Ann Thorac Surg 1995;59:513–515.

182. Sarsam MA, Yonan NA, Beton D, et al. Early pulmonary vein thrombosis after single lung transplantation. J Heart Lung Transplant 1993;12:17–19.

183. Schmid C, Gulba DC, Heublein B, et al. Systemic recombinant tissue plasminogen activator lysis for left atrial thrombus formation after single-lung retransplantation. Ann Thorac Surg 1992;53:338–340.

184. Kroshus TJ, Kshettry VR, Hertz MI, Bolman RM III. Deep venous thrombosis and pulmonary embolism after lung transplantation. J Thorac Cardiovasc Surg 1995;110:540–544.

185. Nalesnik MA, Jaffe R, Starzl TE, et al. The pathology of posttransplant lymphoproliferative disorders occurring in the setting of cyclosporine A-prednisone immunosuppression. Am J Pathol 1988;133:173–192.

186. Maurer JR. Medical complications following lung transplantation. Semin Respir Crit Care Med 1996;17:173–185.

187. Williams TJ, Grossman RF, Maurer JR. Long-term functional follow-up of lung transplant recipients. Clin Chest Med 1990;11:347–358.

188. Miyoshi S, Trulock EP, Schaefers HJ, et al. Cardiopulmonary exercise testing after single and double lung transplantation. Chest 1990;97:1130–1136.

189. Pasque MK, Trulock EP, Kaiser LR, Cooper JD. Single-lung transplantation for pulmonary hypertension: three-month hemodynamic follow-up. Circulation 1991;84:2275–2279.

190. Carere R, Patterson GA, Liu P, et al. Right and left ventricular performance after single and double lung transplantation. J Thorac Cardiovasc Surg 1991;102:115–123.

191. Bando K, Armitage JM, Paradis IL, et al. Indications for and results of single, bilateral, and heart-lung transplantation for pulmonary hypertension. J Thorac Cardiovasc Surg 1994;108:1056–1065.

192. Brunstig LA, Lupinetti FM, Cascade PN, et al. Pulmonary function in single lung transplantation for chronic obstructive pulmonary disease. J Thorac Cardiovasc Surg 1994;107:1337–1345.

193. Briffa NP, Dennis C, Higenbottam T, et al. Single lung transplantation for end stage emphysema. Thorax 1995;50:562–564.

194. Levine SM, Anzueto A, Peters JI, et al. Medium term functional results of single-lung transplantation for end-stage obstructive lung disease. Am J Respir Crit Care Med 1994;150:398–402.

195. Mal H, Sleiman C, Jebrak G, et al. Functional results of single-lung transplantation for chronic obstructive lung disease. Am J Respir Crit Care Med 1994;149:1476–1481.

196. Cooper JD, Patterson GA, Trulock EP. Results of single and bilateral lung transplantation in 131 consecutive recipients. J Thorac Cardiovasc Surg 1994;107:460–471.

197. Griffith BP, Hardesty RL, Armitage JM, et al. A decade of lung transplantation. Ann Surg 1993;218:310–320.

198. Hosenpud JD, Novick RJ, Breen TJ, Daily OP. The Registry of the International Society for Heart and Lung Transplantation: eleventh official report—1994. J Heart Lung Transplant 1994;13:561–570.

199. Spray TL. Transplantation of the heart and lungs in children. Ann Rev Med 1994;45:139–148.

200. Armitage JM, Kurland G, Michaels M, et al. Critical issues in pediatric lung transplantation. J Thorac Cardiovasc Surg 1995;109:60–65.

201. Handelsman H. Single and double transplantation. Health Technol Assess 1991;1–15.

202. Maurer J. Costs of lung transplant in Canada [abstract]. J Heart Lung Transplant 1994;13:S70.

203. Reemtsma K, Gelijns AC, Sisk JE, et al. Supporting future surgical innovation: lung transplantation as a case study. Ann Surg 1993;218:465–475.

204. Korst RJ, McElvaney NG, Chu CS, et al. Gene therapy for the respiratory manifestations of cystic fibrosis. Am J Respir Crit Care Med 1995;151:S75–S87.

205. Shah PL, Scott SF, Fuchs HJ, et al. Medium term treatment of stable stage cystic fibrosis with recombinant human DNase I. Thorax 1995;50:333–338.

206. Range SP, Knox AJ. rhDNase in cystic fibrosis. Thorax 1995;50:321–322.

207. Wilson JM. Cystic fibrosis: strategies for gene therapy. Semin Respir Crit Care Med 1994;15:439–445.

208. Demertzis S, Haverich A, Ziemer G, et al. Successful lung transplantation for posttraumatic adult respiratory distress syndrome after extracorporeal membrane oxygenation support. J Heart Lung Transplant 1992;11:1005–1007.

209. Jurmann MJ, Haverich A, Demertzis S, et al. Extracorporeal membrane oxygenation as a bridge to lung transplantation. Eur J Cardiothorac Surg 1991;5:94–98.

210. Brantigan OC, Mueller E, Kress MB. A surgical approach to pulmonary emphysema. Am Rev Respir Dis 1959;80:194–204.

211. Cooper JD, Trulock EP, Triantafillou AN, et al. Bilateral pneumectomy (volume reduction) for chronic obstructive pulmonary disease. J Thorac Cardiovasc Surg 1995;109:106–119.

212. Gaissert HA, Trulock EP, Cooper JD, et al. Comparison of early functional results after volume reduction or lung transplantation for chronic obstructive pulmonary disease. J Thorac Cardiovasc Surg 1996;111:296–307.

213. Naunheim KS, Keller CA, Krucylak PE, et al. Unilateral video-assisted thoracic surgical lung reduction. Ann Thorac Surg 1996;61:1092–1098.

214. Keller CA, Naunheim KS, Osterloh J, et al. Hemodynamics and gas exchange following single lung transplant and unilateral thoracoscopic lung reduction. J Heart Lung Transplant 1997;16:199–208.

215. Zenati M, Keenan RJ, Landreneau RJ, et al. Lung reduction as bridge to lung transplantation in pulmonary emphysema. Ann Thorac Surg 1995;59:1581–1583.

Chapter 8
Liver Transplantation

Marc St. Amand, Mohammad Al-Sofayan, Cameron Ghent, and William J. Wall

Chapter Plan

History of Liver Transplantation

Dr. T. Starzl and his associates performed the first human liver transplantation at the University of Colorado in 1963.[1] Early experience before the advent of modern antirejection therapy was disappointing, with 1-year survival rates of 24–33%. The poor success produced a major dilemma in that the risks could not be justified for any but the sickest potential recipients. The selection bias in turn ensured that the risks would be higher than if less critically ill patients were selected. This situation continued until the early 1980s, when the effectiveness of cyclosporine as an immunosuppressant was demonstrated in solid organ grafting. By 1983, the results had improved to the point that liver transplantation was a realistic alternative for the treatment of severe and usually fatal types of liver disease. In June of that year, the National Institutes of Health in the United States assembled experts in hepatology, surgery, and pediatrics to develop a consensus on the status of liver transplantation. Their assertion that "liver transplantation is a therapeutic modality for end-stage liver disease that deserves broader application"[2] provided a powerful impetus to the development of more programs, better patient selection, and research leading to improvements in the technical aspects of surgery and postoperative care.

The proliferation of programs and the broadening of indications for liver transplantation after the improved results with cyclosporine led to more transplants for diverse indications in the mid-1980s. Even more significant was the dramatically increased number of patients placed on waiting lists and the intense competition for the limited donor livers available. In

Table 8-1. Common Causes of Acute Liver Failure in Adults

Acute viral hepatitis
Idiosyncratic drug hepatitis
Chemical hepatotoxins (e.g., acetaminophen overdose, carbon tetrachloride, organic solvents)
Biological toxins: *Amanita phalloides*, *Bacillus ceruleus*

Table 8-2. Common Causes of Chronic Liver Failure in Adults

Chronic viral hepatitis (B or C)
Primary biliary cirrhosis
Primary sclerosing cholangitis
Alcoholic liver disease
Chronic autoimmune hepatitis
Chronic Budd-Chiari syndrome
Wilson's disease
Alpha$_1$-antitrypsin deficiency
Hereditary hemochromatosis

1997, nearly 1,000 people died while awaiting liver transplantation in North America. Efforts to increase the number of available organs include the use of donor livers that were not considered suitable previously, such as older donors,[3] the use of split-liver grafting,[4] and living-related partial liver grafting for children.[5] Many countries and some districts within countries have taken political and legal means to increase the number of donor organs, such as the passage of presumed-consent or opting-out legislation, in which donation is assumed unless specifically refused in advance. With the increasing technical expertise, more appropriate candidate selection, better organ preservation, and more drugs to prevent and treat rejection, liver transplantation in most established centers has very good results, with graft and patient survival rates of 80–90%. In the 1990s, attention is increasingly focused on the quality of life after transplantation and the critical discrepancy between the number of candidates and the smaller number of suitable donors. Research efforts are intense in xenotransplantation, to address the shortage of timely donors; in transplantation tolerance, to improve recipients' long-term outcome and quality of life by obviating the need for chronic immunosuppression; and in artificial liver support systems.[6]

Epidemiology

The number of liver transplants performed has increased steadily since the early 1980s to more than 4,000 annually in the United States and a similar number in Europe. In the same period, the number of potential recipients (i.e., registrations on waiting lists) has grown at approximately 30% annually, to more than 7,000 in the United States.[7] The number of patients waiting has increased disproportionately to the number of transplants performed. The risk of dying while on the list for liver transplantation is rea-

sonably constant, at approximately 10%, although waiting times have increased steadily from a mean of 33 days in 1988 to more than 1 year in 1997.[7] The development of artificial liver support systems may soon lead to even larger numbers of critically ill patients waiting for transplantation.

Etiology of Liver Diseases

The list of diseases treatable by liver transplantation has increased steadily during the 1990s. They are conveniently divided into those producing acute liver failure (Table 8-1) and those producing chronic liver failure, or cirrhosis (Table 8-2). The definition of acute liver failure has undergone revision, but the essential feature in all definitions is the development of hepatic encephalopathy within a few weeks of onset of the illness.[8] One of the most common causes is hepatotoxicity from a deliberate overdose of acetaminophen. Transplantation of the liver in this setting is ethically problematic because the patient has no wish to live, and coma prevents the patient from participating in decision making. Other causes of fulminant hepatic failure include viral hepatitis (A, B, or rarely C) and idiosyncratic reactions to medications. In many cases, no cause is determined.

Many chronic liver diseases that lead to decompensated cirrhosis are treatable by transplantation. In most transplant centers, the most common of these are chronic hepatitis C, chronic hepatitis B, primary biliary cirrhosis, primary sclerosing cholangitis, autoimmune hepatitis, alcoholic cirrhosis, and idiopathic cirrhosis. The relative frequency of these diseases varies depending on population demographics and transplant program policies. A few of these diseases merit separate discussion. Chronic hepatitis C is usually traceable to remote street drug use or transfusion before the discovery of the hepatitis C virus in 1989 and screening of blood donors in 1990. In many individuals, cirrhosis develops 20–40 years after acquiring hepatitis C, and patients are asymptomatic for much of the course. Concomitant regular use or abuse of alcohol appears to accelerate the injury due to hepatitis C, although most individuals with hepatitis C and alcohol abuse do not demonstrate histologic features of alcoholic hepatitis. Although the early survival of patients transplanted for chronic hepatitis C is comparable to those transplanted for nonviral diseases, the virus persists, and the major concern is recurrent hepatitis years after grafting.[9] Chronic hepatitis B is equally problematic as an indication for transplantation because early, aggressive recurrence of this infection in the graft in at least 30% of patients adversely affects survival. The routine use of lamivudine preoperatively and postoperatively may greatly reduce this recurrence, although viral resistance has been documented.[10] Primary biliary cirrhosis is one of the best indications for liver transplantation, and there are good prognostic models to aid in the timing of listing.[11] The timing of transplantation for sclerosing cholangitis is more difficult because some individuals develop refractory or recurrent biliary sepsis before developing cirrhosis, and this may be treatable only by transplantation. Both of these chronic cholestatic diseases are commonly complicated by osteopenic bone disease. Recurrence of either disease is uncommon, although biliary tract complications after transplantation for sclerosing cholangitis are commoner than with transplantation for other diseases, even with the type of biliary reconstruction and duration of organ preservation taken into consideration.[12] Autoimmune hepatitis is treatable with corticosteroids and other immunosuppressive agents. Many patients responsive to these agents have nonprogressive disease, even with cirrhosis, and do not require transplantation. When major complications develop, such as variceal bleeding, chronic encephalopathy, refractory ascites, or wasting, transplantation listing is appropriate. Alcoholic liver disease presents a prototypic ethical dilemma for transplant programs. Most centers refuse to transplant patients who are unable to demonstrate abstinence from alcohol for some period, usually 6–12 months. Policies vary, and some programs require completion of an alcohol rehabilitation program before acceptance. The implicit recognition that some patients

Table 8-3. Causes of Liver Failure in Infants and Young Children

Biliary atresia
Alagille syndrome
Nonsyndromatic biliary hypoplasia (Byler's disease)
Neonatal hepatitis
Alpha$_1$-antitrypsin deficiency
Crigler-Najjar syndrome
Glycogen storage diseases
Congenital fructose intolerance
Tyrosinemia
Galactosemia
Wilson's disease
Wolman's disease (cholesterol ester storage disease)

with alcoholic liver disease will die before completing these preconditions complicates the assessments. The Canadian Liver Transplant Study Group has adopted a policy that places the emphasis on a demonstrated ability to comply with reasonable medical advice because it is essential for postoperative survival and rehabilitation.[13]

With the exception of alcoholic cirrhosis, pediatric diseases leading to the need for liver transplantation overlap with those of adult recipients, including all the diseases listed in Tables 8-1 and 8-2. The unique diseases leading to transplantation in young children and infants are listed in Table 8-3, including a variety of inborn errors of metabolism. Biliary atresia and the biliary hypoplasia syndromes are by far the commonest pediatric liver diseases for which transplantation is performed.

Classification of Severity of Disease

Assessing the need for liver transplantation depends critically on knowing the prognosis of the disease under consideration without transplantation. For diseases such as primary biliary cirrhosis and sclerosing cholangitis, disease-specific prognostic models based on logistic regression can predict the prognosis without transplantation.[11] For other diseases, the use of generic prognostic data (e.g., Child-Turcotte or Child-Pugh score) for complications of all types of cirrhosis simplifies the assessment. The prognostic value of these scores was validated in prospective studies before the modern era of liver transplantation.[14] All the data required

Table 8-4. Components of the Child-Turcotte Score*

Component	Score		
	1	2	3
Serum bilirubin (mmol/liter)	<17.1	17.1–51.3	>51.3
Serum albumin (g/liter)	>35	30–35	<30
Ascites	None or minimal	Controllable	Refractory
Nutrition	Normal	Malnourished	Cachexia
Encephalopathy	None	Grade I or II	Grade III or IV

*In the Pugh modification, prothrombin time is substituted for the encephalopathy score. With the adoption of international normalized ratios in place of prothrombin time, the calculation of a Pugh score has become difficult.

to calculate Child-Turcotte or Child-Pugh scores are readily available from simple bedside and laboratory measurements. Table 8-4 details the components of these scores.

Complications of Liver Failure

The common complications of liver failure that are immediately relevant to transplant surgery can be divided into those related to acute and chronic liver failure (Table 8-5). The common complications of acute liver failure are cerebral edema, acute renal failure, and sepsis. Cerebral edema develops in up to 60% of patients with the syndrome of acute liver failure who progress to grade III hepatic encephalopathy.[15] Monitoring of cerebral perfusion pressure, central venous pressure (CVP), and intracranial pressure in the intensive care unit is standard practice. This may include placement of an epidural catheter pressure transducer[16] or use of transcranial Doppler ultrasound to assess cerebral blood flow.[17] Head-up hyperventilation, pressors, and mannitol by bolus injection may avert uncal herniation in these critically ill patients. Of equal importance, such monitoring may identify patients with irretrievable cerebral edema, who should not be transplanted.[18]

Acute renal failure in acute liver failure is similar to that seen with any other critical illness, and it is usually reversible with successful liver transplantation, although temporary dialytic support may be

Table 8-5. Complications of Liver Failure

Acute liver failure
    Cerebral edema
    Acute renal failure
    Sepsis
Chronic liver failure
    Variceal bleeding
    Refractory ascites
    Renal failure
    Hepatic encephalopathy
    Malnutrition

needed. The term *hepatorenal syndrome* (HRS) should be avoided in such patients because it discourages clinicians from searching for reversible and treatable causes of renal dysfunction. The most frequent cause is intravascular volume depletion. Judicious use of colloid and fluids is aimed at maintaining a CVP of 12–15 mm Hg without increasing the risk of cerebral edema.

Sepsis frequently intervenes in the course of acute liver failure, most commonly from aspiration pneumonia, urinary tract infection, or septicemia of unclear origin. A significant percentage of patients develop fungemia. Coverage with broad-spectrum antibiotics and an antifungal may be beneficial while these patients await a suitable donor liver.[19]

Common complications of end-stage cirrhosis include variceal bleeding, refractory ascites, renal failure, hepatic encephalopathy, and malnutrition. Variceal bleeding is best treated by aggressive endoscopic banding or injection sclerotherapy after the first bleed.[20] The risk of variceal bleeding can be predicted from endoscopic appearances and reduced by prophylactic use of beta blockers in high-risk patients.[21] Accordingly, all cirrhotics should undergo periodic assessment by upper gastrointestinal endoscopy and treatment, if high-risk varices are found.

Ascites is almost universal in patients requiring liver transplantation for cirrhosis, but it is usually controllable. Graded salt restriction to as little as 1–2 g of NaCl daily, with careful attention to maintenance of caloric intake, is the first step, followed by diuretics in escalating dosages. Measurement of urine sodium excretion may be helpful in assessing the need for diuretics. A patient who accumulates ascites at the rate of 1 liter per day (as judged by repeated total paracentesis) and excretes 80 mEq of

Na+ per day is assuredly noncompliant with dietary sodium restriction to 88 mEq per day. The use of periodic paracentesis is a safe and effective interim treatment of ascites,[22] but it should not be needed more often than every 2–3 weeks at most. Placement of peritoneovenous shunts is associated with high morbidity and mortality and should seldom be needed in transplant candidates. Infection of ascitic fluid in cirrhosis is very common; the risk of this complication is reduced by routine use of low-dose antibiotic prophylaxis with either norfloxacin or trimethoprim-sulfamethoxazole.[23]

Renal failure in the patient with cirrhosis is an ominous development.[24] The causes include inappropriate fluid restriction in a futile attempt to treat ascites or hyponatremia, drug nephrotoxicity, and coexistent intrinsic renal disease. *HRS* is defined as functional renal failure with oliguria and avid sodium retention without intrinsic renal disease or intravascular volume depletion. Measurements of sodium excretion and CVP are essential to the diagnosis because both drug nephrotoxicity and inapparent volume depletion may mimic this syndrome. As in acute liver failure, dialysis may be needed. Renal function usually recovers after successful liver transplantation in patients who maintain their renal concentrating capacity.

Hepatic encephalopathy may develop slowly and insidiously with subtle personality changes and dulling of mental alertness noted only by the family. It may present as a more obvious neuropsychiatric disorder manifested by sleep reversal, spatial apraxia, tremors, confusion, somnolence, stupor, and coma. There is usually an identifiable precipitant for an episode, such as an infection (especially infected ascites), use of a sedative or hypnotic, or an overload of protein. Whatever the cause or pathophysiology, the graded treatment response is to reduce protein intake to as little as 0.5 g/kg per day and to remove enteric sources of nitrogenous products with the use of cathartics and nonabsorbable antibiotics, such as neomycin. Lactulose has become the favorite cathartic because it reduces the pH of colonic contents, thereby trapping ammonia.

Preoperative malnutrition is predictive of complications after liver transplantation. It is due to altered energy use (fat malabsorption), decreased energy intake, and dietary protein restriction to treat encephalopathy.[25] Vigorous efforts to maintain energy intake are warranted, including nasoduodenal tube feeding of high-caloric supplements and, occasionally, parenteral nutritional support.

Two unusual complications of cirrhosis merit special attention from anesthesiologists involved in liver transplantation: (1) the hepatopulmonary syndrome and (2) pulmonary hypertension secondary to portal hypertension.[26] The hepatopulmonary syndrome is manifested by platypnea (dyspnea when upright, relieved by recumbency), multiple spider nevi, nail clubbing, and orthodeoxia (higher oxygen saturation lying than standing). A mild degree of hepatopulmonary syndrome is quite common in advanced cirrhosis but is of limited significance. The cardinal laboratory feature is upright hypoxemia at least partially correctable with recumbency and an appropriate response to breathing 100% oxygen. Hepatopulmonary syndrome usually resolves slowly after transplantation. Pulmonary hypertension secondary to portal hypertension may not be detected until a pulmonary artery catheter is inserted in preparation for transplantation, but it can usually be suspected with careful cardiac examination (loud pulmonary second heart sound and right ventricular heave). Pulmonary hypertension is readily assessed by echocardiography and is a strong contraindication to transplantation unless it is reversible with pharmacologic treatment preoperatively.[26]

The indications for transplantation have become somewhat simplified with the recognition that this treatment is appropriate for most patients with liver failure, regardless of the etiology, if there are no contraindications. The emphasis now is on identifying contraindications that may not be apparent on initial assessment, especially if the assessment consists of a review of notes, laboratory reports, and various imaging studies rather than an old-fashioned detailed history and physical examination. A list of common contraindications is shown in Table 8-6. Hepatocellular carcinoma is a controversial indication because of the high rates of cancer recurrence. Most centers accept patients with small solitary tumors in decompensated cirrhosis but refuse to do transplants if the tumors are large or multiple or show vascular invasion on imaging studies.

Donor Selection

The excess of potential recipients compared to potential donors has led to efforts to use donated

Table 8-6. Common Contraindications
to Liver Transplantation

Extrahepatic malignancy
Cholangiocarcinoma
Severe disease of other organs limiting life expectancy
Failure to demonstrate an ability to comply with advice and
    treatment regimen
Replicative hepatitis B
Multifocal hepatocellular carcinoma

---

livers from subjects who would not previously have been considered suitable for organ donation. There is now no age limit for liver donation, although older age (older than 60 years) is one factor that increases the risk of initial poor function, in combination with other factors, such as fatty infiltration, prolonged cold ischemia, or prolonged hypotension before retrieval.[27] The use of livers from donors who test positive for hepatitis C is particularly problematic. Many such young brain-dead accident victims are otherwise ideal, with grossly and histologically normal livers. Some programs use livers from these individuals for recipients who are positive for hepatitis C, provided the frozen-section biopsy shows no serious chronic hepatitis. In the authors' program, we require the additional precaution that the potential recipient be made aware of the situation and sign consent to receive a hepatitis C–positive liver. Recurrence of hepatitis C of variable severity is very common in patients transplanted for chronic hepatitis C. There is no evidence that giving hepatitis C–positive recipients a liver from a hepatitis C–positive donor leads to more aggressive disease.

Surgical Considerations

Very few operations require closer collaboration between anesthesiologist and surgeon than liver transplantation. Many times during the operation, there must be mutual anticipation of events to allow safe performance of what is arguably the most unphysiologic of all abdominal operations. Excessive operative mortality in the past was often due to an inability to control bleeding effectively combined with the transplantation of a liver that functioned poorly. Too frequently, organs of questionable via-

bility were transplanted into patients who were cold, acidotic, and hypotensive. Profound coagulopathies worsened bleeding, and even good-quality donor livers were unable to reverse severe metabolic and coagulopathic states in patients who were unstable throughout most of the operation.

The transformation of the operation from a high-risk, desperate procedure into routine surgery was the result of several important advances. Better understanding of the pathophysiology of liver failure and its effect on other organs identified the need to correct deranged physiology in the immediate pretransplant period. This resulted in recipients arriving in the operating room much better prepared to undergo major surgery. Modern intraoperative monitoring had a major impact on the anesthesiologist's ability to control patient stability during surgery. Continuous assessment of oxygenation, hemodynamics, acid-base status, and coagulation profiles provided timely information that was critical for patient management.[28] Surgeons became better at the operation, aided by fixed retractors for good exposure, better techniques for achieving hemostasis, and more technically advanced instruments and sutures for vascular anastomoses. Changing surgical methods and solutions to adapt to inherent complications reduced the magnitude of the operation.[29] Venous bypass undoubtedly provided its greatest advantage soon after its introduction, before other improvements in anesthesia and surgery were established enough to show that venous bypass is not necessary in most cases.[30, 31] The key element to success was, of course, the transplantation of a good liver graft. Today, immediate graft function is confidently relied on because better donor management and superior organ preservation have resulted in the procurement of good-quality organs.[32–34] All these improvements have created a much safer and more controlled recipient operation. Operative disasters can still occur because of the nature of the surgery, but they are infrequent.

The Standard Operation

One of the most important operative principles is to avoid having to play catch-up during the surgery. Close communication between anesthesiologist and surgeon prevents the undesirable circumstance of falling behind in fluid or blood administration or letting a coagulopathy get out of control. Anticipation of events is fundamental to avoiding situations that require constant efforts to correct deficits. The operation can be divided into four practical stages: (1) the recipient hepatectomy, (2) the anhepatic period, (3) the reperfusion period, and (4) the completion stage. Each stage has its own special implications for surgical and anesthetic management.

Recipient Hepatectomy

Removal of the diseased liver is usually the most difficult part of the operation, and it is potentially the most hazardous time for bleeding. Fresh frozen plasma is given simultaneously with the skin incision, aiming to keep the international normalized ratio (INR) close to 2 or less. A bilateral subcostal incision is routine, with an upper midline extension to the xiphoid process if the costal margin is narrow. Virtually all tissues are dissected with electrocautery. Topical hemostatic agents, such as absorbable gelatin sponge (Gelfoam) soaked in topical thrombin, are used to control oozing from raw surfaces. The left lobe is separated from the patient's diaphragm by completely dividing the falciform and left triangular ligaments from their periphery to the suprahepatic vena cava. Then the portal triad structures are dissected. The common duct and right and left branches of the hepatic artery are ligated and divided, exposing the portal vein, which is encircled. Once the inflow to the liver is controlled, the posterior dissection of the right lobe can begin. Manipulation of the patient's liver can compress major vessels and interfere with venous return. At this stage, the surgeon should make the anesthesiologist aware of surgical maneuvers that could alter hemodynamics. The right triangular ligament is divided to separate the right lobe from the patient's diaphragm and retroperitoneum. Isolation of the retrohepatic cava from the suprarenal region to its entrance through the patient's diaphragm is facilitated by keeping the dissection close to his or her liver and the vena cava. The posterior dissection of the right lobe is the most problematic site for bleeding, and wandering into the retroperitoneum invites hemorrhage from venous collaterals. This area is the most difficult to visualize, and no single vessel can be controlled to make the area dry. The right adrenal vein is secured between clips when it is encountered,

and the adrenal gland is disturbed as little as possible. Occasionally, the back wall of the retrohepatic vena cava is left in situ to avoid dissection of retroperitoneal collaterals. In patients with Budd-Chiari syndrome, fibrosis and inflammatory reaction between their diaphragm and suprahepatic cava often obliterates tissue planes.

After the patient's liver has been completely mobilized, it is attached only by the portal vein and vena cava above and below the liver. Bleeding at this point should be minimal. The surgeon should spend as much time as reasonable to obtain a dry field and reduce bleeding to a minimum. The hemodynamics should be stable in preparation for the cardiovascular consequences of cross-clamping the portal vein and vena cava. When there is persistent ooze from the retroperitoneum, good surgical judgment is needed. The choice is between persisting in attempts to obtain hemostasis or waiting until after the patient's liver has been removed and there is better access to this area to control bleeding points. Sometimes it is best to accept minor oozing, covering raw areas with topical hemostatic agents, than to place sutures, which create more bleeding from needle holes. Blood is transfused according to measured losses and the patient's hemodynamics.

Anhepatic Period

The anhepatic period begins with clamping of the portal vein, infrahepatic vena cava, and suprahepatic vena cava and ends with unclamping of these vessels and reperfusion of the donor liver. The period of venous cross-clamping gained the reputation of a crisis period during liver transplantation. Too often, patients entered this stage with unstable hemodynamics and ongoing bleeding. Not surprisingly, they deteriorated dramatically when venous return to their hearts was interrupted by clamping the portal vein and vena cava. The enthusiastic adoption of venous bypass when it was first introduced was therefore very understandable, and there is no doubt that it salvaged many patients.[30] But it is well recognized now that venous bypass is not necessary to perform liver transplantation safely.[31, 35] With modern anesthesia and monitoring, the cardiovascular changes that occur with venous cross-clamping are predictable and well tolerated in the vast majority of patients. It has always been the practice at our center

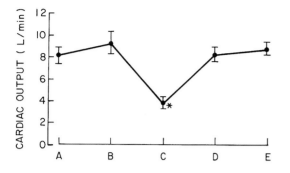

Figure 8-1. Changes in the mean cardiac output in liver transplantation without venous bypass. (A) Start of operation; (B) before venous cross-clamping; (C) anhepatic period; (D) after reperfusion; (E) completion of operation. *p <.01. (Reprinted with permission from WJ Wall, R Mimeault, DR Grant, M Bloch. The use of older donor livers for hepatic transplantation. Transplantation 1990;49:58.)

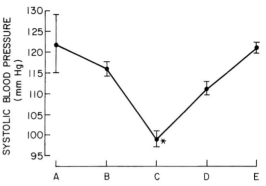

Figure 8-2. Changes in mean systolic blood pressure during liver transplantation without venous bypass. (A) Start of operation; (B) before venous cross-clamping; (C) anhepatic period; (D) after reperfusion; (E) completion of operation. *p <.01. (Reprinted with permission from WJ Wall, R Mimeault, DR Grant, M Bloch. The use of older donor livers for hepatic transplantation. Transplantation 1990;49:58.)

to perform liver transplants without bypass. This approach stems directly from the fact that our program was established before venous bypass was developed and our experience had already proved to us that venous bypass was unnecessary. In our view, there are three prerequisites to performing liver transplantation safely without bypass:

1. The patient should have stable hemodynamics at the end of the recipient hepatectomy.
2. There should be no excessive bleeding that could become worse when the portal vein and vena cava are occluded.
3. The surgical team should have the experience to complete the portal and caval anastomoses in less than 45 minutes.

Performing the operation without venous bypass requires the confidence of both anesthesiologist and surgeon, who must be comfortable with the physiologic changes that occur and understand their respective roles during the period of venous cross-clamping. Preparation and anesthetic management of the patient during this period are discussed under Anesthetic Management. The cardiac output is reduced by approximately one-half, but because the output in cirrhotic patients is usually much higher than in normal subjects, the cardiac output is still adequate (Figure 8-1). It is not possible to return the cardiac output to preclamping levels, and attempts to do so risk fluid overload. The systolic blood pressure stabilizes at approximately 90 mm Hg, accompanied by a dou-

bling of the systemic vascular resistance (SVR) (Figure 8-2). In some cirrhotic patients, the hemodynamic alterations are minimal because many portosystemic collaterals effectively maintain venous return to their hearts in spite of portal and caval occlusion.

We use bypass very infrequently, reserving it for patients with pulmonary hypertension or significant cardiac disease. Venous bypass does not maintain normal hemodynamics, but it reduces considerably the altered physiology during the anhepatic period. If venous bypass is used, it may be started early after the portal structures have been isolated and before the vena cava and retrohepatic tissue is dissected. The portal vein can thus be divided early, allowing added exposure for posterior dissection. Theoretically, the early institution of venous bypass should reduce portal pressure, but there is no evidence that blood loss is reduced when it is used, nor does it result in better renal function.[36] The femoral and jugular catheters can usually be placed percutaneously. Flow rates of 1.5 liters per minute or more should be obtained, and the surgeon and anesthesiologist should know the flow conditions throughout. Complications related to the use of venous bypass (i.e., air embolism, venous thrombosis, and coagulation within the bypass setup) have been reduced to a minimum. In some centers, an altogether different technique is used that avoids either bypass or complete cross-clamping. The piggyback technique occludes the portal vein but maintains caval patency by removing the diseased liver from the intact vena cava of the recipient. Partial venous return is maintained via the patent vena cava, which is only partially occluded when the venous anastomosis is performed.[37–39] Which technique is used is largely one of personal preference; it depends wholly on the routines established in a given center.[40]

Regardless of whether bypass is used, the suprahepatic caval anastomosis is performed first, followed by that of the infrahepatic cava and then the portal vein. Before portal flow to the liver is established, the liver is flushed via the portal vein with 500–1,000 ml of Ringer's lactate to wash out the preservation solution. University of Wisconsin solution, the most widely used liver preservation solution, is hypertonic (osmolarity 320 mOsm) and rich in potassium (125 mEq/liter). It is essential that the highly concentrated potassium be washed out of the graft before reperfusion. We routinely use a second blood flush, temporarily unclamping the portal vein and allowing several hundred milliliters of portal blood to perfuse the liver and escape through the partially open anterior wall of the infrahepatic caval anastomosis, as described by Calne.[41] The blood flush further rids the liver of preservation solution. It also prevents the most stagnated blood from the portal system from entering the systemic circulation. This final maneuver of the anhepatic stage minimizes the influx of potassium and acid metabolites into the right side of the patient's heart when the transplanted liver is perfused.

Reperfusion Phase

The suprahepatic clamp is released first, followed by the portal clamp, thereby revascularizing the graft with portal blood. Before removal of the clamps, calcium and bicarbonate are given, and the volume status of the patient should be optimized. Reperfusion syndrome is characterized by hypotension and a slowing of the heart rate.[42] It occurs immediately after restoration of blood flow to the transplanted liver and the influx of cold, acidotic blood into the patient's heart. If the patient is hemodynamically unstable before release of the clamps, reperfusion may result in marked cardiovascular collapse. It has been shown that discarding the first few hundred milliliters of portal blood that perfuse the transplanted liver decreases the incidence and severity of

the syndrome.[43] In spite of flushing the graft, some degree of transient hyperkalemia can be expected. We normally wait several minutes after removal of the portal vein clamp before releasing the clamp on the infrahepatic cava. Reperfusion syndrome is rarely severe unless the liver is damaged or the patient is hypotensive before reperfusion. Maintenance of body temperature throughout the operation prevents the added effect of hypothermia, which compounds the cardiac effects of acidosis.

Significant anastomotic bleeding from the portal or caval anastomosis after reperfusion puts the patient in double jeopardy. Hypotension from bleeding compounds reperfusion effects by reducing blood flow to the transplanted liver, thus subjecting it to added ischemic injury. Excessive manipulation of the liver at this stage may interfere with graft perfusion, too. At this juncture, it is important to have the patient's coagulation at a reasonable level so that the donor liver is not unfairly burdened with reversing a coagulopathic state. Revascularization of an undamaged donor liver in a physiologically stable recipient virtually guarantees a good immediate outcome.

Completion Stage

During the final stage, the arterial and biliary reconstructions are performed, the operative sites are carefully examined, and the patient's abdomen is closed. This phase should be characterized by patient stability, lack of bleeding, and immediate function of the graft. After venous flow has been restored, the hepatic artery reconstruction should be done expeditiously to provide the transplanted liver with ideal oxygenation. The anastomosis can usually be done in an artery-to-artery fashion, but occasionally it is necessary to use the recipient aorta. The infrarenal site is preferable to the supraceliac position because the latter interrupts splanchnic flow and compromises portal flow to the graft. After completion of the arterial anastomosis, the transplanted liver should be well perfused, although some edema of the graft is common. At this point in the operation, systemic oxygenation and cardiac output should be optimal to promote good liver function and graft recovery from the preservation injury. Avoiding a high CVP prevents harmful venous engorgement of the graft.

During the biliary anastomosis, the color and texture of the transplanted liver, the tension in the portal

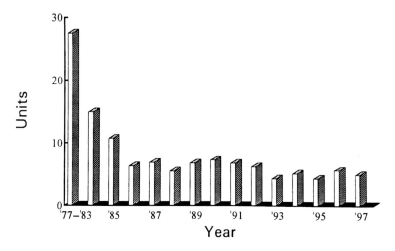

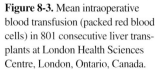

Figure 8-3. Mean intraoperative blood transfusion (packed red blood cells) in 801 consecutive liver transplants at London Health Sciences Centre, London, Ontario, Canada.

vein, and the pulse in the hepatic artery are carefully observed. The gross appearance of the transplanted liver is a good indication of the status of the graft. Either a duct-to-duct reconstruction or a Roux loop anastomosis is performed. The Roux drainage takes slightly longer to perform. When all the anastomoses are completed, raw areas are checked for bleeding. The entire operation takes 5–6 hours on average, and the mean transfusion requirement is 4–5 units of blood (Figure 8-3). Ideal fluid management throughout the operation minimizes the risk of pulmonary edema and increases the likelihood of early extubation in the postoperative period.

Special Considerations

Various abnormal operative findings are commonly encountered that require tailoring or modification of the usual techniques. In general, abnormal findings have one technical implication common to all, namely, the potential for increased bleeding during the transplant. Nearly one-third of patients who undergo liver transplantation have had previous upper abdominal or right upper quadrant surgery. The surgery may have been for independent conditions (e.g., peptic ulcer or gallstones) or conditions related to the underlying liver pathology (e.g., a Kasai procedure for biliary atresia). Regardless, perihepatic adhesions resulting from previous surgery may harbor extensive collaterals after years of portal hypertension. Removal of the patient's diseased liver can be a formidable undertaking. A

longer dissection can be expected, and the anesthesiologist should be prepared for more than the average blood loss. We commonly administer aprotinin in patients who have had previous surgery, although one randomized trial failed to show that it reduced transfusion requirements.[44]

A prior portosystemic shunt is a two-edged sword. Although adhesions are usually created, a decompressed portal system can facilitate removal of the patient's liver. As long as the portal system is patent, a prior shunt usually does not produce serious technical obstacles, although slightly more blood loss can be expected.[45, 46] Central shunts have to be taken down to redirect portal flow to the patient's liver, and they should be left intact until the very end of the recipient hepatectomy to take full advantage of the portal decompression. Selective (Warren) shunts, on the other hand, can usually be left undisturbed, although there are reports of steal syndromes even with selective shunts. Intraoperative Doppler ultrasound studies to measure flow in the portal vein and in the shunt can aid the decision on whether to dismantle a selective shunt at the time of a transplant.[47] It has become increasingly popular to treat portal hypertension in liver transplantation candidates with transjugular intrahepatic portosystemic shunts (TIPS). Occasionally, the wire mesh migrates into the proximal portal vein or, worse, into the suprahepatic vena cava. Extracting malpositioned TIPS at the time of liver transplantation can be tricky and may require extensive vascular exposure.

Thrombosis of the portal vein is found in approximately 5% of transplant recipients. The thrombus may have been detected by preoperative ultrasound, but it may be encountered as an unexpected finding at operation. It is dealt with by either a thromboendarterectomy or ligation of the portal vein and a venous graft from the recipient superior mesenteric vein.[48, 49] In either case, increased bleeding during the portal dissection can be anticipated, and the anhepatic stage may be longer. In situations in which additional blood loss is expected, the Cell Saver autotransfusion system may be useful to salvage and reinfuse lost blood.[50, 51] We reserve the Cell Saver for these special situations, and then we usually set it up only after the operative findings suggest a need for it.

Hepatic retransplantation may be easy or very difficult. When a retransplant is required within days of a primary transplant (e.g., for nonfunction of the liver), the tissue planes are still fresh, and removal of the graft is usually straightforward. In contrast, when retransplantation is performed months or years later, the entire liver and all the anastomoses may be surrounded by dense adhesions and scar tissue. It is usually best to dissect the vessels in virgin tissue planes, either on the recipient side or on the donor side of the vascular anastomoses. Which side is chosen depends on the operative findings and the lengths of the vessels to be secured. A cuff of the first donor's suprahepatic vena cava should always be left in place to ensure adequate length. Unless it is a fresh retransplant, the biliary reconstruction should be done with a Roux loop. Overall survival rates for retransplants have improved, but they are still 20–30% less than primary transplants.[52, 53] Graft and patient survival after retransplantation are significantly affected by the increased complexity of the surgery and whether the need for retransplantation is urgent.[54]

When the liver is transplanted as part of a multivisceral graft, many technical considerations add to the complexity of the operation. Most commonly, the liver and intestine are transplanted together to treat total parenteral nutrition–induced liver failure in patients with short gut syndrome. In these patients, limited venous access is a tremendous practical consideration. The thrombotic consequences of years of central intravenous feeding may have obliterated most of the major veins. Unusual approaches are often needed to secure good venous access and to ensure venous return to the right heart during surgery. It may be necessary to expose the right atrium via a median sternotomy for line insertion. Multivisceral grafts have a huge store of preservation solution that must be thoroughly flushed from the organs before they are revascularized. A segment of donor aorta bearing the composite arterial supply of the liver or intestine graft is anastomosed to the side of the recipient aorta.

Segmental Grafts

Segmental liver grafts were introduced to alleviate the shortage of small livers for children awaiting liver transplantation. There are many technical variations of reduced-size liver grafts, and they are still evolving.[55–57] Typically, the left lateral segment (segments 2 and 3 in the Couinaud classification) of a cadaver liver or the same segment from a living donor is used. The vena cava of the recipient is preserved during the hepatectomy, and the venous outflow from the segmental graft is usually anastomosed to the confluence of the recipient's hepatic veins. The vena cava may be completely occluded when this anastomosis is performed as shown in Figure 8-4. Alternately, only the confluence of the recipient hepatic veins may be occluded by placing an appropriate clamp. Caval patency is thus maintained as with the piggyback technique. Rather than discard the remaining liver in the case of cadaver donors, the right lobe may be used in a second adult recipient. Using segmental liver grafts has two main implications for the recipient surgery. First, spatial orientation of the partial graft and discrepancies in size of donor and recipient vessels usually requires more complex vascular reconstruction than do whole liver grafts. Vascular grafts are needed in most cases, for the portal vein or the hepatic artery, or both. Microsurgical techniques may be needed for small vessels, especially the artery. These features may significantly increase the anhepatic period and prolong the whole operation. Second, segmental grafts have cut surfaces that are additional sites of potential hemorrhage after revascularization. In situ splitting of cadaver livers in the donors gives more secure hemostasis of the cut surfaces and reduces the possibility of bleeding when the grafts are revascularized. The numerous technical variations in segmental liver grafting emphasize the need for anesthesiologist and surgeon to discuss in advance how the operation will proceed and what vascular occlusion will occur.

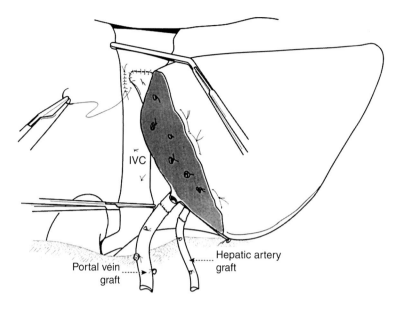

Figure 8-4. A left lateral segmental graft. Venous outflow is to the confluence of the middle and left hepatic veins of the recipient, using complete caval occlusion in this example. (IVC = inferior vena cava.)

IVC

Portal vein graft

Hepatic artery graft

Postoperative Complications

Bleeding is the main operative complication; methods to minimize it during the recipient hepatectomy are discussed in previous sections. Recalcitrant bleeding after completion of all the vascular anastomoses, if it is not "medical" bleeding, is usually from the retroperitoneal area and diaphragm behind the liver. If bleeding from this area continues after reasonable attempts to obtain a dry field, there is a role for packing the area with sponges and planned re-exploration 24 hours later. The packs are removed after local hemostatic mechanisms have been given an opportunity to stop the bleeding. The source of the hemorrhage is usually small vessels on raw surfaces. Packing should be required in fewer than 1% of transplants. It is extremely important to restore the coagulation profile of the recipient to as close to normal as possible when the packs are in place.

Primary nonfunction of the graft occurs in fewer than 5% of cases. It is manifest in the first 24–48 hours by very high aminotransferase levels, coagulopathy, hypoglycemia, and failure of the patient to regain full consciousness, although some patients have deceptively good mentation. Retransplantation is necessary. Risk factors for primary nonfunction are long preservation periods, excessively fatty donor livers, and massive transfusion during the recipient surgery.

Vascular thrombosis is most likely to affect the hepatic artery. When it occurs within the first few days after transplantation, it presents as primary nonfunction or extremely high liver enzymes, or both. If absent hepatic arterial flow is detected in the immediate postoperative period by Doppler ultrasound, prompt reoperation and revision of the arterial anastomosis can salvage some grafts. Otherwise, retransplantation will likely be required, although hepatic artery thrombosis is occasionally a silent event, especially in children. Thrombosis of the portal vein anastomosis is uncommon, and it is more likely to occur in small children. Usually, it presents late with manifestations of portal hypertension and little effect on graft function. Patients with Budd-Chiari syndrome require long-term anticoagulation after transplantation to prevent recurrent hepatic or portal venous thrombosis. Thrombosis of the caval anastomosis is rare.

Of all the anastomoses, the biliary reconstruction is the most prone to complications. Strictures or leaks occur in 9–10% of cases; they occur more commonly in duct-to-duct reconstructions than with Roux loop drainage.[58] Diffuse biliary tract strictures occur late and may be caused by preservation injury, immunologic injury (especially with ABO blood group–incompatible grafts), hepatic artery thrombosis, or recurrence of the primary disease (i.e., sclerosing cholangitis). Early anastomotic strictures may respond to percutaneous or endoscopic drainage and dilation, but more than half require operative revision. Modern methods of imaging have added immeasurably to the early and accurate diagnosis of all technical complications but biliary complications in particular.

Many nonimmunologic factors affect the perioperative morbidity and mortality of liver recipients. Some of the most important are severity of malnutrition, level of coma, and comorbid disease, such as renal failure. Overall, 30-day operative mortality rates of less than 10% are achievable. Death soon after surgery is most often due to sepsis in association with multiple organ failure.

Anesthetic Management

Preoperative Assessment

Evaluation of the recipient's medical condition in preparation for possible transplantation usually takes place shortly after the diagnosis of liver disease has been made. Patients are placed on the waiting list according to the severity of their condition. We use a modification of the United Network for Organ Sharing classification (status 1–4). Status 1 indicates that the patient is able to be maintained at home; status 2, that the patient is hospitalized but stable; status 3, that patients are in the hospital but unstable with varying levels of coma or renal insufficiency; and status 4, that patients are mechanically ventilated in the intensive care unit.

Patients with liver dysfunction undergo a progressive deterioration affecting all organ systems to some degree. Preoperative assessment of patients can therefore be very difficult and may not represent what their condition may be closer to the date of transplantation. Consequently, the assessment of a patient for liver transplantation occurs, at least in part, on two separate occasions.

The first assessment occurs when patients are initially evaluated for potential transplantation. The purpose of this consultation is to rule out any irreversible factors that may increase the risk of surgery to an unacceptable level. The Child-Pugh classification has been successfully used to predict operative deaths and estimate surgical risk in cirrhotic patients undergoing portosystemic shunts. In liver transplantation, however, no consistent correlation has been found between preoperative variables and postoperative outcomes, except perhaps severe encephalopathy. Cuervas-Mons et al. revealed that serum creatinine value was the most accurate predictor of death, with a preoperative level greater than 1.7 mg/dl predicting

death in 79% of cases.[59] They also concluded that ascites, hepatic encephalopathy, elevated white cell count, decreased helper to T cell ratio, and increased plasma creatinine and bilirubin concentrations were associated with increased risk of death, although this was a retrospective analysis. Patients admitted to the intensive care unit before transplant have a higher rate of sepsis and death (32.6%) than inpatients not in the intensive care unit (15.8%) or patients admitted directly from home (11.9%).[60] The consultant must focus on the cardiovascular, respiratory, renal, metabolic, and hematologic disturbances and must separate the factors that are the result of liver dysfunction from coexisting disease. Factors related to liver dysfunction may correct themselves after successful transplantation and must be managed throughout the perioperative period.

The second assessment takes place immediately before transplantation. Long waiting lists usually result in months or years of ongoing liver dysfunction and advancing disease. If the patient has not been reassessed by an anesthesiologist, there may be significant changes in the patient's condition since the initial assessment, although the rate of deterioration is variable. The myriad of systemic derangements associated with liver disease requires that medical management be closely monitored throughout the waiting period. When a donor organ becomes available, the selected recipient must be re-evaluated to ensure optimal medical condition. If a problem is identified and cannot be corrected in time, another recipient may be found. In any unstable patient, sepsis must be ruled out preoperatively because it is almost universally lethal in an immunocompromised host. Clearly, the most favorable option is early transplantation before the onset of multisystem involvement. The shortage of donor organs prolongs the time spent on the waiting list and therefore may result in a significant progression of the liver disease. The most common coexisting medical problems precluding transplantation, excluding hepatobiliary factors, are infection, severe cardiac disease, and respiratory disease unrelated to the liver dysfunction.

Respiratory System

The respiratory system can be affected by hepatic dysfunction in several ways. Large volumes of ascitic fluid reduce diaphragmatic excursion, cause atelectasis, and reduce the functional residual capacity,[61] leading to hypoxemia. Hypoxic pulmonary vasoconstriction may be impaired in patients with cirrhosis. Extensive intrapulmonary shunting is associated with end-stage liver failure,[62] resulting in preoperative hypoxemia at ambient partial pressures of oxygen.[63] It has been said that the inability to achieve a Pao_2 of 200 mm Hg with a fraction of inspired oxygen of 1.0 may be a contraindication to transplantation,[64] although intrapulmonary shunting has been shown to reverse after liver transplantation.[65, 66] Patients also develop restrictive defects that are most commonly due to ascites and pleural effusions, although coexisting disease may also be present. Drainage of effusions may relieve symptoms of dyspnea but are associated with risks of bleeding and infection. Patients may also have coexisting obstructive pulmonary disease that should be treated with bronchodilators and physiotherapy to reduce the risk of infection. Smoking should be stopped when the patient is accepted for transplantation. Chronic liver disease or acute fulminant disease can also produce adult respiratory distress syndrome (ARDS).[67] Although ARDS can resolve after successful transplantation,[68] it greatly increases morbidity by prolonging mechanical ventilation and increasing the risk of infection in the immunocompromised patient. Arterial blood-gas analysis, chest radiograph, and pulmonary function tests are therefore standard in the assessment of these patients.

Up to 2% of patients with portal hypertension have associated pulmonary hypertension.[69, 70] Primary pulmonary hypertension (PPH) is associated with high mortality and morbidity in the liver transplant patient,[71–73] and the presence of pulmonary hypertension in end-stage liver disease is associated with a 6-month mortality of 50%.[74] The etiology and the response to treatment may be variable.[71, 72] Pulmonary hypertension may be due to increased pulmonary vascular resistance, increased pulmonary blood flow, or increased pulmonary venous pressure. In some patients with pulmonary hypertension associated with liver disease, improvement after transplantation may be less likely,[71] and their condition may have reached irreversibility. Nitric oxide, a selective pulmonary vasodilator,[75] has been used in more severe cases,[76] although patients with mild to moderate pulmonary hypertension have undergone orthotopic liver transplantation without difficulty[77] or adverse outcome.[78] Prostacyclin infusions have also been successfully used to control pulmonary pressures.[79] Although the electrocardiogram (ECG) and chest radiograph may suggest pulmonary hypertension, echocardiography is the most useful screening tool. Right ventricular catheterization with a trial of pulmonary vasodilator therapy is required when severe pulmonary hypertension is suspected. Assessment of reversibility establishes the degree of responsiveness to therapy and may influence decisions about management or suitability for transplantation in patients with pulmonary hypertension. Table 8-7 outlines the specific investigations that may be required in liver transplant candidates to rule out disease in respiratory and other systems.

Cardiovascular System

Most patients with end-stage liver disease are in a hyperdynamic cardiovascular state. They typically have increased cardiac index and decreased SVR,[80] which can be confused with septic shock. Adequate cardiovascular reserve is paramount to the successful outcome of transplantation. The dramatic changes in preload that can result from clamping of the major vessels and acute blood loss require that contractility, heart rate, and SVR increase to maintain blood pressure.

Although atherosclerosis may not be prevalent in cirrhotic patients,[81] it and other forms of cardiomyopathy must be ruled out, particularly in patients who are at risk. Dipyridamole-thallium scanning, wall-motion studies, and echocardiography can be helpful in identifying valvular or ventricular dysfunction and the presence of pulmonary hypertension. It must be remembered, however, that assessment is being performed in the setting of reduced SVR, and therefore cardiac function may only appear to be good. An ejection fraction less than 60% may in fact reflect myocardial dysfunction. Abnormal cardiac function does not always preclude successful orthotopic liver transplantation but may significantly increase risk. Transplantation has been reported in two patients with hypertrophic obstructive cardiomyopathy.[82] Alcoholic cardiomyopathy and the cardiac manifestations of hemosiderosis or Wilson's disease may be particularly difficult to identify; endomyocardial biopsy may be the only means of making such a diagnosis. Cardiac stress test and coronary

Table 8-7. Preoperative Systemic Conditions Associated with Liver Disease and Commonly Ordered Tests

System	Condition	Investigations
Respiratory	Atelectasis	Chest roentgenogram
	Pleural effusion	Arterial blood gases
	Decreased FRC secondary to ascites	Pulmonary function tests
	Intrapulmonary shunting	Trial of pulmonary vasodilation
	Increased $\dot{V}/\dot{Q}$ mismatch	
	Pulmonary hypertension	
	Adult respiratory distress syndrome	
Cardiovascular	Increased cardiac output	Electrocardiogram, echocardiogram
	Decreased systemic vascular resistance	Stress test (exercise or thallium)
	Portal hypertension (variable)	Wall-motion studies
	Variceal bleeding	Right heart catheterization
	Pericardial effusions (uncommon)	Cardiac catheterization, with coronary angiogram
		Myocardial biopsy
Renal	Hyponatremia or hypernatremia	Serum electrolytes, creatinine
	Hypokalemia with diuretic use	Urine electrolytes
	Hyperkalemia due to renal failure or elevated aldosterone levels	
	Acute tubular necrosis	
	Hepatorenal syndrome	
Hematologic	Anemia	CBC, INR, PTT, fibrinogen
	Thrombocytopenia	Type and cross-match
	Platelet dysfunction	
	Coagulation-factor deficiency	
	Hypersplenism	
Metabolic	Hypoglycemia in severe liver dysfunction	Glucose, calcium, magnesium, liver function tests
	Hypomagnesemia	Computed tomography scan of the head
	Hypoalbuminemia	
	Metabolic acidosis in severe hepatic dysfunction	
Central nervous	Confusion	
	Encephalopathy	
	Cerebral edema	
	Raised intracranial pressure	

FRC = functional reserve capacity (of lungs); $\dot{V}/\dot{Q}$ = ventilation-perfusion ratio; CBC = complete blood cell count; INR = international normalized ratio; PTT = partial thromboplastin time.

angiogram are not routinely done, but they should be considered in patients with significant risk factors. The typical debilitated state of these patients often precludes exercise stress testing and similarly makes exercise tolerance difficult to ascertain. The hyperdynamic state typically seen in liver disease may result in patients with significant coronary lesions becoming symptomatic, thus serving as its own stress test. These patients would be unable to tolerate the cardiovascular stresses associated with transplantation. Patients who have completed treatment with chemotherapeutic agents known to affect cardiac function should have their cardiac function evaluated before surgery, particularly if the initial assessment is dated. In cases of congenital anomalies affecting liver function, cardiac anomalies, such as pulmonary stenosis or pulmonary hypoplasia, should be evaluated before transplantation.

In patients with reduced cardiac function, venovenous bypass or temporary caval anastomosis with the piggyback technique have been used to maintain preload. Venovenous bypass can reduce the effects of inferior vena caval (IVC) clamping, such as reduced venous return, bowel edema, and increased surgical bleeding.

In our institution, venovenous bypass is used in fewer than 1% of cases. Its use has been reserved for patients with limited cardiac reserve or those responding to a trial of IVC clamping with significant hypotension (i.e., a persistent drop in mean arterial pressure [MAP] of greater than 30%). It is also used in patients who are unresponsive to volume administration, vasopressors, or the manipulation of anesthetic agents. Although bypass of femoral and portal vein to axillary vein has been used, we have also successfully used the right internal jugular as the return limb of the bypass circuit. Percutaneous techniques for establishing venous bypass access have been described.[83]

Renal Function

The presence of preoperative renal failure or severe dysfunction has been shown to significantly increase morbidity and mortality postoperatively, although mild dysfunction may not increase the risk of death.[84] The most frequent causes of renal failure in patients with cirrhosis are acute tubular necrosis and HRS.[84] Decreased fluid intake and excessive use of diuretics for the treatment of ascites can lead to prerenal insufficiency and should be monitored closely. The diagnosis of HRS is based on clinical criteria, including the presence of severe liver disease, absence of proteinuria, oliguria, slowly rising serum creatinine, a urinary sodium less than 10 mEq/liter, sodium retention, decreased free water clearance, and decreased concentrating ability. Diuretic therapy may make the diagnosis more difficult. Although the etiology of HRS is not fully understood, increased sympathetic tone causing renal vasoconstriction, inadequate intrarenal prostaglandins, activation of renin-angiotensin-aldosterone system, and elevation of antidiuretic hormone levels are all thought to play a role in this disorder.[85] In 1969, Koppel et al. published a study showing that transplantation of cadaveric kidneys from patients with HRS resulted in reversal of renal dysfunction.[86]

Some work suggests that HRS can be avoided or reversed.[87] Patients with preoperative renal dysfunction should be managed preoperatively with invasive hemodynamic monitoring and fluid administration to correct any deficits. The presence of ure-

mic symptoms, electrolyte abnormalities, acidosis, and fluid overload may necessitate pretransplant dialysis. Although reversal of HRS with transplantation has been reported,[87, 88] in general, renal dysfunction has been associated with poor posttransplant outcomes. Postoperative renal failure requiring dialysis is associated with a mortality rate of 40–90%.[84, 89, 90] In severe cases of combined liver and renal failure, transplantation of both organs has been undertaken.[91, 92] Although venovenous bypass may be beneficial in some cases, the risks of initiating venovenous bypass strictly for renal protection do not appear to be justified.[93]

Hematologic System

The hematologic and coagulation system must be assessed preoperatively because liver dysfunction is associated with anemia, thrombocytopenia, and coagulopathy. Anemia is commonly seen and may be the result of nutritional and iron deficits, malabsorption, or occult or overt bleeding. These should be corrected or prevented by ensuring adequate nutrition, providing supplemental iron and vitamins, and monitoring the stool for blood loss. The use of erythropoietin has been described and, in particular, used in the successful management of a liver transplant in a Jehovah's Witness.[94] Platelet function may be impaired, and splenic congestion seen with portal hypertension may lead to platelet sequestration and thrombocytopenia. Impaired hepatic synthesis of clotting factors and reduced absorption of vitamin K result in reduced factor levels, and insufficient hepatic clearance leads to increased circulating activated coagulation factors.[95] Defective synthesis of fibrinolytic inhibitors and delayed removal of plasminogen inhibitors lead to ongoing fibrinolysis. Unless the patient is actively bleeding, clotting factors, platelets, or vitamin K is usually not required. Administered immediately preoperatively, however, they may decrease intraoperative bleeding.[96]

Metabolism

Liver transplant candidates can present with mild to severe acid-base, electrolyte, and glucose disturbances due to the underlying liver dysfunction or to the pharmacologic agents used to treat the ascites and portal hypertension. Metabolic alkalosis may be due to hyperaldosteronism or diarrhea and vomiting. Metabolic acidosis secondary to hyponatremia may occur in patients with severe liver failure due to a low-sodium diet, impaired free water excretion, and increased antidiuretic hormonal activity. Chronic hypokalemia results from gastrointestinal losses, diuretic therapy, and poor oral intake, whereas hyperkalemia may result from renal dysfunction. To avoid excessively high potassium levels associated with reperfusion of the donor liver, preoperative hyperkalemia must be treated aggressively using oral and rectal binding resins, diuretics, or dialysis if oliguria is present. Glucose and insulin or bicarbonate are not suitable because they only redistribute potassium rather than eliminate it from body stores.

Despite a high circulating insulin level, glucose intolerance is commonly seen. In patients with severe hepatocellular disease and stored glycogen depletion, severe hypoglycemia may occur and require a dextrose infusion. Inborn errors of metabolism are most common in the pediatric population.

Central Nervous System

The extent of central nervous system (CNS) symptoms depends on the progression of liver disease. Encephalopathy generally occurs later in the disease, or it may be precipitated by bleeding esophageal varices, other gastrointestinal bleeding, or other protein loads. If organic disease is suspected, a computed tomogram of the head may be indicated. The postoperative neuropsychological outcome depends largely on the CNS status at the onset of surgery. Patients with compromised cerebral blood flow secondary to raised intracerebral pressure may experience irreversible injury. Raised intracranial pressure (ICP) secondary to cerebral edema[97] is generally associated with poor outcome, but a timely transplantation can reverse these changes.[98] Preoperatively, raised ICP should be managed with osmotic agents, such as mannitol, steroids, and 30-degree head-up position, and with mechanical hyperventilation if severe. The use of ICP monitors has been described,[98, 99] but the risks of infection and intracranial bleeding must be considered.[100, 101] Using MAP, CVP, and ICP, the goal is to maintain a cerebral perfusion pressure above 40 mm Hg. If a ventriculostomy catheter is used, it can also be used to drain cerebrospinal fluid and

Table 8-8. Preoperative Preparation

Review results of initial assessment.
Repeat blood work and electrocardiogram.
Reassess risk of transplantation.
Optimize volume status before transfer to operating room.
Begin correcting coagulopathy if active bleeding is present.
Inform blood bank.
Send for packed red blood cells before induction.

lower ICP. Patients with reduced levels of consciousness should be considered for endotracheal intubation to protect the airway from aspiration. Clearance of toxic substances from the blood, which can damage the blood–brain barrier, may require plasmapheresis or dialysis.[102]

Preoperative Preparation

Immediately before transplantation, all investigations done during the assessment period should be reviewed, and all laboratory investigations should be repeated (Table 8-8). Although work has been done in an attempt to identify which patients are at higher risk of excessive bleeding,[103] this risk remains highly variable and largely unpredictable. The institution's blood bank should be informed of the planned procedure and arrangements made to meet the needs of a possible massive transfusion. We routinely have a minimum of 6 units of packed red blood cells (pRBCs) sent to the operating room's blood refrigerator before induction of anesthesia. In some cases, additional units of pRBCs are requested in addition to 4–8 units of fresh frozen plasma. In cases of severe anemia or coagulopathy, transfusion of blood products should be started before surgery, and volume status should be optimized. This may require preoperative insertion of a central line for pressure monitoring and a urinary catheter for accurate urine output measurements. Although not routinely done, drainage of ascites can significantly reduce intra-abdominal pressure, improve diaphragmatic excursion, and improve venous return from the IVC. This may lead to a state of hypovolemia, however, and colloids should be administered if paracentesis is performed. Aspiration prophylaxis, such as ranitidine and metoclopramide, can also be given at this time. A list of

Table 8-9. Drugs Typically Used during a Liver Transplantation*

Drug	Induction	Preanhepatic	Anhepatic	Posthepatic
Aprotinin	2 million KIU	150,000 KIU/hr	150,000 KIU/hr	150,000 KIU/hr
Vasopressin	—	0.5 µg/kg/hr	0	0
Fentanyl	4–6 µg/kg	4–6 µg/kg	—	4–6 µg/kg
Midazolam	10–40 µg/kg	0–1 mg	0–1 mg	0–1 mg
Pentothal	4–6 mg/kg	—	—	—
Furosemide	—	10–20 mg	—	—
Mannitol 20%	—	1.0–1.5 g/kg	—	—
Methylprednisolone	—	—	500 mg	—
Magnesium	—	2–4 g	—	—
Calcium chloride	—	2–4 g	1 g	—
Sodium bicarbonate	—	—	0–100 mEq	—
Protamine	—	—	—	0–50 mg
Phenylephrine boluses	—	—	80 µg/bolus	80 µg/bolus
Dopamine (renal)	—	0–2.5 µg/kg/min	0–2.5 µg/kg/min	0–2.5 µg/kg/min
Dopamine vasopressor	—	2.5–10.0 µg/kg/min	2.5–10.0 µg/kg/min	2.5–10.0 µg/kg/min

*Some agents may not be indicated for a given patient and are not always administered. Doses are approximate and vary with the clinical status of the patient.
KIU = kallikrein inactivation units.

drugs typically used throughout the course of a liver transplant is shown in Table 8-9. It is recommended that a supply of all these medications be on hand before induction.

Intraoperative Monitoring

The extent of monitoring depends on the recipient's surgical history, status on arrival to the operating room, surgical technique, and anticipated blood loss. Our average homologous blood transfusion rate is 4 units of pRBCs. Continuous monitoring usually begins in the operating room, although more critically ill patients have monitoring in place before surgery and should be transferred to the operating room with transport monitors. If the invasive monitoring lines have been in place for some time or show evidence of infection, these should be replaced at a clean new site. The standard monitors include pulse oximetry, core body temperature, 5-lead ECG, end-tidal CO_2, and urine output. Leads II and V_5 are routinely monitored, as are ST segments. In most cases, the radial arterial line is inserted after induction of general anesthesia, but, if the patient has been unstable, insertion is done before induction. In our center, one invasive arterial line is used. Some centers routinely use two sites,[104]

one for pressure monitoring and the other for arterial blood sampling. A femoral arterial line may not be useful if the aorta is clamped during hepatic artery anastomosis. If one anticipates using the left axillary vein for venovenous bypass, the radial arterial line should be placed on the patient's right side because the left axilla remains exposed for cannulation. Two 14-gauge peripheral intravenous lines and a 9 French right internal jugular line are inserted. Pulmonary artery catheters are used routinely as a means of measuring CVP, pulmonary artery pressure, pulmonary capillary wedge pressure (PCWP), mixed venous gases, cardiac index, and calculation of SVR. If a percutaneous approach to venovenous bypass is anticipated, the central line is inserted in the left internal jugular vein, leaving the right internal jugular vein available for percutaneous insertion of the bypass circuit return limb. If significant blood loss is anticipated, a second 9 French sheath is inserted in another convenient central site, such as the other jugular vein, cephalic veins, or femoral veins. Subclavian lines are rarely used in patients with preoperative coagulopathies because these vessels are noncompressible. Although prolonged use of femoral lines is avoided, femoral venous lines have been inserted in patients with compromised renal function as a means of monitoring renal perfusion pressure. For example, renal perfusion pressures greater than 60 mm Hg should be maintained during the anhepatic period.

Laboratory investigations are key to safe management of the transplant recipient. We currently use a portable unit that provides results within 2 minutes. Alternatively, we can send our sample to an operating room satellite laboratory for more complete analysis. The values of particular interest include hemoglobin, platelet count, INR, partial thromboplastin time (PTT), calcium, potassium, glucose, and acid-base balance. We also monitor fibrinogen and other coagulation factors, although these are less likely to alter management unless massive blood loss and transfusion have occurred. Samples are drawn after induction, during the dissection period, before applying the caval and portal clamps, early in the anhepatic period, mid-anhepatic period, late in the anhepatic period, after clamps are removed, and during reperfusion. Other tests, such as the Sonoclot and thromboelastography, can be done to assess the coagulation process, including the interaction of coagulation proteins and platelets. Clearly, how closely we monitor the patient's hematologic and metabolic profile depends on his or her preoperative status, hemodynamic stability, rate of blood loss, and products transfused intraoperatively. Core temperature is measured using a pharyngeal or esophageal probe in addition to the pulmonary artery catheter. Convective heat loss, massive transfusions, and a cooled donor organ can lead to hypothermia, which can cause cardiac arrhythmias, contribute to coagulopathy, reduce renal function, and decrease myocardial contractility. The use of warmed rapid-infusion systems, nonconductive head and extremity wraps, and forced-convection air warmer systems may help to maintain and possibly transfer heat to raise body temperature.[105] Forced-air warming has been shown to prevent intraoperative hypothermia during liver transplantation.[106]

Induction and Maintenance

Status 1 and 2 patients have standard monitors applied on arrival to the operating room. A 14-gauge intravenous line is started if there is no established access. End-tidal oxygen levels can be used to ensure adequate preoxygenation before the administration of any pharmacologic agents. Decreased drug-binding protein leads to increased sensitivity to thiopental, and increased volume of distribution leads to increased resistance to muscle relaxants. Drugs acting on the CNS must be titrated carefully to effect, particularly in the presence of encephalopathy. Elimination of midazolam may be delayed,[107] and plasma clearance of fentanyl is decreased[108] in patients with hepatic cirrhosis. A rapid-sequence induction should be used, given the potential for regurgitation and aspiration. Fentanyl, 4–6 µg/kg, is usually administered first to help reduce the response to intubation. The pharmacodynamics are not significantly altered unless liver dysfunction is severe. Midazolam, 10–40 µg/kg, can be used as a co-induction agent. Sodium pentothal, 4–6 mg/kg, followed by 1.5–2.0 mg/kg of succinylcholine is almost always well tolerated with minimal hemodynamic changes. If hemodynamic instability is anticipated, ketamine can be used at a dose of 1–2 mg/kg, although ketamine may also result in cardiovascular depression if the preinduction sympathetic tone is already elevated. Although deficiency in plasma cholinesterase can occur, it is rarely of any clinical importance.

The patient's position must also be carefully checked before draping to ensure that there are no pressure points and that intravenous lines are not occluded. The patient's arms are well padded and generally placed along the body, unless venovenous bypass is anticipated, in which case one of the the patient's arms is positioned to his or her side with the least amount of abduction possible. After the abdominal incision is made, a lubricated nasogastric tube is gently inserted to decompress the patient's stomach and optimize surgical exposure.

Maintenance of anesthesia is achieved using volatile agents, such as isoflurane, which undergoes very little metabolism, and a mixture of air and oxygen. Nitrous oxide is avoided due to its mild myocardial depressant effects and its ability to exacerbate the effects of air emboli, which could occur during the reperfusion phase[109, 110] or as a complication of venovenous bypass.[111, 112] Although drainage of ascites can facilitate abdominal closure, prolonged use of nitrous oxide could make closure more difficult and compromise intra-abdominal blood flow, including hepatic and renal perfusion as a result of bowel distention. In patients with raised ICP, inhaled anesthetic doses should be minimized and anesthesia provided with intravenous agents.

Table 8-10. Relative Changes in Various Parameters during Liver Transplantation*

Variable	Preanhepatic	Anhepatic	Neohepatic
Glucose	+	–/+	++
Hemoglobin	–/– –	–	–/– –
Platelets	–	–	–
Urine output	++	– –	+/++
Cardiac index	++	+	+++
Systemic vascular resistance	– –	++	– – –
Peripheral vascular resistance	+	–	+
Mean arterial blood pressure	–	– –	– – –/– followed by +
Lactate	+	+	+/++
K	+	+	+++ followed by +
Ca	–	– –	–
Mg	–	– –	–
Na	+	+	+
Temperature	–	– – –	+

*The signs reflect a typical change in the direction indicated relative to the value in the preceding stage of the transplant.
+ = mild increase; ++ = moderate increase; +++ = significant increase; – = mild decrease; – – = moderate decrease; – – – = significant decrease.

Muscle relaxation is ensured with long-acting agents, such as pancuronium; if there is coexisting renal dysfunction, vecuronium or rocuronium is most often used. Atracurium is not often used, despite its unique route of Hofmann elimination, because it requires neither hepatic nor renal function for elimination. In addition, laudanosine, its principal metabolite, is converted in the liver for renal excretion, and elevated concentrations of laudanosine in dogs have been associated with CNS stimulation, including seizures. Hepatic disease may reduce metabolism of these drugs, but with proper neuromuscular monitoring, they can be used safely. Antibiotics may require several administrations during long procedures to maintain adequate blood levels in cases of massive blood loss.

Anesthetic Considerations during the Preanhepatic, Anhepatic, and Reperfusion Stages

The anesthetic intraoperative management of the transplant procedure is divided into the preanhepatic, anhepatic, and reperfusion stages, as described under Surgical Considerations. Tables 8-10 and 8-11 summarize the potential changes in biochemistry, hemodynamic parameters, and complications that occur in each stage.

The Preanheptic Stage (Recipient Hepatectomy)

The preanhepatic stage begins with induction of anesthesia and ends with clamping of the portal vein, IVC, and hepatic artery. It is usually associated with constant fluid shifts and blood loss. Vasopressin (0.5 U/kg/hour), used to decrease splanchnic blood flow and portal venous pressure, is infused intravenously from the start, and coagulation factors are transfused as required. Aprotinin can be infused during the entire procedure (150,000 kallikrein inactivation units [KIU]/hour) after a postinduction bolus (2 million KIU). This serine protease inhibitor reduces thrombin and plasmin generation and therefore functions as an antifibrinolytic.[113, 114] It has been shown to reduce blood loss in several studies,[115–118] although it made no difference in another study.[119] The minimum dose required is debatable because no difference in transfusion requirements were found in a study comparing low-dose (500,000 KIU bolus followed by 150,000 KIU/hour infusion) and high-dose aprotinin protocols.[120] Aprotinin may also have anti-inflammatory effects, which may reduce the response to vasoactive substances released during the reperfusion phase, although this needs further study. Alternatively, tranexamic acid, also an antifibrinolytic agent, has also been reported to reduce blood loss in doses of 10–20 g.[121, 122]

Table 8-11. Intraoperative Complications and Management

Complication	Management
Hypothermia	Heat exchanger, fluid warmer, warming blanket, forced-air units, postoperative ventilation, warm blood flush
Hyperkalemia	Binding resins, diuresis, dialysis, hyperventilation, sodium bicarbonate, calcium chloride, insulin or glucose
Hypocalcemia	Calcium chloride or gluconate administered by central line
Oliguria	Maintain adequate volume; increase renal perfusion pressure; mannitol, furosemide, and ethacrynic acid; avoid vasopressor use
Hypotension	Maintain adequate volume, check calcium and magnesium, rule out cardiac dysfunction, administer vasopressors, transfuse blood products if anemic or coagulopathic
Hypertension	Maintain adequate anesthetic depth, reduce filling pressures, avoid long-acting agents to treat hypertension
Postreperfusion syndrome	Anticipate; ensure that volume loading is not excessive; administer calcium, vasopressors

Urinary output must be maintained and may require the use of a dopamine infusion (2 µg/kg/minute),[123] mannitol (1.0–1.5 g/kg), and furosemide, although there is some evidence to suggest that these interventions do not affect postoperative renal function.[124] Cardiac dysrhythmias and episodes of hypotension may be seen as a result of traction during dissection around the IVC. Hemodynamic changes and cardiac arrhythmias may also be due to hypocalcemia or hypomagnesemia, or both.[125] Calcium chloride and magnesium supplements are therefore slowly administered through a central line during this phase in accordance with laboratory results. The vasopressin infusion is discontinued at the end of the dissection. The cardiovascular response to clamping of the major vessels has been used as a marker to determine whether venovenous bypass is required during the anhepatic stage.[126] A decrease in MAP greater than 30% in an appropriately volume-loaded patient or a decrease in cardiac index of more than 50% from preclamp values can be used as a guideline to initiate venovenous bypass. Transesophageal echocardiography (TEE) can be used to monitor filling volumes of ventricles, emboli, and valvular dysfunction, but we have only rarely used it when cardiovascular function was of particular concern. Patients are normally in a reverse Trendelenburg position during the surgery, which can exacerbate hypovolemic states. Renal protection using intravenous mannitol, low-dose dopamine,[127] adequate renal perfusion pressures, and possibly using venovenous bypass[128] must be considered before clamping of the major vessels. In patients without preoperative renal dysfunction who were able to tolerate a trial of clamping, venovenous bypass did not influence postoperative renal function.[128] In this study, the mean renal perfusion pressure was 60 ± 17 mm Hg after clamping and without venovenous bypass. The benefits of routine use of venovenous bypass for renal protection remain unclear, particularly in the patient with preoperative dysfunction.

Clamping of the IVC results in a 50–60% decrease in venous return to the patient's heart, producing substantial decreases in cardiac index, MAP, PCWP, and CVP with increases in heart rate, SVR index, and pulmonary vascular resistance index.[73] MAP is usually partially restored within 10 minutes of IVC clamping through compensatory mechanisms, although CO often remains less than 50% of the preclamp value.

The Anhepatic Stage

The anhepatic stage begins with clamping of the portal venous supply to the native liver and the vena cava, and it ends with unclamping of these vessels and reperfusion of the donor liver. This stage typically lasts 45–60 minutes. It can be marked by significant hemodynamic and acid-base changes. Preparation for the anhepatic stage begins in the preanhepatic stage. If not routinely used, a decision must be made whether venovenous bypass is required. Venovenous bypass is rarely used in our center; it is reserved for patients who do not meet our trial of clamping criteria or are predicted to be unusually difficult to transplant. Clamping the IVC results in a drop in venous return and, consequently, reduced CO and reflex increase in SVR, although the degree of change depends on the extent of collateral venous flow. Cardiac output and arterial pressures can be improved by increasing filling pressures using PCWP and CVP measurements to ensure a controlled volume loading. It is preferable, however, to maintain the filling pressures at or near the reduced levels reached with IVC clamping, which are typically on the order of 2–7 mm Hg. Fluid overload may lead to pulmonary edema when the clamps are removed. Blood pressure is maintained, in part, by an increased SVR and heart rate. If adequate collateral venous channels have not developed as a result of the liver disease, clamping of the IVC may result in significant venous back pressure. The absence of liver metabolism and anaerobic metabolism in tissues below the IVC clamp can lead to lactic acidosis. Consequently, renal perfusion pressure is decreased unless systemic arterial pressure can be raised with slightly higher filling pressures or the judicious use of vasopressors, such as phenylephrine. Urine output is usually reduced during this stage, but continued urine production may be the only indicator of adequate renal perfusion. Core body temperature may decrease by 2–3°C as a result of the absent heat-producing liver, the cold donor organ, massive transfusion, and the extensive abdominal exposure.

The liver is usually first flushed using 750–1,000 ml of a crystalloid solution followed by 300- to 400-ml blood flush, which reperfuses the liver without systemic contamination. This loss of blood volume should be anticipated and replaced as the anastomosis is completed. Preparation for the reperfusion phase necessitates re-evaluation of the acid-base balance, calcium and potassium levels, and volume status. Hyperkalemia may lead to dysrhythmias or a refractory asystolic state. Symptomatic hyperkalemia can be treated with calcium chloride, $NaCO_3$, glucose or insulin administration, and hyperventilation. It is best, however, to minimize the hyperkalemic effect by ensuring adequate diuresis throughout all stages of surgery and raising the threshold to depolarization using intravenous calcium chloride before reperfusion. Ionized calcium is maintained above 1.0 mmol/liter and magnesium levels above 0.5 mmol/liter at all times. Immediately before flushing the donor liver, an arterial blood sample is drawn for acid-base balance, potassium, ionized calcium, and hemoglobin analysis. These results determine what doses of sodium bicarbonate and calcium chloride are to be given before unclamping. Generally, a minimum of 1 g of calcium chloride and 25 mEq of bicarbonate are given to a recipient with a serum potassium level below 4.0 mmol/liter at the end of the anhepatic stage. Hyperventilation is also instituted to minimize the effect of bicarbonate-induced respiratory acidosis.

The Reperfusion Period

This stage coincides with reperfusion of the graft by unclamping the major vessels, which can lead to hypotension, hyperkalemia, lactic acidosis, hypothermia, and coagulopathy. Cardiac arrest has been reported when the clamps are removed, and particular attention must be directed to the ECG. Transient hypotension requiring vasopressors is frequent and likely due to the decrease in peripheral vascular resistance. This transient and reversible relative hypovolemia should not be treated with excessive volume unless a state of true hypovolemia is a suspected contributing factor. It is appropriate to give 40- to 80-μg phenylephrine boluses if systolic pressures decrease by more than 20% or if MAP remains persistently low. Rarely, 100- to 200-μg epinephrine boluses are required. Hyperkalemia, although transient, can lead to dysrhythmias, hypotension, and cardiac arrest. Potassium levels of 7.8 mmol/liter were reported by Carmichael et al.,[127] and levels of 9.5 have been measured (J. Kutt, personal communication, 1997). Cardiovascular collapse resulting from pulmonary thromboembolism has also been reported.[129, 130] Postreperfusion syndrome (PRS) is a transient and occasionally profound cardiovascular collapse that occurs after the release of the portal clamp in 8–30% of cases. PRS was initially defined as a 30% decrease in MAP lasting at least 1 minute within the first 5 minutes after reperfusion.[131] It is characterized by decreased MAP, SVR, and myocardial contractility and increases in pulmonary vascular resistance and pulmonary capillary filling pressures.[132, 133] Severe hypotension usually resolves in the first 5–10 minutes but may persist, requiring the use of inotropic agents and fluid administration. In many cases, cardiac depression attributed to PRS is caused by hypocalcemia.[134] The etiology of PRS is likely multifactorial but has implicated the release of vasoactive substances[135, 136] from the donor liver. Also implicated are transient hyperkalemia, hypothermia, acidosis, hyperosmolality, acute increases in intravascular and left ventricular volume, with left ventricular mechanoreceptor reflex stimulation causing bradycardia and myocardial depression.[127, 137] In one study, hyperkalemia, hypothermia, and acidosis did not appear to play a role in reperfusion hypotension.[95] An acute increase in preload shown by an increase in right ventricular size[134] could lead to right heart strain and hypotension. A TEE study of ventricular function during liver reperfusion found no alteration in left ventricular function to justify PRS, and the hemodynamic changes seemed to be caused by an insufficient increase in preload after unclamping.[138] Also, myocardial depression has not been consistently associated with PRS.[139, 140] Incremental doses of phenylephrine or epinephrine can be used to support MAP and contractility; however, the recipient may have an attenuated response to vasopressors[141] or may be unresponsive to inotropic support if acidosis has not been corrected. The hemodynamic changes associated with PRS appear to be similar whether venovenous bypass is used or not.[142] Estrin et al.[135] found their incidence (7.6%) of PRS to be lower than did Aggarwal et al. (30%).[131] Estrin et al. also found that not using venovenous bypass may have protected against PRS, perhaps because of volume loading required to maintain preload in the absence of venovenous bypass. Martinez et al. have found that the integrity of the vasoconstrictive response, defined as an increase in peripheral vascular resistance greater than 50% as measured immediately after clamping of the IVC, correlates with the occurrence of PRS.[143]

The impact of various flush and reperfusion techniques on PRS suggests that portal vein flush without vena caval venting provides a lower incidence of PRS, although venting does reduce the release of potassium into the circulation. In the same study, postoperative graft function was not significantly affected by flush and reperfusion techniques.[144] The higher incidence of PRS with venting is likely due to a state of hypovolemia created by the venting. One approach is to vent the blood flush, unless the anastomosis has been particularly difficult to complete, and to ensure adequate replacement of the vented volume before removing clamps. In another study, flushing with 500 ml of autologous portal blood resulted in smaller intraoperative shifts in serum potassium, greater hemodynamic stability, better graft function, and improved graft and patient survival.[145] Flushing also helps reduce the toxic substance load (e.g., ammonia), which requires energy for metabolism. Fukuzawa et al. found 3,562 µg of ammonia in the first 500 ml of blood flush.[145] Warming the donor liver with vented blood flush may also minimize hypothermic insult to the heart on reperfusion. This warming technique, by maintaining hemodynamic stability with reperfusion, may help prevent early ischemic injury to the organ, although this has not been proved.

A postreperfusion coagulopathy has also been described. Heparin is generally administered to the organ donor before retrieval, and the possibility of heparin sequestration in the donor liver, with subsequent release in the recipient at reperfusion, has been investigated. Two case reports describing reversal of this coagulopathy using protamine sulfate have been published.[146] Heparin-like activity has been demonstrated in recipients whose donors did not receive heparin, suggesting the presence of an endogenous heparinoid.[147]

Release of glucose from the donor liver because of the stress response to surgery may result in a transient hyperglycemia, with serum levels on the order of 10 mmol/liter. Although mild transient hyperglycemia usually does not need treatment, persistent serum levels above 12 mmol/liter should be closely monitored and treated with an insulin infusion, particularly if there is known CNS compromise.

The Completion Stage

Blood loss during the hepatic artery anastomosis is usually minimal unless there is hidden blood loss at the vena caval and portal anastomoses. During biliary reconstruction and abdominal closure, time is taken to correct metabolic and hematologic abnormalities. A nasojejunal feeding tube is positioned in patients in whom preoperative nutritional status has been very poor, or in those in whom postoperative nutrition may become problematic.

After orthoptic liver transplantation (OLT), patients are admitted to the intensive care unit for monitoring and management of their fluid status and for initiation of immunosuppression. Intermittent positive-pressure ventilation (IPPV) is usually used for ventilatory support rather than treatment of acute respiratory failure. Although immediate extubation is occasionally possible, a short period of ventilation allows for a gradual normothermic emergence. Arguments in favor of IPPV are based on the fact that the prolonged upper abdominal traction required for the procedure can lead to decreased lung volumes, functional residual capacity, and lung compliance and increased work of breathing in a spontaneously breathing patient. In most patients, these parameters return to normal after 18–36 hours of mechanical ventilation, although permanent phrenic nerve injury has been reported. Mechanical ventilation may not be of benefit in all OLT patients. Spontaneous ventilation may be beneficial in the hemodynamically stable patient because reduced intrapleural pressure improves venous return, cardiac output, and hepatic blood flow.[148–150] Immediate tracheal extubation has been reported in approximately 25% of OLT patients.[151] Clearly, more complicated cases, requiring massive transfusion or hemodynamic support, may mandate prolonged ventilation. Some patients may have pleural effusions at the time of transplantation that require drainage and chest tube insertion. Not all effusions may need to be drained, however, and the risk of bleeding and infection should be considered before chest tube insertion. In either case, chest physiotherapy is also an essential part of perioperative respiratory care. After reperfusion of the donor liver or with entrainment of air associated with the use of venovenous bypass, paradoxical air embolism has been described[79] and may contribute to postoperative neurologic deficits.[152]

Once extubated and stable, the patient is transferred to the transplant unit, where he or she continues to be closely monitored. Analgesia is generally provided using intravenous morphine injections. Meperidine is avoided, particularly in patients with compromised renal function, because its metabolite depends on renal excretion. Patient-controlled analgesia has been used in a few patients who are fully oriented.

Fluid Management: Types and Amounts

Appropriate fluid management begins in the preoperative period. Patients should be well hydrated before surgery, as determined by adequate urine output or CVP. In more critically ill patients, pulmonary artery catheters may be used early. Electrolytes should be checked and the choice of crystalloid based on those results. Hyponatremia is associated with liver disease and is particularly common in patients with HRS. Sodium correction should be carried out slowly to avoid central pontine myelinolysis associated with rapid correction. In patients with significant renal dysfunction and decreased urine output, preoperative hemodialysis may be required to correct electrolyte and volume status. Fluid management is perhaps the most challenging aspect of this procedure because it is unpredictable and variable, depending on the extent of portal hypertension, coagulation profile, and the difficulty of dissection. The goals of fluid management are to maintain normovolemia, oxygen-carrying capacity, and hemostasis. Although most of the fluid given consists of crystalloid and blood products, albumin can be used to maintain oncotic pressure in the hypoalbuminemic patient. Disturbances in acid-base balance and coagulation, sudden massive blood loss, variable renal function, and potentially impaired cardiac function require ongoing reassessment. Ringer's solution may cause serum lactate levels to rise, and normal saline may cause metabolic acidosis. Rapid-transfusion devices, which permit large volumes of warm products to be safely administered, should be used.

Patients may need to be rehydrated after induction and after drainage of ascites. If required, part of this rehydration can be accomplished using fresh frozen plasma, if coagulation has not been corrected. The dissection is usually associated with slow but constant blood loss. Occasionally, significant blood loss may occur, particularly in the presence of severe portal hypertension. Although measured blood and fluid losses are usually good indicators of transfusion requirements, these losses tend to be so great that it may be difficult to estimate volumes accurately. For this reason, central pressures, hemodynamic profile, and urine output are used to monitor volume status. In other areas of anesthesia, the current acceptable practice is to lower the transfusion triggers and perfuse with lower hematocrits. With the risk of sudden massive blood loss, however, it is preferable to keep the hematocrit and blood volume slightly above the lower acceptable levels to serve as a buffer. We generally aim for hemoglobin levels between 9 and 10 g/dl, with a hematocrit between 28% and 32%, and

PCWP in the range of 15–20 mm Hg. The PCWP at the end of the procedure should be less than 15 mm Hg in most cases. Higher pressures may be necessary to ensure that urine output is maintained. Overtransfusion and elevated hematocrits should be avoided due to the increased risk of antibody sensitization, infection, and hepatic artery thrombosis. Microfilters of 80 microns or so should be used to clear microaggregates from the blood being transfused. After 3–4 units, the filters should be replaced to minimize resistance to flow.

Before clamping, there should be satisfactory surgical hemostasis, and blood volume should be optimized. Rarely, in difficult cases, the clamps may have to be applied before full dissection to achieve surgical hemostasis. Filling pressures should be high normal (15–20 mm Hg) before clamping if venovenous bypass is not used. A trial clamping of the IVC is then done. A greater than 30% decrease in MAP may reflect inadequate volume or the need for vasopressor use or venovenous bypass. Blood, plasma, or crystalloid is usually required only in small volumes during the anhepatic time. Transfusion may then again be required with the 300- to 400-ml blood flush and reperfusion phase. Although infrequent, a technically difficult anastomosis may lead to significant blood loss after the clamps are removed, and volume should be prepared to infuse readily before removing the clamps.

The use of recovered blood through a Cell Saver unit has become more common. One study showed that the use of 6.2 erythrocyte units per case was cost-effective, reduced the exposure to homologous blood and blood components,[153] and reduced the blood bank usage. The salvaged blood is washed and centrifuged, producing a suspension of red cells with a hematocrit in excess of 55%. The major weakness of cell saving is the fact that processing of salvaged blood requires at least 1,000 ml of collected blood before the 5- to 8-minute washing procedure can begin. In cases of massive blood loss, this rate of retransfusion is inadequate, and homologous transfusions are usually required. The use of fresh frozen plasma should also be increased to compensate for the absence of factors in the washed cells.

Coagulopathy is often present before transplant and is characterized by decreases in coagulation factors, qualitative and quantitative platelet defects, and fibrinolysis. Surgical bleeding commonly leads to dilutional coagulopathy in addition to pre-existing problems. During the anhepatic stage, coagulation factors are further depleted, and clearance of activated factors and inhibitors is impaired. The use of venovenous bypass can result in a small heparin effect caused by the heparin used in the bypass priming solution. With reperfusion, coagulation is impaired further as a result of tissue plasminogen activator and heparin released from the donor liver, hypothermia, and additional dilutional effects.

Transfusion of fresh frozen plasma is generally required to replace that which is lost during the surgical procedure. It is surprisingly difficult to fully normalize PTT and INR using fresh frozen plasma, and its use should be based on a clinical need. Liver transplantation without the use of fresh frozen plasma has been reported in a subgroup of recipients.[154]

Platelets should also be available and transfused as required. In the presence of hypersplenism, platelet transfusions may not be effective. Desmopressin (DDAVP) may help improve platelet function. Cryoprecipitate is rarely used to treat a coagulopathy in our patients unless the fibrinogen levels are particularly low. During the neohepatic stage, overtransfusion or volume loading should be avoided because it may lead to pulmonary edema, decreased oxygenation, and prolonged mechanical ventilation.

Special Cases

The patient undergoing retransplantation is a special case. In addition to all the usual considerations, these patients are immunosuppressed; have likely been sensitized to antibodies, which makes crossmatching more difficult; and may have acquired hypertension and renal dysfunction as a result of cyclosporine toxicity. These patients are considered steroid dependent and should receive 500 mg of methylprednisolone before induction of anesthesia. Aseptic technique must be followed strictly. In some cases, particularly if the original surgery was recent, the dissection may be easier than the original.

Simultaneous transplantation of liver and kidney may be necessary in patients with end-stage disease of both organs. When both organs are from the same donor, the liver protects the kidney from antibody-mediated injury. Primary hyperoxaluria is a particular indication for combined liver and kidney transplantation,[155] although combined procedures for other indications have been reported.

Intraoperative Use of Immunosuppressive Agents

Immunosuppression has been the single most important factor in improving patient outcomes after liver transplantation. Intravenous corticosteroids, such as methylprednisolone, are generally administered during the transplant. OKT3 monoclonal antibody may be used for induction immunosuppression in the perioperative period. OKT3 administration should be undertaken only after the patient has been hemodynamically stabilized, typically in the completion stage of surgery, because its use has been associated with unpredictable acute side effects, such as fever, bronchospasm, hypotension, hypertension, and pulmonary edema. We currently administer H_1-receptor antagonists (diphenhydramine, 50 mg) and H_2-receptor antagonists (ranitidine, 50 mg) in conjunction with corticosteroid (methylprednisolone, 500 mg) before giving OKT3. Postoperative hypoxemia and ARDS may be seen secondary to OKT3 and may be due, in part, to overzealous fluid administration.

References

1. Starzl TE, Marchioro TL, von Kaulla K, et al. Homotransplantation of the liver in humans. Surg Gyn Obstet 1963;117:659–674.
2. National Institutes of Health Consensus Conference Statement: liver transplantation—June 20–23, 1983. Hepatology 1984;4:107S–110S.
3. Wall WJ, Mimeault R, Grant DR, Bloch M. The use of older donor livers for hepatic transplantation. Transplantation 1990;49:377–384.
4. Otte JB, deVille de Goyet J, Sokal E, et al. Size reduction of the donor liver is a safe way to alleviate the shortage of size-matched organs in pediatric liver transplantation. Ann Surg 1990;211:146–157.
5. Broelsch CE, Burdelski M, Rogiers X, et al. Living donor for liver transplantation. Hepatology 1994;20:49–55.
6. Watsnsbe FD, Mullon CJP, Hewitt WR, et al. Clinical experience with a bioartificial liver in the treatment of severe liver failure. Ann Surg 1997;225:484–494.
7. United Network for Organ Sharing. Annual Report of the U.S. Scientific Registry for Organ Transplantation and the Organ Procurement and Transplantation Network. Richmond, VA: UNOS; and Rockville, MD: the Division of Transplantation, Bureau of Health Resources Development, Health Resources and Service Administration, U.S. Department of Health and Human Services, 1997.
8. Williams W. Classification, etiology, and considerations of outcome in acute liver failure. Semin Liver Dis 1996;4:343–348.
9. Boker KHW, Dalley G, Bahr MJ, et al. Long-term outcome of hepatitis C virus infection after liver transplantation. Hepatology 1997;25:203–210.
10. Bartholomew MM, Jansen RW, Jeffers LJ, et al. Hepatitis B virus resistance to lamivudine given for recurrent infection after orthotopic liver transplantation. Lancet 1997;349:20–22.
11. Pasha TM, Dickson ER. Survival algorithms and outcome analysis in primary biliary cirrhosis. Semin Liver Dis 1997;17:147–158.
12. Fisher A, Miller CM. Ischemic type biliary strictures in liver allografts: the Achilles heel revisited [editorial]? Hepatology 1995;21:589–591.
13. Ghent CN, Grant DR, Wall WJ. Letter to the editor. CMAJ 1994;151:509.
14. Christensen E, Schlichting P, Fauerholdt L, et al. Prognostic value of Child-Turcotte criteria in medically treated cirrhosis. Hepatology 1984;4:430–435.
15. Cordoba J, Blei AT. Brain edema and hepatic encephalopathy. Semin Liver Dis 1996;16:271–280.
16. Ellis JA, Wendon J, Williams R. Efficacy and safety of intracranial pressure monitoring in fulminant hepatic failure. J Hepatol 1994;21:S51.
17. Morgan MY. Noninvasive neuroinvestigation in liver disease. Semin Liver Dis 1996;16:293–314.
18. McCashland TM, Shaw BW, Tape E. The American experience with transplantation for acute liver failure. Semin Liver Dis 1996;16:427–434.
19. Rolando N, Phipott-Howard J, Williams R. Bacterial and fungal infection in acute liver failure. Semin Liver Dis 1996;16:389–402.
20. Steigmann GV, Goff JS, Onody PA, et al. Endoscopic sclerotherapy as compared to endoscopic ligation for bleeding esophageal varices. N Engl J Med 1992;326:1527–1532.
21. Beppu K, Ionkuchi K, Koyanagi N, et al. Prediction of variceal hemorrhage by esophageal endoscopy. Gastrointest Endosc 1981;27:213–218.
22. Gines P, Arroyo V, Vargas V, et al. Paracentesis with intravenous infusion of albumin as compared with peritoneovenous shunting in cirrhosis with refractory ascites. N Engl J Med 1991;325:829–835.
23. Singh N, Gayowski T, Yu VL, Wagener M. Trimethoprim-sulfamethoxazole for the prevention of spontaneous bacterial peritonitis in cirrhosis. A randomized controlled trial. Ann Intern Med 1995;122:595–598.
24. Cuevras-Mons V, Millan I, Gavaler JS, et al. Prognostic value of preoperatively obtained clinical and laboratory data in predicting survival following orthotopic liver transplantation. Hepatology 1986;6:922–927.
25. Pikul J, Sharpe MD, Lowndes R, Ghent CN. Degree of preoperative malnutrition is predictive of postoperative morbidity and mortality in liver transplant recipients. Transplantation 1994;57:469–472.
26. Ghent C. Overall evaluation: screening and assessment

of risk factors. Liver Transplant Surg 1996;2(5)(Suppl 1): 2–8.

27. Strasberg SM, Howard JK, Molmenti EP, Hertl M. Selecting the donor liver. Risk factors for poor function after orthotopic liver transplantation. Hepatology 1994; 20:829–838.

28. Carmichael FJ, Lindop MJ, Farman JV. Anaesthesia for hepatic transplantation: cardiovascular and metabolic alterations and their management. Anaesth Analg 1985;64:108–116.

29. Starzl TE, Demetris AJ. Liver transplantation: a 31-year perspective. Part I. Curr Probl Surg 1990;27:72–116.

30. Shaw BW, Martin DJ, Marquez JM, et al. Venous bypass in clinical liver transplantation. Ann Surg 1984;200:524–534.

31. Wall WJ, Grant DR, Duff JH, et al. Liver transplantation without venous bypass. Transplantation 1987;43: 56–61.

32. Jamieson NV, Sundberg R, Lindell S, et al. Preservation of the canine liver for 24–48 hours using simple cold storage with UW solution. Transplantation 1988; 46:517–525.

33. Stratta RJ, Wood PR, Langnas AN, et al. The impact of extended preservation on clinical liver transplantation. Transplantation 1990;50:438–443.

34. Kalayaglu M, Sollinger HW, Stratta RJ, et al. Extended preservation of the liver for clinical transplantation. Lancet 1988;1:617–619.

35. Stock PG, Payne WD, Ascher NL, et al. Rapid infusion technique as a safe alternative to venovenous bypass in orthotopic liver transplantation. Transplant Proc 1989;21:2322–2325.

36. Grande L, Rimola A, Cugat E, et al. Effect of venovenous bypass on perioperative renal function in liver transplantation: results of a randomized controlled trial. Hepatology 1996;23:1418–1428.

37. Calne RY. Surgical aspects of clinical liver transplantation in 14 cases. Br J Surg 1969;56:729–734.

38. Tzakis A, Todo S, Starzl TE. Piggyback orthotopic liver transplantation with preservation of the inferior vena cava. Ann Surg 1989;210:649–652.

39. Jovine E, Mazziotti A, Grazi GL, et al. Piggy-back versus conventional technique in liver transplantation: report of a randomized trial. Transpl Int 1997;10: 109–112.

40. Shaw BW Jr. Just winging it [editorial]. Liver Transplant Surg 1997;3:190–193.

41. Calne RY. Recipient Operation. In RY Calne (ed), Liver Transplantation. New York: Grune & Stratton, 1983; 155–173.

42. Aggarwal S, Kang Y, Freeman JA, et al. Postperfusion syndrome: cardiovascular collapse following hepatic reperfusion during liver transplantation. Transplant Proc 1987;19(Suppl 3):54–55.

43. Brems J, Takiff H, McHutchison J, et al. Systemic versus nonsystemic reperfusion of the transplanted liver. Transplantation 1993;55:527–529.

44. Garcia-Huete L, Domenech P, Sabate A, et al. The prophylactic effect of aprotinin on intraoperative bleeding in liver transplantation: a randomized clinical study. Hepatology 1997;26:1144–1148.

45. Aboujaoude MM, Grant DR, Ghent C, et al. Effect of portosystemic shunts on subsequent liver transplantation. Surg Gynecol Obstet 1991;172:215–219.

46. Mazzaferro V, Todo S, Tzakis AG, et al. Liver transplantation in patients with previous portosystemic shunt. Am J Surg 1990;160:111–116.

47. Shapiro RS, Varma CVR, Schwartz ME, Miller CM. Splenorenal shunt closure after liver transplantation: intraoperative Doppler assessment of portal hemodynamics. Liver Transplant Surg 1997;3:641–642.

48. Shaw BW, Iwatsuki S, Bron K, Starzl TE. Portal vein grafts in hepatic transplantation. Surg Gynecol Obstet 1985;161:66–68.

49. Kirsch JP, Howard TK, Klintmalm GB, et al. Problematic vascular reconstruction in liver transplantation. Part II. Portovenous conduits. Surgery 1990;107:544–548.

50. Dzik WH, Jenkins R. Use of intraoperative blood salvage during orthotopic liver transplantation. Arch Surg 1985;120:946–948.

51. Kristianson M, Lantz B, Gulliksson H, et al. Autotransfusion in liver transplantation. Transplant Proc 1989; 21:3537.

52. Shaw BW, Gordon RD, Iwatsuki S, Starzl TE. Retransplantation of the liver. Semin Liver Dis 1985;3:394–398.

53. D'Alessandro AM, Ploeg RJ, Knechtle SJ, et al. Retransplantation of the liver—a seven year experience. Transplantation 1993;55:1083–1086.

54. Mora HP, Klintmalm GB, Cofer JB, et al. Results after liver retransplantation: a comparative study between "elective" vs "nonelective" retransplants. Trans Proc 1990;22:1509–1512.

55. Broelsch CE, Emond JC, Whitington MD, et al. Application of reduced-size liver transplants as split grafts, auxiliary orthotopic grafts and living related segmental transplants. Ann Surg 1990;212:368–375.

56. Inomoto T, Nishizawa F, Hirokazu S, et al. Experiences of 120 microsurgical reconstructions of hepatic artery in living related liver transplantation. Surgery 1996; 119:20–26.

57. Azoulay D, Astarcioglu I, Bismuth H, et al. Split-liver transplantation. The Paul Brousse Policy. Ann Surg 1996;224:737–748.

58. Verran DJ, Asfar SK, Ghent CN, et al. Biliary reconstruction without T-tubes or stents in liver transplantation: report of 502 consecutive cases. Liver Transplant Surg 1997;3:365–369.

59. Cuervas-Mons V, Millan I, Gavaler JS, et al. Prognostic value of preoperatively obtained clinical and laboratory data in predicting survival following orthotopic liver transplantation. Hepatology 1986;6:922–927.

60. Baliga P, Merion RM, Turcotte JG, et al. Preoperative risk factor assessment in liver transplantation. Surgery 1992;112:704–711.

61. Craig DB. Postoperative recovery of pulmonary function. Anaesth Analg 1981;60:46–52.

62. Keren G, Boichis H, Zwas TS, Frand M. Pulmonary arterio-venous fistulae in hepatic cirrhosis. Arch Dis Child 1983;58:302–304.

63. Rodriguez-Roisen R, Roca J, Agusti AG, et al. Gas exchange and pulmonary vascular reactivity in patients with liver cirrhosis. Am J Med Sci 1984;287:10–13.

64. Krowka MJ, Cortese DA. Hepatopulmonary syndrome: an evolving perspective in the era of liver transplantation [editorial]. Hepatology 1990;11:138–142.

65. Stoller RW, Moodie D, Shiquone WA, et al. Reduction of intrapulmonary shunt and resolution of digital clubbing associated with primary biliary cirrhosis after liver transplantation. Hepatology 1990;11:54–58.

66. Laberge JM, Brandt ML, Lebeaque P, et al. Reversal of cirrhosis-related pulmonary shunting in two children by orthotopic liver transplantation. Transplantation 1992;53:1135–1138.

67. Bell RC, Coalson JJ, Smith JD, Johanson WG. Multiple organ system failure and infection in adult respiratory distress syndrome. Ann Intern Med 1983;99:293–298.

68. Matuschak GM, Rinaldo JE, Pinsky MR, et al. Effect of end-stage liver failure on the incidence and resolution of adult respiratory distress syndrome. J Crit Care Med 1987;2:162–171.

69. Lebrec D, Capron J, Dhumeaux D, Benhamou J. Pulmonary hypertension complicating portal hypertension. Am Rev Respir Dis 1979;120:849–856.

70. Hadengue A, Benhayoun MK, Lebrec D, Benamou JP. Pulmonary hypertension complicating portal hypertension: prevalence and relation to splanchnic hemodynamics. Gastroenterology 1991;100:520–528.

71. Prager MC, Cauldwell CA, Ascher NL, et al. Pulmonary hypertension associated with liver disease is not reversible after transplantation. Anesthesiology 1992;77:375–378.

72. Cheng EY, Woehlck HJ. Pulmonary artery hypertension complicating anesthesia for liver transplantation. Anesthesiology 1992;77:389–392.

73. Mortier E, Ongenae M, Poelaert J, et al. Rapidly progressive pulmonary artery hypertension and end-stage liver disease. Acta Anaesthesiol Scand 1996;40:126–129.

74. Robalino BD, Moodie DS. Association between primary pulmonary hypertension and portal hypertension. Analysis of its pathophysiology and clinical, laboratory and hemodynamic manifestations. J Am Coll Cardiol 1991;17:492–498.

75. Frostell C, Fratacci MD, Wain JC, et al. Inhaled nitric oxide: a selective pulmonary vasodilator reversing hypoxic pulmonary vasoconstriction. Circulation 1991; 83:2038–2047.

76. Mandell MS, Duke J. Nitric oxide reduces pulmonary hypertension during hepatic transplantation. Anesthesiology 1994;81:1538–1542.

77. Plevak D, Krowka M, Rettke S, et al. Successful liver transplantation in patients with mild to moderate pulmonary hypertension [letter]. Transplant Proc 1993;25: 1840.

78. Taura P, Garcia-Valdecasas JC, Beltran J, et al. Moderate primary pulmonary hypertension in patients undergoing liver transplantation. Anesth Analg 1996;83:675–680.

79. Liu G, Knudsen KE, Secher NH. Orthotopic liver transplantation in a patient with primary pulmonary hypertension. Anaesth Intensive Care 1996;24:714–716.

80. Gelman S. Hemodynamic support in patients with liver disease. Trans Proc 1996;23:1899–1901.

81. Rappaport E. Cardiopulmonary Complications of Liver Disease. In D Zakim, TD Boyer (eds), Hepatology: A Textbook of Liver Disease. Philadelphia: Saunders, 1982.

82. Harley ID, Jones EF, Liu G, et al. Orthotopic liver transplantation in two patients with hypertrophic obstructive cardiomyopathy. Br J Anaesth 1996;77:675–677.

83. Oken AC, Frank SM, Merritt WT, et al. A new percutaneous technique for establishing venous bypass in orthotopic liver transplantation. J Cardiothorac Vasc Anesth 1994;8:58–60.

84. McCauley J, Van Thiel DH, Starzl TE, Puschett JB. Acute and chronic renal failure in liver transplantation. Nephron 1990;55:121–128.

85. Epstein M. Hepatorenal syndrome: emerging perspectives of pathophysiology and therapy. J Am Soc Nephrol 1994;4:1735–1753.

86. Koppel MH, Coburn JW, Mims MM, et al. Transplantation of cadaveric kidneys from patients with hepatorenal syndrome. Evidence for the functional nature of renal failure in advanced liver disease. N Engl J Med 1969;280:1367.

87. Gonwa TA, Morris CA, Goldstein RM, et al. Long-term survival and renal function following liver transplantation in patients with and without hepatorenal syndrome—experience in 300 patients. Transplantation 1991;51:428–430.

88. Iwatsuki S, Popovtzer M, Corman J, et al. Recovery from "hepatorenal syndrome" after orthotopic liver transplantation. N Engl J Med 1973;289:1155–1159.

89. Kirby RM, McMaster P, Clemons D, et al. Orthotopic liver transplantation: postoperative complications and their management. Br J Surg 1987;74:3–11.

90. Ishitani M, Wilkowski M, Stevenson W, Pruett T. Outcome of patients requiring hemodialysis after liver transplantation. Transplant Proc 1993;25:1762–1763.

91. Starzl TE, Iwatsuki S, Malatack JJ, et al. Liver and kidney transplantation in children receiving cyclosporine A and steroids. J Pediatr 1982;100:681–686.

92. Gil-Vernet S, Prieto C, et al. Combined liver-kidney transplantation. Transplant Proc 1992;24:128–129.

93. Grande L, Rimola A, Cugat E, et al. Effect of venovenous bypass on perioperative renal function in liver transplantation: results of a randomized, controlled trial. Hepatology 1996;23:1418–1428.

94. Snook NJ, O'Beirne HA, Enright S, et al. Use of recombinant erythropoietin to facilitate liver transplantation in a Jehovah's Witness. Br J Anaesth 1996;76:740–743.

95. Ragni MV, Lewis JH, Spero JA, et al. Bleeding and coagulation abnormalities in alcoholic cirrhotic liver disease. Clin Exp Res 1982;6:267–274.

96. Lichtor JL, Emond J, Chung MR, et al. Pediatric orthotopic liver transplantation: multifactorial predictions of blood loss. Anesthesiology 1988;9:710–714.

97. Ware AJ, D'Agostino AN, Combes B. Cerebral edema: a major complication of massive hepatic necrosis. Gastroenterology 1971;61:877–884.

98. Brajtbord D, Parks RI, Ramsay MA, et al. Management of acute elevation of intracranial pressure during hepatic transplantation. Anesthesiology 1989;70:139–141.

99. Keays R, Potter D, O'Grady J, et al. Intracranial and cerebral perfusion pressure changes before, during and immediately after orthotopic liver transplantation for fulminant hepatic failure. QJM 1991;79(289):425–433.

100. Chapin JW, Morgan JB, Shaw BW, et al. Monitoring of intracranial pressure (ICP) during liver transplantation. Anesth Analg 1992;74:S41.

101. Potter D, Peachy T, Eason J, et al. Intracranial pressure monitoring during orthotopic liver transplantation for acute liver failure. Transplant Proc 1989;21:3528.

102. Ede RJ, Williams R. Hepatic encephalopathy and cerebral edema. Semin Liver Dis 1986;6:107–118.

103. Motschman TL, Taswell HF, Brecher ME, et al. Intraoperative blood loss and patient and graft survival in orthotopic liver transplantation: their relationship to clinical and laboratory data. Mayo Clin Proc 1989;64:346–355.

104. Begliomini B, De Wolf A, Snyder J, et al. Is radial arterial pressure monitoring accurate during liver transplantation? Eur J Anaesth Rel Special 1990;2:13.

105. Müller CM, Gabriel A, Langenecker S, et al. Effectiveness of rapid infusion and Bair hugger systems in maintaining normothermia during orthotopic liver transplantation. Transplant Proc 1993;25(2):1833–1834.

106. Müller CM, Langenecker S, Andel H, et al. Forced-air warming maintains normothermia during orthotopic liver transplantation. Anaesthesia 1995;50:229–232.

107. MacGilchrist AJ, Birnie GC, Cook A, et al. Pharmacokinetics and pharmacodynamics of intravenous midazolam in patients with severe alcoholic cirrhosis. Gut 1986;27:190.

108. Kang YG, Uram M, Shin GK, et al. The pharmacokinetics of fentanyl and end-stage liver disease. Anesthesiology 1984;61:A380.

109. Kutt JL, Gelb AW. Air embolism during liver transplantation. Can Anaesth Soc J 1984;31:713–715.

110. Prager MC, Gregory GA, Ascher NL, Roberts JP. Massive venous air embolism during orthotopic liver transplantation. Anesthesiology 1990;72:198–200.

111. Khoury GF, Mann ME, Porot MJ, et al. Air embolism associated with venovenous bypass during orthotopic liver transplantation. Anesthesiology 1987;67:848–851.

112. Bohrer H, Luz M. Bypass-associated air embolism during liver transplantation. Anaesth Intensive Care 1990;18:265–280.

113. Cottam S, Hunt B, Segal H, et al. Aprotinin inhibits tissue plasminogen activator-mediated fibrinolysis during orthotopic liver transplantation. Transplant Proc 1991;23:1933.

114. Hunt BJ, Cottam S, Segal H, et al. Inhibition by aprotinin of TPA-induced fibrinolysis during orthotopic liver transplantation. Lancet 1990;336:381.

115. Mallett S, Rolles K, Cox D, et al. Intraoperative use of aprotinin (Trasylol) in orthotopic liver transplantation. Transplant Proc 1991;23:1931–1932.

116. Mallett S, Cox D, Burroughs AK, Rolles K. Aprotinin and reduction of blood loss and transfusion requirements in orthotopic liver transplantation. Lancet 1990;336:886–887.

117. Grosse H, Lobbes W, Frambach M, et al. The use of high dose aprotinin in liver transplantation: the influence on fibrinolysis and blood loss. Thromb Res 1991;63:287–297.

118. Scudamore CH, Randall TE, Jewesson PJ, et al. Aprotinin reduces the need for blood products during liver transplantation. Am J Surg 1995;169:546–549.

119. Welte M, Groh J, Kazad S, et al. No beneficial effect of aprotinin on blood loss and coagulation in liver transplantation. Anesthesiology 1992;77:A225.

120. Soilleux H, Gillon MC, Mirand A, et al. Comparative effects of small and large aprotinin doses on bleeding during orthotopic liver transplantation. Anesth Analg 1995;80:349–352.

121. Boylan MB, Sandler AN, Sheiner P, et al. Reduced blood product usage with tranexamic acid prophylaxis in primary liver transplantation. Anesthesiology 1992;77:A1092.

122. Boylan JF, Klinck JR, Sandler AN, et al. Tranexamic acid reduces blood loss, transfusion requirements and coagulation factor use in primary orthotopic liver transplantation. Anesthesiology 1996;85:1043–1048.

123. Polson RJ, Park G, Lindop MJ, et al. The prevention of renal impairment in patients undergoing orthotopic liver grafting by low dose dopamine. Anaesthesia 1987;42:15–19.

124. Swygert TH, Roberts LC, Valek TR, et al. Effect of intraoperative low-dose dopamine on renal function in liver transplant recipients. Anesthesiology 1991;75:571–576.

125. Ranasinghe DN, Mallett SV. Hypomagnesemia, cardiac arrhythmias and orthotopic liver transplantation. Anaesthesia 1994;49:403–405.

126. Shaw BW. Some further notes on venous bypass for orthotopic transplantation of the liver. Ann Surg 1984;200:524–533.

127. Carmichael FJ, Lindop MJ, Farman JV. Anesthesia for hepatic transplantation: cardiovascular and metabolic alterations and their management. Anesth Analg 1985;64:108–116.

128. Veroli P, El Hage C, Ecoffey C. Does adult liver transplantation without venovenous bypass result in renal failure? Anesth Analg 1992;75:489–494.

129. Ellis JE, Lichtor JL, Feinstein SE, et al. Right heart dysfunction, pulmonary embolism, and paradoxical

embolization during liver transplantation. A transesophageal two-dimensional echocardiographic study. Anesth Analg 1989;68:777–782.

130. Navalgund AA, Kang Y, Sarner JB, et al. Massive pulmonary thromboembolism during liver transplantation. Anesth Analg 1988;67:400.

131. Aggarwal S, Kang Y, Freeman JA, et al. Postreperfusion syndrome: cardiovascular collapse following hepatic reperfusion during liver transplantation. Transplant Proc 1987;19(4 Suppl 3):54.

132. Goode HF, Webster NR, Howdle PD, et al. Reperfusion injury, antioxidants and hemodynamics during orthotopic liver transplantation. Hepatology 1994;19(2):354.

133. Emery RW, Estrin JA, Wahler GM, et al. Reflex hypotension due to regional activation of left ventricular mechanoreceptors to explain hypotension noted in clinical myocardial ischemia or reperfusion. Cardiovasc Res 1986;20(3):161.

134. Martin DJ, Marquez JM, Kang YG, et al. Liver transplantation: hemodynamic and electrolyte changes seen immediately following revascularization. Anesth Analg 1984;63:246.

135. Estrin JA, Belani KG, Ascher NL, et al. Hemodynamic changes on clamping and unclamping of major vessels during liver transplantation. Transplantation Proc 1989;21:3500–3505.

136. Gabriel A, Muller C, Tuchy G, et al. Reperfusion during orthotopic liver transplantation: analysis of right ventricular dynamics. Transplant Proc 1993;25:1811–1812.

137. Kang YG, Freeman JA, Aggarwall S, et al. Hemodynamic instability during liver transplantation. Transplant Proc 1989;21:3489–3492.

138. de la Morena G, Acosta F, Villegas M, et al. Ventricular function during liver reperfusion in hepatic transplantation. Transplantation 1994;58:306–310.

139. DeWolf AM, Begliomini B, Gasior TA, et al. Right ventricular function during orthotopic liver transplantation. Anesth Analg 1993;76:562–568.

140. Aggarwal S, Kang Y, Freeman JA, et al. Postreperfusion syndrome: hypotension after reperfusion of the transplanted liver. J Crit Care 1993;8:154–160.

141. Lunzer MR, Mewman SP, Bernard AG, et al. Impaired cardiovascular responsiveness in liver disease. Lancet 1975;2:382–385.

142. Jugan E, Albaladejo P, Jayais P, Ecoffey C. The failure of venovenous bypass to prevent graft liver postreperfusion syndrome. Transplantation 1992;54:81–84.

143. Martinez IG, Olmedilla L, Perez-Peña JM, et al. Response to clamping of the inferior vena cava as a factor for predicting postreperfusion syndrome during liver transplantation. Anesth Analg 1997;84:254–259.

144. Millis JM, Melinek J, Csete M, et al. Randomized controlled trial to evaluate flush and reperfusion techniques in liver transplantation. Transplantation 1997;63:397–403.

145. Fukuzawa K, Schwartz ME, Acarli K, et al. Flushing with autologous blood improves intraoperative hemodynamic stability and early graft function in clinical hepatic transplantation. J Am Coll Surg 1994;178:541–547.

146. Bayly PJM, Thick M. Reversal of post-reperfusion coagulopathy by protamine sulphate in orthotopic liver transplantation. Br J Anaesth 1994;73:840–842.

147. Bakkar CM, Stibbe J, Gomes MJ, et al. The appearance of donor heparin in the recipient after reperfusion of a liver graft. Transplantation 1993;56:327–329.

148. Higgins JE. Pro: early endotracheal extubation is preferable to late extubation in patients following coronary surgery. J Cardiothorac Vasc Anesth 1992;6:488–493.

149. Jullien T, Valtier B, Hongnat JM, et al. Incidence of tricuspid regurgitation and vena caval backward flow in mechanically ventilated patients. A color Doppler and contrast echocardiographic study. Chest 1995;107:488–493.

150. Ben-Haim SA, Amar R, Shofty R, Dinnar U. Low positive end expiratory pressures improve left ventricular workload versus coronary blood flow relationship. J Cardiovasc Surg 1991;32:239–245.

151. Mandell MS, Lockrem J, Kelley SD. Immediate tracheal extubation after liver transplantation: experience of two transplant centers. Anesth Analg 1997;84: 249–253.

152. Starzl TE, Schneck SA, Mazzoni G, et al. Acute neurologic complications after liver transplantation with particular reference to intraoperative cerebral air embolism. Ann Surg 1978;187:236–240.

153. Williamson KR, Taswell HF, Rettke SR, Krom RAF. Intraoperative autologous transfusion: its role in orthotopic liver transplantation. Mayo Clin Proc 1989;64: 340–345.

154. Dupont J, Messiant F, Declerck N, et al. Liver transplantation without the use of fresh frozen plasma. Anesth Analg 1996;83:681–686.

155. Jamieson NV. The results of combined liver/kidney transplantation for primary hyperoxaluria (PH 1) 1984–1997. The European PH 1 transplant registry report. J Nephrol 1998;11:36–41.

Chapter 9
Small Bowel Transplantation

Judith Kutt, Sami Asfar, Cameron Ghent, and David R. Grant

Chapter Plan

Before small bowel transplantation (SBT), total parenteral nutrition (TPN) was the only therapy available that would enable long-term survival for patients with short gut syndrome (SGS). The numerous complications of TPN, including liver failure, served as an impetus to consider SBT for patients requiring long-term TPN. Initially, SBT had poor success due to the inability to prevent graft rejection and graft-versus-host disease (GVHD). The improved success of SBT with the introduction of the new immuno-suppressive agent tacrolimus (FK506) has provided a second impetus to investigate SBT as a viable therapeutic option for patients with SGS.

Epidemiology

Few data have been generated on the incidence of SGS suitable for treatment by SBT. This is analogous to the situation of liver transplantation in the early 1980s. When the indications for the procedure become standardized and then liberalized, the number of people who are suitable candidates increases dramatically. The incidence of SGS is best derived from data about the long-term use of TPN for its treatment. In various university centers, the number of patients on home TPN is approximately 5–10 per million population.[1-4] This number does not include patients who have developed SGS but die in hospital or who have concomitant conditions that preclude home TPN as a treatment. Furthermore, these are prevalence data and, for SBT planning, the incidence is more important than prevalence data.

Not all patients on long-term TPN are suitable candidates for SBT because of concomitant serious problems, particularly cardiovascular disease in adults with SGS due to mesenteric vascular disease.

Table 9-1. Etiology of Short Gut Syndrome

Children
    Intestinal atresia
    Necrotizing enterolysis
    Midgut volvulus
    Gastroschisis
    Microvillus inclusion disease
Adults
    Crohn's disease
    Ischemia
    Desmoid tumors
    Intestinal pseudo-obstruction

Etiology of Short Gut Syndrome

The causes of SGS differ in adults and children (Table 9-1). In young children, the causes (in order of frequency) are intestinal atresia, necrotizing enterolysis, midgut volvulus, gastroschisis, and microvillus inclusion disease. Familial microvillus inclusion disease, found in certain geographic areas, particularly in Quebec, often affects several children in a family and presents with massive malabsorption and diarrhea in infancy. Crohn's disease in older children, although uncommon, may lead to the need for enterectomy and SGS. Surgical misadventures in children who have had delayed recognition of the problem may lead to intestinal gangrene and the need for total enterectomy.

In adults, aggressive Crohn's disease resistant to medical therapy may lead to the need for resections over a period of years, leaving the patient with insufficient gut to survive without continuous TPN. Ischemic disease, usually due to superior mesenteric artery (SMA) occlusion from embolism or thrombosis, is the most common underlying problem in older adults that requires massive resection of small bowel. These individuals are problematic candidates for SBT because they commonly have associated cardiac, cerebral, or peripheral vascular disease. These associated conditions, independently of the SGS, limit survival to the point that the benefits of SBT cannot be realized. A careful assessment of the vascular system is required before recommending SBT for such individuals. Systemic sclerosis (scleroderma) with predominant gastrointestinal manifestations often leads to TPN dependence but has a poor prognosis when other organs are involved, particularly if pulmonary hypertension is present.[5] Only

rarely should SBT be considered in these people, and only after very careful evaluation of renal and pulmonary function. A similar situation occasionally arises in patients who develop small bowel infarction as a complication of nephrotic syndrome. In these individuals, consideration should be given to a "medical nephrectomy" followed by combined SBT and renal transplantation.

Desmoid tumors in the retroperitoneum, usually associated with Gardner's syndrome, are very slow growing but may result in invasion or compression of major abdominal vessels.[6] Very careful imaging of the vasculature is required before recommending SBT in these individuals because the tumor may involve renal vessels, ureters, or an extensive portion of the abdominal wall. Furthermore, with desmoid tumors, polyposis may develop in the portions of the gastrointestinal tract left after SBT, especially the duodenum. Some such individuals may require a cluster transplant, including the duodenum, pancreas, stomach, and liver as well as the small bowel. Use of a scarce resource, such as a donor liver, for this type of experimental surgery becomes problematic because of the greater success of isolated liver transplantation and the number of individuals, often desperately ill, who are awaiting liver transplants.

Intestinal pseudo-obstruction in adults includes a heterogeneous group of patients who have in common a failure of gut motility so severe that the gut cannot be used for nutritional support. Familial visceral myopathy involves not only atony of the entire gastrointestinal tract but also of the ureters (megaureter) and urinary bladder.[7] A subgroup of patients with failure of gut motility are narcotic dependent, and it is often difficult to determine with confidence the role of narcotics in adult-acquired idiopathic intestinal pseudo-obstruction. Our center has accepted that many patients being considered for SBT are dependent on narcotics by the time they are referred. If addiction is not the primary problem and is acknowledged by the patient, our center accepts the patient for SBT. We prefer to treat narcotic addiction in these patients after successful SBT.

Surgical misadventures occasionally result in SGS in adults as well as children. This is probably more common than is reported. It involves not only technically poor surgery but also delays in diagnosis, resulting in irretrievable ischemia of gut, and poor judgment in deciding to undertake resection of a large portion of small bowel for Crohn's disease. One patient awaiting intestinal retransplantation at our center as of this writing originally presented with complicated appendicitis.

Medical Management of Short Gut Syndrome

It is important to recognize that the gut has a remarkable capacity to adapt to resection. Some infants have been able to survive completely on enteral feeding, after a period of TPN support, with as little as 12 cm of jejunum left after massive resection.[8, 9] This may require aggressive nutritional support consisting of nasogastric feeding overnight with calorie-rich low-volume supplements, such as glucose polymers and medium-chain triglycerides. This regimen is particularly useful in children with SGS from extensive surgical resection. It is much less effective in patients with concomitant colonic resection, who often cannot tolerate the osmotic diarrhea with high enterostomy output.

Complications of Short Gut Syndrome

Systemic complications of SGS, apart from specific deficiencies, are listed in Table 9-2.

Enteric oxalosis results from excessive absorption of dietary oxalate, which is usually excreted in stool bound to calcium. The exact mechanisms are disputed, but the common factor appears to be fat malabsorption, with calcium being unavailable in the gut to bind to oxalate.[10] Treatment is reduction of oxalate intake.

Bile salt deficiency, with ensuing formation of cholesterol stones in the biliary tree, results from enteric loss of bile salts in excess of the liver's ability to synthesize and secrete them.[11] This excess loss of bile salts must exceed approximately 1,500 mg per day before biliary concentrations are depressed. Because bile salt is mainly reabsorbed in the terminal ileum, this is a particular problem in patients with no ileum left in situ. The deficiency also can result from use of bile salt sequestrants, such as cholestyramine and colestipol, used to reduce the diarrhea resulting from large amounts of bile salts reaching the colon. At this level, bile salt excesses produce a secretory diarrhea, and sequestrants can

Table 9-2. Complications of Short Gut Syndrome

Malnutrition
Enteric oxalosis
Calcium oxalate nephrolithiasis
Bile salt deficiency resulting in diarrhea and cholesterol
  cholelithiasis
Metabolic bone disease
Peptic ulcer disease

be very effective in reducing the volume of stool produced. Use of these agents is fraught with hazards, however, such as cholelithiasis, metabolic acidosis due to fecal bicarbonate loss, and deficiencies of other lipid-soluble nutrients that are also bound to these anion exchangers.[12] In some individuals with TPN-associated cholestasis, the 7 beta-hydroxy bile acid ursodeoxycholic acid (a bile acid analogue that is well absorbed in the proximal gut and undergoes enterohepatic cycling) may be beneficial in treating fat malabsorption and cholestasis.[11]

Metabolic bone disease associated with SGS is complicated and relatively poorly understood. Normal human subjects are not dependent on dietary sources for vitamin D and can produce all the necessary vitamin D in skin in response to ultraviolet irradiation. It has been said that it is impossible to be vitamin D deficient if one has a tan, a liver, and a kidney. Nevertheless, calcium malabsorption results in negative calcium balance in subjects with SGS, and calcium removal from bone to maintain serum acid-base balance is very common. Metabolic acidosis resulting from use of anion exchange resins, which effectively promote fecal excretion of bicarbonate, probably contributes to the rapid loss of bone minerals.[13]

Peptic ulcer disease is theoretically a complication of SGS because almost all subjects with SGS have hypergastrinemia.[14] With the extensive use of H_2-blockers and proton-pump inhibitors, this complication is now uncommon.

Complications of Total Parenteral Nutrition

The common serious complications of TPN are infections, vascular occlusions, and hepatobiliary dysfunction. Infections are usually related to central venous catheters, and the very best catheter care and aseptic technique are still associated with frequent need for catheter changes due to bacteremia. A wide variety of organisms, mostly bacterial, are responsible for line sepsis.

Vascular access problems are common in patients on long-term TPN. An extensive Doppler ultrasound search may be necessary to find a suitable vein for catheter insertion when both subclavian veins are occluded. Innovative techniques include direct percutaneous cannulation of the inferior vena cava[15] and transhepatic placement of a catheter in the right hepatic vein (D. R. Grant, personal communication, 1997). Surgically created arteriovenous fistulas may be necessary to provide access for some patients.

In neonates, hepatobiliary complications of TPN are frequent, often progressive, and sometimes fatal.[16] The spectrum of histopathologic disease in both infants and adults ranges from reversible fatty liver to a severe cholestasis with bile ductule proliferation and progressive periportal fibrosis leading to cirrhosis.[17] The development of liver complications is directly related to the duration of TPN, and various other factors have been hypothesized to account for them. Current evidence does not support a direct role for any particular component of the TPN solution in causing these changes.[18, 19] The progressive forms of cholestasis appear to be more likely to develop when there is total reliance on TPN, no remaining gut, associated sepsis, and prematurity in infants.[20]

With the poorly understood pathophysiology of cholestasis associated with TPN, it is not surprising that there are a large number of proposed treatments, none of which has been subjected to a controlled trial.[21] With what is known about this disorder, it seems important to try to prevent it by use of any remaining gut to supply as much nutrition as possible, to limit the duration of TPN as much as possible, and to monitor the serum liver enzymes to detect the problem at an early stage. Less well-documented strategies include glutamine supplementation, either orally or as part of the TPN[20, 22]; taurine supplementation[23, 24]; cyclical rather than continuous administration of TPN[25]; and routine administration of metronidazole,[26] ursodeoxycholic acid,[11, 27] or somatostatin.[28–30] All these agents have theoretical support for their use but do not have proved clinical benefit. Isolated liver transplantation has also been successful in the treatment of severe cholestasis

associated with SGS and TPN.[31] It is clear from our review of the literature that every effort should be made to limit the volume and duration of TPN and to maximize the enteral administration of nutrients in the treatment of this serious problem.

Indications for Transplantation and Recipient Selection

There are no currently recognized standardized indications for SBT, which is still considered an experimental procedure. The high morbidity and mortality of the alternative treatments of SGS with complications of TPN make SBT a reasonable consideration for those who have no hope of freedom from TPN dependence. This excludes many neonates with SGS, who may be able to adapt and survive without TPN if they are supported through the first few months of life.[16] Nonscientific issues frequently arise as well, and some third-party insurers view SBT as a less costly alternative to an indefinite outlay for TPN. Quality of life must be taken into account, and patients whose life situation makes TPN unacceptable because of interference with work or family obligations are generally good candidates for SBT. The importance of informed consent cannot be overstressed: Patients must be willing to accept the risks of SBT after extensive discussion of risks and potential benefits.

The investigations that precede acceptance of a patient as a candidate for SBT vary from patient to patient. The physical examination of the whole body must be detailed: It determines what other investigations are needed. Barium studies of the remaining gut should be reviewed to assess the anatomy and the feasibility of enteral feeding. A very careful search for femoral, carotid, or coronary artery disease is needed in the older individual with a mesenteric arterial occlusion. Routine repetitive abdominal imaging is probably not warranted, although some determination of the potential size of a shrunken abdominal cavity would be welcome.

In many individuals with SGS, serious consideration of combined liver transplantation and SBT may be needed, or even liver transplantation alone if there is hope of getting the patient off TPN. Routine review of potential candidates by an experienced hepatologist is strongly recommended by this unbiased, experienced hepatologist (C. Ghent). It is probably not necessary to routinely assess the liver by biopsy in patients who have normal liver chemistry and no independent risk factors or clinical signs of chronic liver disease. For those with cholestasis associated with TPN, a liver biopsy and a cholangiogram are essential for choosing between isolated SBT and SBT plus liver transplantation. In general, the presence of extensive fibrosis on biopsy or the presence of any clinical signs of portal hypertension dictates a combined transplant, including the liver.

Early referral is essential if the results of SBT are to improve beyond the current level. It is generally accepted that the ideal patient for this procedure is a well-motivated, otherwise healthy young person with no hope of ever being free of TPN who is willing to accept the risks involved when realistically informed of their magnitude. If there are life-threatening reversible complications of TPN, the arguments for offering such an individual SBT become compelling.

Donor Selection and Management

Intestinal grafts are usually procured from cadaveric solid-organ donors with the same blood group as the recipient. The use of ABO-compatible intestinal grafts can result in severe hemolysis,[32] but experience in Omaha suggests that this may be avoided by transfusing donor-type blood (A. Lagnas, personal communication, 1995). The abdominal cavity becomes smaller after massive intestinal resections; it is therefore desirable to use donors who are 20–30% smaller than the recipient.

Antibiotics are given to decontaminate the gastrointestinal tract before organ removal. Our current regimen includes erythromycin (1 g orally q4h × 3), neomycin (1 g orally q4h × 3), intravenous cefotaxime (1 g), and intravenous metronidazole (500 mg). Some centers also use mechanical bowel preparations and antilymphocyte agents for procurement of the small intestine.

The use of living-related SBTs may be a partial solution to the shortage of donor organs. The terminal ileum, ileocecal valve, cecum, and ascending colon can provide good graft function with little disability to the donor. Moreover, the use of major histocompatibility complex (MHC)-matched grafts may reduce the risk of rejection.[33]

Donor Surgery

The types of intestinal grafts include the small bowel alone, the small bowel and colon (ascending and transverse colon), or composite grafts with the liver or other solid organs.

A cruciate incision is used to expose the donor's abdomen. The right colon is mobilized medially, and the small bowel with its mesentery is mobilized to the duodenojejunal junction. The greater omentum is detached from the transverse colon, preserving the mesocolon. The common hepatic artery is identified and encircled with vascular tape. The gastroduodenal artery is ligated and cut to bring the portal vein into view, which is then dissected and encircled with vascular tape. The lesser omentum is opened. The pancreas is identified. The first part of the duodenum is mobilized and transected with a GIA stapler. A finger is passed along the front of the portal vein and behind the neck of the donor's pancreas to its lower edge. The pancreas is then transected with the stapler to expose the retropancreatic portal vein and the confluence of the splenic and superior mesenteric veins. All tributaries to the portal vein in this area are carefully dissected, ligated, and cut, preserving the superior mesenteric and splenic veins. Branches of the SMA to the pancreas and duodenum in this area are likewise carefully dissected, ligated, and cut. The transverse colon is divided just to the left of the middle colic artery using a linear cutting stapler (if the colon is not procured with the small bowel, the terminal ileum is divided just proximal to the ileocecal junction). The donor's small bowel is divided just beyond the duodenojejunal junction using a linear cutting stapler. At the end of this dissection, the small bowel, cecum, ascending colon, and the right side of the colon are attached only by the portal vein and the SMA.

When composite small bowel and liver grafts are procured, the donor's liver is dissected from the diaphragm by cutting the falciform and right and left triangular ligaments using electrocautery. The phrenic veins are suture ligated with 2-0 silk sutures. The distal common bile duct is dissected, ligated, and cut. The infra- and retrohepatic inferior vena cava (IVC) is mobilized to the level of the renal veins. The right lobe of the donor's liver is turned to the left side to expose the retrohepatic IVC. The right adrenal vein is dissected, ligated, and cut to free the IVC from the retroperitoneum (Figure 9-1).

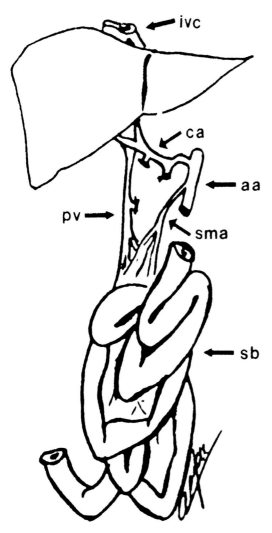

Figure 9-1. En bloc small bowel and liver graft with a segment of the abdominal aorta (aa) containing both the celiac axis (ca) and the superior mesenteric artery (sma). Inferior vena cava (ivc), small bowel (sb), and portal vein (pv) are also shown.

Twenty thousand to 30,000 units of intravenous heparin are given to the donor. A cannula is inserted into the distal abdominal aorta. Another cannula is inserted into the IVC just above the confluence of the iliac veins to collect 1 unit of donor blood and to decompress the liver. The abdominal organs are flushed with 1–3 liters of University of Wisconsin (UW) solution. The donor gut should blanch uniformly after perfusion with the preservation solution. The viscera are packed in ice. The SMA is then dissected down to its origin from the aorta.

Lymphatic channels and nodes in this area are secured with clips or ligatures to prevent a chyle leak in the recipient. A patch of the aorta is removed together with the origin of the SMA. When the liver is procured with the bowel, a segment of the thoracic and abdominal aorta is excised that includes the origins of the celiac artery and SMA.

The organs are placed in a container full of cold UW solution and stored on ice. This technique permits approximately 10 hours of cold ischemia with satisfactory function after transplantation.[34]

Recipient Surgery

Most SBT candidates have undergone several laparotomies by the time they are referred for assessment. Hours of tedious dissection are sometimes required to divide adhesions within the peritoneal cavity and remove the diseased native bowel. We try to coordinate the donor and recipient surgeries so that the graft can be transplanted as soon as it arrives in the operating room to reduce the total ischemia time.

Portal venous drainage provides first-pass delivery of the hepatotropic substances to the liver and allows the liver to filter translocated organisms and toxins from the bowel.[35–37] Therefore, it is preferable to obtain portal venous drainage of the bowel whenever possible using (1) an end-to-end anastomosis with the native superior mesenteric vein at the root of the mesentery or (2) an end-to-side anastomosis with the native portal vein at the porta hepatis. If a portal venous anastomosis is not possible, the portal vein can be anastomosed to the vena cava (Figure 9-2).[38]

A conduit of the donor aorta containing the origin of the SMA (and the celiac axis, if the liver is simultaneously transplanted) can be anastomosed to the recipient's infrarenal aorta. Alternatively, the SMA with an aortic cuff can be anastomosed to the native SMA or the aorta. Before completing the arterial anastomosis, the graft is flushed with approximately 300 ml of Ringer's lactate solution at room temperature to wash out the UW solution. The arterial clamps are released, and approximately 300 ml of portal venous blood is vented via the stump of the splenic vein, which is ligated afterward to restore portal flow to the liver. The graft should perfuse uniformly and turn pink.

Figure 9-2. Isolated small bowel transplant with ileostomy (*open arrow*). **A.** Donor portal vein (dpv) is anastomosed to the side of the recipient's portal vein (rpv) **B.** Donor's superior mesenteric artery (dsma) with an aortic patch is anastomosed end-to-side to the recipient's aorta (ra) below the renal vessels (rv).

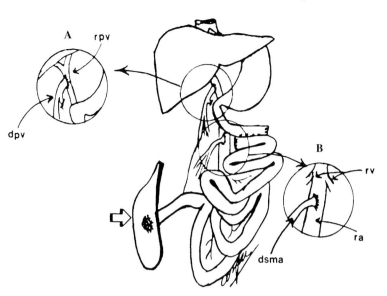

After revascularization, the proximal donor small bowel is anastomosed to the native intestine just distal to the ligament of Treitz as a side-to-side anastomosis using a linear cutting stapler. Different techniques are used to manage the distal end of the graft, which can either be (1) brought out as a terminal ileostomy or (2) anastomosed to the native bowel (colon or small intestine) with a proximal loop ileostomy or as a Bishop-Koop Cheminey procedure (Figure 9-3). If the colon is transplanted in continuity with the small intestine, it is exteriorized as a terminal colostomy or anastomosed with the native colon, and a loop ileostomy is performed.

Before the abdomen is closed, a feeding tube is passed through the nose into the stomach and manipulated to well beyond the proximal anastomosis.

Anesthetic Management

Preoperative Assessment

Patients presenting for SBT have usually undergone a long trial of conventional therapy that has failed. The major issues to consider during the initial assessment of these patients are their degree of debilitation secondary to malnutrition, accessibility of peripheral and central veins, and hepatobiliary function, which may be compromised as a result of long-term TPN. This necessitates a careful examination of all organ systems. Usually, these patients do not have significant cardiorespiratory disease, but if abnormalities of cardiac function are detected, then further testing may include echocardiography, radionuclide angiography, dipyridamole or thallium scanning, or cardiac catheterization. The presence of pulmonary disease may also necessitate pulmonary function studies. Table 9-3 lists routine investigations at our institution. In particular, both synthetic (international normalized ratio, partial thromboplastin time, albumin, serum protein) and metabolic (bilirubin, aspartate aminotransferase, alanine aminotransferase, glucose) hepatic functions are determined. A combined liver transplant and SBT may be planned if significant liver dysfunction is present. (See Chapter 8 for a more detailed discussion of the principles of anesthesia for liver transplantation.)

In the immediate preoperative period, hematology, coagulation, and serum chemistry, including tests of liver function, electrocardiogram, chest x-ray, and blood gases, are repeated.

Evaluation of venous access is particularly important during initial assessment of the patient. Venous access is sometimes limited to central veins because of obliteration of peripheral veins by previous multiple intravenous sites. These patients may present with thrombosis of one or more central veins. Ultrasonography and venous angiography are often helpful to assess patency of central veins and to place central venous catheters before surgery.

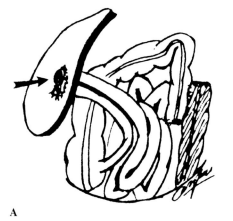

A

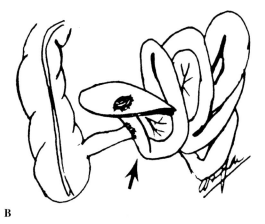

B

Figure 9-3. Small bowel and colon transplant, distal anastomosis of transplant bowel. **A.** Side-to-side transplant colon to native colon (*shaded*) and loop ileostomy (*arrow*). **B.** Bishop-Koop Cheminey procedure connecting native terminal ileum to transplant terminal ileum (*arrow*) and ileostomy.

Table 9-3. Preoperative Investigations

Complete blood count (hemoglobin, white blood cell count, platelets)
Serum electrolytes (sodium, potassium, chloride, calcium, magnesium)
Creatinine, blood urea nitrogen
International normalized ratio, partial thromboplastin time
Glucose
Albumin, serum protein
Liver function tests: aspartate transaminase, alanine amino transferase, bilirubin, alkaline phosphatase
Electrocardiogram
Chest radiograph
Blood gas
Pulmonary function tests*
Echocardiogram*
Radionuclide myocardial scan*
Angiography*

*If clinically indicated.

Intraoperative Monitoring

Routine monitors, including noninvasive blood pressure measurement, continuous electrocardiography (leads II and V), pulse oximetry, capnography, and end-tidal gas analysis, are applied before induction of anesthesia. Rectal and esophageal temperature probes and a Foley catheter are inserted postinduction to monitor core temperature and urine output. Invasive blood pressure monitoring (radial or femoral arterial catheters) are usually established postinduction. If a central vein catheter has not already been established, a large-bore (9 French) intravenous cannula is inserted into either the internal jugular or subclavian vein, or if necessary, the femoral vein. Peripheral and central veins of the patient's lower limbs are acceptable because the IVC blood flow is usually not compromised during surgery. If significant underlying cardiac dysfunction is present, a pulmonary arterial catheter is inserted. Otherwise, measurement of the central venous pressure (CVP) via a double- or triple-lumen catheter usually suffices to monitor fluid status.

Intraoperative Management

Usually, patients have had an adequate period of fasting preoperatively, but there may be delayed gastric emptying as a result of their underlying disease. A rapid-sequence induction of anesthesia is therefore required due to the potential for aspiration.

General anesthesia is used because of the long duration of the surgery and the extent of the abdominal incision and exposure, which lends itself to hypothermia. Anesthesia is induced usually with a narcotic (fentanyl 4–5 µg/kg) and sodium thiopental (3–6 mg/kg) or propofol (1–2 mg/kg) technique. Muscle relaxation is obtained with a nondepolarizing muscle relaxant. There is no one particular agent of benefit, but an agent that does not require renal function for metabolism and excretion may be indicated for patients who present with renal dysfunction (e.g., hepatorenal syndrome) associated with hepatic failure. Succinylcholine (1.5–2.0 mg/kg) is used for rapid-sequence inductions. All patients are orally intubated. Maintenance of anesthesia proceeds using a balanced technique of a volatile agent (usually isoflurane), narcotic (e.g., fentanyl, sufentanil) and nondepolarizing muscle relaxant (e.g., vecuronium, pancuronium, rocuronium). Nitrous oxide is avoided because of the potential for bowel distention. Often, the recipient's peritoneal cavity is small, and abdominal closure may be difficult due to the relatively large size of the donor graft. Therefore, increases in intra-abdominal pressure may necessitate postoperative assisted ventilation, although the anesthetic technique is usually directed toward early extubation. Ringer's lactate solution is used to maintain CVP in the range of 10–15 mm Hg. Albumin may be used if the serum albumin is low, but pentastarch may be preferable to assist in maintaining filling pressures, especially if there has been some blood loss. If urine output is less than 1 ml/kg per hour despite a CVP of at least 10 mm Hg, mannitol, furosemide, or dopamine (2–3 μg/kg/minute) may be necessary.

The decrease in venous return to the heart and hypotension associated with caval clamping is anticipated. Before clamping, colloid (albumin, pentastarch) is administered to ensure a CVP greater than 10 mm Hg. The volatile agent is also reduced to allow the systemic pressure to rise and to reduce the vasodilation induced by isoflurane, for instance. These maneuvers usually suffice to maintain an appropriate mean blood pressure. Occasionally, vasopressors such as phenylephrine (50–100 mg) may be administered intermittently for hypotension.

Steps should be taken to maintain body temperature because these patients are prone to develop hypotension during the course of the long procedure. These include blood and fluid warmers, warming blankets, and, if necessary, raising the room temperature of the operating theater.

Adequate fluid balance is maintained during the procedure by monitoring CVP and urine output (1–2 ml/kg/hour). Compared to liver transplantation, blood loss is usually not significant during SBT, although multiple previous abdominal surgeries potentially increase the intraoperative transfusion requirements due to multiple adhesions. Fresh frozen plasma is administered if an underlying coagulopathy exists. Otherwise, colloid (albumin, pentastarch) is administered with judicious use of Ringer's lactate to minimize tissue edema.

The venous anastomosis is usually superior mesenteric vein to portal vein because this restores hepatic blood flow, and intestinal toxins are first passed through the liver. If a portal anastomosis is not feasible, an anastomosis to the IVC may be made; this anastomosis may involve temporary occlusion of the IVC, which decreases venous return to the heart and may lead to hypotension. This is preceded by fluid resuscitation and a reduction in volatile agents before clamping.

During the arterial anastomosis, which is usually with the SMA conduit to the infrarenal aorta, the side-biting clamp used may be an actual cross-clamp of the aorta. The anesthesiologist must be prepared to deal with the consequences of aortic cross-clamping. Controlling the increase in systemic vascular resistance caused by aortic cross-clamping necessitates the use of a technique opposite to that used for caval cross-clamping. Deep anesthesia and the use of vasodilators (nitroglycerin or nitroprusside) may be necessary to control blood pressure.

Routine monitoring of hematology and blood chemistry should be continued throughout the procedure. Hemoglobin, hematocrit, and platelet count should be monitored before vascular clamps are applied, during the clamp period, and after the vascular clamps have been removed. Serum sodium, potassium, calcium, and magnesium are also determined during these periods. Because acid-base status may change during the periods of vascular occlusion, blood gases are also determined during these periods. Because intravenous hyperalimentation has been stopped preoperatively, rebound hypoglycemia can occur; therefore, blood glucose levels should be checked regularly.

During the period of graft reperfusion, hemodynamic instability[39] may occur due to acute changes in potassium, acid-base status, and temperature as the preservative solution is flushed out of the graft or relative to aortic unclamping. The UW solution used as a preservative is very high in potassium. With a portal anastomosis, the liver normally buffers the effect of the cold, high-potassium fluid on the heart. If a caval anastomosis has been done, however, an effect similar to the metabolic abnormalities seen with reperfusion of a transplanted liver is possible. The patient's temperature usually decreases during the period of vascular anastomosis as the cold intestinal graft sits in the abdominal cavity. A fall of 0.5°C may be seen, with a further acute fall of another 0.5°C associated with graft reperfusion. The major consequences of graft reperfusion on the heart are arrhythmias and asystole, which are due to acute hyperkalemia or hypothermia. Calcium chloride may be given if measured calcium levels are low or if a caval anastomosis has been used. In addition, sodium bicarbonate may be used if a metabolic acidosis has developed. It is important to maintain hemodynamic stability to ensure adequate graft perfusion.

Intraoperatively, further antibiotic coverage may be needed because of the long duration of the surgery. Infection is a major postoperative complication because of the intense immunosuppression induced.

With SBT, immunosuppression is started intraoperatively. Intravenous OKT3 is given with reperfusion of the graft. After OKT3 administration, T cells are opsonized by the reticuloendothelial system, resulting in the release of lymphokines and other substrates, which can cause hemodynamic instability and increased capillary permeability.[40] Pretreatment with H_1- and H_2-receptor blockers (diphenhydramine, 50 mg, and ranitidine, 50 mg), as well as methylprednisolone, 500 mg, may help decrease these effects. Ranitidine, diphenhydramine, and methylprednisolone should be given 30–60 minutes before OKT3 administration.

A continuous infusion of prostaglandin E_1 (PGE_1) (0.6–0.8 mg/kg/day) is also started at the time of reperfusion or shortly thereafter. PGE_1, a potent vasodilator, is administered to enhance graft perfusion. There is evidence to suggest that PGE_1 may protect against the nephrotoxic effects of immunosuppressive agents. For instance, the renal dysfunction seen with cyclosporine and FK506 may be due in part to a redistribution of blood flow within the kidney due to release of thromboxane A_2, PGE_2, and endothelin causing afferent arteriolar vasoconstriction. Furthermore, endogenous prostaglandin synthesis may also be reduced during perioperative renal ischemia.[41–43] Therefore, it is postulated that PGE_1 protects the kidneys by counteracting the deleterious effects of these changes in intrarenal vasoactive substances. The systemic hypotension associated with the perioperative use of PGE_1 is offset by adequate fluid replacement and reducing the volatile anesthetic.

At our institution, a transfusion of whole blood from the donor is also part of the immunosuppression technique. Although the blood should be ABO compatible, a brief cross-match of the donor's blood with the recipient's blood adds a safety precaution.

Postoperatively, patients are transferred to the intensive care unit. Hypothermia or high intra-abdominal pressures, due to a relatively large graft (with edema) placed in a small abdominal cavity, may require assisted positive-pressure ventilation for a short period. Postoperative analgesia is provided with intravenous narcotics; patient-controlled analgesia is used once the patient is awake. Epidural catheter infusions have not been used routinely for postoperative analgesia in these patients, partly because there is often liver dysfunction associated with intravenous alimentation, with an associated coagulopathy.

Immune Suppression

With cyclosporine immune suppression, SBT was successful in dogs and pigs,[44, 45] but most human grafts were lost because of intractable rejection or severe systemic infections.[32, 46–49]

The results of SBT improved with the use of FK506.[34] Our immune-suppressive protocol includes the following:

1. Three daily doses of OKT3, 5 mg
2. PGE_1, 0.6–0.8 mg/kg per day intravenous continuous infusion starting on release of vascular clamps and continued for 2 weeks, followed by oral misoprostol, 200 mg 3–4 times a day for an additional 4–6 weeks to protect against FK506 nephrotoxicity
3. Enteral tacrolimus (orally or via feeding tube) is started as early as possible, usually within 24 hours at 0.3 mg/kg per day in two divided doses
4. Methylprednisolone (1 mg/kg/day) orally, tapered to 0.2 mg/kg per day within 2 weeks
5. One unit of donor blood (collected during organ procurement) given during surgery

Tacrolimus whole blood levels are measured daily for the first 2 weeks and then two to three times per week thereafter. To avoid side effects,[50] the tacrolimus levels should be kept at a lower range than originally recommended by the Pittsburgh Transplant Institute.[34] Our center currently aims for the following levels: 15–25 ng/ml during the first week reduced to 5–15 ng/ml during the first month, then 5 ng/ml thereafter.

Complications

Graft-versus-Host Disease

Large numbers of lymphocytes and dendritic cells in the regional mesenteric lymph nodes, lamina propria, and Peyer's patches are transplanted with the intestinal graft. These cells are a major target for immune attack by the host in the form of graft rejection. In rare situations, the roles may be reversed and the graft cells react against the recipient, causing GVHD. Mild GVHD manifests as erythema of the palms, soles, and ears and occasionally with a maculopapular eruption, asymptomatic increases in serum bilirubin, and diarrhea. Severe GVHD may involve liver (hepatic failure, coagulopathy) and abdominal pain and diarrhea, causing severe electrolyte and fluid abnormalities.

The clinical syndrome of GVHD has been rare after SBT in humans. Only two cases of GVHD have been reported so far.[34, 51] Both of these patients received combined small bowel and liver transplants. The donor lymphocytes appeared in the recipient's peripheral circulation concurrently with the appearance of the typical rash of GVHD. The condition resolved spontaneously in both patients. One survived for 5 years; the other died later of sepsis.

Graft Rejection

The small bowel graft provides a strong stimulus for rejection because of massive expression of MHC class II antigens on mucosal enterocytes,[52–54] trafficking of donor lymphocytes from the graft into the recipient,[55] and nonspecific immune stimulation by micro-organisms in the lumen of the bowel.[56]

The clinical signs and symptoms of rejection are nonspecific and may include any combination of the following: abdominal pain, sudden increase of stoma output, fever, nausea, and vomiting. In severe cases, abdominal distention and metabolic acidosis with or without leukocytosis may result. Daily inspection of the stoma is important. Within the first few days, some edema of the stoma is expected, but changes in the color of the stoma from a rosy pink to a cyanotic or dusky appearance should raise the suspicion of rejection and initiate an immediate biopsy.

Endoscopic biopsies are standard for diagnosing graft rejection. Small bowel rejection is patchy.[46, 57]

At least 10–20 cm of the graft lumen should be visualized and biopsies taken from abnormal as well as normal areas. The endoscopic findings of acute rejection include mucosal edema, hyperemia, and loss of mucosal pattern. Severe cases may show ulceration, friable mucosa, and loss of peristalsis. At the London Health Sciences Centre, London, Ontario, Canada, SBT patients get weekly protocol endoscopic biopsies for the first 4 weeks; thereafter, biopsy is repeated on clinical suspicion of a rejection episode. Because changes in permeability precede the clinical features of rejection,[51] the entire graft is also screened for rejection weekly by measuring gut barrier function using orally administered chromium-labeled ethylenediaminetetra-acetic acid (^{51}Cr-EDTA).

At the Pittsburgh Transplant Institute, the incidence of acute graft rejection was 93% in isolated SBTs compared to 62% in combined SBT-liver transplants under tacrolimus immune suppression.[58] Twenty-five percent (4 of 16) of isolated SBTs were removed because of severe rejection, whereas only 4.5% (1 of 22) combined small bowel–liver grafts were lost for this reason.

At the London Health Sciences Centre, we have performed 16 intestinal transplants: six were treated with cyclosporine and 10 were treated with tacrolimus. Five of the seven isolated small bowel grafts (71.4%) had one or more episodes of graft rejection, whereas two rejection episodes occurred in seven combined small bowel–liver transplants (28.5%). These findings are consistent with other experimental and clinical reports showing protection of kidney, heart, and intestinal grafts from rejection by concurrent liver transplants.[59–63]

Infection

There is a high rate of infections after SBT due to the use of intense immune suppression and bacterial translocation from the lumen of the small bowel graft.[56, 58, 64] Despite selective decontamination of the graft for 4–6 weeks, the Pittsburgh group reported an infection rate of 90.5% of their recipients with a mean of 3.5 infections per patient.[65] The majority of infections (88%) were polybacterial, but 44% were fungal infections.[58]

At the London Health Sciences Centre, where no routine gut decontamination is practiced, we had 40 culture-proved infections in five of six recipients who received cyclosporine immune suppression (eight infections per patient). The last 10 patients on tacrolimus therapy had 13 culture-proved infections (1.6 episodes per patient). Most were polybacterial (63.6%) with only one fungal infection. Measures that we currently use to reduce bacterial and fungal sepsis include

1. Prophylactic broad-spectrum antibiotics for 48–72 hours after transplantation; thereafter, specific antibiotics as indicated by culture and sensitivity results
2. Antifungal prophylaxis with fluconazole until discharge from hospital
3. Discontinuing central lines as early as possible
4. Providing early enteral feeds to enhance gut barrier function

Cytomegalovirus (CMV) infections are a major cause of graft loss and patient death after SBT. Pittsburgh reported 37% incidence of CMV infection, which caused the loss of three grafts.[58] At the London Health Sciences Centre, four of six patients on cyclosporine therapy developed CMV infections, and one patient died of this complication. Of the 10 recipients in our tacrolimus group, two developed a CMV enteritis in the transplanted bowel. One infection was intractable and required removal of the graft; the other responded to treatment with ganciclovir. To reduce the risk of CMV infections, we take the following measures:

1. Try to transplant CMV-negative organs into CMV-negative recipients whenever possible.
2. Administer oral acyclovir prophylaxis as soon as enteral feeds are started.
3. Give pre-emptive treatment with ganciclovir whenever immune suppression is increased (i.e., during rejection treatment).

Posttransplantation Lymphoproliferative Disease

Epstein-Barr virus (EBV) infections or reactivation combined with excessive immune suppression and intense antilymphocyte therapy are risk factors for posttransplantation lymphoproliferative disease (PTLD).[66, 67] Patients may present with an unexplained fever, a mononucleosis-like illness, an enlarged lymph node, or an intra-abdominal mass. PTLD can involve any organ, including the central nervous system.

The incidence of PTLD was high during the early experience of SBT with cyclosporine immune suppression.[68, 69] With tacrolimus therapy, the Pittsburgh group reported PTLD in 12 of 63 (19%) SBT recipients with 66% (8 of 12) mortality.[70] The majority (11 of 12) of these recipients had received antilymphocyte therapy in the posttransplant period. At the London Health Sciences Centre, PTLD was the cause of death in two adult recipients of multivisceral grafts under cyclosporine immune suppression. After switching to tacrolimus therapy, only one child of 10 recipients developed PTLD, and her tumors resolved after temporary withdrawal of immune suppression and treatment with acyclovir. The low incidence of PTLD in our last 10 SBT patients may be due to our policy of avoiding excessive immune suppression by waiting for histologic confirmation of graft rejection and giving oral acyclovir prophylaxis to all patients once enteral feeding starts.[71]

Graft Function

Gastrointestinal dysfunction early after transplantation can be due to preservation injury, vascular compromise, rejection, infection, or GVHD. However, the available tests are crude and do not help to differentiate between these causes. Moreover, there is no simple, reliable serologic or blood test for monitoring graft function or indicating the onset of a rejection episode. Serial D-xylose absorption studies have been used by the Pittsburgh group to monitor intestinal graft function, but the results are unreliable in the presence of impaired renal function or abnormal gastrointestinal motility, which are common after transplantation.[72]

Small bowel function is usually impaired immediately after transplantation due to denervation and disruption of lymphatics.[73] Gut-barrier function may be enhanced by early enteral feeding[74] and by providing specific cytoprotective nutrients (e.g., glutamine) that are essential for metabolism of the gut mucosa.[75, 76] High ileostomy output is common early in the postoperative period and may result in electrolyte imbalances, dehydration, and acidosis. When this happens, patients usually respond to prompt treatment with intravenous fluids, sodium bicarbonate infusion, and oral codeine.

Poor gastric emptying sometimes occurs, particularly in patients who had a gastrostomy tube draining their stomach for a long time before transplantation. Usually, these patients respond to prokinetic agents, but sometimes surgical drainage procedures, such as a gastroenterostomy, are required to alleviate symptoms.

Most intestinal recipients maintain normal nutrition on an unrestricted oral diet despite minor abnormalities in gut absorption. Fat absorption remains abnormal for more than a year after transplantation, and the D-xylose absorption test is normal in only 50% of recipients at 22 months.[34]

The blood levels of oral tacrolimus may be used as an indication of the absorptive function of the transplanted bowel. However, significant mucosal damage may occur before there is any discernible change in absorption.[77–79]

Graft and Patient Survival

The largest series reported so far is from the University of Pittsburgh, where 66 patients received intestinal transplants. The overall actuarial patient and graft survival at 1 year was 74% and 68%, and at 4 years was 46% and 38%, respectively.[70] The causes of death were technical complications, opportunistic infections, uncontrolled rejection, and PTLD. Fifty-four percent of the recipients died during the first 3 months after transplantation, whereas the rest died well beyond the first posttransplant year. Intractable rejection resulted in loss of 25% of isolated small bowel grafts and 4.5% of combined small bowel–liver transplants. One graft was lost to chronic rejection caused by noncompliance.[58]

At the London Health Sciences Centre, cyclosporine immune suppression was used in six patients. Two of three combined small bowel–liver recipients survived for more than 5 years but eventually died of thromboembolism and atypical pneumonia, respectively. The third combined transplant patient died at 2.5 months because of severe CMV enteritis. Two multivisceral recipients died at 7 and 9 months because of lymphoma. Ten patients at the center have been treated with tacrolimus. Two children died, one with viral gastroenteritis at 11 months, the other from cardiomyopathy due to tacrolimus toxicity at 21 days after transplantation. Eight patients are alive as of this writing. Five are off TPN and eating normal meals; two recipients still need supplementary TPN due to prolonged gastroparesis. The eighth patient is waiting for retransplantation (her first isolated small bowel graft was removed because of severe CMV enteritis). The actuarial survival rate for intestinal grafts treated with tacrolimus in our series is 67%, with 80% of patients alive at a median follow-up of 14 ± 7.5 months (range, 3–24 months).

Conclusions

SBT has become a life-saving procedure for patients with intestinal failure who have failed on conventional therapies. The outcomes of SBT have improved since the introduction of tacrolimus; they are expected to further improve with the earlier referral of patients and better immunosuppressive protocols.

References

1. Jeejeebhoy KN. Therapy of short-gut syndrome. Lancet 1983;1(8339):1427–1430.
2. Steiger E, Srp F. Morbidity and mortality related to home parenteral nutrition in patients with gut failure. Am J Surg 1983;145:102–105.
3. Kirkman RL. Small bowel transplantation. Transplantation 1984;37:429–433.
4. Grouttebel M, Saint-Aubert B, Astre C, Joyeux H. Total parenteral nutrition needs in different types of short bowel syndrome. Dig Dis Sci 1986;31:718–722.
5. Gilliand BC. Systemic Sclerosis. In JD Wilson, E Braunwald, KJ Isselbacher, et al (eds), Harrison's Principles of Internal Medicine (12th ed). New York: McGraw-Hill, 1991;1443–1448.
6. Jones IT, Jozelman DG, Fazio VW, et al. Desmoid tumors in familial polyposis coli. Ann Surg 1986;204: 94–97.
7. Schuffler MD, Jonak Z. Familial visceral myopathy. Chronic intestinal pseudo-obstruction caused by a degenerative disorder of the myenteric plexus: the use of Smith's method to define the neuropathology. Gastroenterology 1982;82:476–481.
8. Weser E. Nutritional aspects of malabsorption. Short gut adaptation. Am J Med 1979;67:1014.
9. Surana R, Quinn FM, Puri P. Short-gut syndrome: intestinal adaptation in a patient with 12 cm of jejunum. J Pediatr Gastroenterol Nutr 1994;19:246–249.
10. Dobbins JW, Bindner HJ. Importance of the colon in enteric hyperoxaluria. N Engl J Med 1977;296:298–302.
11. Hoffman AF. Defective biliary secretion during total parenteral nutrition: probable mechanisms and possible solutions. J Pediatr Gastroenterol Nutr 1995:20: 376–390.

12. Hoffman Af, Poley JR. Cholestyramine treatment of diarrhea associated with ileal resection. N Engl J Med 1969;281:397–402.

13. Ghent CN. The liver transplant candidate. In WC Maddrey (ed), Transplantation of the Liver. New York: Elsevier, 1988;59–85.

14. Williams NS, Evans P, King RFGJ. Gastric acid secretion and gastrin production in the short bowel syndrome. Gut 1985;26:914–918.

15. Kenney PR, Dorfmann GS, Denny DF. Percutaneous inferior vena cava cannulation for long-term parenteral nutrition. Surgery 1985;97:602–605.

16. Caniano DA, Starr J, Ginn-Pease ME. Extensive short-gut syndrome in neonates: outcome in the 1980s. Surgery 1989;105:119–124.

17. Mullick FG, Moran CA, Ishak KG. Total parenteral nutrition: a histopathologic analysis of the liver changes in 20 children. Mod Pathol 1994;7:190–194.

18. Klein S, Fleming CR. Enteral and Parenteral Nutrition. In M Feldman, B Scharschmidt, B Sleisenger, S Klein (eds), Sleisenger and Foitran's Gastrointestinal and Liver Disease (6th ed). Philadelphia: Saunders, 1998; 254–277.

19. Fleming CR. Hepatobiliary complications in adults receiving nutritional support. Dig Dis Sci 1994;12:191–198.

20. Moss RL, Das JB, Raffensperger JG. Total parenteral nutrition-associated cholestasis: clinical and histopathologic correlation. J Pediatr Surg 1993;28:1270–1275.

21. Frankel WL, Zhang W, Afonzo J, et al. Glutamine enhancement of structure and function in the transplanted small intestine in the rat. JPEN J Parenter Enteral Nutr 1993;17:47–55.

22. Yang RR. The effect of glutamine on cholestasis caused by total parenteral nutrition. Chung Hua Wai Ko Tsa Chih 1993;31:94–96.

23. Guertin F, Roy CC, Lepage G, et al. Effect of taurine on total parenteral nutrition-associated cholestasis. JPEN J Parenter Enteral Nutr 1991;15:247–251.

24. Howard D, Thompson DF. Taurine: an essential amino acid to prevent cholestasis in neonates? Ann Pharmacother 1992;26:1390–1392.

25. Takehara H, Hino M, Kameoka K, Komi N. A new method of total parenteral nutrition for surgical neonates: is it possible that cyclic TPN prevents intrahepatic cholestasis? Tokushima J Exp Med 1990;37:97–102.

26. Kubota A, Okada A, Imura K, et al. The effect of metronidazole on TPN-associated liver dysfunction in neonates. J Pediatr Surg 1990;25:618–621.

27. Beau P, Labat-Labourdette J, Ingrand P, Beauchant M. Is ursodeoxycholic acid an effective therapy for total parenteral nutrition-associated liver disease? J Hepatol 1994;20:240–244.

28. Rosenberg L, Brown PA. Sandostatin in the management of nonendocrine gastrointestinal and pancreatic disorders: a preliminary study. Can J Surg 1991;34:223–229.

29. Rintala RJ, Lindahl H, Pohjavuori M. Total parenteral nutrition-associated cholestasis in surgical neonates may be reversed by intravenous cholecystokinin: a preliminary report. J Pediatr Surg 1995;30:827–830.

30. Teitelbaum DH, Han-Narkey T, Schumacher RE. Treatment of total parenteral nutrition-associated cholestasis with cholecystokinin-octapeptide. J Pediatr Surg 1995; 30:1082–1085.

31. Lawrence JP, Dunn SP, Bilmire DF, et al. Isolated liver transplantation for liver failure in patients with short gut syndrome. J Pediatr Surg 1994;29:751–753.

32. Cohen Z, Silverman RE, Wassef R, et al. Small intestinal transplantation using cyclosporine. Report of a case. Transplantation 1986;42:613–621.

33. Fortner JG, Sichuk G, Litwin SD, et al. Immunological responses to an intestinal allograft with HLA-identical donor-recipient. Transplantation 1972;14:531–535.

34. Todo S, Tzakis AG, Abu-Elmagd K, et al. Intestinal transplantation in composite visceral grafts or alone. Ann Surg 1992;216:223–234.

35. Beeson PB, Brannon ES, Warren JV. Classics in infectious diseases. Observations on the sites of removal of bacteria from the blood of patients with bacterial endocarditis. Rev Infect Dis 1985;7:565–573.

36. Schraut WH, Abraham VS, Lee KK. Portal versus caval venous drainage of small bowel allografts: technical and metabolic consequences. Surgery 1986;99:193–198.

37. Starzl TE, Porter KA, Francavilla A. The Eck fistula in animals and humans. Curr Probl Surg 1983;20: 687–752.

38. Calne RY, Pollard SG, Jamieson NV, et al. Intestinal transplant for recurring mesenteric desmoid tumor. Lancet 1993;342:58–59.

39. Noli S, Bellinzono G, Spada M, et al. Haemodynamic changes during experimental small bowel transplantation. Transplant Proc 1994;26:1667–1669.

40. Busing M, Mellert J, Greger B, Hopt UT. Acute pulmonary insufficiency due to OKT3 therapy. Transplant Proc 1990;22:1779–1781.

41. Klein AS, Cofer JB, Pruett TL, et al. Prostaglandin E_1 administration following orthotopic liver transplantation: a randomized prospective multicenter trial. Gastroenterology 1996;111(3):710–715.

42. Henley KS, Lucey MR, Normolle DP, et al. A double-blind, randomized, placebo-controlled trial of prostaglandin E_1 in liver transplantation. Hepatology 1995; 21(2):366–372.

43. Oishi M, Tanaka N, Orita K. Beneficial effects of prostaglandin E1 on hemodynamic changes during liver transplantation in pigs. Transpl Int 1996;9(Suppl 1):S100–104.

44. Reznick RK, Craddock GN, Langer B, et al. Structure and function of small bowel allografts in the dog: immunosuppression with cyclosporin A. Can J Surg 1982;25:51–55.

45. Grant D, Duff J, Zhong R, et al. Successful intestinal transplantation in pigs treated with cyclosporin. Transplantation 1988;45:279–284.

46. Grant D, Sommerauer J, Mimeault R, et al. Treatment

with continuous high dose intravenous cyclosporine following intestinal transplantation. A case report. Transplantation 1989;48:151–152.

47. Revillon Y, Jan D, Goulet O, Ricour C. Small bowel transplantation in seven children: preservation technique. Transplant Proc 1991;23:2350–2351.

48. Schroeder P, Goulet O, Lear P. Small bowel transplantation: European experience. Lancet 1990;336:110–111.

49. Tattersall C, Gebel H, Haklin M, et al. Lymphocyte responsiveness after irradiation in canine and human intestinal allografts. Curr Probl Surg 1989;46:16–19.

50. Atkison P, Joubert G, Barron A, et al. Hypertrophic cardiomyopathy associated with tacrolimus in paediatric transplant patients. Lancet 1995;345:894–896.

51. Grant D, Wall W, Mimeault R, et al. Successful small-bowel/liver transplantation. Lancet 1990;335:181–184.

52. Monchik GJ, Russel PS. Transplantation of small bowel in the rat: technical and immunological considerations. Surgery 1971;70:693–702.

53. Quan D, Grant D, Zhong R, et al. Patterns of cytokine transcripts in intestinal allograft rejection. Transplant Proc 1994;26:1530.

54. Schmid T, Oberhuber G, Korozsi G, et al. Altered distribution of MHC class II antigens on enterocytes during acute small bowel allograft rejection in rats. Transpl Int 1990;3:73–77.

55. Iwaki Y, Starzl TE, Yagihashi A, et al. Replacement of donor lymphoid tissue in small-bowel transplants. Lancet 1991;337:818–819.

56. Grant D, Hurlbut D, Zhong R, et al. Intestinal permeability and bacterial translocation following small bowel transplantation in the rat. Transplantation 1991;52:221–224.

57. Madara JL, Kirkman RL. Structural and functional evolution of jejunal allograft rejection in rats and the ameliorating effects of cyclosporine therapy. J Clin Invest 1985;75:505–512.

58. Abu-Elmagd K, Todo S, Tzakis A, et al. Three years' clinical experience with intestinal transplantation. J Am Coll Surg 1994;179:385–400.

59. Calne RY, White HJO, Binns RM, et al. Immunosuppressive effects of the orthotopically transplanted porcine liver. Transplant Proc 1969;1:321–324.

60. Wall WJ, Stiller CR, Wright FF, et al. Experimental and clinical liver transplantation. Transplant Proc 1982;15:724–729.

61. Zhong R, He G, Sakai Y, et al. Combined small bowel and liver transplantation in the rat: possible role of the liver in preventing intestinal allograft rejection. Transplantation 1991;52:550–552.

62. Gonwa TA, Nery JR, Husberg BS, Klintmalm GB. Simultaneous liver and renal transplantation in man. Transplantation 1988;46:690–693.

63. Rasmussen A, Davies H, Jamieson NV, et al. Combined transplantation of liver and kidney from the same donor protects the kidney from rejection and improves kidney graft survival. Transplantation 1995;59:919–921.

64. Starzl TE, Todo S, Tzakis A, Murase N. Multivisceral and intestinal transplantation. Transplant Proc 1992;24:1217–1223.

65. Kusne S, Manez R, Bonet H, et al. Infectious complications after small bowel transplantation in adults. Transplant Proc 1994;26:1682–1683.

66. Swinnen LJ, Costanzo-Nordin MR, Fisher SG, et al. Increased incidence of lymphoproliferative disorder after immunosuppression with monoclonal antibody OKT3 in cardiac transplant recipients [abstract]. N Engl J Med 1990;323:1723–1738.

67. Randhawa PS, Jaffe R, Demetris AJ, et al. Expression of Epstein-Barr virus-encoded small RNA (by the EBER-1 gene) in liver specimens from transplant recipients with post-transplantation lymphoproliferative disease [abstract]. N Engl J 1992;327:1710–1714.

68. Starzl TE, Rowe MI, Todo S, et al. Transplantation of multiple abdominal viscera. JAMA 1989;261:1449–1457.

69. Williams JW, Sankary HN, Foster PF, et al. Splanchnic transplantation: an approach to the infant dependent on parenteral nutrition who develops irreversible liver disease. JAMA 1989;261:1458–1462.

70. Todo S, Reyes J, Furukawa H, et al. Outcome analysis of 71 clinical intestinal transplantations. Ann Surg 1995;222:270–282.

71. Kuo PC, Dafoe DC, Alfrey EJ, et al. Posttransplant lymphoproliferative disorders and Epstein-Barr virus prophylaxis. Transplantation 1995;59:135–138.

72. Kadry Z, Furukawa H, Abu-Elmagd K, et al. Use of the D-xylose absorption test in monitoring intestinal allografts. Transplant Proc 1994;26:1645.

73. Quigley EMM, Thompson JS, Rose SG. The long-term function of canine jejunoileal autotransplants—insights into allograft physiology. Transplant Proc 1992;24:1105–1106.

74. Moore FA, Feliciano DV, Andrassy RJ, et al. Early enteral feeding, compared with parenteral, reduces postoperative septic complications. The results of meta-analysis. Ann Surg 1992;216:172–183.

75. Lee TK, Cardona MA, Kurkchubasche AG, et al. Mucosal glutamine utilization after small-bowel transplantation: an electrophysiologic study. J Surg Res 1992;52:605–614.

76. Frankel WL, Zhang W, Afonso J, et al. Glutamine enhancement of structure and function in transplanted small intestine in the rat. JPEN J Parenter Enteral Nutr 1993;17:47–55.

77. Cohn WB, Hardy MA, Quint J, State D. Absorptive function in canine jejunal autografts and allografts. Surgery 1969;65:440–446.

78. Stamford WP, Hardy MA. Fatty acid absorption in jejunal autograft and allograft. Surgery 1974;75:496–501.

79. Toledo-Pereyra LH, Simmons RL, Najarian JS. Absorption of carbohydrates and vitamins in the preserved and transplanted small intestine. Am J Surg 1975;129:192–197.

Chapter 10
Pancreas Transplantation

David S. Beebe, David M. Kendall,
Rainer W. G. Gruessner, and Kumar G. Belani

Chapter Plan

History of Pancreas Transplantation

At the turn of the century, before the isolation of insulin, grafting of portions of the pancreas to treat diabetes was actually attempted.[1, 2] In 1929, Banting proposed transplantation of the insulin-producing tissue of the pancreas.[3] Lillehei and colleagues performed the first pancreas transplant to treat diabetes in humans in 1966 at the University of Minnesota, as reported by Kelly et al.[4] They did a combined pancreas and kidney transplant in two patients with long-standing diabetes and far-advanced secondary complications. One patient died of complications related to surgery. The other had satisfactory graft function and remained normoglycemic and insulin independent for nearly 6 months posttransplant. The success rate for pancreas transplantation was initially very low, but it has constantly improved due to better surgical techniques and the introduction of cyclosporine. Approximately 1,000 cadaveric transplants are now done yearly in 150 centers internationally. One-year graft and patient survival rates are now 70% and 91%.[5]

The restoration of normoglycemia after pancreas transplantation reduces the rate of secondary diabetic complications. Further benefits include correction of defects in glucose counterregulation and improvements in quality of life. The limitations of pancreas transplantation include the morbidity and mortality associated with the surgery, the morbidity and cost of lifelong immunosuppression, and the

Table 10-1. Benefits of Pancreas Transplantation

Elimination of exogenous insulin requirements
Euglycemia
Prevention of nephropathy
Stabilization of neuropathy
Prevention or reduction of atherosclerosis

significant financial costs. Patients must be carefully selected so that the benefits of a transplant meet or exceed those of standard insulin treatment in terms of glucose metabolism, quality of life, and secondary complications (Table 10-1).

Currently, the most common surgical options are simultaneous pancreas and kidney transplantation (SPK) for uremic patients, pancreas after kidney transplant (PAK) for chronically immunosuppressed recipients, and pancreas transplantation alone (PTA) for nonuremic, nonkidney recipients.

Simultaneous Pancreas and Kidney Transplantation for Uremic Patients

SPK is the most common pancreas transplantation performed worldwide. Of the 5,807 transplants performed between January 1968 and April 1994 reported to the International Pancreas Transplant Registry, 80% were SPK. Before transplantation, these patients have severe secondary complications of diabetes, many of which are permanent and not likely to be reversed by a transplant. Adding a pancreas graft to a kidney graft is justified for three reasons:

1. Patients are already obligated to immunosuppression due to the kidney transplant, and it is generally accepted that quality of life is better when immunosuppressed and dialysis free than when nonimmunosuppressed and dialysis dependent.[6]
2. It may prevent recurrence of diabetic nephropathy in the allograft.[7]
3. Quality of life improves even if insulin independence is the only benefit achieved other than reversal of uremia, with only minimal additional surgical risk.

Disadvantages of adding a pancreas graft include the additional surgical procedure, the potential for complications related to the pancreas graft alone (such as graft pancreatitis or difficulties with man-

agement of exocrine secretions), and slightly higher rates of kidney graft loss.[6] A simultaneous transplant improves survival of the pancreas graft because the kidney, by virtue of serum creatinine measurements, serves as an indirect marker of rejection in both organs.[7]

Pancreas after Kidney Transplantation for Chronically Immunosuppressed Recipients

Secondary complications are also usually far advanced in this category. Pancreas transplantation is done primarily to improve quality of life by obviating the diabetic control problem. In regard to kidney graft survival, PAK recipients have an advantage over SPK recipients if the kidney is from a living-related donor (LRD): The long-term outcome with kidney grafts from LRDs continues to be significantly better than with cadaver kidneys.[6]

Pancreas Transplantation Alone for Nonuremic, Nonkidney Recipients

Unlike SPK and PAK, posttransplantation immunosuppression in pancreas transplantation alone is given only to correct diabetes with the pancreas rather than treating renal failure as well. It is not known if the risk of immunosuppression exceeds the risk of developing secondary complications from diabetes. Therefore, offering pancreas transplants to the entire nonuremic diabetic population for the sake of diabetic control alone awaits the development of tolerance or of less toxic immunosuppression. However, the situation is different for diabetic patients with extreme lability of metabolic control and low quality of life. For them, the problems of diabetes likely exceed those of immunosuppression, so a pancreas transplant should be done.[6]

Diabetes Mellitus

Diabetes mellitus is a disorder of carbohydrate, fat, and protein metabolism that is characterized by hyperglycemia. Surveys from the United States suggest that diabetes affects approximately 1–2% of the population. An additional 1–2% who have not been diagnosed with diabetes demonstrate abnormal glucose tolerance. Diabetes results from either an absolute or a relative deficiency of insulin secretion or action.[8]

Type 2, or non–insulin-dependent diabetes mellitus (NIDDM) results from a relative deficiency of insulin. The most common type of diabetes, NIDDM usually develops after age 30 years. A combination of insulin resistance and defects in insulin secretion are required for NIDDM to develop. NIDDM is managed by a diabetic diet, oral hypoglycemic agents, or exogenous supplemental insulin. Pancreas transplantation is not performed for this disorder.[8]

Type 1, or insulin-dependent diabetes mellitus (IDDM), is caused by complete destruction of pancreatic beta cells. These patients secrete little or no insulin. Approximately 1.5 million individuals in the United States have type 1 diabetes (IDDM); 12,000–20,000 new cases develop annually. Most cases of IDDM occur in children and young adults, with the peak incidence in the midteens.[9]

The destruction of beta cells in patients with IDDM is now thought to be immune mediated.[10, 11] Destruction results from activation of subsets of T lymphocytes, which affect a cytotoxic response directed specifically against the pancreatic beta cells.[12] The disruption in self-recognition (which gives rise to the autoimmune process in type 1 diabetes) likely results from a combination of genetic and environmental factors. In addition to cytotoxic T-cell responses, a number of specific "autoantigens" are associated with type 1 diabetes (insulin, pancreatic beta cells, glutamic acid decarboxylase). Although these autoantigens can serve as markers for individuals at risk for type 1 diabetes, their specific pathogenetic role is not fully defined.[11, 13]

Some evidence for the autoimmune origin of IDDM comes from the experience of Sutherland et al. with living-related pancreas transplantation between identical twins.[14] They transplanted a section of the pancreas (more than 50%) from a nondiabetic twin into an identical twin with IDDM. In the first three patients in their series, immunosuppression was not used; diabetes recurred 6–12 weeks posttransplantation. Graft biopsies showed isletitis with selective beta cell destruction. In subsequent transplants between identical twins, immunosuppression was provided; diabetes did not recur. In cadaver pancreas transplantation, immunosuppression is always provided; isletitis in the transplanted graft recurs rarely, if ever.

Insulin, an anabolic hormone, is essential for survival. It promotes glucose uptake and glycogen synthesis in the liver and muscles. It also stimulates triglyceride synthesis in adipose tissue, enhances amino acid transport for protein synthesis in cells, and inhibits glycogenolysis, gluconeogenesis, lipolysis, proteolysis, and ketogenesis. During hypoglycemia and fasting, insulin release is suppressed. Catabolic, counterregulatory hormones (such as glucagon, catecholamines, growth hormone, and glucocorticoids) are secreted to overcome hypoglycemia and to continuously supply glucose, fatty acids, and ketone bodies for energy use by the brain and other organs.[15]

Hyperglycemia is due to inadequate insulin replacement. Glucose cannot enter the cells without insulin. The result is cellular starvation despite hyperglycemia. The counterregulatory hormones initiate lipolysis of adipose tissue, raising the free fatty acid and glycerol levels in the blood. Furthermore, during insulin deficiency, glucagon stimulates the production of ketone bodies in the mitochondria, which may lead to severe diabetic ketoacidosis.[15]

Patients with type 1 diabetes mellitus produce little or no insulin. Therefore, either exogenous insulin or a functioning pancreas transplant is necessary for survival.[15] The discovery of insulin by Banting and Best in 1922 made it possible to prevent many metabolic consequences of type 1 diabetes.[16] Subcutaneous injections of insulin are effective in controlling gross hyperglycemia and other metabolic complications in patients with IDDM. Despite modern formulations and dosing regimens, however, control of blood sugar remains imperfect. Many patients still require treatment for ketoacidosis if their insulin dose is inadequate. Conversely, many patients have hypoglycemic episodes due to excessive insulin treatment.[17]

Chronic hyperglycemia plays a major role in the pathogenesis of diabetic complications, and genetic and other environmental factors are believed to contribute. Even with intensive insulin management techniques, most patients with IDDM have relative, chronic hyperglycemia.[18] Chronic hyperglycemia is thought to be a major cause of diabetic vascular complications.[19] These complications (nephropathy, retinopathy, neuropathy) affect up to 50% of patients with diabetes of 20 years' duration or longer. The average life span of patients with dia-

Table 10-2. Complications of Type 1
Diabetes Mellitus

Nephropathy
Retinopathy
Neuropathy
Coronary artery disease
Cardiomyopathy
Peripheral vascular disease
Gastroparesis
Ketoacidosis
Chronic hyperglycemia
Hypertension

betes is markedly shorter than that of the general population, which is due, in great part, to the increased incidence of cardiovascular disease.[20]

Several theories explain how chronic hyperglycemia may cause cellular damage:

1. Chronic hyperglycemia leads to the production of sorbitol by the enzyme aldose reductase. Sorbitol accumulation exerts osmotic changes in vascular, neuronal, and other tissues, possibly causing cellular damage.
2. Elevated glucose and sorbitol levels may compete with the cellular uptake of myoinositol. The reduction of myoinositol may cause cellular dysfunction.
3. Hyperglycemia may alter the redox potential and adversely affect cellular function.
4. Hyperglycemia activates the diacylglycerol and protein kinase pathway involved in the synthesis and turnover of basement membranes.
5. A chronically elevated blood sugar may lead to the formation of abnormal covalent products by nonenzymatic processes with various proteins (such as hemoglobin, albumin, low-density lipoproteins, collagen, and perhaps even DNA). The result may be thickening of the basement membrane and vascular dysfunction.
6. Finally, glycosylated products released into the circulation may bind as well to macrophages to release tumor necrosis factor, interleukin-1, and other cytokines, all associated with chronic hyperglycemia and ultimately, vascular damage.[21, 22]

The universal nature of vascular injury, affecting both large and small vessels, is responsible for the multiorgan involvement in patients with IDDM (Table 10-2). For example, both peripheral and autonomic diabetic neuropathy is a result of microvascular disease.[20] Autonomic neuropathy is particularly ominous in patients with diabetes mellitus because it is associated with increased mortality.[23] Diabetic nephropathy, a result of microvascular disease in the renal glomerulus, develops in the setting of hypertension, poor glucose control, and unknown genetic factors.[20, 24] Retinopathy is a direct result of vascular injury.[25] The incidence of coronary and peripheral vascular disease is also very high in patients with type 1 diabetes.[26] Silent myocardial ischemia or infarction is common because many of these patients have peripheral neuropathies.[27]

Patients with type 1 diabetes mellitus may develop cardiomyopathy even in the absence of coronary artery disease. Pathologic studies of the heart in patients with type 1 diabetes mellitus who develop cardiomyopathy reveal (1) microvascular disease (similar to that in the retina or kidney); (2) hyaline thickening in the coronary arteries (with or without endothelial cell proliferation); and (3) interstitial infiltration with periodic acid Schiff–positive material, fibrosis, degeneration, and fragmentation of myocytes.[28, 29] These changes are responsible for the diminished left ventricular compliance and ejection fraction, particularly with exercise, seen in patients with IDDM.[30, 31]

At present, medical management of type 1 diabetes is directed at control of blood glucose (in an attempt to reduce the deleterious effects of hyperglycemia) and at treatment and prevention of secondary complications. The focus is on improving and even normalizing blood glucose levels. With multiple daily insulin injections and subcutaneous insulin pumps, some individuals have achieved impressive improvements in blood glucose control.

In 1993, results of the Diabetes Control and Complications Trial clearly showed that intensive glycemic control could significantly reduce the incidence of diabetic retinopathy, microalbuminuria, and neuropathy.[19] Even with very tight glucose control (near-normal glycemia), however, secondary complications did develop. The benefits of improved control came at the expense of dangerous increases in the incidence of iatrogenic hypoglycemia. Insulin reactions were three times more likely in the intensive treatment cohort of the trial. Patients also had to increase the number of blood samples and insulin injections from two to four times a day to accomplish the intensive therapy.

Other therapies are available that, in addition to controlling blood glucose, reduce the morbidity associated with diabetes complications. Laser photocoagulation therapy reduces the incidence of vision loss in patients with proliferative diabetic retinopathy. Antihypertensive treatment, particularly with angiotensin-converting enzyme inhibitors, reduces urinary protein excretion and stabilizes serum creatinine levels in many patients. The result may be lower rates of progression to end-stage renal disease.[32] Finally, treatment with tricyclic antidepressants can reduce the symptoms of diabetic neuropathy.

Although medical management has improved since the 1960s, the goal of finding a cure for type 1 diabetes has not yet been realized. Only by reconstituting intact, functional beta cells can the treatment of diabetes possibly restore long-standing normoglycemia. It is with this goal in mind that pancreas transplantation was developed.

Successful pancreas transplantation effectively normalizes serum glucose levels in patients with type 1 diabetes (see Table 10-1). Other benefits are:

1. The need for daily insulin injection is eliminated, with most transplant recipients reporting a significant improvement in lifestyle.[33]
2. Euglycemia is more effectively maintained than with exogenous insulin administration, which may benefit patients who have frequent, severe hypoglycemic episodes and hypoglycemic unawareness.[5]
3. Diabetic nephropathy is prevented in both native and transplanted kidneys.[7]
4. Somatic and autonomic nerve function is stabilized and possibly reversed, thus decreasing the high incidence of sudden death in diabetic patients with autonomic neuropathy.[34, 35]
5. Atherosclerosis may be prevented or reduced because the serum lipid profile is favorably altered, even though insulin is delivered systemically (rather than via the portal venous system).[36]

These advantages are likely to make pancreas transplantation more common in the future.

Indications for Transplantation and Recipient Selection

If diabetic patients hope to achieve and maintain normal blood glucose levels, therapeutic alterna-

Table 10-3. Indications for Pancreas Transplantation

Extremely labile diabetes mellitus with frequent hypoglycemia
Poor quality of life
Diabetic complications exceed side effects of immunosuppression
End-stage renal disease, with renal transplantation planned or already done

tives to standard insulin treatment must be sought. Pancreas transplantation is the only current method that consistently normalizes serum glucose levels.[5] Table 10-3 lists the indications for pancreas transplantation.

The restoration of normoglycemia after pancreas transplantation reduces the rate of secondary diabetic complications. Further benefits include correction of defects in glucose counterregulation and improvements in quality of life. The limitations of pancreas transplantation include the morbidity and mortality associated with the surgery, the morbidity and cost of lifelong immunosuppression, and the significant financial costs. Patients must be carefully selected so that the benefits of a transplant meet or exceed those of standard insulin treatment in terms of glucose metabolism, quality of life, and secondary complications.

Protocol for Pretransplantation Evaluation

Before the anesthesiologist sees them, patients scheduled for a pancreas or combined pancreas-kidney transplantation undergo a thorough assessment by an endocrinologist and transplant surgeon (Table 10-4). At our institution, this assessment includes (1) confirmation of presence of type 1 diabetes, (2) standard tissue typing and pretransplantation education, (3) pretransplantation evaluation for ischemic heart disease, and (4) documentation and evaluation of secondary diabetic complications.

To confirm the presence of type 1 diabetes (defined as an absolute deficiency of endogenous insulin production), simple measurements of basal and stimulated C peptide are made. C peptide (the portion of the proinsulin molecule cleaved to produce circulating insulin) is cosecreted with insulin by functional pancreatic beta cells. The absence of C

Table 10-4. Protocol for Pretransplantation Evaluation of Pancreas Candidates

---

Confirm presence of type 1 diabetes mellitus
Do standard tissue and blood typing
Begin pretransplantation education
Evaluate for secondary diabetic complications
    Ischemic heart disease
    Renal failure
    Autonomic and peripheral neuropathy
    Retinopathy
    Other

Table 10-5. Concerns Requiring Preoperative Assessment

Potential difficult airway
Functional and anatomic status of cardiopulmonary
    systems
Severity of autonomic neuropathy
Presence of gastroparesis
Extent of motor and sensory neuropathy
Metabolic status
    Insulin dose
    Glucose level
    Electrolyte levels
    Acid-base abnormality

---

peptide confirms loss of endogenous insulin production and thus confirms absolute insulin deficiency.

Preoperative evaluation for coronary heart disease is essential. Ischemic heart disease is common in diabetic patients referred for transplantation. It is the chief cause of both morbidity and mortality in those with end-stage renal disease. Silent coronary disease is common in diabetic patients with autonomic neuropathy, however, particularly those with uremia. Therefore, cardiac disease is often not detected during the preoperative history and physical examination or by an electrocardiogram.[37]

To detect signs or symptoms suggestive of coronary heart disease, exercise or dipyridamole cardiac stress testing using thallium radionuclide imaging is done in addition to a thorough history and physical examination. If coronary vascular disease is suggested, or if the patient is older than 35 years old, is a smoker, or has an abnormal electrocardiogram, angiography is done. Appropriate coronary revascularization (angioplasty or coronary artery bypass grafting) is completed before a pancreas transplant is considered; this has resulted in a decrease in posttransplantation incidence of cardiac complications.[38–41]

All patients considered for a pancreas transplant are also evaluated for the presence of other secondary diabetic complications, including retinopathy, nephropathy, and neuropathy. Such evaluation establishes the need for pretransplantation intervention. Renal function is of particular importance because SPKs are available for patients with progressive diabetic renal disease. Renal function is assessed by using standard measurements of serum creatinine and creatinine clearance and by evaluating for the presence of pathologic levels of urinary protein excretion.

If there is doubt about the diagnosis of diabetic nephropathy, a renal biopsy is done. Medical management of hypertension is also optimized. Diabetic retinopathy is documented by routine ophthalmologic examination; proliferative retinopathy often requires photocoagulation therapy. Diabetic peripheral and autonomic neuropathy are assessed by electromyographic studies, neurologic examination, and measurement of cardiac autonomic nerve function.

Preoperative Evaluation

Except in the rare case of living-related segmental pancreas donation, pancreas transplantation is performed soon after a cadaver organ is available. Because preservation time is usually limited to less than 24 hours,[42] anesthesiologists must work under emergent or semiurgent conditions. In spite of time constraints, a thorough presurgical evaluation is essential before administering the anesthetic (Table 10-5). Most patients undergoing pancreas, islet cell, or combined kidney-pancreas or islet cell transplantation have severe systemic complications of long-standing diabetes mellitus, including coronary artery disease, severe hypertension, renal insufficiency, autonomic and systemic neuropathy, and gastroparesis (see Table 10-2). In a review of 55 patients who underwent pancreas or combined kidney-pancreas transplantation at the University of Minnesota, 29% had significant coronary artery disease; most had retinopathy, neuropathy, and nephropathy (Table 10-6); and 62% had hypertension.[43]

Evaluation of the airway should be given special consideration in patients undergoing a pancreas

Table 10-6. Concurrent Diseases in 55 Pancreas Recipients, University of Minnesota (1990 and 1991)

Disease	Number	Percentage
Coronary artery disease by angiogram	16	29
Prior myocardial infarction	4	7
Retinopathy	53	96
Neuropathy		
Peripheral	50	89
Autonomic	5	9
Nephropathy	52	95
Nephropathy with dialysis	14	25
Gastroparesis	13	24
Hypertension	34	62
Peripheral vascular disease	7	13

Source: Reprinted with permission from DS Beebe, KG Belani, M Yoo, et al. Pancreas transplantation: anesthetic considerations based upon a one year review. Am J Anesth 1995;22:239.

transplant.[43] Hogan et al. found that, of 125 patients with long-standing diabetes undergoing a pancreas or kidney transplant, 30% were difficult to intubate, and two required an emergency tracheostomy.[44] Similarly, Beebe et al. found that 13% of patients undergoing a pancreas transplant were difficult to intubate.[43] The risk of difficult intubation in the control population is less than 3%.[44] Difficulty with intubation increases the risk for permanent tracheal damage and aspiration, particularly in the diabetic patient with gastroparesis.[45]

The cause of increased difficulty with intubation in diabetic patients is not known. One reason may be that abnormal cross-linking of collagen via nonenzymatic glycosylation occurs with chronic hyperglycemia.[44] Renal insufficiency potentiates this collagen cross-linking.[46] Diabetic patients therefore often develop waxy skin, contractures, and general stiffness of their joints (stiff joint syndrome). Stiff joint syndrome usually involves the joints of the patient's head and neck, particularly the atlantooccipital joint, which may limit visualization of the trachea during laryngoscopy. The patient's inability to oppose his or her palms due to stiffness of the interphalangeal joints is predictive of difficult tracheal intubation in patients with long-standing diabetes.[44]

The immediate pretransplantation status of cardiac and pulmonary systems must be studied. Car-

diac disease can affect both hemodynamic stability and long-term patient and allograft survival. For example, in their study of 155 SPK transplant recipients, Gruessner et al. found that the death rate from myocardial infarction or stroke in the first year after an SPK transplant was four times greater (18%) in patients with known coronary disease than in those without.[41] The choice of anesthetic, intraoperative monitoring, and postoperative respiratory support is influenced by the severity of diabetic cardiopulmonary involvement.

Neuropathy, both systemic and autonomic, is common in pancreas transplant recipients (see Table 10-6).[43] Autonomic neuropathy significantly increases the risk for perioperative morbidity and mortality.[47, 48] Such patients often develop severe hypotension during anesthetic administration because of the impaired function of their sympathetic nervous systems.[48] Several diabetic patients with autonomic neuropathy have died suddenly during recovery from anesthesia, possibly due to an altered autonomic response to hypoxia.[47] Denervation hypersensitivity of cardiac acetylcholine receptors may also develop in diabetic patients with autonomic neuropathy. One patient developed refractory bradycardia after neostigmine administration, presumably from denervation hypersensitivity.[49] Therefore, anesthesiologists should specifically inquire about symptoms of autonomic dysfunction (i.e., dizziness on standing, hypotension on initiating dialysis, esophageal dysmotility, nausea, and intermittent diarrhea). Orthostatic blood pressure and pulse measurements obtained before anesthesia may also suggest autonomic dysfunction.[50]

Electrocardiograms should also be examined for resting tachycardia, which may indicate vagus nerve dysfunction. A change in the resting heart rate, on deep inspiration, of 5 beats per minute or less (normal is more than 15 beats/minute) indicates significant autonomic neuropathy.[47]

Neuropathy of the vagus nerve induces gastroparesis, which increases the risk of aspiration of gastric contents.[50, 51] Heartburn, bloating, and explosive diarrhea indicate intestinal autonomic dysfunction; symptomatic patients may be on gastric motility agents. If gastroparesis or intestinal autonomic dysfunction is present, then proper aspiration precautions must be taken.[51]

Motor and sensory peripheral neuropathy are quite common.[29, 43] Severe motor neuropathy from diabetes or uremia may increase the risk for hyperkalemia after succinylcholine administration.[52] In addition, the risk for postoperative neuropraxias is increased, probably relative to impaired vascular supply to the peripheral nerves.[53] Accurate preoperative neurologic examination is essential to document preexisting pathology; this step is helpful if a nerve injury after surgery is alleged and litigation ensues.

Evaluation of the preoperative metabolic status is essential because many pancreas transplantation patients have extremely brittle diabetes or renal insufficiency. For proper metabolic management during anesthesia, it is important to know details of insulin therapy in pancreas recipients. A baseline blood glucose level must be obtained before transplant. Hyperglycemia has been shown to be harmful to islet cells and must be avoided during revascularization of the graft or infusion of the islet cells.[43] If a patient is extremely hyperglycemic (blood sugar greater than 500 mg/dl) and has not received insulin recently, blood gases should be measured and the blood and urine analyzed for ketones to rule out existing diabetic ketoacidosis.[54] In the rare event of extreme hyperglycemia, surgery may have to be delayed until the patient's metabolic status is stabilized.

Renal insufficiency is common, occurring in 95% of our pancreas transplantation patients.[43] It is important to obtain preoperative electrolytes and serum creatinine levels as well as the timing of the last dialysis in dialysis-dependent patients. Hyperkalemia (potassium greater than 5.5 mmol/liter) should be treated pretransplant either with insulin (if associated with hyperglycemia); with ion exchange resins, such as sodium polystyrene (Kayexalate) (if dialysis is not an option); or with dialysis (if the patient is in renal failure). Finally, a hemoglobin level should be obtained to help plan fluid and transfusion management intraoperatively. All patients should have blood typed and crossmatched in case transfusion is required.

Surgical Considerations

Refinements in organ procurement, preservation, and surgical technique have all helped to achieve the current transplantation success rates. Most multiorgan donors in the United States now serve as both liver and pancreas donors; reconstruction of the arterial blood supply to the pancreas has been standardized, with few technical complications. The introduction of University of Wisconsin solution

Table 10-7. Exocrine Drainage of Pancreas Grafts: Surgical Considerations

Drainage Type	Considerations
Enteric drainage	Most physiologic (mimics normal pancreatic drainage); difficult to identify rejection
Duct injection with synthetic polymer	Results in exocrine fibrosis; difficult to identify rejection
Bladder drainage	Technically easy; urinary amylase levels useful in detecting rejection

allows preservation times of up to 30 hours, though early transplantation is still desirable.[42]

A point of controversy is drainage of the exocrine pancreas (Table 10-7). Several surgical techniques have been used to manage these graft secretions, which is a key issue in preventing surgical complications. These techniques include (1) enteric drainage, which is the usual drainage of the pancreas (this technique would mimic the normal physiology of pancreatic drainage); (2) duct injection using a synthetic polymer, which causes exocrine fibrosis but leaves the endocrine function of the pancreas intact; and (3) urinary drainage.[55–57] Enteric drainage and duct injection remain popular in many European centers, but urinary drainage is now used in more than 90% of pancreas transplantations in the United States.[58] Originally, secretions were drained through the ureter,[59] but in the early 1980s, surgical practice changed to connecting the pancreas directly to the bladder (duodenocystostomy).[55] The pancreas secretes numerous digestive enzymes, which can impede the healing of anastomoses and cause wound breakdown and abscess formation. The bladder is well vascularized; it heals well in spite of the presence of pancreatic secretions. Urinary drainage also allows detection of pancreas rejection episodes at an early stage through the monitoring of urinary amylase levels.[55, 59, 60] Both clinically and experimentally, exocrine rejection (i.e., decrease in urinary amylase levels) precedes endocrine rejection (i.e., hyperglycemia).[60, 61] When exocrine pancreas function is monitored, antirejection treatment can be started before hyperglycemia, thereby successfully reversing most rejection episodes.[62]

Monitoring urinary amylase levels is particularly important for PTA and PAK recipients.[63] For SPK

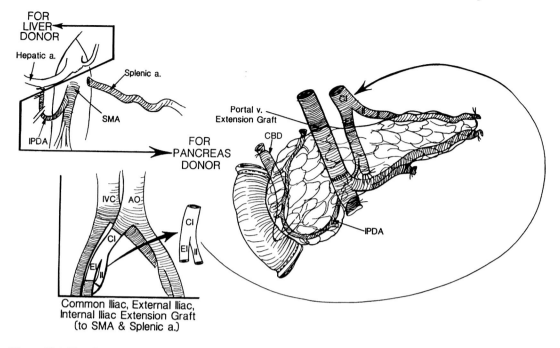

Figure 10-1. Vessels, entire pancreas, and part of duodenum that should be harvested during combined whole pancreas and liver removal from a cadaver donor. *Upper left inset*: celiac plexus, arterial supply to the liver and the pancreas. *Lower left inset*: iliac vessels to be removed for use as a Y graft for the vascular anastomoses in the recipient. (a. = artery; SMA = superior mesenteric artery; IPDA = inferior pancreaticoduodenal artery; CBD = common bile duct; Ao = abdominal aorta; IVC = inferior vena cava; v. = vein; CI = common iliac [artery]; EI = external iliac [artery]; II = internal iliac [artery].)

recipients, whose grafts both come from the same donor, a rise in serum creatinine levels, which is a renal manifestation of rejection, usually occurs before any demonstrable changes in exocrine pancreas function.[61, 63] Therefore, in SPK, the method of pancreas graft duct management is not as critical as for PTA and PAK recipients because the kidney can be used as a surrogate indicator of rejection.

The venous drainage of the transplanted pancreas is to the systemic venous system rather than to the liver via the portal vein. Drainage through the portal vein is possible but is technically more difficult. The metabolic advantage over portal venous drainage is also not apparent. Although insulin levels are higher with systemic venous drainage, euglycemia is accomplished with either systemic or portal drainage.[64]

Surgical Technique

The following description of surgical technique is based on whole pancreaticoduodenal transplantation via bladder drainage (duodenocystostomy)

from a combined pancreas-liver cadaver donor (Figures 10-1 and 10-2). Variants of this technique are published elsewhere.[65]

Most pancreases are procured along with the liver from multiorgan donors, and both organs share a blood supply. Thus, vascular reconstruction is necessary. Bench preparation of the pancreas can be done before the recipient vessels and bladder are dissected and exposed (or at the same time if a second surgical team is available). The standard bench vascular reconstruction technique uses an arterial extension iliac Y graft of donor common, external, and internal iliac artery.[66] The internal iliac artery of the donor Y graft is end-to-end anastomosed to the splenic artery, as is the external iliac artery to the superior mesenteric artery. Various modifications of this standard reconstruction technique have been described.[67] Bench preparation of the pancreas also involves removing the spleen (usually attached), closing the proximal duodenum in two or three layers, shortening the mesenteric root, and carefully ligating its vessels.

In the recipient, the pancreas graft is usually placed in the right side of the patient's lower abdomen

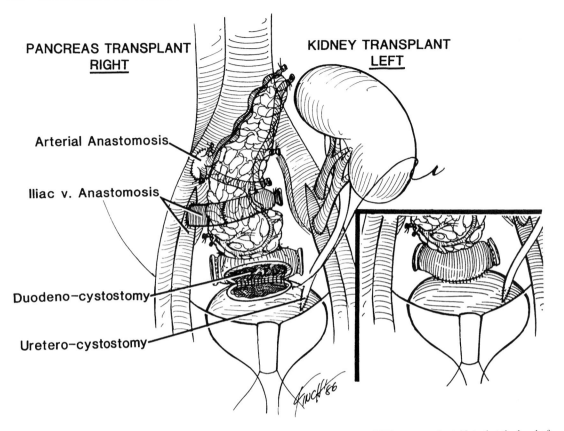

Figure 10-2. Vascular and bladder anastomoses of a combined cadaver pancreas and kidney transplant. Note that the head of the pancreas is pointed toward the dome of the bladder, where the duodenum is anastomosed to allow exocrine drainage of the pancreas. Preferably, the kidney is transplanted in the left iliac fossa. (v. = vein.)

(where the dissection of the common iliac vessels is easier than the left side). In addition, the natural position of the right iliac vessels (vein lateral to artery) does not require vascular realignment, though on the left side it might (see Figures 10-1 and 10-2).

The patient's abdominal cavity is entered through a midline incision, extending from midway between the xiphoid process and umbilicus down to the pubic bone. To create a comfortable bed for the pancreaticoduodenal graft, the cecum is mobilized first. The right common, external, and internal iliac artery and veins are identified and dissected free. All hypogastric vein branches, including the first lumbar vein, are ligated and divided for complete mobilization of the vein from the vena cava to the inguinal ligament. This dissection technically facilitates the venous anastomosis. It also prevents tension on, and possible tears at, the anastomosis; theoretically, it decreases the risk of venous thrombosis.

The dissection is completed by mobilizing the bladder and taking down its lateral attachments (and in women, the round ligaments). Anterior and lateral mobilization of the bladder allows later creation of a duodenocystostomy without tension.

For nonuremic PTA and PAK recipients, once the vascular structures and the bladder are properly exposed, intravenous heparin (70 units/kg) is given to decrease the risk of clot formation during the vascular anastomosis. For uremic SPK recipients, heparin is not given because uremia itself acts as a sufficient anticoagulant.

The iliac arteries and veins are clamped. Before engraftment, a venotomy is made, followed by an arteriotomy cephalad to the venous anastomosis. For anatomic and technical reasons, the venotomy and arteriotomy should not overlap. The arteriotomy is usually made in the common iliac artery; any plaques or intestinal flaps are tacked at this time.

The donor pancreas is brought over to the operative field. The venous end-to-side anastomosis between the graft portal vein and the recipient common iliac vein is completed first, in a running fashion. The end-to-side arterial anastomosis between the donor Y graft and the iliac artery is completed in identical fashion. After the vascular anastomoses are done, the duodenum and head of the pancreas point toward the bladder, and the tail of the pancreas points toward the recipient's liver or stomach. The native ureter is left proximal and medial to the arterial anastomosis to prevent impingement on the venous graft anastomosis.

During the arterial anastomosis, 25 g of mannitol is given intravenously to minimize reperfusion edema. Limiting crystalloid fluid during the operation may also diminish the risk of edematous pancreatitis. Before clamp removal, it is important to check central venous pressure and blood pressure. We recommend maintaining a systolic blood pressure of 120–140 mm Hg and a central venous pressure of approximately 14 mm Hg to ensure adequate volume status and to establish good blood flow to the pancreas graft.

When the clamps are removed, bleeding sites are identified and controlled. In case of severe edematous pancreatitis, additional mannitol may be given intravenously. When the graft is revascularized, the duodenal stump is cultured for aerobic, anaerobic, and fungal organisms.

The donor duodenum-to-recipient bladder anastomosis (duodenocystostomy) can be either hand-sewn or done with the EEA (end-to-end anastomosis) stapler (United States Surgical Corporation, Norwalk, CT). For the hand-sewn anastomosis, a horizontal cystotomy on the posterior aspect of the bladder and a horizontal duodenotomy are made; a two-layer anastomosis is created between the bladder and the duodenum.

With the EEA stapler, different sizers are used to determine the size of the anastomosis. A curved EEA stapler with its anvil removed is inserted into the open, distal end of the duodenum. The rod is punched through the antimesenteric wall of the duodenum with the aid of the cautery opposite the papilla. The bladder is opened anteriorly to create the anastomosis under direct vision. The rod of the EEA stapler is punched through the posterosuperior wall of the bladder; the anvil is now placed on the stapler from within the bladder. The stapler is tightened, and the walls of the duodenum and bladder are

stretched over the ends of the stapler. The stapler is fired, creating a circular staple line. The EEA stapler is examined for intactness of both rings. To facilitate hemostasis, a continuous 4-0 absorbable suture is used to oversew the completed duodenocystostomy circular staple line from inside the bladder.

Once the hand-sewn or EEA stapler duodenocystostomy is completed, the open distal end of the duodenum is closed with a TA-55 stapler (Minnesota Mining and Manufacturing, St. Paul, MN). The staple line is inverted with interrupted Lempert sutures. If the EEA stapler is used, the anterior cystotomy is closed in three layers, after first irrigating the bladder with antifungal antibiotic solution.

Finally, the patient's abdomen is irrigated with 4 liters of antibiotic solution (e.g., cephalothin sodium, 1 g/liter of saline) and 4 liters of antifungal solution (e.g., amphotericin B, 10 mg/liter of sterile water). The midline abdominal incision is closed in layers. The Foley catheter previously inserted through the urethra is left in the bladder for 7–10 days after transplant.

Anesthetic Management

Induction

A pancreas transplant, particularly if combined with a renal transplant, can be a long (8–9 hours) and arduous procedure. For this reason, general anesthesia is always used. Anesthesia is usually induced intravenously with a small dose of narcotic (fentanyl or alfentanil) and either a barbiturate (thiopental) or etomidate.[43] Etomidate is preferred over thiopental in case of significant cardiac disease or autonomic neuropathy because it causes minimal cardiac depression and maintains autonomic tone. Adrenal suppression has been reported after etomidate administration[68]; however, transplant recipients receive relatively high doses of corticosteroids for immunosuppression. After the hypnotic agent is administered, a skeletal muscle relaxant that does not depend on renal excretion (e.g., vecuronium or atracurium) is administered. The patient is orotracheally intubated. Selick's maneuver should always be applied before intubation because patients may have gastroparesis but be unaware of it. If the patient has not been NPO (nothing by mouth for 8 hours), has a known history of gastroparesis, is obese, or has other risk factors for aspiration, rapid-sequence induction should be performed. These patients should receive a nonparticulate antacid, such as sodium citrate, preoperatively. In a review of our experience, a formal rapid-sequence induction was done for 44% of pancreas transplantations.[43]

Anesthesiologists should have available all the tools necessary for difficult intubation. If the preoperative physical examination or history identifies a difficult airway, a fiberoptic intubation should be done under topical sedation.

In some patients, a difficult airway may not be recognized until general anesthesia has been induced. If intubation has not occurred after several attempts, the recipient should be allowed to recover from general anesthesia and skeletal muscle relaxation and then given an awake fiberoptic intubation. Persisting with unsuccessful intubation attempts risks the loss of the airway due to edema, increases the chances for aspiration, and may permanently injure the laryngeal structures.

If mask ventilation cannot be performed, transtracheal jet ventilation or establishment of a surgical airway via a cricothyroidotomy may be necessary.[45] The laryngeal mask has been successfully used to ventilate patients who were impossible to ventilate by face mask, but it is imperative to establish a protected airway. A new technique uses the laryngeal mask as a conduit for fiberoptic bronchoscopy to facilitate endotracheal intubation.[69] Consequently, the laryngeal mask should be readily available.

Maintenance

After tracheal intubation, general anesthesia is maintained most often with isoflurane, a low-dose narcotic, and a skeletal muscle relaxant. Nitrous oxide may be used concurrently with isoflurane, allowing rapid adjustment of anesthetic depth during any period of potential hemodynamic instability (such as revascularization). The muscle relaxant chosen should take into account the degree of renal impairment. Drugs such as atracurium or vecuronium, which do not depend significantly on the kidney for elimination, should be chosen for patients with renal impairment. Most patients can then be extubated after surgery.[43]

In addition to the standard anesthetic agents and intravascular fluids, all patients receive broad-spectrum antibiotics throughout surgery and a low dose (70 units/kg) of intravenous heparin 5 minutes before clamping the major vessels. A variety of immunosuppressive agents (including intravenous prednisolone and azathioprine) are also administered. Cyclosporine may be given as well, but it is often begun after surgery. Most of these agents cause minimal changes in hemodynamics during surgery.[43] The monoclonal antibody OKT3 may sometimes be required for immunosuppression, but it has resulted in hypotension and pulmonary edema in some patients.[43, 70]

Monitoring

Standard monitoring includes pulse oximetry, noninvasive blood pressure, esophageal temperature probe, continuous electrocardiography, capnography, and end-tidal gas analysis. In addition, pancreas transplantation patients need central venous pressure monitoring to assess their intravascular volume status and provide central intravenous access for immunosuppressive drugs, inotropic support if required, blood sampling, and hyperalimentation for patients who cannot attain adequate enteric intake. In patients with a history of cardiac disease or autonomic instability, an arterial catheter is placed before anesthesia to allow rapid detection of changes in blood pressure (during anesthesia induction and other critical phases of surgery, such as clamping of vessels and reperfusion of the graft). Perfusion pressure and cardiac output must be normal during graft reperfusion. Reduced cardiac output can result in poor graft perfusion and subsequent graft thrombosis. Therefore, we recommend pulmonary artery thermodilution catheters in all patients with significant cardiac or pulmonary disease. Cardiac output and intravascular volume status can then be optimized before graft perfusion with intravenous fluids, vasodilators, or inotropes.[43] Similar aggressive monitoring and hemodynamic management reduces the incidence of graft thrombosis in diabetic patients undergoing peripheral vascular surgery.[71]

Metabolic Status

Monitoring metabolic status is important in pancreas or islet cell transplantation. Serum glucose

Table 10-8. Blood Glucose Level Protocol for Pancreas Recipients, University of Minnesota

Blood Glucose Level (g/dl)	Insulin Infusion Rate (units/hr)	5% Dextrose in Water Infusion Rate (ml/hr)
>350	3–5[a]	0
250–350	2[a]	0
150–250	2[a]	0
100–150	2	20
70–100	1–2	20–100
<70	0	100[b]

[a]Boluses of insulin (5–10 units) may be necessary to treat hyperglycemia.
[b]Boluses of dextrose (5–25 g 50% dextrose in water) may be necessary to treat hypoglycemia.

levels must be checked at least hourly throughout surgery and every half-hour if significant adjustments are made. Glucose determinations should be made every half-hour immediately after allograft reperfusion, both to optimize the glucose level during this critical period and to help determine if the islet cells are functioning.[43]

Pancreas recipients often become hyperglycemic from the metabolic response to stress, the reduced effect of insulin during anesthesia and surgery, the hyperglycemic effect of corticosteroids or cyclosporine, the metabolism of lactate from intravascular fluids, and administration of dextrose as a component of urine replacement after renal revascularization.[72–75] Glucagon from reperfused pancreas allografts may induce hyperglycemia.[76]

Experimentally, hyperglycemia induces islet cell dysfunction and structural lesions in rats, dogs, and cats.[77–79] Also, the growth and function of fetal islet cell isografts in mice is impaired with chronic hyperglycemia.[80] In humans, sustained remissions of type 1 diabetes have been achieved by preventing hyperglycemia.[81] It is therefore prudent to treat hyperglycemia during revascularization.

To prevent hyperglycemia, some authors suggest withholding dextrose-containing solutions throughout surgery unless the blood sugar level falls below 70 mg/dl. If the patient becomes hyperglycemic even when dextrose is withheld, insulin may be infused. Hypoglycemia (glucose <50 mg/dl) is common with this technique, however.[76] On the other hand, intraoperative ketosis has developed in diabetic patients who were not given dextrose solutions in spite of normal glucose levels.[82] Inadequate dextrose administration may also increase levels of free fatty acids.[82] Experimentally, free fatty acids increase the oxygen consumption of the myocardium and may precipitate cardiac arrhythmias.[83, 84] We therefore recommend continuous administration of dextrose during the operative procedure.

Table 10-8 describes the blood glucose protocol of the University of Minnesota. Concurrent with an insulin infusion, dextrose is begun at low infusion rates when the serum glucose level falls below 150 mg/dl; it is increased if the serum glucose stays below this level.[43] The optimal rate of glucose infusion during surgery has not been determined. In a review of anesthesia for patients with diabetes undergoing general surgery, however, a dextrose infusion rate of 5 g per hour (72 mg/kg/hour) for an average (70-kg) adult was recommended, along with insulin infusion, to prevent the accumulation of free fatty acids.[72]

We have found that metabolic acidosis (pH less than 7.30) is common in pancreas transplantation patients. In a review, it was noted during surgery 29% of the time.[43] An obvious reason may be inadequate systemic perfusion. Occasionally, if the patient has not received optimum diabetic care, metabolic acidosis may be due to ketosis. Most often, however, it is due to renal insufficiency or renal failure. Many patients have a chronic metabolic acidosis well compensated by hyperventilation in the awake state. It is helpful, therefore, to periodically monitor arterial or central venous blood gases along with the blood glucose levels. A small degree of acidosis may not require any treatment other than increasing minute ventilation. Significant acidosis (pH less than 7.30) despite mild hyperventilation may require sodium bicarbonate (1–2 mmol/kg).[43]

Hemodynamic status must be optimal before and after perfusion of the pancreas allograft. Reduction

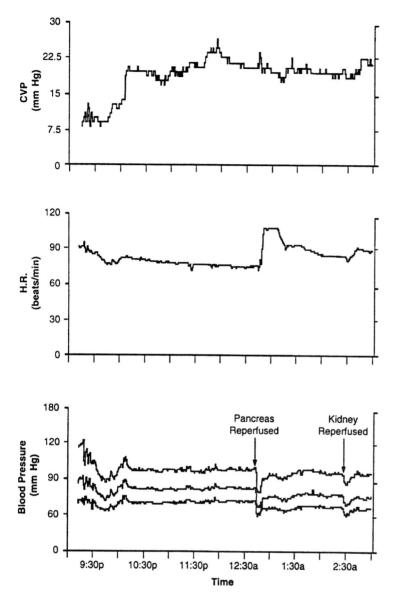

Figure 10-3. Real-time tracing of central venous pressure (CVP), heart rate (H.R.), and blood pressure (systolic, diastolic, mean) in a 36-year-old man with type 1 diabetes mellitus. Note the sudden hypotension with increase in heart rate during unclamping of the arterial and venous anastomoses to the transplanted pancreas graft. In addition to administration of packed red blood cells (pRBCs), dopamine infusion was started to improve blood pressure. The hemoglobin before unclamping was 7.5 g/dl. Transfusion of 2 units of pRBCs improved the hemoglobin to 10.0 g/dl. Later unclamping of renal vessels to the newly transplanted kidney also resulted in hypotension, but it was less severe than the hypotension during pancreas vessel unclamping. Serum electrolytes were within normal limits. Postoperatively, dopamine was tapered, and the patient was successfully extubated.

in graft flow and the release of thrombotic factors from the transplanted pancreas may result in vascular thrombosis.[85] Graft vessel thrombosis is one of the most common reasons for graft failure, causing up to 23% of graft losses.[43] Reperfusion of the pancreas allograft was demonstrated to cause a significant (more than 25%) fall in systolic blood pressure in 18% of recipients. This is probably due primarily to release of cardiovascular dilatory substances or ischemic by-products from the allograft into the circulation (Figure 10-3).[43]

To ensure adequate perfusion and prevent hypotension with reperfusion, patients must have an adequate circulating blood volume when the vascular clamps are released. In younger patients without significant cardiac disease, blood volume can be expanded with normal saline, colloids (e.g., 5% albumin or 6% hetastarch), or packed red blood cells until the central venous pressure is at least 14 mm Hg at the time of reperfusion. Hypotension, if it still occurs, may be treated with vasopressors, such as ephedrine, phenylephrine, or dopamine.[43]

Simple volume expansion before reperfusion may not be adequate for patients with serious cardiovascular disease. In such patients, central venous pressure may not be an accurate index of volume status and

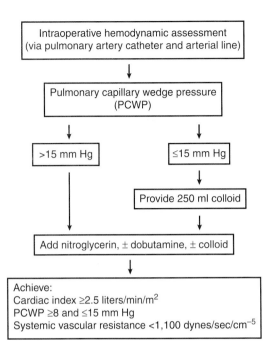

```
┌─────────────────────────────────────────┐
│   Intraoperative hemodynamic assessment  │
│ (via pulmonary artery catheter and arterial line) │
└─────────────────────────────────────────┘
                    ↓
┌─────────────────────────────────────────┐
│   Pulmonary capillary wedge pressure     │
│                (PCWP)                     │
└─────────────────────────────────────────┘
        ↓                      ↓
┌──────────────┐       ┌──────────────┐
│  >15 mm Hg   │       │  ≤15 mm Hg   │
└──────────────┘       └──────────────┘
        │                      ↓
        │              ┌──────────────────────┐
        │              │  Provide 250 ml colloid │
        │              └──────────────────────┘
        │                      ↓
┌─────────────────────────────────────────┐
│ Add nitroglycerin, ± dobutamine, ± colloid │
└─────────────────────────────────────────┘
                    ↓
┌─────────────────────────────────────────┐
│ Achieve:                                  │
│ Cardiac index ≥2.5 liters/min/m²          │
│ PCWP ≥8 and ≤15 mm Hg                      │
│ Systemic vascular resistance <1,100 dynes/sec/cm⁻⁵ │
└─────────────────────────────────────────┘
```

Figure 10-4. Protocol for maximizing cardiovascular performance of pancreas recipients. The increase in cardiac index with an optimal systemic vascular resistance ensures adequate graft perfusion on unclamping of vessels, which helps prevent graft thrombosis in the newly reperfused graft.

does not guarantee that cardiac output is adequate for perfusion. Thus, a pulmonary artery catheter should be used. An intraoperative protocol for maximizing cardiovascular performance is shown in Figure 10-4.[43, 71]

Edema of the pancreas allograft after reperfusion can also cause vascular insufficiency and graft thrombosis. Crystalloid fluid overload should be avoided. An adequate hemoglobin level (10 g/dl) must be ensured by including packed red blood cells during fluid expansion before reperfusion. Some authors recommend using only colloids (rather than crystalloids) concurrently with packed red blood cells to maintain colloid osmotic pressure and prevent graft edema.[85] Sodium mannitol (25 g) before reperfusion may also help decrease intracellular edema and prevent graft thrombosis.[43]

Postoperative Care

After surgery, most pancreas recipients can be extubated after reversal of neuromuscular blockade, provided they are alert and hemodynamically stable.

Serum glucose, electrolytes, hemoglobin, and arterial blood gases should be measured when patients arrive in the recovery room. Dextrose and insulin infusions should be maintained in the recovery room and adjusted based on the serum glucose and electrolyte levels.[43]

Patients continue on intravenous dextrose infusions after discharge from the recovery room until they begin taking adequate nutrition orally, usually within 10 days after surgery. However, patients with poor nutritional status at the time of surgery may benefit from intravenous hyperalimentation. An insulin infusion is continued if serum glucose levels remain above 150 mg/dl.[43]

Patients often require supplemental sodium bicarbonate to treat metabolic acidosis because bicarbonate is lost from the pancreatic secretions into the bladder and urine. For the same reason, adequate fluid intake is essential during the postoperative period because loss of pancreatic secretions in urine may result in dehydration.[86] These complications generally resolve with time, but occasionally, patients may require conversion to enteric drainage because of metabolic acidosis and dehydration.[87]

Pancreas graft function is assessed by tracking serum glucose and urinary amylase levels (Figure 10-5). Recipients are also examined for signs of acute graft dysfunction or rejection, such as abdominal pain, a fall in urinary amylase levels, or an increase in serum glucose levels. Open or transcystoscopic biopsies of pancreas may be done (Figure 10-6 and Color Plate 10-6). Patients can be discharged home when their wounds are healed and they are eating normally with no sign of infection or rejection.[43]

Postoperative Immunosuppression

Principles of immunosuppression for pancreas recipients are basically the same as those for other solid organ transplants. The amount of immunosuppression required, however, appears to be more than for liver, heart, or kidney transplants alone, based on a higher number of pancreas rejection episodes. Rejection is the most common cause of graft failure, accounting for up to 30% of graft losses in the first year after transplantation.

Combination immunotherapy has been the mainstay of clinical immunosuppression since the first pancreas transplantations in the 1960s. Since the early 1990s, convincing data have accumulated in support

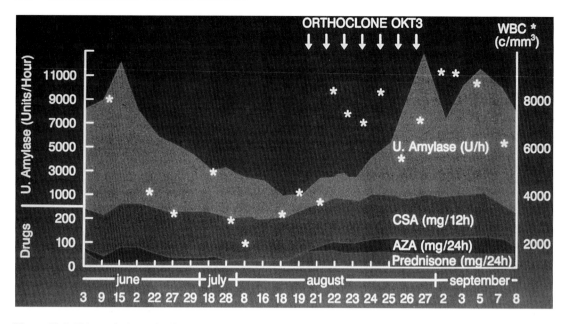

Figure 10-5. This graph shows the diminution of urinary amylase (U. amylase) in a pancreas transplantation patient undergoing rejection and recovery with increased immunosuppression (OKT3). (WBC = white blood cell count; CSA = cyclosporin A; AZA = azathioprine.) (Courtesy of RW Gruessner, personal communication, 1997.)

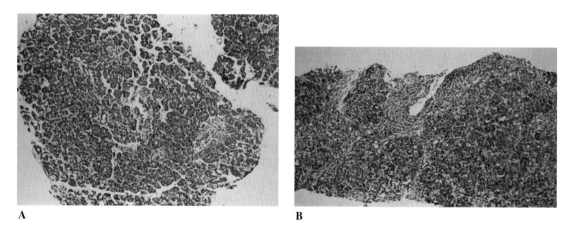

A   B

Figure 10-6. Biopsy specimens showing (**A**) a normal transplanted pancreas and (**B**) one undergoing rejection. Note the infiltration of white blood cells in the specimen undergoing rejection.

of quadruple immunosuppression for induction therapy. A randomized, multicenter Scandinavian study compared triple ($n = 28$) to quadruple ($n = 22$) induction in SPK recipients. It showed that quadruple-induction therapy with polyclonal antibody therapy not only postponed the first rejection episode but also reduced the number of rejection episodes.[88]

PTA recipients are more prone to (reversible) rejection episodes and graft loss from (irreversible) rejection than are SPK recipients. This finding has led to the following protocol at the University of Minnesota: anti–T-cell therapy is given to SPK recipients for 10 days and to PTA and PAK recipients for 14 days during induction. For PTA and

PAK recipients only, cyclosporine is given intravenously immediately after transplant (starting at 3 mg/kg). For SPK recipients, cyclosporine is not started until posttransplant day 5 to circumvent drug-related nephrotoxicity (so-called sequential immunosuppression). Thereafter, the dose is tapered to maintain cyclosporine blood levels at 200–300 ng/ml for the first 6 months, 150–200 ng/ml for the second 6 months, and 100–150 ng/ml thereafter. Azathioprine is started at 2.5 mg/kg per day and adjusted to maintain a whole white blood cell count greater than 3×10^9 cells/liter. The initial methylprednisolone dose is 2 mg/kg per day, which is tapered to 0.5 mg/kg per day by 1 month and 0.2 mg/kg per day by 1 year.[36]

More recently, FK506 (tacrolimus, Prograf) has replaced cyclosporine for maintenance therapy at some centers. In a multicenter study of 75 pancreas recipients at five institutions, FK506 was given for induction (quadruple) therapy and maintenance (triple) therapy. The median starting dose was 4 mg/kg per day; the median FK506 blood level was 12 ng/ml. The most common side effects were neurotoxicity (16%), nephrotoxicity (13%), and gastrointestinal toxicity (9%). New-onset diabetes mellitus requiring insulin therapy (a potential side effect of FK506) did not occur. The multicenter study showed a low rate of graft loss from rejection when FK506 was used for induction therapy, but the results were tarnished by three posttransplant lymphomas in the induction group. Further studies are necessary to analyze the long-term risk-benefit ratio of FK506.[89]

The advent of new immunosuppressive drugs (e.g., rapamycin, mycophenolate, mofetil) may further improve the safety and efficacy of immunosuppression.

Rejection

The features of rejection, with interstitial and vascular white blood cell infiltration, are similar in the pancreas as in other solid organs (see Figure 10-6 and Color Plate 10-6). In SPK recipients, the kidney is more susceptible to end-stage rejection than is the pancreas: 50% of all rejection episodes involve the kidney alone, 40% the kidney and pancreas, and 10% the pancreas alone.[90] In PTA recipients, the incidence of rejection is high, perhaps because a kidney graft is not there to serve as a surrogate marker

for pancreas rejection. Biochemical markers show exocrine dysfunction several days before endocrine dysfunction, but no markers are specific or sensitive enough to preclude confirmatory biopsies. In clinical practice, serial urinary amylase measurements are the standard laboratory test: A decrease in urinary amylase activity (relative hyperamylasuria) is the most common biochemical marker of acute rejection (see Figure 10-5). When urine amylase levels are monitored, antirejection treatment can begin before hyperglycemia occurs. Urine amylase measurements are simple and inexpensive and can be done in any laboratory. Pancreas graft biopsies can be done either percutaneously (under computed tomographic guidance) or transcystoscopically (using specially designed biopsy needles under intraoperative ultrasound guidance).[91] Pancreas rejection episodes are most frequent in the first year posttransplant. They are often steroid resistant but usually are reversible with anti–T-cell therapy.

Postoperative Complications

The major postoperative complications are listed in Table 10-9.

The most common causes of technical failure posttransplant are thrombosis (8%), infection (8%), and pancreatitis (6%). Other surgical complications include anastomotic leakage (2%) and bleeding (1%).

Table 10-9. Major Postoperative Complications of 73 Living Pancreas Donors

Complication	N (%)
Pancreatitis	1 (1.4)
Splenectomy*	1 (1.4)
Abdominal fluid collection	4 (5.5)
Atelectasis	25 (34)
Pleural effusion	25 (34)
Reoperation for sponge retrieval	1 (1.4)
Wound infection	1 (1.4)
Persistent ileus	1 (1.4)
Transient ischemic attack	1 (1.4)
Long-term chronic incisional pain	1 (1.4)
Mortality	0

*Required for splenic infarction.
Source: Reprinted with permission from KG Belani, DS Beebe, B Thyr, DER Sutherland. Perioperative outcome for living related pancreas donation. Am J Anesth 1996;23:121.

Table 10-10. Risk Factors for Vascular Thrombosis and Intra-Abdominal Infections after Pancreas Transplantation

Vascular thrombosis
    Donor age (≥45 yrs)
    Preservation time (≥24 hrs)
    Cause of death (cerebrovascular disease)
    Implantation site (left side)
    Type of arterial reconstruction (other than Y graft)
Intra-abdominal infection
    Donor age (≥45 yrs)
    Preservation time (≥24 hrs)
    Recipient age (≥50 yrs)

Vascular thrombosis and intra-abdominal infections are the leading cause of nonimmunologic, technical graft failure. A multivariate analysis has identified risk factors related to each complication (Table 10-10).[92, 93] Intra-abdominal infections are associated with decreased patient and graft survival. In a retrospective study of 445 pancreas recipients, the mortality of patients with intra-abdominal infections was 12%,[93] and only one-third of these maintained pancreas graft function. Graft pancreatitis can be the result of an intra-abdominal infection or cause an intra-abdominal infection.

The incidence of operative reintervention in the early posttransplant period (first 3 months) is high: 15–25% of recipients require at least one relaparotomy. Vascular graft thrombosis, infection, and pancreatitis are the most common causes for intervention. The early relaparotomy incidence is not significantly different by transplant category (primary versus retransplant) or by recipient category (SPK, PTA, or PAK). Posttransplant laparotomy

was associated with a decrease in patient survival at 1 year from 93% to 78% and a decrease in graft survival from 72% to 28%.[94]

Transplant pancreatectomy is necessary for 15–25% of pancreas recipients. The most frequent indications are vascular graft thrombosis, rejection, and infection. In absolute numbers, rejection is the most common cause of graft loss, yet only 25% of pancreas grafts require removal. In contrast, transplant pancreatectomy after graft thrombosis is virtually unavoidable.[95]

Outcome

For all type 1 diabetic SPK transplants ($n = 3,224$) using cadaver donors in the United States between October 1, 1987, and May 31, 1995, recipient survival rates were 91% at 1 year, 87% at 2 years, and 84% at 3 years (Figure 10-7). Pancreas graft survival rates were 77%, 75%, and 70% (Figure 10-8). The outcome is similar in European centers. Graft survival rates at 1 year were significantly higher for primary (versus retransplant) recipients and for SPK (versus PAK or PTA) recipients. The results of HLA, A, B, and DR mismatching on outcome were best for the 6-antigen match, followed by the 1-antigen mismatch. It was least favorable for two to six mismatches.[58]

Living-Related Donors

LRDs were first used for renal transplantations. Their increasing popularity in the United States is due to consistently high graft and patient survival rates and a shortage of cadaver donors. Transplan-

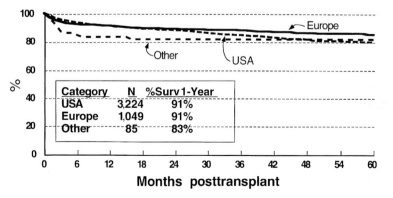

Figure 10-7. Actuarial worldwide survival of patients after a simultaneous pancreas and kidney transplantation using a cadaver donor from October 1, 1987, to May 31, 1995. (Surv = survival.) (Data courtesy of AC Gruessner, Scientific Director, International Pancreas Transplant Registry, Minneapolis, MN.)

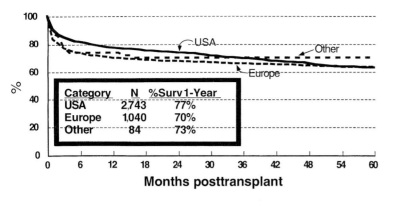

Figure 10-8. Actuarial worldwide graft survival using cadaver-donor pancreas grafts after simultaneous pancreas and kidney transplantation from October 1, 1987, to May 31, 1995. (Surv = survival.) (Data courtesy of AC Gruessner, Scientific Director, International Pancreas Transplant Registry, Minneapolis, MN.)

tation of the distal half of the pancreas from LRDs has also been successful. In general, LRD (versus cadaver) pancreas recipients have fewer episodes of rejection and may require less immunosuppression. This is an important consideration because rejection is the chief cause of pancreas graft loss.[96]

Nonetheless, LRD pancreas transplantations are not as popular as LRD renal transplantations for these reasons:

1. Because of the smaller number of pancreas transplantations done, there is no shortage of cadaver donors, as there is for renal transplantations.
2. Only a segment of the pancreas is transplanted; the vessels used for engraftment (splenic artery and vein) are small in diameter and short. Thus, LRD (versus cadaver) pancreas transplantations are more prone to arterial and venous thrombosis.[96]
3. For donors, there is a definite morbidity, although small, from hemipancreatectomy and postoperative complications (see Table 10-9).[97]
4. Donors must have adequate beta-cell reserve to tolerate the loss of half of their pancreas.[7, 96]

Four groups of patients are considered potential candidates for LRD pancreas transplantation at the University of Minnesota.

1. Recipients who are highly sensitized and have a low probability of receiving a cadaveric graft
2. Recipients who must avoid high-dose immunosuppression
3. Recipients with nondiabetic identical twins or with 6-antigen–matched siblings
4. Recipients who accept a higher technical failure rate as a tradeoff for less immunosuppression

In all cases, the donor, the recipient, and the entire family must understand all risks and benefits.[96]

Although anesthesia for LRD and cadaver pancreas recipients is the same, the surgical technique is slightly different. The splenic vein and artery are harvested en bloc, along with the distal pancreas from the donor (to provide circulation to this segment). These vessels are anastomosed to the external or common iliac arteries and veins. The cut end of the pancreas is then either sewn directly to the bladder or to a Roux-en-Y loop of jejunum (to provide exocrine drainage).[7]

At the University of Minnesota, before undergoing hemipancreatectomy, potential donors must meet these criteria to ensure that diabetes does not develop in the donor:

1. At the time of donation, donors must be at least 10 years older than the recipient's age at onset of diabetes (and the onset of diabetes in the recipient must have been at least 10 years before transplant).
2. For sibling donors, no family members other than the recipient can be diabetic. All potential donors must also undergo a thorough endocrine workup to determine their suitability for hemipancreatectomy.

In the early experience with LRDs, a few donors with normal glucose tolerance tests before transplantation did not remain normoglycemic after surgery. Since 1984, an intravenous glucose tolerance test is given to all potential donors. Only those with a postintravenous glucose-stimulatory, first-phase insulin level above the thirtieth percentile of the normal range are now accepted as donors. None of the donors who have met this criterion have become hyperglycemic after hemipancreatectomy.[96]

In general, living donors are healthy patients and easily tolerate standard anesthetic techniques. However, hemipancreatectomy is a major intra-abdominal operation. Blood transfusions are occasionally required. Atelectasis and pleural effusions are the most common serious perioperative complications, which increase the risk for postoperative hypoxemia and pneumonia. Vigorous pulmonary physiotherapy and optimal analgesia to ensure adequate coughing are essential.[97]

Islet Cell Transplantation

Islet cells alone can be transplanted with low morbidity. In 90% of all islet transplants between 1990 and 1994, the implantation site was the liver. Islets can be implanted either surgically or percutaneously (using radiologic intervention by injection into the portal venous system). As of December 1995, a total of 305 adult islet cell transplantations had been attempted at 36 different institutions.[98] In contrast to solid pancreas transplantations, long-term results of islet transplants for diabetes have remained disappointing, with only a few documented cases of insulin independence at 1 year.[98, 99] However, when a basal C-peptide level greater than 1 ng/ml at 1 month is used in place of the more rigorous end-point of insulin independence, success rates have gradually improved from 5% (1974–1984) to more than 25% (1985–1989) to 57% (1990–1994).[98] Thus, human islet cell transplantation is clearly feasible.

Three problems prevent stable engraftment of islets:

1. The number of viable islets may be insufficient to achieve insulin independence. Some reports from the International Islet Transplant Registry (administered by Bernard J. Hering, M.D., Department of Medicine, Justice-Liebig University of Giessen, Rodthol 6, D-35385 Giessen, Germany) suggest that more than 6,000 islet cells/kg of body weight must be transplanted to achieve insulin independence.[98] However, this number may be difficult to obtain with a single donor. Although the use of multiple donors has been tried, it exposes the patient to increased antigenicity and poses severe logistical problems.

2. Infused islet cells may elicit a greater immunologic response than when transplanted as part of a whole organ; at least initially, they require more immunosuppression.[99]

3. Experimental evidence suggests that metabolic exhaustion may occur, and then islet cell death, if hyperglycemia is present posttransplantation.[77, 80]

Other agents may also prove toxic to islet cells in the initial vulnerable period before complete engraftment occurs.

According to the Islet Registry, the following criteria must be met for successful engraftment of islet cells:

1. The yield from the donor must be more than 6,000 islet equivalents/kg body weight.
2. The purity of transplanted islets must be at least 50%.
3. The liver, not subcutaneous tissue or peritoneal cavity, must be the implantation site.
4. Preservation time must be less than 8 hours.
5. Anti–T-cell treatment must be used for induction therapy.

When all these criteria were met, the number of patients whose C-peptide level was greater than 1 ng/ml at 1 year was 27%, in contrast to zero when at least one of the criteria was not fulfilled.[98] The success rate is higher if a simultaneous kidney transplant is performed.

Technique

The technique for islet cell transplantation is as follows: Through a hockey-stick incision in the right or left lower abdominal quadrant (for retroperitoneal engraftment of the kidney), the peritoneum is opened. A loop of bowel with its mesenteric vessels is identified. A mesenteric vein is dissected free and ligated distally; a No. 18 angiocatheter is placed proximally. The portal vein pressure is measured; in the absence of portal hypertension, heparin is given intravenously (70 units/kg body weight). Purified cells or dispersed pancreatic tissue is transfused via the mesenteric vein into the liver. Portal vein pressure, measured throughout, should not exceed 33 cm H_2O at the end of the procedure.

For combined kidney-islet recipients, the islets are usually transplanted first. For systemically heparinized islet recipients, meticulous hemostasis is required during the subsequent kidney transplantation to avoid complications from bleeding. During the islet transplantation, coagulation parameters and platelet counts should be checked to avoid disseminated intravascular coagulation–related complications perioperatively.[99, 100]

Anesthetic Considerations

In a review of 26 patients undergoing an autologous islet cell transplant for pancreatitis, Farney and Sutherland found that the infusion of islet cells raised the mean portal pressure from 10 to 27 cm of H_2O. This rise was often accompanied by a fall in central venous pressure and systemic hypotension. By the end of surgery, however, portal pressures declined to near normal, and systemic hemodynamics improved.[100] Similar hemodynamic changes were seen in two islet cell allograft recipients with type 1 diabetes.[101]

To prevent hypotension, circulatory volume status must be adequate before islet cells are injected. Vasopressors and inotropic agents (such as phenylephrine, calcium, and epinephrine) must be ready; hypotension can be quite rapid and profound during islet cell infusion. Increasing injection time to at least 10–15 minutes decreases the likelihood of hypotension. Finally, communication between the anesthesiologist and surgeon is essential during islet cell infusion. The surgeon must be prepared to periodically and rapidly halt injection until hemodynamic stability has been achieved.[100, 101]

As with whole-organ transplantations, meticulous glucose control to avoid hyperglycemia is essential. Such control may be even more important in islet cell transplantations. It may be several days before islets are fully revascularized, leaving islet cells more susceptible to damage from hyperglycemia than are whole organs.[77, 80]

Conclusions

Pancreas transplantation promises to benefit many patients with IDDM, primarily by improving lifestyle but also by possibly preventing some of the secondary complications of disease. Results continue to improve with advances in surgical technique, perioperative care, and immunosuppression.

Islet ceil transplantation is also promising. It may become more common as problems with islet cell storage, purification, and immunogenicity are solved. Pancreas recipients may be difficult to care for perioperatively because of the severe nature of their underlying disease. By thoroughly evaluating them preoperatively and by optimizing their metabolic and hemodynamic status, however, anesthesi-ologists can help ensure graft function, prevent perioperative mortality, and minimize morbidity.

Acknowledgments

The authors acknowledge the editorial support of Mary E. Knatterud and the secretarial assistance of Nadine A. Hanson in the preparation of this chapter.

References

1. Hedon E. Griffe souscutanee du pancreas: ses resultats au pointe do one do la theoria du diabete pancreatique. Compt Rend Soc Biol 1892;44:678–730.
2. Ssobolew LW. Zur normalen und pathologischen morphologie der inneren secretion der bauchspercheldruse. Virchows Arch [A] 1902;168:91–128.
3. Banting FG. The history of insulin. Edinb Med J 1929;36:118.
4. Kelly WD, Lillehei RC, Merkel FK, et al. Allotransplantation of the pancreas and duodenum along with the kidney in diabetic nephropathy. Surgery 1967;61:827–837.
5. Sutherland DER. Pancreatic transplantation: state of the art. Transplant Proc 1992;24:762–766.
6. Gruessner RWG, Sutherland DER. Clinical Diagnosis in Pancreatic Allograft Rejection. In K Solez, LC Racusen, ME Billingham (eds), Pathology and Rejection Diagnosis in Solid Organ Transplantation. New York: Marcel Dekker 1996;455–499.
7. Bilous RW, Mauer SM, Sutherland DER, et al. The effects of pancreas transplantation on the glomerular structure of renal allografts in patients with insulin-dependent diabetes. N Engl J Med 1989;321:80–85.
8. Foster DW. Diabetes Mellitus. In KJ Isselbacher, E Braunwald, JD Wilson, et al. (eds), Harrison's Principles of Internal Medicine. New York: McGraw-Hill, 1994;1979–2000.
9. Melton LJ, Polumbo PJ, Chu CP. Incidence of diabetes mellitus by clinical type. Diabetes Care 1983;6:75–86.
10. Naji N, Silvers WK, Barker CF. Autoimmunity and type 1 (insulin-dependent) diabetes mellitus. Transplantation 1983;36:355–361.
11. Barbosa J, Bach F. Cell-mediated autoimmunity in type I diabetes. Diabetes Metab Rev 1987;3:981–1004.
12. Buschard K, Ropke C, Madsbad S. T lymphocyte subsets and activation in patients with newly diagnosed type I (insulin-dependent) diabetes: a prospective study. Diabetalogia 1983;25:247–251.
13. Irvine WJ, Gray RS, Steel JM. Islet Cell Antibody as a Marker for Early Stage Type I Diabetes Mellitus. In WJ Irvine (ed), Immunology of Diabetes. Edinburgh: Teviot Scientific Publications, 1980;117–154.
14. Sutherland DER, Gruessner RW, Dunn DL, et al. Pancreas transplants from living-related donors. Transplant Proc 1994;26:443–445.

15. Kitabachi AE, Fischer JN, Murphy MB, Rumbak MJ. Diabetic Ketoacidosis and the Hyperglycemic Hyperosmolar Nonketotic State. In CR Kahn, GE Weir (eds), Joslin's Diabetes Mellitus (13th ed). Philadelphia: Lea & Febiger, 1994;748–794.

16. Banting FG, Best C. The internal secretion of the pancreas. J Lab Clin Med 1922;7:251–266.

17. DCCT Research Group. Diabetes control and complications trial (DCCT): update. Diabetes Care 1993;13:427–433.

18. Singer DE, Coley CM, Samet JH, Nathan DM. Tests of glycemia in diabetes mellitus: their use in establishing a diagnosis and treatment. Ann Int Med 1989;100:125–137.

19. DCCT Research Group. The effect of intensive treatment of diabetes on the development and progression of long-term complications in insulin-dependent diabetes mellitus. N Engl J Med 1993;329:977–986.

20. Pirart J. Diabetes mellitus and its degenerative complications: a prospective study of 4,400 patients observed between 1947 and 1973. Diabetes Care 1978;1: 168–188.

21. King GL, Banskota NK. Mechanism of Diabetic Microvascular Complications. In CR Kahn, GC Weir (eds), Joslin's Diabetes Mellitus (13th ed). Philadelphia: Lea & Febiger, 1994;631–647.

22. Brownlee M. Glycosylation products as toxic mediators of diabetic complications. Ann Rev Med 1991;42: 159–166.

23. Ewing DJ, Campbell IW, Clarke BF. Mortality in diabetic autonomic neuropathy. Lancet 1976;1:601–603.

24. Christlieb AR, Krowlewski AS, Warren JH. Hypertension. In CR Kahn, GC Winer (eds), Joslin's Diabetes Mellitus (13th ed). Philadelphia: Lea & Febiger, 1994;820–823.

25. Krolewski AS, Barzilay J, Warram JH, et al. Risk of early onset proliferative retinopathy in IDDM is closely related to cardiovascular autonomic neuropathy. Diabetes 1992;41:430–435.

26. Crall FV, Roberts WC. The extramural and intramural coronary arteries in juvenile diabetes mellitus: analysis of nine necropsy patients aged 19 to 38 years with onset of diabetes before age 15 years. Am J Med 1978;64:221–230.

27. Nesto RW, Watson FS, Kowalchuk GJ, et al. Silent myocardial ischemia and infarction in diabetics with peripheral vascular diseases: assessment by dipyridamole thallium-201 scintigraphy. Am Heart J 1990;120:107–137.

28. Zoneraich S, Silverman G, Zoneraich O. Primary myocardial disease, diabetes mellitus and small vessel disease. Am Heart J 1980;10:754–755.

29. Ledet T. Histological and biochemical changes in the coronary arteries of old diabetic patients. Diabetologia 1968;70:268–272.

30. Vered Z, Battler A, Segal P, et al. Exercise-induced left ventricular dysfunction in young men with asymptomatic diabetes mellitus (diabetic cardiopathy). Am J Cardiol 1984;54:633–637.

31. Shapiro LM, Leatherdale BA, Mackinnon J, Fletch RF. Left ventricular function in diabetes mellitus. II. Relation between clinical features and left ventricular function. Brit Heart J 1981;45:129–132.

32. Lewis E, Unsicker L, Bain R, et al. The effect of angiotensin-converting enzyme inhibition on diabetic nephropathy. New Engl J Med 1993;329:1456–1462.

33. Zehrer CL, Gross CR. Quality of life of pancreas transplant recipients. Diabetologia 1991;34:S145–S149.

34. Kennedy WR, Navarro X, Goetz FC, et al. Effects of pancreatic transplantation on diabetic neuropathy. New Engl J Med 1990;322:103–117.

35. Navarro X, Kennedy WR, Sutherland DER. Autonomic neuropathy and survival in diabetes mellitus: effects of pancreas transplantation. Diabetologia 1991;34(Suppl 1):S108–S112.

36. Katz HH, Nguyen TT, Velosa JA, et al. Effects of systemic delivery of insulin on plasma lipids and lipoprotein concentrations in pancreas transplant recipients. Mayo Clin Proc 1994;69:231–236.

37. Weinrauch L, D'Elia EA, Healy RW, et al. Asymptomatic coronary artery disease: angiographic assessment of diabetics evaluated for renal transplantation. Circulation 1978;58:1184–1190.

38. Lemmers MJ, Barry JM. Major role for arterial disease in morbidity and mortality after kidney transplantation in diabetic recipients. Diabetes Care 1991;14:295–301.

39. Morrow CE, Schwartz JS, Sutherland DER, et al. Predictive value of thallium stress testing for coronary and cardiovascular events in uremic patients before renal transplantation. Am J Surg 1983;146:331–335.

40. Boudreau RJ, Strony JT, du Cret RP, et al. Perfusion thallium imaging of type I diabetic patients with end-stage renal disease: comparison of oral and intravenous dipyridamole. Radiology 1990;175:120–135.

41. Gruessner RWG, Dunn DL, Gruessner AC, et al. Recipient risk factors have an impact on technical failure and patient and graft survival rates in bladder-drained pancreas transplants. Transplantation 1994;57:1–7.

42. D'Alessandro AM, Sollinger HW, Hoffman RM, et al. Experience with Belzer UW cold storage solution in simultaneous pancreas-kidney transplantation. Transplant Proc 1990;22:532–534.

43. Beebe DS, Belani KG, Yoo M, et al. Pancreas transplantation: anesthetic considerations based upon a one year review. Am J Anesth 1995;22:237–243.

44. Hogan K, Rusy D, Springman SR. Difficult laryngoscopy and diabetes mellitus. Anesth Analg 1988;67:1162–1165.

45. Benumof JL. Management of the difficult adult airway with special emphasis on awake tracheal intubation. Anesthesiology 1991;75:1087–1110.

46. Makita Z, Bucala R, Rayfield EJ, et al. Reactive glycosylation end-products in diabetic uraemia and treatment of renal failure. Lancet 1994;343:1519–1522.

47. Page M, Watkins PJ. Cardiorespiratory arrest and diabetic autonomic neuropathy. Lancet 1978;1:146.

48. Burgos LG, Ebert TJ, Asiddao C, et al. Increased intraoperative cardiovascular morbidity in diabetics with autonomic neuropathy. Anesthesiology 1989;70:591–597.

49. Triantafillou AN, Tsueda K, Berg J, et al. Refractory bradycardia after reversal of muscle relaxant in a diabetic with vagal neuropathy. Anesth Analg 1986;65:1237–1241.

50. Ciccarelli LL, Ford CM, Tsueda K. Autonomic neuropathy in a diabetic patient with renal failure. Anesthesiology 1986;64:283–287.

51. Ishihara H, Singh H, Giesecke AH. Relationship between diabetic autonomic neuropathy and gastric contents. Anesth Analg 1994;78:943–947.

52. Walton JD, Farman JV. Suxamethonium hyperkalemia in uremic neuropathy. Anaesthesia 1973;28:666–668.

53. Navalgund AA, Jahr JS, Gieraerts R, et al. Multiple nerve palsies after anesthesia and surgery. Anesth Analg 1988;67:1002–1004.

54. Kreisberg RA. Diabetic ketoacidosis: new concepts and trends in pathogenesis and treatment. Ann Int Med 1978;88:681–695.

55. Sollinger HW, Cook K, Kamps D. Clinical and experimental experience with pancreaticocystostomy for exocrine pancreatic drainage in pancreas transplantation. Transplant Proc 1984;16:749–751.

56. Dubernard JM, Traeger J, Neyra P, et al. A new method of preparation of segmental pancreatic grafts for transplantation: trials in dogs and in man. Surgery 1978;84:633–640.

57. Tyden G, Tibell A, Bolinder J, et al. Pancreatic transplantation with enteric exocrine diversion: experience with 120 cases. Transplant Proc 1992;24:771–773.

58. Gruessner A, Sutherland DER. Pancreas Transplant Results in the United Network for Organ Sharing (UNOS). United States of America (USA) Registry Compared with Non-USA Data in the International Registry. In PI Terasaki, JM Cecka (eds), Clinical Transplants. Los Angeles: UCLA Tissue Typing Laboratory, 1994;47–68.

59. Gliedman ML, Gold M, Whittaker J, et al. Clinical segmental pancreatic transplantation with ureter-pancreatic duct anastomosis for exocrine drainage. Surgery 1973;74:171–180.

60. Prieto M, Sutherland DER, Fernandez-Cruz L, et al. Experimental and clinical experience with urine amylase monitoring for early diagnosis of rejection in pancreas transplantation. Transplantation 1987;43:71–79.

61. Gruessner RWG, Nakhleh R, Tzardis P, et al. Rejection patterns after simultaneous pancreaticoduodenal-kidney transplants in pigs. Transplantation 1994;57:756–760.

62. Prieto M, Sutherland DER, Goetz FC, et al. Pancreas transplant results according to technique of duct management: bladder versus enteric drainage. Surgery 1987;102:680–691.

63. Gruessner RWG, Dunn DL, Tzardis PJ, et al. Simultaneous pancreas and kidney transplants versus single kidney transplants and previous kidney transplants in uremic patients and single pancreas transplants in nonuremic diabetic patients: comparison of rejection, morbidity and long-term outcome. Transplant Proc 1990;22:622–623.

64. Rosenlof LK, Earnhardt RC, Pruett TL, et al. Pancreas transplantation: an initial experience with systemic and portal drainage of pancreatic allografts. Ann Surg 1992;215:586–595.

65. Gruessner RWG, Sutherland DER. Pancreas transplantation. Part II—the recipient operation. Surgical Rounds 1994;17:383–391.

66. Marsh CL, Perkins JD, Sutherland DER, et al. Combined hepatic and pancreaticoduodenal procurement for transplantation. Surg Gynecol Obstet 1989;168: 254–258.

67. Gruessner RWG, Sutherland DER. Pancreas transplantation. Part I—The donor operation. Surgical Rounds 1994;17:311–324.

68. Wagner RL, White PF, Kan PB, et al. Inhibition of adrenal steroidogenesis by the anesthetic etomidate. N Engl J Med 1984;310:1415–1421.

69. Benumof JL. Use of the laryngeal mask airway to facilitate fiberoptic-aided tracheal intubation. Anesth Analg 1992;74:313–315.

70. Roth S, Kupferberg JP. Adverse responses following intraoperative administration of Orthoclone OKT3. Anesth Analg 1989;69:822–825.

71. Berlauk JF, Abrams JH, Gilmour IJ, et al. Preoperative optimization of cardiovascular hemodynamics improves outcome in peripheral vascular surgery: a prospective, randomized clinical trial. Ann Surg 1991;214:289–299.

72. Hirsch IB, McGill JB, Cryer PE, et al. Perioperative management of surgical patients with diabetes mellitus. Anesthesiology 1991;74:346–359.

73. Weissman C. The metabolic response to stress: an overview and update. Anesthesiology 1990;73:308–327.

74. Baumgartner D, Schlumpf R, Largiader F. Cyclosporine A interferes with postoperative blood glucose control after clinical pancreas transplantation. Transplant Proc 1987;19:4009–4010.

75. Gliedman ML, Tellis V, Soberman R, et al. The clinical use of steroids in pancreatic transplantation. Transplant Proc 1975;7:93–98.

76. Perkins JD, Fromme GA, Narr BJ, et al. Pancreas transplantation at Mayo. II. Operative and perioperative management. Mayo Clin Proc 1990;65:483–495.

77. Clark A, Bown E, King T, et al. Islet changes induced by hyperglycemia in rats: effect of insulin or chlorpropamide therapy. Diabetes 1982;31:319–325.

78. Imamura T, Koffler M, Helderman JH, et al. Severe diabetes induced in subtotally depancreatized dogs by sustained hyperglycemia. Diabetes 1988;37:600–609.

79. Dohan FC, Lukens FDW. Lesions of the pancreatic islets produced in cats by administration of glucose. Science 1947;105:183.

80. Cutherbertson RA, Koulmanda M, Mandel TE. Detri-

mental effect of chronic diabetes on growth and function of fetal islet isografts in mice. Transplantation 1988;46:650–654.

81. Mirouze J, Selam JL, Pham TC, et al. Sustained insulin-induced remissions of juvenile diabetes by means of an external artificial pancreas. Diabetologia 1978;14:223–227.

82. Alberti KGMM, Thomas DJB. The management of diabetes during surgery. Br J Anaesth 1979;51:693–710.

83. Challoner DR, Steinberg D. Effect of free fatty acid on the oxygen consumption of perfused rat heart. Am J Physiol 1966;210:280–286.

84. Tansey MJ, Opie LH. Relation between plasma free fatty acids and arrhythmias within the first twelve hours of acute myocardial infarction. Lancet 1983;2:419–421.

85. Nader A, Büsing M, Blumenstock I, et al. Coagulation disorders after reperfusion of pancreatic allografts. Transplant Proc 1993;25:1174–1175.

86. Ketel B, Elkhammas EA, Tesi RJ, et al. Metabolic complications in combined kidney/pancreas transplantation. Transplant Proceed 1992;24:774–775.

87. Burke GW, Gruessner RW, Dunn DL, et al. Conversion of whole pancreaticoduodenal transplants from bladder to enteric drainage for metabolic acidosis or dysuria. Transplant Proceed 1990;22:651–652.

88. Wadstrøm J, Brekke B, Wrammer L, et al. Triple versus quadruple induction immunosuppression in pancreas transplantation. Trans Proc 1995;27:1317–1318.

89. Gruessner RW, Burke GW, Stratta R, et al. A multicenter analysis of the first experience with FK506 for induction and rescue therapy after pancreas transplantation. Transplantation 1996;61:261–273.

90. Gruessner RW, Dunn DL, Tzardis PJ, et al. Simultaneous pancreas and kidney transplants versus single kidney transplants and previous kidney transplants in uremic patients and single pancreas transplants in non-uremic diabetic patients: comparison of rejection, morbidity and long-term outcome. Transplant Proc 1990;22:622–623.

91. Jones JW, Nakkleh RE, Casanova D, et al. Cystoscopic transduodenal pancreas biopsy: a new needle. Transplant Proc 1994;26:527–528.

92. Troppmann C, Gruessner AC, Benedetti E, et al. Vascular graft thrombosis after pancreas transplantation: uni- and multivariate surgical and nonsurgical risk factor analysis. J Am Coll Surg 1996;182:285–316.

93. Benedetti E, Gruessner AC, Troppmann C, et al. Intra-abdominal fungal infections after pancreatic transplantation: incidence, treatment, and outcome. J Am Coll Surg 1996;183:307–316.

94. Troppman C, Dunn DL, Najarian JS, et al. Operative re-intervention following early complications after pancreas transplantation. Trans Proc 1994;26:454.

95. Troppman C, Gruessner RW, Dunn DL, et al. Is transplant pancreatectomy after graft failure necessary? Transplant Proc 1994;26:445.

96. Gruessner RW, Najarian JS, Gruessner AC, Sutherland DER. Pancreas Transplants from Living Related Donors. In JL Touraine (ed), Organ Shortage: The Solutions. Dordrecht, the Netherlands: Kluwer Academic Publishers, 1995;77–83.

97. Belani KG, Beebe DS, Thyr B, Sutherland DER. Perioperative outcome for living related pancreas donation. Am J Anesthesiol 1996;23:119–123.

98. Hering BJ, Geier C, Schultz AO, et al. International Islet Transplant Registry. Newsletter No. 7 1996;6:1–20.

99. Gores PF, Najarian JS, Stephanian E, et al. Insulin independence in type I diabetes after transplantation of unpurified islets from a single donor using 15-deoxyspergualin. Lancet 1993;341:19–21.

100. Farney AC, Sutherland DER. Islet Autotransplantation. In C Ricordi (ed), Pancreatic Islet Cell Transplantation. Austin, TX: RG Landes, 1992;291–312.

101. Torres LE, Traverso LW, Sohn YZ. Intraoperative hemodynamic changes in patients undergoing mixed-cell intraportal autotransplantation of pancreatic tissue. Anesthesiology 1980;53:427–429.

Chapter 11
Renal Transplantation

Carol Stockall, Angel J. Amante, Barry D. Kahan,
J. Jastrzebski, and Paul A. Keown

Chapter Plan

History of Renal Transplantation

Since the 1960s, kidney transplantation has emerged as the preferred treatment for patients with end-stage renal disease (ESRD). Although Carrel[1] and Guthrie[2] described the requisite vascular anastomotic techniques for transplantation in the early 1900s, they recognized that host "biological factors" caused long-term failure of transplanted organs. In 1905, Floresco[3] described the present surgical technique of implantation in the recipient iliac fossa site with ureteroneocystostomy. However, fear of anastomotic disruption of a ureteroureterostomy or a ureteroneocystostomy led to a prolonged period during which ureters were implanted cutaneously. The first transplantation procedure in humans was performed in 1906 by Jaboulay,[4] who anastomosed the brachial vessels of a human recipient with acute nephritis to pig kidneys, each of which functioned for approximately 1 hour.

For several decades, clinical transplantation was attempted with minimal success until 1955, when Hufnagel, Landsteiner, and Hume connected a human pediatric cadaver donor kidney to the brachial vessels of a young woman dying of acute renal failure. The graft initially functioned but had to be removed after 2 days. Hume et al. then used anastomoses to the femoral vessels and cutaneous ureterostomies in a series of cadaver donor kidney transplantations.[5, 6] Although none of the kidneys exhibited long-term function, a few grafts displayed significant diuresis for more than a month. The procedure described by Lawler,[7] in which a renal transplant was placed orthotopically, was probably a technical failure. When the graft was removed at 7 months, it was the size of a walnut. The retroperitoneal technique was rediscovered by Dubost and Kuss and then used by Murray et al.[8] to perform transplants between monozygotic twins that resulted in excellent long-term graft survival rates.

Between 1959 and 1964, Murray et al.[9] and Hamburger et al.[10] used total body irradiation as a cytotoxic immunosuppressive regimen for mismatched grafts. Franksson[11] depleted lymphocytes by thoracic duct drainage, and Starzl[12] performed splenectomy or thymectomy to debulk the reticulo-endothelial system surgically. However, the nonselective effects of these approaches produced a high incidence of serious infections that limited patient and graft survival.

The chemical era of immunosuppression began with the findings of Schwartz and Dameshek,[13] which led to the introduction of azathioprine by Hitchings and Elion in 1962.[14] Shortly thereafter, Woodruff and Anderson[15] introduced antilymphocyte sera, and Starzl et al.[16] used it in clinical transplantation. By 1980, it was recognized that the most effective form of immunosuppression would inhibit T cells selectively. Cyclosporine, discovered by Borel et al.[17] and first used by Calne et al.,[18] was the first chemical agent of this type, and the murine monoclonal antibody OKT3 was the first such biological agent.

These improvements in immunosuppressive therapy increased the 2-year survival rates of cadaveric and live-donor renal transplants to 80% and 90%, respectively, and the overall patient survival rate to 95%. It is difficult to compare the morbidity and mortality figures for patients who remain on chronic dialysis with those of patients who receive transplants because there is some bias toward selecting younger and healthier patients for transplantation. However, a cross-sectional study of more than 68,000 patients followed for 1 calendar year showed that transplant recipients had a lower mortality rate than did dialysis patients.[19] Because the procedure is economical and improves the quality of life for patients, the number of kidney transplantations performed in the United States increased from 4,500 in 1975 to 11,390 in 1995.[20] A study of a cohort of 226 transplant recipients found that patients whose transplantation procedures were successful reported an improved level of general health. Of the patients with functioning transplants, 64% were capable of working part- or full-time; only 32% of the patients with failed transplants were so classified. If the patients with failed transplants successfully received new transplants, however, the percentage of those who could work rose to 73%.[21]

Renal transplantation is now recognized as the optimal therapy for almost all patients with chronic renal failure, achieving greater long-term survival with superior quality of life and lower maintenance cost than any other therapy. More than 20,000 kidney transplantations per year are now performed worldwide. Despite these advantages, transplantation is not fully exploited as a therapeutic option in most countries: Only 5–27% of patients with renal disease in Japan, Eastern Europe, Germany, and the United States are maintained by this treatment. Only in Canada, Denmark, Australia, and the United Kingdom are more patients (45–62%) maintained with a functioning transplant than with any form of dialysis therapy. Although these transplantation rates parallel the relative availability of organs from both cadaver and living donor sources, they also reflect the inherent treatment bias of many countries. In these countries, dialysis is preferred as the initial form of therapy, and patients are selected from this pool for subsequent transplantation. This practice is gradually changing as patients, physicians, and payers realize the social and economic costs of this approach and insist on transplantation as the primary treatment.

Chronic Renal Failure

Epidemiology and Etiology

Since the late 1980s, an alarming growth in the problem of ESRD in industrialized countries has occurred. The number of new patients accepted for renal replacement therapy has risen at a compound rate of 5–10% per year and ranges between 60 and 220 patients per million population, depending on the country.[22, 23] In parallel, the number of patients receiving therapy has almost doubled, reaching 420 patients per million in the United Kingdom, 570 in Canada, 807 in the United States, and 990 in Japan.[22] Men slightly outnumber women patients in most countries. Older people account for an increasing proportion of patients and exhibit a greater frequency of comorbid disorders, including ischemic heart disease, cerebrovascular disease, and chronic pulmonary disease. Patients older than age 65 years now have an incidence of disease four times that of the overall population, and the fastest growing subgroup is among those older than 75 years.[22, 23]

The major causes of chronic renal failure are shown in Table 11-1. Diabetes mellitus is the principal cause of renal insufficiency, accounting for 20–30% of new cases. Renal failure occurs in up to 40% of patients with type 1 (juvenile-onset) diabetes mellitus with a mean interval of 15–18 years from diagnosis. Although the incidence of renal failure is lower in type 2 (adult-onset) diabetes, this probably reflects the high cardiac mortality before the development of ESRD. Glomerulosclerosis is generally accompanied by retinopathy, neuropathy, and coronary and peripheral vascular disease and has a poor prognosis for long-term survival.[24–26] Primary oxalosis is a rare hereditary disorder of oxalate metabolism that results in renal failure, vascular disease, and bone marrow dysfunction.[27] Patients present clinically in the first three decades with recurrent calculi and hyperoxaluria. Progressive oxalate accumulation in the kidney results in interstitial fibrosis, thus decreasing oxalate clearance and increasing deposition in the blood vessels and bone marrow. Other metabolic disorders, including cystinosis, Fabry's disease, and amyloidosis, may also lead to renal failure, although the incidence of these diseases is low.

Glomerulonephritis is the second most prevalent etiology, responsible for approximately 20% of patients who require renal replacement therapy. Idiopathic progressive forms include membranous and membranoproliferative disease, focal glomerulosclerosis, postinfectious glomerulonephritis, and immunoglobulin (Ig) A nephropathy. Secondary glomerulonephritis may occur in

Table 11-1. Major Causes of Chronic Renal Failure

Metabolic disorders
    Diabetes mellitus
    Primary oxalosis
    Cystinosis
    Fabry's disease
    Amyloidosis
Glomerulonephritis
    Primary
        Membranous or membranoproliferative disease
        Focal glomerulosclerosis
        Postinfectious glomerulonephritis
        Immunoglobulin A nephropathy
    Secondary
        Systemic lupus erythematosus
        Polyarteritis nodosum
        Wegener's granulomatosis
Chronic tubulointerstitial disease
    Analgesic nephropathy
    Chronic pyelonephritis
    Vesicoureteric reflux
    Renal calculi
    Urethral valves
    Neurogenic bladder
Hereditary renal disease
    Alport's disease
    Polycystic disease
    Medullary cystic disease
Arterial disease
    Atherosclerosis
    Renal thromboembolism
    Systemic inflammatory disease
    Malignant hypertension

metabolic disorders and certain forms of collagen vascular disease, including systemic lupus erythematosus, polyarteritis nodosum, and Wegener's granulomatosis.[28]

Chronic tubulointerstitial disease is distinguished from the preceding disorders by mild proteinuria of the tubular variety, loss of concentrating ability, and natriuresis or kaliuresis.[29] Analgesic nephropathy is now rare after the withdrawal of phenacetin, but it is occasionally encountered in patients taking large amounts of analgesics for rheumatic diseases.[30] Chronic pyelonephritis is characterized by a history of recurrent bacterial infections and often accompanies structural abnormalities of the genitourinary tract. Sterile vesicoureteric reflux may produce a similar renal injury, with small, unequal kidneys, cortical scarring, and calyceal deformities. Differentiation is not always easy. Complicating the confusion is that reflux may resolve spontaneously during childhood or adult life, but the deterioration in renal function may progress due to the development of secondary IgM nephropathy.[31] Renal calculi, urethral valves, and neurogenic bladder dysfunction may predispose to obstruction and infection with secondary tubulointerstitial disease.

Hereditary renal disease presents in three typical forms. Alport's disease is a familial disorder associated with a structural abnormality of the glomerular basement membrane that results in glomerulosclerosis and interstitial fibrosis. Transmission is predominantly X-linked, with an increased penetrance in men.[32] Hematuria and proteinuria may be associated with high-tone neurosensory deafness and ocular defects. Renal insufficiency develops in the second to fourth decade in men and in the third to sixth decade in women. Adult polycystic disease is an autosomal dominant trait, though recessive and sporadic forms have been described. Cysts of varying size distort the normal renal architecture, and the kidneys may be grossly enlarged, leading to renal failure in the fourth to sixth decade of life. Medullary cystic disease, a form of microcystic disease of the kidney, is less common but more rapidly destructive, frequently causing renal failure in the first to second decade of life.[33–35]

Arterial disease of the kidney may present with a wide variety of symptoms, ranging from atherosclerotic narrowing to renal thromboembolism, microvascular injury associated with systemic inflammatory disease, or malignant hypertension. Disease of the major renal vessels is uncommon in younger patients but increases slowly with age, reaching 10–15% by age 65 years. The cause of renal disease remains unknown in 7–15% of cases.[22, 23]

Complications of Chronic Renal Failure

The metabolic consequences of renal failure contribute to dysfunction in many organ systems, resulting in neurologic disorders and cognitive impairment, anemia, accelerated cardiovascular disease, metabolic bone disease, gastrointestinal dysfunction, and malnutrition. Acute and potentially life-threatening conditions, such as hyperkalemia, metabolic acidosis, pulmonary edema, pericarditis, encephalopathy, and bleeding diatheses, may be superimposed on this clinical tableau. Finally, the kidney is the principal route of elimination of many therapeutic agents, and drug toxicity may readily occur unless dosage or timing of administration is adjusted according to the glomerular filtration rate.[36]

Neuropsychiatric Disease

Organic mental disorders are common in patients with chronic renal failure. They range from subtle disorders of cognitive impairment to clinical depression, anxiety, psychoses, and suicidal behavior.[37] Many variants of these present as noncompliance with therapy, leading to dietary indiscretion, missed treatments, and medication avoidance. Uremic encephalopathy may commence with lassitude and confusion and proceed to stupor with fasciculation, asterixis, and seizures. The electroencephalogram may be grossly abnormal, with a frequency less than 5 Hz. Peripheral uremic neuropathy is present to some degree in approximately 65% of patients receiving dialysis. It may occur in two clinical forms: as a symmetric combined sensorimotor polyneuropathy or as an isolated mononeuritis.[38] The former is the more severe, involving both lower and upper limbs in a glove-and-stocking distribution. It may proceed to paralysis, confining the patient to a wheelchair or bed. Both forms have been attributed to uremic toxins in the middle molecular weight range of 500–2,500 daltons, which are poorly cleared by dialysis. Finally, dialysis dementia is a particularly severe and progressive complication leading to dysarthria, apraxia, personality changes, seizures, and death, usually within 6 months of onset. Aluminum toxicity has been implicated in many cases of this disease, although other etiologies are certainly involved.[39]

Anemia

The anemia of chronic renal failure is characterized by diminished red cell production, hyperfragility, and shortened survival.[40] Hemoglobin levels may fall to less than 60 g/liter, producing profound fatigue, weakness, malaise, and cognitive impairment. Many factors contribute to the genesis of this anemia, including malnutrition, chronic disease, bone marrow fibrosis (particularly in patients with hyperparathyroidism), blood loss, and the presence of uremic toxins. The principal cause, however, is deficiency of the glycoprotein erythropoietin secreted by specialized cells in the renal interstitial space.[41] Precise regulation of red cell production in the marrow, controlled by oxygen delivery to renal tissue sensors, is lost in parallel with the decrease in functioning glomerular mass. Recombinant human erythropoietin 50–100 units/kg administered parenterally two to three times per week produces a significant rise in hemoglobin after 4–8 weeks of therapy.[40] There is no consensus regarding the ideal target hemoglobin, although a range of 105–115 g/liter is accepted in most renal centers. Correction of anemia (with the accompanying improvement in oxygen transport) improves energy level, decreases left ventricular mass, reduces the symptoms of angina and congestive heart failure, and increases cognitive function and quality of life. Erythropoietin also increases the platelet count and improves platelet function, thereby reducing blood loss. Despite the obvious benefits, this therapy carries certain risks. The rise in hemoglobin is accompanied by an increase in viscosity and a rise in peripheral vascular resistance related to increased peripheral tissue oxygenation. These factors may precipitate hypertension, angina, and acute cerebrovascular or cardiovascular events, especially when the rise of hematocrit is rapid, requiring phlebotomy and a reduction in dose.[40]

Vascular Disease

Accelerated atherosclerosis involves the cardiac, cerebral, or peripheral vessels. It is the most common and serious comorbid condition associated with renal failure.[42] Ischemic heart disease occurs in 25% of patients on dialysis, whereas frank myocardial infarction, angina, or acute pulmonary edema present with an incidence of approximately 10% per year. Cerebrovascular accidents are an important cause of morbidity and mortality, with intracranial hemorrhage being more frequent in patients on hemodialysis. Both large and small peripheral vessels may show typical "tram-tracking" on radiographs due to calcific deposits. Stenosis or occlusion of the iliofemoral-popliteal vessels is common and may require bypass, thereby prejudicing renal transplantation. Cardiac disease of nonischemic origin is also increased. Uremic cardiomyopathy is a well-established entity, although its pathogenesis remains obscure.[43] Independent of the cause, myocardial failure is responsible for up to 45% of long-term mortality, especially in the diabetic population. Sudden death of uncertain etiology is the predominant form of cardiac failure. The prognosis for individuals with persistent heart failure is poor, with survival of only 53% at 2 years.[44]

Accelerated vascular disease reflects the combined influences of hyperglycemia, hyperlipidemia, and hypertension.[45] Thirty percent to 50% of patients with chronic renal failure have clinical evidence of glucose intolerance. This is due to diabetes mellitus as the origin of their renal failure or as a secondary complication of peritoneal dialysis, aging, or reduced exercise tolerance and consequent weight gain. Patients with renal failure demonstrate alterations in the lipid metabolism most consistent with type IV hyperlipidemia. Moderate hypertriglyceridemia occurs in up to 80% of uremic patients, due to the accumulation of very-low-density lipoproteins (VLDLs), intermediate-density lipoproteins, and residual particles of intestinal origin. Cholesterol is mildly elevated and low-density lipoprotein (LDL) is normal, whereas high-density lipoprotein is decreased, so that cholesterol is redistributed to VLDL and LDL. Homocysteine clearance is also decreased, which has been implicated as a major risk factor for accelerated atherosclerosis and frequent thrombotic events.[46] Hypertension affects up to 80% of patients on dialysis. It is multifactorial in origin, though predominantly due to salt and volume overload associated with increased activity of the autonomic system and persistent activation of the renin-angiotensin system due to local renal ischemia.[45] Careful management of volume status is required to maintain dry weight. Aggressive treatment of hyperparathyroidism is also important because parathormone (PTH) appears to play a major role in triggering smooth muscle proliferation in the peripheral vessels.

Renal Osteodystrophy

Metabolic bone disease accompanying renal failure reflects a profound disturbance in calcium and phosphorus metabolism leading to osteitis fibrosa, osteoporosis, osteomalacia, and osteosclerosis. It may present with pruritus and soft-tissue calcification, tissue necrosis, skeletal pain, joint erosions, or fractures and deformity with severe limitation of mobility. The pathophysiology of renal osteodystrophy is complex. Reduced glomerular filtration causes significant phosphate retention with a decrease in intestinal calcium absorption. The compensatory elevation of serum PTH level enhances osteoclast and osteoblast activity and accelerates bone remodeling. This activity further suppresses renal tubular 1-hydroxylation of vitamin D already impaired by reduced nephron mass. Metabolic acidosis potentiates bone calcium loss by use of calcium carbonate as a buffer; aluminum-containing phosphate binders reduce bone turnover and increase the volume of demineralized bone. Finally, *adynamic bone disease* describes a reduction in bone formation, which is not accompanied by an increase in osteoid formation. This disorder appears in patients with relatively low levels of PTH and may be related to overaggressive treatment of osteitis fibrosa.[47] Management of renal osteodystrophy requires dietary control and the use of phosphate binders to reduce phosphate absorption, along with administration of vitamin D, usually in the form of 1-hydroxycholecalciferol. Resulting hypercalcemia must be managed with modifications of intake of calcium preparations and reductions in dosing of calcitriol. If hypercalcemia persists, tertiary hyperparathyroidism must be considered. This complication probably arises due to adenomatous change within the parathyroid glands, and it does not regress after renal transplantation.[48]

Medical Management

Initiation of Renal Replacement Therapy

Symptomatic progression of chronic renal failure is generally slow, with increasing weakness and fatigue, anorexia, sleep disturbances, and muscle cramps or bone pain. Supportive therapy should commence early to minimize renal osteodystrophy, prevent anemia, and ensure nutrition. Definitive therapy is not usually required until the glomerular filtration rate falls to 5% of normal (5 ml/minute), although earlier intervention may be required in diabetics, the elderly, or those with multisystem disease. Uncontrollable hyperkalemia, pulmonary edema, pericarditis, encephalopathy, and bleeding are life-threatening problems that necessitate urgent dialysis. They may occur at the onset of treatment or at any point during care, and they usually signal inadequate clearance or uncontrolled dietary intake.[49]

Two principal forms of dialysis are available for chronic renal failure: hemodialysis and peritoneal dialysis. The appropriate therapy should be selected with the patient as early as possible. Preparations should commence at least 3 months before the anticipated start of treatment to permit detailed patient education, the placement and maturation of all access sites, and immunologic evaluation and donor selection for subsequent transplantation.

Hemodialysis

Hemodialysis is the most common form of therapy for chronic renal failure worldwide and is applied in 20% of patients in the United Kingdom and 60% of patients in the United States. It can be performed in a hospital setting, a community unit, or at home. Hemodialysis requires a vascular access permitting high-volume flow through an extracorporeal circulation. This can be achieved in the short term via a special single- or twin-lumen catheter placed in the subclavian, internal jugular, or femoral veins. Longer-term care requires the creation of an arteriovenous fistula or the placement of a bridge graft. Bridge grafts are increasingly common, particularly in elderly or diabetic patients whose peripheral vessels do not permit satisfactory flow through an autogenous fistula at the wrist or other site.

Hemodialysis is normally performed for a period of 4 hours, three times per week. The duration of therapy, blood flow, membrane characteristics, and dialysate composition are adjusted to maintain optimal homeostasis. Three types of dialysis are currently performed. Conventional hemodialysis uses a blood flow rate of 200–300 ml per minute and a dialysate flow of 500 ml per minute, with a 0.8–1.3 m^2 low hydraulic permeability membrane. High-efficiency dialysis, in contrast, permits shorter treatment times (approximately 3 hours) but requires sophisticated technology for ultrafiltration control. This technique uses a blood flow rate of 350–500 ml per minute and a dialysis flow rate of 600–800 ml per minute, with a large surface area membrane of 1.5–2.2 m^2. High-flux dialysis resembles the latter approach but uses highly permeable membranes to achieve higher solute clearance.[50, 51]

Therapy is adjusted according to clinical features, volume status, and laboratory data. The long-term adequacy of therapy may be monitored by urea kinetic modeling. Intradialytic morbidity, due predominantly to the profound osmotic fluxes and intercompartmental volumetric changes that occur during therapy, commonly presents as transient hypotension, leg cramps, fatigue, arrhythmias, angina, or, occasionally, seizures. Maintenance of plasma volume through careful control of ultrafiltration and the use of a bicarbonate dialysate with an elevated dialysate sodium concentration all help to minimize these problems. Febrile reactions may occur due to pyrogen exposure or to the so-called first-use syndrome, representing the clinical expression of bioincompatibility with the dialyzer membrane, resulting in complement activation and cytokine release into the systemic circulation.[52, 53]

Peritoneal Dialysis

Peritoneal dialysis is an important alternative to hemodialysis, particularly in elderly or diabetic patients whose peripheral vessels do not permit satisfactory arteriovenous access. It is less widely used than hemodialysis in most countries, accounting for approximately 10% of patients in Europe and the United States, and no more than 35% in the United Kingdom and Canada. Acute peritoneal dialysis is generally performed in a hospital setting, whereas chronic dialysis is usually performed at home. Both forms of dialysis require continuous sterile access to the peritoneal cavity. This can be achieved in the short term via a special semirigid, single-lumen catheter placed through the anterior abdominal wall. Chronic dialysis requires the insertion of a permanent Tenckhoff-type polymeric silicone (Silastic) catheter. The catheter is tunneled through the subcutaneous tissue and anchored by one or more fibrous cuffs before being inserted into the peritoneum. Between treatments, it can be capped to preserve sterility.

Peritoneal dialysis requires the repeated instillation of dialysis solution into the peritoneum, with a variable dwell to allow for fluid removal and solute exchange. Homeostatic control is achieved by varying the cation and anion concentrations of the dialysate, and ultrafiltration is obtained by increasing dialysate osmolality through the use of glucose at 1.5–4.5 g/dl producing an osmolality of 350–500 mOsm/liter. The two most common forms of dialysis are continuous ambulatory peritoneal dialysis (CAPD) and continuous cycling peritoneal dialysis (CCPD), although alternative options of nightly peritoneal dialysis and tidal peritoneal dialysis also exist. CAPD is the simplest and most widely used; it can be performed by the patient alone. A volume of 1–3 liters of dialysate is inserted into the peritoneal cavity every 6 hours, then drained and replaced. CCPD requires six exchanges of 2 liters to be performed using a special machine during the night, with a similar volume left in situ throughout the daylight hours. In both cases, the rate and volumes of exchange and the dialysate composition must be adjusted according to the measured adequacy of dialysis and the residual renal function of the patient.[54]

The consequences of acute volumetric change are rarely seen on peritoneal dialysis, and cardiovascular events normally reflect chronic disease rather than treatment-related complications. Painful abdominal distension or hernias (e.g., ventral, inguinal, rectal prolapse) may occur in up to 25% of patients due to increased intra-abdominal pressure, requiring discontinuation of therapy. Infections in the catheter tunnel or at the skin exit site occur on average once every 2–3 years and may require changing the catheter site or conversion to hemodialysis if chronic and refractory to therapy. Peritonitis is the most serious complication of chronic peritoneal dialysis, however. The immune depression of uremia and the inhibitory influence of peritoneal solutions on phagocytic cell function impair peritoneal defenses. Peritonitis occurs with an average frequency of one episode every 30–50 months, although certain patients are particularly susceptible for technical or medical reasons. Contamination may be exogenous or endogenous, and gram-positive and gram-negative organisms may be responsible, depending on the source. The appearance of cloudy peritoneal drainage with more than 100 leukocytes/µl is followed rapidly by abdominal pain and tenderness, nausea, vomiting, fever, and deterioration in dialysis efficiency. Immediate therapy with intraperitoneal antibiotics is required, and long-term consequences may include sclerosing peritonitis with loss of filtration capacity.[54]

Renal Transplantation

Selection and Preparation of the Recipient

The increasing success of transplantation has resulted in a gradual relaxation of the selection criteria. As a result, the majority of patients with chronic renal failure can now be considered candi-

Table 11-2. Exclusion Criteria for Renal Transplantation

Absolute contraindications
    Unresolved malignancy
    Ongoing metabolic disorders (oxalosis)
    Active tuberculosis
    Active acquired immunodeficiency syndrome or hepatitis
    Severe vascular disease
    Active intravenous drug abuse
    Life expectancy <5 years
    Active lupus erythematosus
    Recent myocardial infarction
    Other end-stage organ diseases (cardiac, pulmonary, hepatic)
Relative contraindications
    Fabry's disease
    Sickle cell disease
    Obesity or malnutrition
    Recurrent, intractable urinary tract infection
    Peripheral vascular disease
    Poorly controlled diabetes
    Prior malignancy
    History of noncompliance
    Inadequate social support
    Primary renal disease with high postoperative recurrence rate (e.g., immunoglobulin A nephropathy, anti-glomerular basement membrane disorders, focal glomerulosclerosis)
    Severe chronic obstructive lung disease
    Cytomegalovirus or hepatitis seropositivity
    Extremes in age
    Emotional instability, particularly psychosis
    Decreased mental capacity

Table 11-3. Recipient Screening Procedure for Renal Transplantation

Procedure	Tests
History and physical examination	
Dental	Full evaluation; oral surgery (extractions) when indicated
Pulmonary	Chest radiography; spirometry when indicated
Cardiac	Electrocardiogram; stress test, echocardiography, coronary angiography, angioplasty, or surgical correction when indicated
Gastrointestinal	Stool guaiac; contrast studies or endoscopy when indicated
Genitourinary	Voiding cystourethrogram; nephrectomy for significant reflux associated with urinary infection
Vascular	Complete examination to identify significant disease; treatment if indicated
Laboratory tests	
Calcium	Severe hypercalcemia; consider pretransplant parathyroidectomy
Complete blood count	Epogen or iron for significant anemia
Nutritional panel	Supplementation when indicated
Liver panel	Imaging or biopsy for abnormalities
Amylase	If elevated, lipase; computed tomography of pancreas
Serology	Cytomegalovirus, human immunodeficiency virus, hepatitis B and C
Psychosocial assessment	Full evaluation by social worker; further evaluation when indicated
Immunologic assessment	ABO, HLA typing, panel-reactive antibody
Financial assessment	Evaluation of resources; assistance to obtain public aid if qualified

dates for transplantation. Chronologic age is no longer a rigid selection criterion, and patients in their seventh or eighth decade may now be successfully transplanted. Morbid obesity and the presence of comorbid diseases, such as diabetes, play an important role in determining risk and long-term outcome. Patients with a body mass index greater than 30 or severe systemic disease are often not accepted as suitable candidates for treatment.[55–57] Absolute and relative contraindications to renal transplantation are listed in Table 11-2.

    Clinical assessment is normally performed on an outpatient basis. The original renal disease must be clearly defined and symptoms of cardiovascular disease, urinary tract infection, bladder dysfunction and other systemic disease elicited. Careful physical examination is mandatory to document coexisting cardiovascular, gastrointestinal, or genitourinary disease; to assess respiratory reserve; and to define potential sources of infection, including dental caries. The laboratory evaluation should include routine hematology to document thrombocytopenia or leukopenia, which may prejudice surgery or immunosuppressant use. Liver function tests identify patients with active hepatitis or possible abnormal drug metabolism. Table 11-3 contains a summary of the recipient screening procedure.

Urinary tract infection is excluded by routine cultures before inclusion on the transplantation list. Voiding cystourethrography, measurement of residual urine volume, and full cystometric evaluation are performed on patients with suspected or overt bladder dysfunction due to mechanical or neurogenic causes. Lower urinary tract abnormalities are corrected when possible before transplantation. A contracted bladder may be expanded by hydrodilation; it generally enlarges satisfactorily after transplantation. In the small proportion of patients with irreversible structural or neurogenic dysfunction, transplantation may be performed into an ileal conduit fashioned before transplantation.[58]

Bilateral nephrectomy is now rarely performed because of the substantial morbidity and mortality of this procedure. The only definitive indications are grossly enlarged polycystic kidneys and persistent upper urinary tract infection: Uninfected vesicoureteric reflux is no longer considered a requirement for removal of the kidneys. When required, nephrectomy is generally performed by a bilateral posterior approach that offers more rapid patient recovery and decreased operative morbidity. An anterior midline approach may be performed in small patients or patients requiring ureterectomy, and laparoscopic techniques are gradually being adopted to minimize surgical intervention.[59]

Severe atheromatous disease of the aorta or iliac vessels may jeopardize the technical feasibility of transplantation or predispose to ischemia or infarction of the lower limbs in the event of a steal syndrome through the transplanted organ.[60] Hypertension must be managed aggressively to reduce left ventricular hypertrophy and myocardial oxygen demand, which may lead to ischemic complications. Patients with symptomatic ischemic heart disease and those at high risk, such as those with diabetes or elderly patients, may be evaluated noninvasively by echocardiography and exercise radioisotopic angiography to define ventricular contractility and cardiac ejection fraction.[61] Subjects with demonstrable abnormalities should proceed to further invasive evaluation by cardiac catheterization.[62] Because limited exercise tolerance reduces the diagnostic accuracy of thallium scintigraphy in a significant proportion of patients, some transplantation centers require mandatory angiography in high-risk individuals before activation on the transplantation waiting list. Coronary artery bypass or balloon dilation should be performed before transplantation for correctable lesions, although the implications of this approach are significant in patients with silent lesions.

The lethal consequences of peptic ulceration have been revolutionized by current medical therapy. Although gastric *Helicobacter pylori* contamination is more common in patients with renal disease, the proportion of infected patients who develop clinical ulceration is less than in normal subjects.[63] Nonetheless, patients with established or suspected peptic ulceration should undergo endoscopy to define the site, activity, and nature of the ulcer. Surgical therapy is now rarely required, but aggressive medical therapy should be commenced, healing confirmed by repeat endoscopy, and treatment continued throughout the period of transplantation and for 3–6 months postoperatively.

Active infection and malignancy still constitute absolute contraindications to transplantation until appropriately treated. Patients should be free from peritoneal infection and tunnel infection for at least 2 weeks before surgery. Transplantation may be performed in patients receiving antituberculous therapy, but careful follow-up is required to ensure compliance and to document recrudescence of the disease.[64] Viral hepatitis is increasingly common among patients awaiting transplantation, and liver biopsy is often required to assess disease severity.[65] Persistent hepatitis or mild changes in patients with either hepatitis B or C virus are not contraindications to transplantation, although acute exacerbations may occur or progression to terminal injury may intensify under immunosuppression.[66] More severe changes of chronic active hepatitis or frank cirrhosis are considered serious adverse prognostic factors, usually precluding transplantation.

Immunosuppression greatly increases the risk of lymphoreticular neoplasms, but the incidence of epithelial malignancies is only slightly increased.[67] Tumors with low metastatic risk, such as non-melanomatous skin or prostatic carcinoma, require appropriate medical or surgical therapy before transplantation. Patients with adequately treated primary tumors at other sites may also be considered for transplantation after a tumor-free period of at least 2 years. Metastatic disease or the continued presence of a primary tumor is normally an absolute preclusion to transplantation.

The ABO blood group is determined at the time of initial assessment, and complete HLA typing is performed at both class I (HLA-A, -B, -C) and class II (HLA-DR) loci. Serologic techniques are still used for class I typing, but DNA-based typing methods using the polymerase chain reaction are increasingly used for class II testing. The DNA methods have greatly enlarged the allele specificities at this locus.[68] Cytotoxic antibodies in the recipient serum are measured monthly or bimonthly using a panel of T- and B-lymphocytes or an enzyme-linked immunosorbent assay method to determine the degree of anti-HLA sensitization.[69] A high degree of sensitization decreases the probability of a negative donor cross-match, thereby prolonging the waiting time for cadaveric transplantation. Most centers no longer practice routine pretransplantation blood transfusion because of the risks of viral infection; the high risks of sensitization, particularly in children, blacks, multiparous women, and previous graft recipients; and the gradual reduction in measurable benefit on long-term outcome.[70, 71]

Psychosocial evaluation of the recipient is critical to identify patients in whom serious problems may develop as a result of stress or surgery, to ensure an adequate environment for psychological and physical recovery, and to uncover emotional or psychiatric disorders that may prejudice long-term outcome.[72] Patient education is vital to ensure comprehension of the procedure, improve compliance, and decrease anxiety. Patients in whom compliance with dialysis therapy has been problematic present a very special problem; they must be clearly informed of the consequences of discontinuation of immunosuppression. Such patients may even be excluded from transplantation until greater commitment is ensured.[73]

Donor Selection

Living-Related Donor

The use of living donors for kidney transplantation is justified on three grounds:

1. Graft survival is superior, exceeding that obtained with cadaveric transplants by 5–10% at 1 year and increasing over time.
2. Transplantation can be performed expeditiously and at an optimum moment, thereby facilitating recipient preparation when surgical intervention is required.

3. It circumvents the chronic failure of cadaver donation to meet the increasing demand for organ transplantation.[22]

Despite these compelling reasons and the psychological benefit obtained in many cases, the use of a live donor is acceptable only if significant morbidity or mortality does not accompany this altruistic act. Survival studies indicate that unilateral nephrectomy in the healthy adult has a mortality risk of less than 0.1%, with a 5-year life expectancy comparable to that of the normal population.[74, 75] The possibility that continued hyperfiltration in the remaining kidney may jeopardize long-term renal function, as in the remnant kidneys of experimental animals, has been a concern. Follow-up studies over 10–15 years in large numbers of kidney donors have provided no evidence of such functional deterioration, however.[76, 77]

Selection of the donor is based on clinical, immunologic, and emotional criteria.[78] The donor is normally between the ages of 18 and 65 years (although both younger and older individuals may be accepted in special circumstances), is in excellent physical health, and has no evidence of structural or functional renal disease. Hypertension, diabetes, and other systemic disorders contraindicate donation due to excessive risk to the donor. ABO compatibility (not identity) between donor and recipient is essential. Although success is greatest with HLA-identical siblings, graft survival of 90% or greater may now be obtained between genetically unrelated HLA-incompatible subjects with the use of current immunosuppression, thus permitting the use of the emotionally related donor, as in spousal transplantation.[79, 80] Finally, the donor must be emotionally stable, highly motivated, and free from coercion.

A preliminary physical, immunologic, and psychological assessment is performed to identify the most suitable donor candidate. Intensive evaluation is then undertaken to examine general clinical status, to eliminate unsuspected hypertension or subclinical diabetes, and to confirm normal renal function using measured creatinine clearance and radionuclear measurement of glomerular filtration rate.[81] An intravenous pyelogram and renal angiogram with selective catheterization of the renal vessels, computed tomography, or magnetic resonance imaging are performed last to demonstrate renal morphology and vasculature before surgery.[82, 83]

Table 11-4. Contraindications for Cadaver
Organic Procurement

Absolute contraindications

Prolonged hypotension

Prolonged hypothermia

Poorly treated or untreated hypertension

Systemic lupus erythematosus and other collagen disorders

Congenital or acquired metabolic disorders

Sickle cell anemia and related hemoglobinopathies

Malignancy other than confined to the central nervous
system or the skin

Generalized viral or bacterial infections

Hepatitis B or human immunodeficiency virus carrier state

Disseminated intravascular coagulation

Relative contraindications

Diabetes mellitus

Physiologic age >70 years

History or evidence of renal disease

Pathologic urine analysis (severe vascular diseases,
proteinuria)

High or rising terminal serum creatinine level (>2.3 ng/dl)

Preterminal urine output not exceeding 0.5 ml/kg/hr

Profound preterminal use of inotropic vasoconstrictor
drugs

Cadaver Donor

For more than 75% of patients, however, no suitable living donor can be identified, and cadaveric donation is required. After declaration of brain death, multiple criteria are considered to determine the suitability of cadaver kidneys (Table 11-4). The kidneys are preferably removed en bloc, flushed with refrigerated preservation solution to permit core cooling, and stored by simple hypothermic preservation at 4°C. Rarely, kidneys are preserved by pulsatile perfusion, which appears valuable in determining the suitability of older kidneys.[84]

Recipient selection is based on clinical urgency, ABO compatibility, HLA match, and a negative cross-match against donor T cells using recipient serum stored at monthly intervals while the patient is on the waiting list. Clinical urgency is normally determined by the degree of anti-HLA sensitization or overriding clinical complications. Patients who have antibodies to more than 60–80% of the population panel are often given elevated priority status, as are those with a rapid deterioration in clinical status, advancing neuropathy, or loss of dialysis access sites. Transplantation is normally performed

within blood group to avoid selection bias against group O recipients, but it may occur between any compatible groups (e.g., O to B, B to AB). HLA matching at A, B, and DR loci is considered extremely important in Europe; national or international organ sharing programs exist to distribute kidneys to the most appropriately matched patients.[85] In North America, the impact of matching is more hotly debated. Although the value of a six-antigen or "full-house" match is clearly proved, the value of lesser degrees of compatibility is questioned.[86] As a result, kidneys are often transplanted in-center without a high degree of HLA compatibility. Primary transplantation may be performed with good outcome when the T-cell cross-match is negative on current serum, despite positivity in a previous sample. In previously grafted or sensitized subjects, however, historic positivity is associated with an increased incidence of graft loss and should be avoided.[87] Additional assays are used in many centers to increase the sensitivity of the cross-match, including the antiglobulin-enhanced microcytotoxicity assay or fluorescent cell cytometry techniques.[88] Finally, the kidney may be allocated according to donor and recipient cytomegalovirus status in certain centers to minimize the risk of viral transmission with the transplanted organ.[89] This step detracts from the ability to ensure a close HLA match, however, and the introduction of new antiviral agents has diminished the need for this precaution.

Preoperative Preparation and Dialysis

Patients may remain on the transplantation list for several months or years, during which they may not be closely followed by the transplantation team. Scrupulous clinical re-evaluation is therefore essential when the patient presents for transplantation to exclude new evidence of cardiovascular disease, lower limb arteriopathy, subclinical infection, or other systemic illnesses. A decision regarding preoperative dialysis must be made quickly for patients who are already maintained on this therapy and those with advanced failure. This decision depends on the timing and efficiency of the preceding dialysis, the interdialytic volume gain, and the metabolic status of the patient. In general, the same criteria used to commence dialysis are applied. A short dialysis run is generally sufficient. Patients are brought to within 0.5 kg of their ideal weight. Acute hypotension is strenuously avoided to minimize the risk of intraoperative collapse and prevent volume depletion in the early postoperative phase, which could lead to acute tubular necrosis in the graft.

Hyperkalemia

The most serious risk is that of acute hyperkalemia, which may be exacerbated intraoperatively. Certain drugs may also accentuate this risk, including potassium supplements, potassium-sparing diuretics, angiotensin-converting enzyme inhibitors, nonsteroidal anti-inflammatory drugs, and cyclosporine.[90] The toxicity of hyperkalemia is due to sodium channel inactivation resulting in partial membrane depolarization, decreased neuronal excitability, and impaired neuromuscular transmission in cardiac and skeletal muscle. Hyperkalemia may be particularly dangerous when accompanied by hypocalcemia and metabolic acidosis, which accentuate potassium toxicity. The diagnosis depends primarily on the biochemical observation of potassium elevation. Changes in the electrocardiogram (ECG), including loss of P waves, peaked T waves, a widened QRS complex, or a decrease in muscular strength, are also important indicators of serious intoxication.[91] However, they may be present only preterminally, and they are unlikely to be evident if the serum K^+ concentration is less than 7 mmol/liter.

Treatment of acute hyperkalemia has three objectives: to reverse the membrane effects resulting in impaired neurotransmission, to lower the serum potassium concentration, and to enhance potassium elimination.[92] Intravenous calcium gluconate is most commonly used to stabilize neurotransmission, 10 ml of 10% solution being infused slowly over 3 minutes. This effect lasts for approximately 30–60 minutes, providing a temporary respite for second- and third-line therapies. Infusion of 10 units of regular insulin with 25 g dextrose to prevent hypoglycemia activates the sodium- and potassium-activated adenosine triphosphate pump in skeletal muscles, and results in a 0.5–1.5 mmol/liter-fall in potassium concentration within 15–60 minutes. Administration of 0.45 mmol of sodium bicarbonate potentiates this decrease within approximately 30 minutes by stimulating hydrogen

ion movement from the cell and causing an intracellular shift of potassium. The cation exchange resin sodium polystyrene (Kayexalate), which exchanges sodium for potassium ions, is effective only for the subacute control of hyperkalemia. Administration of a single dose (30–50 g, orally or as an enema) decreases potassium concentration by 0.5–1.0 mmol/liter within 2 hours. Long-term use of this agent may lead to secondary acute fluid overload in patients with renal failure. Care must be used in the perioperative period after intra-abdominal surgery due to the risk of ischemic bowel necrosis. In general, dialysis should be performed in all patients with a serum potassium level greater than 5.5 mmol/liter before transplantation.

Transplantation Procedure

Preparation of the Transplantation Bed

After induction of anesthesia, a 22 French urethral catheter is inserted into the bladder aseptically; any urine obtained is sent for analysis and culture. The bladder is then distended with antibiotic solution (50,000 units of bacitracin/1 g kanamycin/liter normal saline) to facilitate intraoperative identification. The site for the renal allograft is chosen based on avoiding the presence of a previously failed transplant or existence of peripheral vascular disease. If there is no contraindication, the right iliac fossa is generally preferred over the left iliac fossa because the right iliac vein runs a more superficial and horizontal course. The most widely used approach is the standard pelvic Gibson technique (Figure 11-1). The internal oblique, transversus abdominis, and rectus muscles are divided to obtain adequate exposure of the patient's bladder and iliac vessels within the iliac fossa (Figure 11-2). Retractor blades are padded to prevent traction injuries to the patient's femoral or superficial femoral nerves. Typically, the symptoms of quadriceps weakness or painless cutaneous numbness of the lateral thigh, respectively, present within the first 2–5 postoperative days and resolve within 2–12 months.

Revascularization of the Kidney

The transplantation procedure starts when the flushed, cooled kidney is brought to the operative

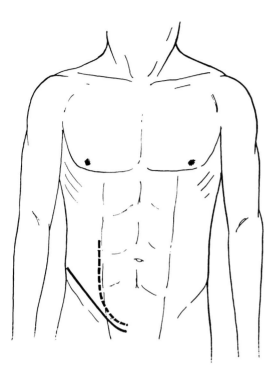

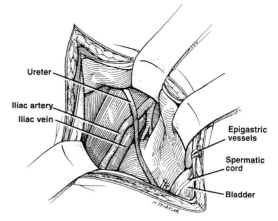

Figure 11-2. The allograft bed showing epigastric vessels controlled by ligatures, iliac artery or vein, and host ureter. Note that the spermatic cord is reflected medially.

Figure 11-1. Incisions for recipient renal transplantation operation. Hockey-stick incision (*dotted line*) and the usual Gibson incision (*solid line*).

field. The kidney is placed where it lies most naturally with the renal pelvis and ureter oriented distally. Unless the artery is particularly short or the anastomosis is deemed difficult, the deeper venous anastomosis between renal and external iliac vein is usually performed first. Variations of the arterial supply to the donor kidney (e.g., internal or external iliac artery, hypogastric artery) are determined at this time. In situations in which there is extensive atherosclerosis of the hypogastric artery, as in diabetic patients, an end-to-side or end-to-end arterial anastomosis (Figure 11-3) is performed either to the common iliac or external iliac artery. Other situations that preclude the use of the hypogastric artery include when there is significant disparity in caliber of the renal and hypogastric arteries, when there are multiple donor renal arteries that are readily encompassed by a Carrel aortic patch, or in male patients who have undergone previous transplants in which the contralateral hypogastric artery was used and who are at risk of postoperative impotence. During the vascular anastomoses, the kidney must be kept cold by continuous surface irrigation with ice-cold saline.

At the completion of the arterial anastomosis, the vascular clamps are removed in quick succession. First, the low-pressure clamps, the superior venous clamp, and inferior arterial clamp are removed. Then the high-pressure clamps, the inferior venous clamp, and the upper arterial clamp on the external iliac artery are removed, and hemostasis is ensured. The kidney should regain its normal pink color and turgor. It is important at this time to ensure adequate circulating volume and hydration. Mottling of the graft surface due to arterial spasm sometimes occurs but generally resolves within 30 minutes. Occasionally, dramatic improvement in the mottled look is attained by topical application of 1% lidocaine (Xylocaine) solution (without epinephrine) on the renal artery.

Sometimes the allograft fails to reperfuse well intraoperatively because of problems with arterial inflow, including dissection under an intimal flap, technical misadventures, or twisting of the vessels. In these cases, the arterial anastomosis must be immediately revised. After systemic heparinization (1 mg/kg) and establishment of proximal and distal vascular control over both iliac artery and vein, the allograft is reflushed through the renal or external iliac artery. Room-temperature and then chilled solution is used, with venous venting via a tributary of the renal vein, such as the gonadal or adrenal branches, so that one avoids disrupting the venous anastomotic suture line. After the arterial anastomosis has been corrected, the organ is reperfused after closure of the vein tributary.

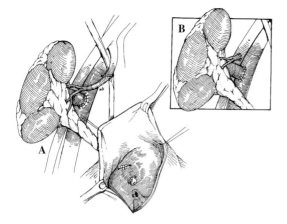

Figure 11-3. Vascular anastomoses of renal transplantation artery. **A.** End-to-end renal to internal iliac artery. **B.** End-to-side renal to external iliac artery.

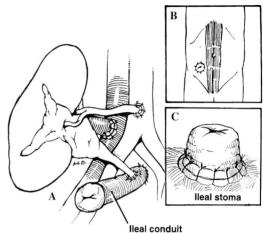

Figure 11-4. Use of a straight ileal segment to construct a urinary conduit. **A.** Ureter anastomosed to proximal end of ileal conduit and distal portion of ileum fashioned into a stoma. **B.** Position of ileal stoma on abdominal wall. **C.** Maturing Brook ileostomy sutures.

Re-Establishment of Urinary Tract Continuity

Continuity of the urinary tract is usually established with a ureteroneocystostomy technique. In the Leadbetter-Politano method, an anterior cystotomy is performed to make visible the interior of the bladder. A 2- to 3-cm submucosal tunnel is created so that the transplant ureter can be implanted into the bladder mucosa near the trigone.[93]

The surgical approach to urinary drainage must be modified in patients experiencing the abnormalities of a pathologically scarred bladder resulting from chronic infection (e.g., tuberculous cystitis). It also is changed in multiple previous surgical procedures; long-standing neurogenic detrusor dysfunction secondary to meningomyelocele, spinal cord trauma, and other neurologic diseases; or bladder neck contractures or urethral strictures secondary to prostatic disease, vesicoureteral reflux, bladder exstrophy, and posterior urethral valves. Although it is preferable to detect and correct these bladder abnormalities before transplantation, they must be addressed postoperatively with treatments ranging from intermittent clean self-catheterization to supravesical urinary diversion.[94]

If pretransplantation evaluation reveals a noncompliant and nondistensible bladder that is not suitable for use after transplantation, bladder augmentation, bladder substitution, or urinary diversion is required. Augmentation cystoplasty with isolated bowel segments (e.g., ileocecal, sigmoid patch, ileal patch, tubular portion of sigmoid colon, or an isolated segment from the greater curvature of the stomach)[95, 96] increases bladder capacity and decreases intravesical pressure, thereby protecting the upper calyceal tract. Substitution cystoplasty replaces most of the bladder with bowel, leaving only the vesicle trigone and bladder neck.

If bladder augmentation or substitution is not possible, supravesical urinary diversion is necessary. In 1966, Kelly applied ureteroileal cutaneous urinary diversion in renal transplantation.[97] The conduit is constructed at least 4–6 weeks before transplantation by using a short, straight ileal segment of approximately 10–15 cm fed by at least two large branches of the superior mesenteric artery. The stoma of the ileal conduit is placed in the right lower quadrant just medial to the lateral border of the rectus muscle (Figure 11-4).

Urinary tract infection is the most common complication after conduit drainage of kidney transplants.[98] Other complications are upper tract deterioration, stenosis of the stoma, parastomal hernia, calculus formation, ureterointestinal stenosis, pyocystis of the isolated bladder, small bowel fistula, bowel obstruction, and electrolyte abnormalities.[99] These are particularly common among pediatric recipients.

Table 11-5. Postoperative Surgery-Related Complications

Vascular
  Renal artery thrombosis
  Renal artery stenosis
  Renal vein thrombosis
  Arterial or venous anastomotic hemorrhage
Urinary tract
  Ureteral devascularization
  Ureteral leakage or ureterocutaneous fistula
  Ureteral obstruction
  Bladder fistulas
Renal pelvis
  Urine leakage
Transplantation bed
  Lymphoceles
  Perinephric hemorrhage or hematoma
Scrotum
  Hydrocele
  Testicular atrophy or necrosis
  Acute bacterial epididymitis
  Recurrent scrotal pain
  Acute bacterial prostatitis

Surgery-Related Postoperative Complications

The incidence and severity of technical complications after kidney transplantation have decreased since the 1960s because of improved surgical, diagnostic, and immunosuppressive tools. However, complications resulting from misadventures, albeit infrequent, may cause renal dysfunction, graft loss, and even death. Although most complications occur in the early postoperative period, some may not be detected until several years after transplantation. Table 11-5 summarizes potential surgery-related complications. Management of these complications may include surgical intervention in the early postoperative period.

Anesthetic Management

Preoperative Assessment

Patients undergoing cadaveric renal transplantation arrive in hospital after receiving notification that a kidney is available. It is therefore common that these patients are seen only shortly before surgery. A careful history and physical examination along with a review of the laboratory investigations are essential. If there are concerns about cardiovascular function, pericardial effusion, uncontrolled hypertension, unstable angina, or other medical problems, these should be optimized when the patient is selected as a candidate for transplantation.

Patients may be very anxious; they may have been waiting months for transplantation. The purpose of the preoperative visit is to establish a rapport with the patient and to explain the intraoperative routines, including monitors, central line insertion, and the possible need for blood transfusion. It is also useful to discuss preoperative sedation, anesthetic technique, and postoperative pain management.

A review of body systems is necessary because these patients often have a variety of medical problems associated with their renal failure (Table 11-6).

Fluid, Electrolyte, and Acid-Base Balance

Before preoperative dialysis was routine, earlier reviews of anesthesia for renal transplantation reported a 16% perioperative mortality.[100] Today, perioperative mortality has been reduced to less than 1% in most series, and some have reported no immediate perioperative mortality.[101–103]

Fluid and electrolyte imbalances must be corrected before surgery. It is impossible to overemphasize the role of preoperative dialysis in improving the safety of anesthesia and surgery.[104] Dialysis returns the profound metabolic derangement of renal failure to a normal or near-normal state. This is especially important for potassium, acid-base balance, and overall volume status. With modern organ-preservation techniques, the window of opportunity for transplantation after organ harvesting leaves ample time to optimize the patient, including dialysis.

Anemia

The anemia of chronic renal failure can be severe, with hemoglobin levels 6–8 g/100 ml and hematocrits of 20–25%. Various physiologic mechanisms help these patients to compensate. Severe anemia reduces oxygen-carrying capacity by approximately 50%, which results in an increase in cardiac output. Levels of 2,3-diphosphoglycerate are increased to shift the oxyhemoglobin dissociation curve to the

Table 11-6. Assessment and Preparation of the Patient for Renal Transplantation

System	Possible Problems	Investigations	Interventions
Respiratory	Fluid overload, pulmonary edema, hypoxemia, pleural effusion	Body weight, blood gases	Dialysis, supplemental oxygen
Cardiovascular	Hypertension	ECG, chest x-ray	Dialysis, antihypertensives
	Ischemic heart disease	ECG, stress test Angiography	Antianginals
	Uremic pericarditis	ECG, chest x-ray, echocardiogram	Dialysis, surgery, pericardial window
Neurologic	Peripheral neuropathy	EMG	Avoid succinylcholine
Hematologic	Anemia	Hemoglobin, hematocrit	Judicious transfusion
	Coagulopathy	INR, PTT	Dialysis
	Impaired platelet function	Bleeding time	—
	Immunosuppression	Cultures, if clinically indicated	Aseptic technique, prophylactic antibiotics
Renal	Uremia	Serum urea	Dialysis, serum creatinine
	Hyperkalemia	Serum electrolytes	Dialysis, sodium polystyrene (Kayexalate), sodium bicarbonate, insulin and glucose, calcium, avoid potassium-containing fluids, avoid succinylcholine
	Hyponatremia	Serum electrolytes	Dialysis, avoid hypotonic fluids
	Hypermagnesemia	—	Avoid magnesium-containing antacids
Musculoskeletal	Renal osteodystrophy	Serum calcium, phosphorus	Oral replacement
Endocrine	Hyperparathyroidism	Hypocalcemia	Calcium supplementation, surgery, parathyroidectomy
	Diabetes	Serum glucose	Insulin and glucose as indicated

ECG = electrocardiogram; EMG = electromyography; INR = international normalized ratio; PTT = partial thromboplastin time.

right, which produces improved oxygen delivery to the tissues. Metabolic acidosis shifts the curve even further.[105]

Erythropoietin

Before erythropoietin, approximately 25% of dialysis patients required intermittent (or even regular) blood transfusions for relief of anemia-related symptoms.[106] With erythropoietin, hemoglobin levels can be normalized in several months. Patients treated with erythropoietin have less fatigue, less psychological depression, and improved exercise tolerance than do untreated patients. However, there may be a higher incidence of hypertension and clotting of vascular access sites in patients treated with erythropoietin.[107]

Transfusion

There has been considerable debate over the effects of blood transfusion on renal graft survival. Transfusion was initially discouraged due to the fear of sensitization against further renal grafts. It was later shown that transfusion improved renal graft survival, which led to the recommendation for pregraft transfusion weeks or months before transplantation.[108, 109] However, immediate preoperative or intraoperative transfusion has never been shown to improve graft survival.

Cyclosporine and modern immunosuppression techniques have improved graft survival to such an extent that it is now difficult to find a beneficial effect related to blood transfusions.[110, 111] Current enthusiasm for pregraft transfusions is further limited by the fear of acquiring hepatitis or human immunodeficiency virus.

Intraoperative blood loss is usually less than 500 ml. Aldrete et al. reported average blood loss as 175 ml; therefore, perioperative transfusion is not indicated routinely.[112] Blood loss of up to 8,000 ml has been reported. As with any vascular procedure, the loss may be rapid and massive.[113] Blood should therefore be available for intraoperative transfusion and administered if indicated rather than routinely.

Coagulation

Chronic renal failure is associated with a tendency toward increased bleeding. Platelet count may be mildly depressed, and platelet function is typically abnormal. However, platelet function may be partially corrected by dialysis.[114, 115] Bleeding time is usually prolonged, but prothrombin and partial prothrombin times are usually normal.

Fasting

The duration of preoperative fasting must be determined. Uremic patients have a variety of reasons for inadequate gastric emptying, including anxiety, autonomic neuropathy, diabetes, dialysis, and inadequate duration of preoperative fasting. Reissell et al. found that residual gastric volumes were greater in diabetic than in nondiabetic patients with renal failure, but they found no delay in gastric emptying for nondiabetic uremic patients.[116]

Some authors suggest the routine preoperative administration of nonparticulate antacid, such as sodium citrate; of an H_2-receptor antagonist, such as ranitidine; or of gastrointestinal prokinetic agents, such as metoclopramide.[105] Alternatively, or in addition, cricoid pressure and a rapid-sequence induction can be used.

Anesthetic Technique

Both regional and general anesthesia have been successfully used for renal transplantation.[101, 117–120] The advantages of regional anesthesia include avoidance of intravenous agents that require renal excretion, such as muscle relaxants and opiates.

Theoretic disadvantages of regional anesthesia are many. Neurologic complications, epidural hematoma, and postdural puncture headache are potential limitations. It should be noted, however, that 146 cases of regional anesthesia were reported without evidence of these complications. Patients arriving for transplantation may be very anxious, and the duration of surgery varies between 2.5 and 7.0 hours. Therefore, it may be difficult for patients to endure long procedures under regional anesthesia.[100] Furthermore, central venous pressure lines, and if necessary, arterial lines, must be inserted while the patient is awake. Many authors have described the need for excessive supplementation with intravenous or inhalational agents.[119] Linke and Merin reported five patients with epidural anesthesia, four of whom eventually required general anesthesia.[117] Aldrete et al. described 22 patients with epidural anesthesia; all but one patient required general anesthesia.[112]

If regional anesthesia is used, fluid loading before the block must be done cautiously, and it is complicated by chronic hypertension and the possibility of overhydration. Regional anesthesia may produce hypotension, which must be considered, particularly during the revascularization of the new renal graft, when perfusion of the new kidney is of paramount importance.[117, 121] One study linked hypotension to cardiac arrest, suggesting that regional anesthesia not be used.[121]

For these reasons, general anesthesia has become the technique of choice for renal transplantation. In seven retrospective reviews of renal transplantation summarizing 2,133 cases, not a single patient received regional anesthesia.[100, 103, 113, 120, 122–124] In the 13 papers reviewed, only 146 of 3,282 (4%) patients received regional anesthesia, and 60 of these 146 (41%) eventually required general anesthesia.

General anesthesia is typically induced with propofol or thiopentone and a narcotic, such as fentanyl or sufentanil. Endotracheal intubation is facilitated using either succinylcholine or an intermediate-acting muscle relaxant, such as atracurium or vecuronium. Fentanyl, nitrous oxide, isoflurane, and atracurium are commonly used to maintain anesthesia.

Intraoperative Management of the Transplant Recipient

Monitoring and Equipment

In monitoring the patient during renal transplantation, it is important to remember that ESRD results in multiple medical problems. The patient is placed on the operating room table with a warming blanket. Because the surgery may last several hours and large volumes of fluid may be required, a fluid warmer is required. Special care must be taken during positioning to ensure adequate protection of the dialysis fistula to ensure continued function. The blood pressure cuff, intravenous lines, and arterial lines should not be placed on the same extremity as the fistula. Intermittent auscultation or palpation of the fistula to document fistula patency is advised. Monitors should be applied and baseline measures recorded before the induction of anesthesia (Table 11-7).

Uremic patients have an impaired immune response and are susceptible to infection. This is aggravated in transplant recipients due to the use of immunosuppressants. Sepsis remains an important cause of death in these patients; therefore, aseptic technique should be observed during intubation and insertion of invasive monitors.[125]

Intraoperative Fluid Therapy

Maximal hydration during renal transplantation is of utmost importance. The new kidney must have adequate perfusion to ensure optimal function. A central venous pressure line is an essential intraoperative and postoperative monitor. Some authors recommend the use of pulmonary artery catheters

Table 11-7. Intraoperative Monitors and Equipment

Stethoscope
Temperature probe
Pulse oximeter
Electrocardiogram (optional 5 leads to monitor cardiac ischemia)
Noninvasive blood pressure monitor (optional arterial line)
Peripheral nerve stimulator
End-tidal carbon dioxide monitor
Central venous pressure line (optional pulmonary artery catheter)
Urinary catheter
Warming blanket and fluid warmer
Laboratory requisitions and blood sample tubes for blood gases, electrolytes, hemoglobin, and glucose
Armboard and padding for fistula

and arterial lines routinely.[126, 127] For most patients without evidence of left ventricular failure, central venous pressure is an adequate reflection of pulmonary artery diastolic pressure. Similarly, most patients without evidence of cardiac dysfunction do not require an arterial line for blood pressure monitoring.

Delayed primary function of the transplanted kidney has been studied extensively. There is overwhelming consensus that the "filling effect" is important for immediate graft function. Usually, anesthesiologists manage patients with chronic renal failure by keeping them "dry" to prevent fluid overload and to avoid the need for postoperative dialysis. In contrast, the transplant patient must be "wet," with a supernormal intravascular volume to ensure luxury flow to the new renal graft. Anesthesia for the uremic patient undergoing transplantation is unique in this respect, and the anesthesiologist must be aware of this extremely important difference.

Intraoperative fluid balance is important because adequate intravascular volume is essential for maintaining perfusion to the new kidney.[126–129] There is a definite relationship between renal graft perfusion and the incidence of acute tubular necrosis.[130–132] A central venous pressure of 10 mm Hg at the time the arterial clamps are released is recommended.

Carlier et al. suggested that patients with diastolic pulmonary artery pressures less than 15 mm Hg had a 36% incidence of acute tubular necrosis, whereas only 6% of patients with pulmonary artery pressures greater than 15 mm Hg developed acute tubular necrosis.[126] Typically, the transplantation patient received 90–100 ml/kg, or just over 5 liters of intravenous fluid, during the procedure. Patients received on average of 2 units of packed red blood cells and 600 ml of whole blood. This amount of fluid approximately doubled the central venous pressure, from an initial value of 6–12 mm Hg. In a study by Davidson et al., patients received approximately 60 ml/kg of intravenous fluid, 1.2 g/kg of albumin, and 1 unit of blood.[128] Administration of albumin was associated with a reduced incidence of delayed graft function.

To further stimulate urine production and promote immediate function of the transplanted kidney, mannitol, furosemide, and dopamine have been used. Mannitol is frequently used in doses of 20–50 g.[126, 128, 129, 133, 134] Furosemide in doses varying from 200 to 500 mg has been recommended before unclamping the newly grafted kidney.[126, 128] Dopamine has been used to maintain blood pressure at or above 140 mm Hg to ensure adequate flow to the graft.[126, 135]

Before administering mannitol to patients in renal failure, the anesthesiologist must appreciate the subsequent alterations in fluid and electrolyte balances. Mannitol is an osmotic diuretic and, when given to patients with normal renal function during neurosurgical procedures, results in hyponatremia, a transient increase in potassium (0.5 mmol/liter), and a reduction in serum bicarbonate.[136] Mannitol administered during renal transplantation has been associated with hyperkalemia.[137] The average maximal change in serum potassium is 0.7 mmol/liter.[133, 134] In one study, 4 of 13 patients who received mannitol developed a rise of potassium exceeding 1 mmol/liter. This may be of clinical importance and suggests that some patients are at risk for significant hyperkalemia after mannitol. In this study, an additional patient who did not receive mannitol also had an increase in serum potassium greater than 1 mmol/liter. This observation simply reminds us that all patients in renal failure are at risk for developing hyperkalemia.

Intraoperative rises in serum potassium have also been associated with the use of Collins solution and with the release of vascular clamps.[133, 134, 138, 139] It may be difficult to determine the factors responsible for the rise in potassium because these events occur simultaneously.

Table 11-8. Treatment of Intraoperative Hyperkalemia

Electrocardiogram Changes Associated with Hyperkalemia	Treatment
Potassium >5.0: No electro-cardiogram changes	Discontinue potassium-containing fluids Monitor glucose and arterial blood gases Observation
Potassium >6.0: Tall, peaked T waves	Sodium polystyrene (Kayexalate) Hyperventilation Sodium bicarbonate 50 ml 50% glucose and 5 units insulin
Potassium >7.0: Loss of P waves, widening of QRS complex, ventricular fibrillation	Calcium gluconate 1 g intravenously slowly Dialysis

Because patients with renal failure are unable to excrete free water, mannitol may produce a profound reduction in serum sodium. Postoperative hyponatremia below 120 mmol/liter may be associated with convulsions. Isotonic saline 0.9% NaCl is theoretically the ideal fluid to administer during renal transplantation because it contains no lactate or potassium and has a high sodium content.

Potassium

Preoperative dialysis has made the problem of preoperative hyperkalemia far less common. Surgery should be postponed until potassium values are normalized. Patients with diabetes or predialysis hyperkalemia may be at greater risk of developing intraoperative hyperkalemia; intraoperative potassium should be regularly monitored.

Intraoperative hyperkalemia can be treated in several ways, depending on its severity (Table 11-8). Generally, potassium levels less than 6 mEq/liter rarely result in ECG change. Potassium levels greater than 6 mEq/liter may produce tall, peaked T waves. Higher levels are associated with loss of P waves, widening of the QRS complex, and, ultimately, ventricular fibrillation.

The ECG should be observed frequently for changes in the waveform, which may indicate hyperkalemia. An ECG monitor with a paper printout is ideal. A baseline strip can be made before induction of anesthesia and used for comparison later, if hyperkalemia is suspected. Serum potassium levels should be checked if hyperkalemia is questioned. The central venous pressure line can be used to obtain blood samples for potassium analysis.

Glucose, insulin, bicarbonate, and hyperventilation lower serum levels by shifting potassium intracellularly, but the effect is only temporary. Intravenous calcium does not lower potassium levels but blocks the effects of potassium at the cell membrane. Levels below 6.0 mEq/liter should be monitored closely; levels greater than 6.0 should be treated with glucose, insulin, and bicarbonate. Levels greater than 7.0 should be treated with calcium and hyperventilation. The results of either therapeutic intervention should be monitored closely. Postoperatively, dialysis may be required to remove potassium because these therapies merely shift potassium into the cells. The patient should remain intubated and ventilated until metabolic and hemodynamic stability can be maintained.

Patients with insulin-dependent diabetes may be at greater risk of developing hyperkalemia due to diabetic ketoacidosis.[138] Intravenous glucose and insulin infusions should be adjusted as required. Glucose levels should be monitored hourly and maintained within the normal range.

Acidosis

Patients with renal failure have varying degrees of metabolic acidosis. A minimum pH of 7.25 is advisable before surgery.[114] The problem of preoperative acidosis is best corrected by preoperative dialysis. Bicarbonate therapy corrects acidosis until the donor kidney begins to function or until dialysis can be performed. Deliberate hyperventilation can be used to temporarily compensate for metabolic acidosis. Careful attention should be given to ventilation and acid-base balance because hyperventilation may shift the oxyhemoglobin dissociation curve to the left, thereby decreasing the ability of hemoglobin to release oxygen to the peripheral tissues. This may be undesirable in severely anemic patients.

Anesthetic Agents and Special Considerations in Renal Transplantation

Induction Agents

No anesthetic agent stands alone as the induction agent of choice. A variety of induction agents have been used, including barbiturates (thiopentone and methohexitone), benzodiazepines (diazepam and midazolam), althesin, ketamine, droperidol, and propofol.

Lindahl-Nilsson et al. described neurolept anesthesia for renal transplantation in 176 operations.[103] Anesthesia was induced with either droperidol or barbiturates; they concluded that the barbiturate was preferable. Morgan and Lumley described their experience in 941 anesthetics given to patients with renal failure.[113] Droperidol and fentanyl were used in 19% of patients, providing slow but smooth induction with minimal postoperative nausea and vomiting. Neurolept anesthesia has also been advocated as the preferred technique by Trudnowski et al.[121] Weir and Chung suggest that high-dose fentanyl technique should be limited to patients with minimal cardiac reserve.[105]

In the early years of transplantation, inhalational inductions with halothane or cyclopropane were common.[100, 113] Inhalational inductions were particularly useful in patients with poor venous access and for intubating without muscle relaxants.

Thiopentone

Thiopentone has been the most popular induction agent for renal transplantation. The dose of thiopentone and its duration of action in renal failure have been debated. The protein binding of thiopentone is altered in renal failure because albumin levels are decreased in uremia.[140] In healthy volunteers, 28% of thiopentone remains unbound, but 56% is unbound in uremic patients. Acidosis further increases the amount of nonionized drug available.[141]

It has been suggested that the blood-brain barrier may not be intact in patients with uremia, which would make these patients particularly sensitive to lipid-soluble agents, such as thiopentone.[142] It was therefore postulated that uremia results in an increased sensitivity to thiopentone; hence the recommendation for reduced doses.[143]

Burch and Stanski and Christensen et al. have challenged this recommendation.[144, 145] Burch and Stanski found that when total drug concentrations were used in calculations, decreased protein binding resulted in altered clearance and total volume of distribution at steady state, but after adjusting for the reduction in protein binding, the unbound volume of distribution and tissue binding were unchanged. Thus, they suggested that the rate of administration should be slower, but the total dose of thiopentone is not different.

Similarly, Christensen et al. compared patients with renal failure to healthy controls and found reduced protein binding of thiopentone but no reduction in sleep dose and no difference in hemodynamic response, stroke volume, or cardiac output.[145] The arterial and venous sleep concentrations were similar, with no evidence to support increased brain sensitivity to thiopentone. Therefore, thiopentone should be titrated slowly and carefully while hemodynamic parameters are closely monitored.

Propofol

Propofol is a unique intravenous agent suitable for both induction and maintenance of anesthesia. Propofol has no adverse effects on renal function and may be used in patients with renal failure. Studies of propofol in uremic patients indicate no alteration in terminal half-life or clearance.[146] Clearance of propofol is primarily metabolic; less than 0.3% is excreted unchanged in the urine.[147]

Clearance values for propofol are 30% greater than hepatic blood flow. Extensive extrahepatic metabolism has been suggested.[148, 149] Gray et al. have confirmed this while studying propofol metabolism during the anhepatic phase of liver transplantation.[150] Pulmonary extraction contributes to the elimination of propofol in sheep; this has also been postulated in humans but was not confirmed in the study by Gray et al. during hepatic transplantation.[151, 152] Both rat and human studies suggest that the gut wall also participates in the extrahepatic metabolism of propofol.[150, 153]

Use of propofol for total intravenous anesthesia during renal transplantation has also been reported.[154, 155] Compared to inhalational anesthesia, the incidence of postoperative nausea and vomiting was reduced after propofol; otherwise, recovery was very similar with the two techniques. It is unlikely that the reduction in nausea and vomiting alone can justify the increased cost of propofol for total intravenous anesthesia.

Opiates

Patients with renal failure are typically hypertensive and on a variety of medications. Intravenous opioids, such as fentanyl, are commonly used to blunt the hemodynamic response to tracheal intubation. Overall, fentanyl has been the most commonly used intraoperative opioid, and morphine has been the most commonly used postoperative opioid.[103, 121, 123]

Fentanyl

Fentanyl has been used extensively in renal transplantation. The elimination of fentanyl is mainly due to hepatic metabolism, and only approximately 10% is excreted by the kidneys.[156] A radioimmunoassay technique has demonstrated that only 21% of the initial dose of fentanyl is excreted within 50 hours.[157]

Uremia has no influence on the binding of fentanyl.[158] The pharmacokinetics of fentanyl during anesthesia is not altered in patients with renal failure. The pharmacokinetics of fentanyl studied in patients during dialysis showed an increase in volume of distribution and systemic clearance.[159]

Morphine

Prolonged and profound analgesia, sedation, and respiratory depression have been reported in uremic patients receiving morphine.[160–164] Cancer patients with increased plasma creatinine concentrations, when allowed to titrate their analgesia, require only one-fourth of the average dose of morphine.[165] Yet, the literature on the pharmacokinetics of morphine in renal failure is conflicting and confusing.

Early studies found alterations in morphine pharmacokinetics. Olsen found reduced protein binding of morphine in patients with renal failure: 25–30% compared to 35% for healthy controls.[166] In a study of morphine kinetics during renal transplantation, Moore et al. found that although the terminal half-life of morphine was no different, the plasma morphine concentrations were higher.[167] After transplantation, when the creatinine concentrations fell, the morphine concentrations also fell. Therefore, they concluded that morphine kinetics were different during transplantation in anesthetized and nonanesthetized controls. Other studies concluded that the kinetics of morphine were altered in uremia.[168] Later studies found conflicting results. Using gas chromatography and mass spectrometry, no alteration in drug disposition was observed when morphine was administered to patients with chronic renal failure compared to healthy controls.[169, 170] They concluded that renal failure does not impair the elimination of morphine. Similarly, radioimmunoassay techniques have also shown unaltered morphine disposition in patients with chronic renal failure undergoing arteriovenous fistula creation.[171] Sawe and Odar-Cederlof found that pharmacokinetic data were no different for patients with normal and abnormal renal function.[172] However, the concentrations of active morphine metabolites were increased. Osborne et al., Chauvin et al., and Aitkenhead et al. concluded that renal failure did not alter elimination of unchanged morphine, but it did cause accumulation of the morphine metabolites.[163, 169, 171] Sear et al. assayed the two glucuronide metabolites separately.[173] They gave uremic patients undergoing transplantation 10 mg morphine. Elimination half-life for the active metabolites was 2–4 times longer in uremic patients than in healthy anesthetized controls. This study reaffirmed that renal failure does not impair the clearance of morphine but does alter clearance of the active glucuronide metabolites.

Therefore, earlier studies that concluded that renal failure impairs the clearance of morphine had unintentionally measured active morphine metabolites.[167, 168] It is postulated that the metabolites of morphine are eliminated slowly, are both physiologically and analgesically active, and are responsible for the prolonged duration of action observed clinically in patients with renal failure.[174] It is prudent to anticipate a greater degree and duration of effect, as well as prolonged side effects for a given dose. Opioid analgesia should be carefully titrated to effect in each patient.

Meperidine

Repeated doses of meperidine result in the accumulation of the active metabolite normeperidine.[175] This may result in irritability, twitching, and, ultimately, seizures; therefore, it has potentially serious consequences for patients with renal failure.[176] Due to the toxicity of its metabolites, meperidine is not the preferred analgesic for postoperative pain.

Alfentanil

Studies of the pharmacokinetics of alfentanil in renal failure have reported an increase in the free fraction of alfentanil and a larger total drug volume of distribution.[177, 178] However, there were no differences in free drug volume or systemic clearance.[179] Continuous infusions of alfentanil have been successfully combined with propofol for total intravenous anesthesia during renal transplantation.[155]

Sufentanil

Sufentanil has a high hepatic extraction ratio and requires little renal involvement in drug clearance.[180, 181] In studies by Fyman et al. and Sear, there were no apparent differences in the concentration-effect relationship between normal patients and those with renal failure.[182, 183] There also were no differences in elimination half-life, clearance, volume of distribution, or binding to plasma proteins. Pharmacokinetic data suggest that sufentanil is suitable for uremic patients and that a reduction of sufentanil dose is unnecessary in uremic patients undergoing renal transplantation. Nevertheless, prolonged ventilatory depression with altered drug kinetics has been reported when sufentanil was given to patients with renal failure.[184]

Muscle Relaxants

First, are muscle relaxants necessary at all? Renal transplantation is a lower-abdominal extraperitoneal procedure, and for decades it has been known that minimal relaxation is required.[118, 124, 185] In 3 of 19 patients described by Wyant, general anesthesia with nitrous oxide and inhalational agents alone produced sufficient relaxation.[119] Furthermore, the use of inhalational agents, such as isoflurane, significantly reduces the dose of muscle relaxants required for adequate surgical conditions.[186, 187]

Neuromuscular blocking drugs can be divided by their mode of excretion[188]:

1. Entirely by the kidney (e.g., gallamine)
2. Predominantly by the kidney but also by the liver (e.g., pancuronium)
3. Predominantly by the liver but also by the kidney (e.g., D-tubocurarine, vecuronium, rocuronium)
4. Removed by other metabolic pathways (e.g., succinylcholine, atracurium, mivacurium)

Prolonged paralysis after nondepolarizing muscle relaxants was first described in patients receiving gallamine.[189] Pancuronium is associated with persistent block in 7% of patients with renal failure.[122] Morgan and Lumley found that 1% of patients who received nondepolarizing muscle relaxants (D-tubocurarine and pancuronium) failed to breathe adequately.[113] Rouse et al. surveyed 247 patients undergoing renal transplantation and found that 7 of the 65 patients who had received either pancuronium or D-tubocurarine required ventilation (up to 6 days).[190] Difficulty has been encountered with as little as 15 mg of D-tubocurarine or 4 mg of pancuronium. Therefore, any neuromuscular blocking agent or active metabolites that accumulate increase the risk of prolonged neuromuscular block in patients with renal failure.

Various neuromuscular blocking agents have been used successfully in patients with renal failure. Problems with relaxants can be avoided by using smaller doses, avoiding repeated incremental dosing (particularly toward the end of surgery), using inhalational agents to reduce the requirement for muscle relaxation, and closely monitoring the neuromuscular blockade. Muscle relaxants of intermediate duration of action offer a greater margin of safety and therefore offer a significant advantage in uremia. Furthermore, agents not requiring renal function for their elimination are optimal for these patients. Consequently, the most popular neuromuscular blocking agent for use in renal transplantation is atracurium.

Succinylcholine

Succinylcholine is not dependent on renal excretion and has the most rapid onset of action of all muscle relaxants. It is the agent of choice for rapid endotracheal intubation. Concerns in renal failure include reduced pseudocholinesterase activity and hyperkalemia. Succinylcholine has been used without the report of prolonged paralysis or hyperkalemia in six reviews of 818 patients with renal failure.[112, 185, 186, 191, 192]

Pseudocholinesterase.   Evidence conflicts on whether pseudocholinesterase is reduced in renal failure. Wyant described a reduction in pseudocholinesterase activity in patients after hemodialysis.[119] Pseudocholinesterase levels were measured in 18 patients; 11 patients had pretransplant nephrectomy, 3 of the 11 patients had low pseudocholinesterase activity, and in two of these three patients, the levels had returned to normal at the time of transplantation. The remaining seven patients underwent nephrectomy at the time of transplantation, and two of the seven had low levels. In contrast, Ryan measured serum cholinesterase concentrations in 81 patients with chronic renal failure and did not find significant differences in cholinesterase concentrations in patients undergoing dialysis.[193]

These findings are supported by Desmond and Gordon, who found that hemodialysis had no effect on pseudocholinesterase levels in 17 patients with chronic renal failure.[194] Thomas and Holmes found similar results, comparing pseudocholinesterase levels pre- and postdialysis in 100 patients; 31 were less and 64 greater after dialysis.[195] They concluded that patients who require hemodialysis tend to have lower pseudocholinesterase values. These values did not fall to critically low levels, however, and the reduction in pseudocholinesterase was more likely due to renal failure rather than dialysis. Although the activity of plasma cholinesterase may be lower in uremic patients than in patients with normal renal function, this seems to be of minimal clinical importance because it does not appear to significantly prolong the duration of action of succinylcholine.[195] The early cellophane types of membranes did lower the serum cholinesterase, but newer dialysis membranes do not cause this problem. Therefore, succinylcholine is not contraindicated because of prolonged paralysis.

Hyperkalemia.   An intubating dose of succinylcholine increases serum potassium by an average of 0.5 mEq/liter due to leakage of potassium from the muscle membrane.[196] The largest rise in serum potassium after succinylcholine was 0.7 mEq/liter.[192] The rise in potassium may not be attenuated by precurarization and is unpredictable.[196]

Compamanes et al. reported three cardiac arrests in patients with known hyperkalemia who received succinylcholine.[197] Hampers et al. reported one patient with a potassium value of 6.1 mEq/liter who received succinylcholine and had a fatal cardiac arrest.[198] Roth and Wuthrich described two cases of succinylcholine-induced hyperkalemia and cardiac arrest.[199] Both patients had significantly elevated serum potassium values preoperatively: 6.2 and 6.5 mEq/liter. In another case, succinylcholine-induced hyperkalemia was blamed for ventricular tachycardia.[200] This patient was a 44-year-old woman with a preoperative potassium value of 4.1 mEq/liter. She received 50 mg of succinylcholine before endotracheal intubation. Anesthesia was maintained with halothane and nitrous oxide. When she was transferred onto the operating room table, she coughed and received another 20 mg of succinylcholine. Ten minutes later, after skin incision, she received an additional 20 mg of succinylcholine. Three doses were given, totaling 90 mg of succinylcholine. She developed ventricular tachycardia, and her potassium level was 6.9 mEq/liter. Despite treatment with sodium polystyrene, 6 hours postoperatively her potassium rose to 7.5 mEq/liter. The hyperkalemia was persistent, lasting 24 hours. Typically, the rise in potassium due to succinylcholine is transient, lasting only 15 minutes.[192] Koide and Waud reported another uremic patient with normal potassium value who experienced an increase of 0.2 mEq/liter with the first dose of succinylcholine but a rise of 1.0 mEq/liter with the second dose.[196] Therefore, successive doses of succinylcholine may be important. However, Katz et al., in a series of cases, used succinylcholine for intubation followed by an infusion and reported no problems.[185]

Hyperkalemia is not the only biochemical abnormality in uremic patients. Nevertheless, succinylcholine-induced hyperkalemia seems to be associated with a higher probability of cardiac arrest. Therefore, succinylcholine should be avoided in patients with pre-existing hyperkalemia greater than 5.5 mEq/liter.[201] Repeated doses of succinylcholine may cause marked increases in serum potassium levels. Succinylcholine should also be avoided in patients with uremic neuropathy because of the potential risk of profound hyperkalemia due to an exaggerated release of potassium in patients with nerve injury.[202]

D-Tubocurarine

As much as 20% of D-tubocurarine is excreted by the liver.[203, 204] Because it is less dependent on renal excretion than pancuronium, D-tubocurarine has been used extensively in patients with renal failure. However, there are numerous case reports of prolonged neuromuscular blockade in patients with renal failure given D-tubocurarine.[100, 122, 190, 205, 206] Other disadvantages include slow onset time and its propensity to cause ganglionic blockade, resulting in hypotension.

Pancuronium

Renal excretion accounts for up to 80% of pancuronium elimination, whereas biliary excretion accounts for only 10%.[203] Prolonged paralysis is therefore not unusual after the administration of pancuronium in patients with renal failure, despite the use of relatively small doses.[207–211] The prolonged duration of action of pancuronium and accumulation of active metabolites (3,OH-pancuronium), coupled with a significant incidence of residual paralysis (21–42%) due to inadequate reversal in patients with normal renal function, and numerous case reports of prolonged paralysis in patients with chronic renal failure make pancuronium a poor choice. Intermediate-acting relaxants, such as vecuronium or atracurium, are preferable.[212–215]

Vecuronium

Prolonged paralysis has been described in uremic patients during short- and long-term administration of vecuronium.[216, 217] Vecuronium is a monoquaternary homologue of pancuronium but has no significant cardiac effects, unlike pancuronium, which produces tachycardia. Both pancuronium and vecuronium are metabolized in the liver by the same deacetylation reaction. Vecuronium is deacetylated, producing 3-desacetyl, 17-desacetyl, and 3,17-desacetyl vecuronium; all three metabolites are active neuromuscular blocking compounds and depend on renal function for their elimination. The main metabolite is 3-desacetyl vecuronium; it has been implicated in prolonged paralysis.[218]

Initial studies found no difference in vecuronium metabolism in renal failure.[219–221] Hunter et al. found no difference in duration of action and no evidence of accumulation, but administration of vecuronium was limited to several hours.[220] It is important to consider the potential for accumulation of the active metabolites of vecuronium in patients with renal failure, particularly during prolonged administration. Bevan et al. studied the administration of repeated doses of vecuronium in uremic patients and in normal patients.[222] Uremic patients receiving more than 10 top-up doses (usually over 2 hours) showed a 50% increase in the duration of action of vecuronium. This was not seen in patients with normal renal function. Nevertheless, all patients were easily reversed, with no evidence of reparalysis.

Bencini et al. also found that renal failure decreases the plasma clearance of vecuronium.[223] The duration of action and the recovery rate as well as the pharmacokinetics of vecuronium only marginally alter the pharmacokinetics of vecuronium in renal failure. Repeated doses of vecuronium given to patients in renal failure result in a prolonged duration of action due to accumulation of vecuronium metabolites.[224, 225]

Beauvoir et al. performed a meta-analysis of studies examining the pharmacodynamics of vecuronium in patients with renal failure. They found no differences in onset time or in the recovery index, but the duration of action was longer in renal failure.[226] Pollard et al. suggested that vecuronium should be used with caution in patients with renal failure due to the possibility of prolonged paralysis.[227]

Rocuronium

Rocuronium is similar to vecuronium with respect to the variables derived from the plasma concentration decay curves and the proportion excreted renally.[228] Rocuronium is mainly excreted by the liver. Pharmacokinetic and pharmacodynamic studies in humans suggest that its duration of action may be more prolonged in patients with hepatic disease than in patients with renal disease. The effect is likely to be modest and not a contraindication to its use.[188]

Atracurium

Atracurium is the ideal neuromuscular blocking agent for patients with chronic renal failure.[220, 229] It is broken down by Hofmann elimination and nonspecific esterases, as well as nonenzymatic decomposition.[230] Neither the liver nor the kidney plays a major role in its metabolism or elimination. The pharmacokinetics and pharmacodynamics of atracurium are therefore not altered by renal failure.[229] Several studies have shown no prolongation of effect or evidence of accumulation in patients with renal failure.[224, 231, 232]

One of the major metabolites of atracurium is laudanosine, which is a central nervous system stimulant. Laudanosine has produced seizures in dogs, but its seizure threshold for humans is unknown. Fahey found the concentration of laudanosine elevated in patients with renal failure.[233] However, levels have not been sufficient to elicit seizure activity and are far less than the levels required to produce seizures in dogs. Approximately 4–9% of laudanosine is excreted by the kidneys; the remaining portion depends on hepatic metabolism. Consequently, the elimination half-life of laudanosine is similar in uremic patients and patients with normal renal function.[233, 234]

Possible histamine release and concomitant hypotension are theoretic concerns with atracurium. Hunter et al. found a small decrease in blood pressure with atracurium compared to vecuronium in anephric patients.[220] Hypotension can be reduced significantly by avoiding rapid bolus injection of large doses.

Cisatracurium

Cisatracurium, a stereoisomer of atracurium, is approximately three to four times as potent, has a similar duration of action, and has none of the histamine-releasing properties of atracurium.[235, 236] It also undergoes Hofmann elimination and ester hydrolysis and is therefore independent of renal or hepatic function for its metabolism.[237, 238] Due to its increased potency, a smaller amount of mass of drug is given. As a result, significantly less laudanosine will be produced.[239]

Mivacurium

Mivacurium is a new short-acting nondepolarizing muscle relaxant. Cook et al. studied the pharmacokinetics of mivacurium in patients with renal failure and found that duration of neuromuscular blockade was 1.5 times longer in patients with renal failure.[240]

The dose of mivacurium necessary to maintain 95% neuromuscular block was similar in patients with normal and abnormal renal function. After continuous infusion of mivacurium, recovery from neuromuscular block is significantly prolonged in patients with renal failure. The pharmacodynamics of mivacurium is closely correlated to pseudocholinesterase activity but not to creatinine clearance.[241]

Potentiation of Muscle Relaxants by Inhalational Agents

A dose-dependent potentiation of the effects of neuromuscular blocking agents is observed when inhaled anesthetics are used.[242] Isoflurane and enflurane are more potent than halothane, which is in turn more potent than nitrous oxide-narcotic anesthesia in augmenting the neuromuscular blocking agents.[187] Isoflurane potentiates the effect of atracurium but potentiates vecuronium less than do other nondepolarizing muscle relaxants.[243] Both atracurium and vecuronium are less affected by inhaled anesthetics than are long-acting neuromuscular blocking agents, such as pancuronium.[244] During isoflurane anesthesia (compared to a narcotic-nitrous oxide technique), the effective dose (ED) values of atracurium and vecuronium are reduced approximately 20%, but the ED values of D-tubocurarine and pancuronium are reduced as much as 50%.[245] It is therefore important to continuously monitor the degree of neuromuscular block with a peripheral nerve stimulator.

Reversal of Neuromuscular Blocking Agents

Patients with renal failure are at increased risk for developing postoperative respiratory complications due to accumulation of muscle relaxants or their metabolites that require renal function for their elimination. Great care must be taken to ensure that muscle relaxants are adequately reversed, as determined by the peripheral nerve stimulator and clinical signs of adequate reversal, such as sustained head lift.

Neostigmine, edrophonium, or pyridostigmine can all be used in uremic patients. Pyridostigmine undergoes only 25% hepatic metabolism, whereas neostigmine is 50% metabolized. In uremic patients, pyridostigmine therefore has a longer duration of action. Absence of renal function decreases excretion of all acetylcholinesterase inhibitors to a similar extent.[246, 247] The duration of action of neostigmine, edrophonium, and pyridostigmine are therefore all prolonged in renal failure.[248] The renal clearance of the anticholinesterase is reduced even more than with pancuronium and D-tubocurarine; therefore, the antagonist should outlast the muscle relaxant. Residual blockade or recurarization likely indicates accumulation of either the relaxant or its active metabolites, or both.

Inhalational Agents

Inhalational agents are rapidly eliminated from the body by the lungs, independent of renal function. An important advantage of inhalational agents is that they reduce or eliminate the need for muscle relaxants.[119, 124, 185, 187]

Enflurane

Approximately 2% of enflurane is metabolized by the liver. The inorganic fluoride levels seldom exceed the nephrotoxic threshold of 20 μm/liter.[249–251] Peak fluoride levels above 25 μm/liter are seldom achieved with enflurane, unless its metabolism is increased by enzyme induction, as seen during isoniazid therapy.[249] Case reports do exist, however, of renal failure associated with high fluoride levels after enflurane anesthesia.[252–254]

In renal transplantation patients who were given enflurane, no untoward effects on graft function could be detected in two separate studies.[255, 256] However, Wickstrom showed that patients undergoing renal transplantation who received enflurane had increases in serum organic fluoride levels approaching 75% of the nephrotoxic threshold.[257] They concluded that "enflurane should not be routinely used for renal transplantation."

Halothane

Approximately 10–20% of halothane is metabolized by the liver but produces negligible amounts of fluoride. Halothane has been used extensively in renal transplantation.[100, 112, 119] Patients with renal failure may also have known hepatic impairment; the use of halothane in these individuals is controversial. Halothane hepatitis has been reported after renal transplantation, but the issue is complicated by the hepatotoxicity of immunosuppressive agents.[258] Halothane may be more depressing to the cardiovascular system than is isoflurane. It is also associated with a higher incidence of cardiac arrhythmias. Patients with renal failure may present with alterations in fluid and electrolyte balance that augment the arrhythmogenic potential of halothane. In Aldrete's series, six of the seven patients who developed severe arrhythmias were receiving halothane.[112]

Isoflurane

Isoflurane is metabolized to a lesser extent (0.2%) than its isomer enflurane (2%) or halothane (20%).[259] The inorganic fluoride levels produced are of insufficient magnitude to cause renal dysfunction.[260] Although halothane and enflurane have been used extensively in renal transplantation, isoflurane is the inhalational agent of choice due to the reduced incidence of cardiac arrhythmias, minimal hepatic effects, and lack of nephrotoxic metabolites.

Postanesthesia Care

The majority of patients are extubated awake in the operating room. They are transferred to postanesthesia care for continuous monitoring of temperature, oxygen saturation, ECG, noninvasive blood pressure monitoring, and central venous pressure. Postoperative measurements include serum electrolytes, glucose, blood gases, and hemoglobin. Analgesia is provided using intravenous opiates, usually morphine. Renal perfusion is enhanced by maintaining central venous pressure at approximately 10 mm Hg. It is important to maintain adequate central venous pressure in the immediate postoperative period to prevent acute tubular necrosis and delayed graft function. If these patients are overhydrated, however, they may develop hypoxemia and respiratory distress, requiring reintubation and dialysis. The urinary catheter is monitored closely for urine output as evidence of early graft function. Patients typically remain in the recovery room for several hours.

If severe fluid and electrolyte imbalance is experienced intraoperatively (e.g., hyperkalemia, hyponatremia, or acidosis) it may be prudent to transfer the patient directly from the operating room to the intensive care unit instead of the recovery room for immediate dialysis and monitoring. In patients with hyperkalemia and acidosis, ventilation should be maintained. This will allow hyperventilation to compensate for metabolic acidosis and prevent further increases in serum potassium. Patients who experience both metabolic acidosis and hyperkalemia, if extubated, may be unable to compensate

for metabolic acidosis by increasing their respiratory rate (compensatory respiratory alkalosis).[261] This could result in further acidosis and hyperkalemia, which could ultimately be fatal.

Conclusions

Renal transplantation has become a relatively common procedure. It is now offered to patients with an increasingly challenging array of medical problems, and yet the mortality associated with anesthesia for renal transplantation remains low. Preoperative dialysis is of fundamental importance because it reverses many of the biochemical abnormalities caused by uremia. Modern anesthetic agents provide a greater margin of safety. There is no single or correct anesthetic for all patients with renal failure. With a clear understanding of the pharmacokinetics of anesthetic agents and an appreciation of the changes incurred by renal failure, many agents are being used successfully. During renal transplantation, the anesthesiologist must optimize volume status, perfusion pressure, and other factors that affect the function and survival of the renal graft.

References

1. Carrel A. La technique operatoire des anastomoses vascularis, et la transplantation des visceres. Lyon Med 1902;98:859–880.
2. Guthrie CC. Blood Vessel Surgery and its Application. New York: Longmans Green, 1912.
3. Floresco M. Transplantation des organs; conditions anatomiques et techniques de la transplantation du rein. J Physiol Path Gen 1905;7:27–31.
4. Jaboulay M. Greffe de reins sau pli du conde sor dures arterielles et veinuses. Lyon Med 1906;107:575–576.
5. Hume DM, Merrill JP, Harrison JH. Homologous transplantation of human kidneys. J Clin Invest 1952;31:640.
6. Hume DM, Merrill JP, Miller BF, Thorn GW. Experiences with renal homotransplantation in the human: report of nine cases. J Clin Invest 1955;34:327–382.
7. Lawler RH, West JM, McNulty PH, et al. Homotransplantation of the kidney in humans. JAMA 1950;144:844–845.
8. Murray JE, Merrill JP, Harrison JH. Renal homotransplantation in identical twins. Surg Forum 1955;6:432–436.
9. Murray JE, Merrill JP, Dammin GJ, et al. Study on transplantation immunity after total body irradiation: clinical and experimental investigation. Surgery 1960;48:272–284.
10. Hamburger J, Vaysse J, Crosnier J, et al. Renal homotransplantation in man after radiation of the recipient:

experience with six patients since 1959. Am J Med 1962;32:854–871.

11. Franksson C. Letter to the editor. Lancet 1964;1: 1331–1332.

12. Starzl TE, Marchioro TL, Waddell W, et al. Splenectomy and thymectomy in human renal transplantation. Proc Soc Exp Biol Med 1963;113:929–937.

13. Schwartz RS, Dameshek W. Drug-induced immunological tolerance. Nature 1959;183:1682.

14. Elion GB. The George Hitchings and Gertrude Elion Lecture, The pharmacology of azathioprine. Ann N Y Acad Sci 1993;685:400–407.

15. Woodruff MFA, Anderson NF. Effect of lymphocyte depletion by thoracic duct fistula and administration of antilymphocyte serum on the survival of skin homografts in rats. Nature 1963;200:702.

16. Starzl TE, Marchioro TL, Porter KA, et al. The use of heterologous antilymphoid agents in canine renal and liver homotransplantation and in human renal transplantation. Surg Gynecol Obstet 1967;124:301–318.

17. Borel JF, Feurer C, Gubler HU, et al. Biological effects of cyclosporine A: a new antilymphocyte agent. Agents Actions Suppl 1976;6:468–475.

18. Calne RY, Rolls K, White DJG. Cyclosporine A initially as the only immunosuppressant in 34 recipients of cadaveric organs: 32 kidneys, 2 pancreas, and 2 livers. Lancet 1979;2:1033–1036.

19. United States Renal Data System (USRDS). 1992 annual data report. Mortality rate comparison of never, previously, and currently transplanted ESRD patients. Am J Kidney Dis 1992;20(Suppl 2):55–60.

20. U.S. Scientific Registry for Transplant Recipients. 1995 Annual Report: Organ Procurement and Transplantation Network, transplant data: 1988–1994. Richmond, VA: United Network for Organ Sharing and Division of Transplantation, Bureau of Health Resources Development, Health Resources and Services Administration. Rockville, MD: U.S. Department of Health and Human Services.

21. Manninen DL, Evans RW, Dugan MK, et al. The costs and outcomes of kidney transplant graft failure. In RW Evans, DL Manninen, FB Dong (eds). The National Cooperative Transplantation Study: Final Report. Seattle: Batelle-Seattle Research Center, 1991.

22. Canadian Institute for Health Information. Canadian Organ Replacement Register Annual Report. Toronto: Canadian Institute for Health Information, 1997.

23. Disney AP. Demography and survival of patients receiving treatment for chronic renal failure in Australia and New Zealand: report on dialysis and renal transplantation treatment from the Australia and New Zealand Dialysis and Transplant Registry. Am J Kidney Dis 1995;25:165–175.

24. United States Renal Data System (USRDS). 1994 annual report. Am J Kidney Dis 1994;24(Suppl 2):S48–S56.

25. Ritz E, Keller C, Bergis K, et al. Pathogenesis and course of renal disease in IDDM/NIDDM: differences and similarities. Am J Hypertens 1997;10(9 Pt 2):202S–207S.

26. Lloyd CE, Becker D, Ellis D, et al. Incidence and complications in insulin dependent diabetes mellitus, a survival analysis. Am J Epidemiol 1996;143:431–434.

27. Latta K, Brodehl J. Primary oxaluria type I. Eur J Pediatr 1990;149:518–520.

28. Anganco R, Thiru S, Esnault VLM, et al. Does truly idiopathic crescentic glomerulonephritis exist? Nephrol Dial Transplant 1994;9:630–636.

29. Eknoyan G, McDonald MA, Appel D, Truong LD. Chronic tubulointerstitial disease. Correlation between structural and functional finding. Kidney Int 1990;38: 736–743.

30. De Broe ME, Elseviiers MM. Analgesic Nephropathy. N Engl J Med 1998;338:446.

31. Pascai RR, Sian CS, Brensiiver JM, Lefavour GS. Demonstration of an antibody to tubular epithelium in glomerulonephritis associated with obstructive uropathy. Am J Med 1980;69:944.

32. Trygvasson K, Zhou J, Hostikka SL, Shoows TB. Molecular genetics of Alport syndrome. Kidney Int 1993; 43:38–40.

33. Parfrey PS, Bear JC, Morgan J, et al. The diagnosis and prognosis of autosomal dominant polycystic kidney disease. N Engl J Med 1990;323:1085–1089.

34. Gabow PA, Johnson AM, Kachny WD, et al. Factors affecting the progression of renal disease in autosomal-dominant polycystic kidney disease. Kidney Int 1992;41:1311-1319.

35. Dedeouglu IO, Fisher JE, Springale JE, et al. Spectrum of glomerulocystic kidneys: a case report and a review of the literature. Pediatr Pathol Lab Med 1996;16:941–949.

36. Bennett WM, Aronoff GR, Golper TA, et al. Drug Prescribing in Renal Failure: Dosing Guidelines for Adults (3rd ed). Philadelphia: American College of Physicians, 1994.

37. Cloonan CC, Gatrell CB, Cushner HM. Emergencies in continuous dialysis patients: diagnosis and management. Am J Emerg Med 1990;8:134–148.

38. Bicknell JM, Lim AC, Rarogue HG. Carpal tunnel syndrome, subclinical median mononeuropathy and peripheral polyneuropathy: common early complication of chronic peritoneal dialysis and hemodialysis. Arch Phys Med Rehabil 1991;72:378–381.

39. Fraser CL, Arieff AI. Nervous system complications in uremia. Ann Intern Med 1988;109(15):143–153.

40. Muirhead N, Bargman J, Burgess E. Evidence-based recommendations for the clinical use of recombinant human erythropoietin. Am J Kidney Dis 1995;26(2 Suppl 1):S1–S24.

41. Loya F, Yang Y, Lin H, et al. Transgenic mice carrying the erythropoietin gene promoter linked to lacZ express the reporter in proximal convoluted tubule cells after hypoxia. Blood 1994;84:1831–1836.

42. Parfrey PS. Cardiac and cerebrovascular disease in chronic uremia. Am J Kidney Dis 1993;21:77–80.

43. Parfrey PS, Harnett JD. The management of cardiac disease in chronic uremia. Curr Opin Nephrol Hypertens 1994;3:145–154.

44. Parfrey PS, Harnett JD, Griffiths SM, et al. The clinical course of left ventricular hypertrophy in dialysis patients. Nephron 1990;55:114–120.

45. Epstein M. Proceedings from renal and metabolic considerations in hypertension: recent advances. Am J Kidney Dis 1993;21(6):S3.

46. Dennis VW, Robinson K. Homocystinemia and vascular disease in end stage renal disease. Kidney Int 1996; 57(Suppl):S11–S17.

47. Olaizola I, Asnarez A, Jorgesti V, et al. Are there any differences in the parathyroid response to the different types of renal osteodystrophy? Nephrol Dial Transplant 1998;13(Suppl 3):15–18.

48. Miles AM, Markell MS, Sumrani N. Severe hyperparathyroidism associated with prolonged hungry bone syndrome in a renal transplant recipient. J Am Soc Nephrol 1997;8:1626–1631.

49. Hakim RM, Lazarus JM. Initiation of dialysis. J Am Soc Nephrol 1995;6:1319–1328.

50. Dumler F, Stalla K, Mohim R, et al. Clinical experience with short-term hemodialysis. J Am Soc Nephrol 1992;19:49–56.

51. Collins DM, Lamber MB, Tannelbaum JS, et al. Tolerance of dialysis: a randomized prospective trial of high-flux versus conventional high-efficiency hemodialysis. J Am Soc Nephrol 1993;4:148–154.

52. Daugirdas JT, Ing TS. First-use reactions during hemodialysis: a definition of subtypes. Kidney Int 1988;24(Suppl):S37–S43.

53. Hertel J, Kimmel PL, Phillips TM, Bosch JP. Eosinophilia and cellular cytokine responsiveness in hemodialysis patients. J Am Soc Nephrol 1992;3:1244–1252.

54. Twardowski ZJ. Peritoneal dialysis glossary III. Perit Dial Int 1990;10:173–175.

55. Drafts HH, Humphries AL, Bowley JN, et al. The impact of pre-transplant obesity on renal transplant outcomes. Clin Transplant 1997;11(5 Pt 2):493–496.

56. Modlin CS, Novick AC, Mastroianni B, et al. Should obese patients lose weight before receiving a kidney transplant? Transplantation 1997;64:599–604.

57. Halme L, Salmela K, Kyllonen L, Eklund B. Is obesity still a risk factor in renal transplantation? Transpl Int 1997;10:284–288.

58. Glass NR, Uehling D, Sollinger H, Belzer F. Renal transplantation using ileal conduits in 5 cases. J Urol 1985;133:666–668.

59. Fornara P, Doehn C, Frick L, et al. Laparoscopic bilateral nephrectomy: results in 11 cases. J Urol 1997:157:445–449.

60. Hubert J, Blum A, Renoult E, et al. Three-dimensional computed tomography scan and maximum intensity projection reconstruction in the pretransplant evaluation of patients at risk of vascular disease. Transplant Proc 1995;27:2433–2434.

61. Mistry BM, Bastani B, Solomon H, et al. Prognostic value of dipyridamole thallium-201 screening to minimize perioperative cardiac complications in diabetics undergoing kidney or kidney-pancreas transplantation. Clin Transplant 1998;12:130–135.

62. Murphy SW, Parfrey PS. Screening for cardiovascular disease in dialysis patients. Curr Opin Nephrol Hypertens 1996;5:532–540.

63. Hruby Z, Myszka-Bijak K, Gosciniak G, et al. *Helicobacter pylori* in kidney allograft recipients: high prevalence of colonization and low incidence of active inflammatory lesions. Nephron 1997;75:25–29.

64. Aguado JM, Herrero JA, Gavalda J, et al. Clinical presentation and outcome of tuberculosis in kidney, liver, and heart transplant recipients in Spain. Spanish Transplantation Infection Study Group, GESITRA. Transplantation 1997;63:1278–1286.

65. Boletis J, Delladetsima J, Psimenou E, et al. Liver biopsy is essential in anti-HCV(+) renal transplant patients irrespective of liver function tests and serology for HCV. Transplant Proc 1995;27:945–947.

66. Pereira BJ, Levey AS. Hepatitis C virus infection in dialysis and renal transplantation. Kidney Int 1997;51:981–999.

67. Penn I. The effect of immunosuppression on pre-existing cancers. Transplantation 1993;55:742–747.

68. Bunce M, Young NT, Welsh KI. Molecular HLA typing—the brave new world. Transplantation 1997;64:1505–1513.

69. Worthington JE, Thomas AA, Dyer PA, Martin S. Detection of HLA-specific antibodies by PRA-STAT and their association with transplant outcome. Transplantation 1998;65:121–125.

70. Scornik JC, Pfaff WW, Howard RJ, et al. Increased antibody responsiveness to blood transfusions in pediatric patients. Transplantation 1994;58:1361–1365.

71. Opelz G, Vanrenterghem Y, Kirste G, et al. Prospective evaluation of pretransplant blood transfusions in cadaver kidney recipients. Transplantation 1997;63:964–967.

72. Soos J. Psychotherapy and counseling with transplant patients. In J Craven, GM Rodin (eds), Psychiatric Aspects of Organ Transplantation. Oxford, UK: Oxford University Press, 1992;89–107.

73. Douglas S, Blixen C, Bartucci MR. Relationship between pretransplant noncompliance and posttransplant outcomes in renal transplant recipients. J Transpl Coord 1996;6:53–58.

74. Johnson EM, Remucal MJ, Gillingham KJ, et al. Complications and risks of living donor nephrectomy. Transplantation 1997;64:1124–1128.

75. Fehrman-Ekholm I, Elinder CG, Stenbeck M, et al. Kidney donors live longer. Transplantation 1997;64:976–978.

76. Borchhardt KA, Yilmaz N, Haas M, Mayer G. Renal function and glomerular permselectivity late after living related donor transplantation. Transplantation 1996;62:47–51.

77. Eberhard OK, Kliem V, Offner G, et al. Assessment of long-term risks for living related kidney donors by 24-h blood pressure monitoring and testing for microalbuminuria. Clin Transplant 1997;11:415–419.

78. Kasiske BL, Bia MJ. The evaluation and selection of living kidney donors. Am J Kidney Dis 1995;26:387–398.

79. Binet I, Bock AH, Vogelbach P, et al. Outcome in emotionally related living kidney donor transplantation. Nephrol Dial Transplant 1997;12:1940–1948.

80. Terasaki PI, Cecka JM, Gjertson DW, Takemoto S. High survival rates of kidney transplants from spousal and living unrelated donors. N Engl J Med 1995;333:333–336.

81. Gaspari F, Perico N, Remuzzi G. Measurement of glomerular filtration rate. Kidney Int 1997;63(Suppl):S 151–S154.

82. Low RN, Martinez AG, Steinberg SM, et al. Potential renal transplant donors: evaluation with gadolinium-enhanced MR angiography and MR urography. Radiology 1998;207:165–172.

83. Cochran ST, Krasny RM, Danovitch GM, et al. Helical CT angiography for examination of living renal donors. AJR Am J Roentgenol 1997;168:1569–1573.

84. Burdick JF, Rosendale JD, McBride MA, et al. National impact of pulsatile perfusion on cadaveric kidney transplantation. Transplantation 1997;64:1730–1733.

85. Smits JM, De Meester J, Persijn GG, et al. Long-term results of solid organ transplantation. Report from the Eurotransplant International Foundation. Clin Transpl 1996; :109–127.

86. Takemoto S, Terasaki PI, Gjertson DW, Cecka JM. Equitable allocation of HLA-compatible kidneys for local pools and minorities. N Engl J Med 1994;22(331): 760–764.

87. Speiser DE, Jeannet M. Renal transplantation to sensitized patients: decreased graft survival probability associated with a positive historical crossmatch. Transpl Immunol 1995;3:330–334.

88. Scornik JC, Brunson ME, Schaub B, et al. The crossmatch in renal transplantation. Evaluation of flow cytometry as a replacement for standard cytotoxicity. Transplantation 1994;57:621–625.

89. Schnitzler MA, Woodward RS, Brennan DC, et al. Impact of cytomegalovirus serology on graft survival in living related kidney transplantation: implications for donor selection. Surgery 1997;121:563–568.

90. Bacon NC. Hospital-acquired hyperkalaemia. Postgrad Med J 1997;73:433–434.

91. Kuvin JT. Images in clinical medicine. Electrocardiographic changes of hyperkalemia. N Engl J Med 1998;338:662.

92. Greenberg A. Hyperkalemia: treatment options. Semin Nephrol 1998;18:46–57.

93. Leadbetter GW, Monaco AP, Russell PS. A technique for reconstruction of the urinary tract in renal transplantation. Surg Gyne Obst 1966;123:839–841.

94. Barnett MG, Bruskewitz RC, Belzer FO, et al. Ileocecocystoplasty bladder augmentation and renal transplantation. J Urol 1987;138:855–858.

95. Sagalowsky AI, Kennedy TJ, Davidson I, Peters PC. Pretransplant bladder rehabilitation in patients with abnormal lower urinary tracts. Clin Transplant 1989;3:198–203.

96. Buerton D, Vu P, Terdjman S, et al. Derivations urinaires et greffens intestinaux en transplantation renale chez l'enfant. Rapport de huit case. Ann Urol 1987;21: 49–54.

97. Kelly WD, Merkel FK, Markland C. Ileal urinary diversion in conjunction with renal homotransplantation. Lancet 1966;1:222–226.

98. Hatch DA, Belitsky P, Barry JM, et al. Kidney transplantation in patients with an abnormal lower urinary tract. Urol Clin North Am 1994;21:311–320.

99. Hatch DA, Belitsky P, Barry JM, et al. Fate of renal allografts transplanted in patients with urinary diversion. Transplantation 1993;56:838–842.

100. Strunin L. Some aspects of anaesthesia for renal homotransplantation. Br J Anaesth 1966;38:812–822.

101. Heino A, Orko R, Rosenberg PH. Anaesthesiological complications in renal transplantation: a retrospective study of 500 transplantations. Acta Anaesthesiol Scand 1986;30:574–580.

102. Marsland AR, Bradley JP. Anaesthesia for renal transplantation—5 years' experience. Anaesth Intensive Care 1983:11:337–344.

103. Lindahl-Nilsson C, Lundh R, Groth CG. Neurolept anaesthesia for the renal transplant operation. Acta Anaesthesiol Scand 1980;24:451–457.

104. Bastron RD. Anesthetic considerations for patients with ESRD. In PG Barash (ed), Refresher Course in Anesthesiology. Philadelphia: Lippincott, 1985;13.

105. Weir PH, Chung FF. Anaesthesia for patients with chronic renal disease. Can Anaesth Soc J 1984;31:468–481.

106. Eschbach JW, Egrie JC, Downing MR, et al. Correction of the anemia of ESRD with recombinant human erythropoietin. N Engl J Med 1987;316:73–78.

107. Group CES. Association between recombinant human erythropoietin and quality of life and exercise capacity of patients receiving haemodialysis. Canadian Erythropoietin Study Group. BMJ 1990;300:573–578.

108. Opelz G, Terasaki PI. Improvement of kidney-graft survival with increased numbers of blood transfusions. N Engl J Med 1978;299:799–803.

109. Opelz G, Terasaki PI. Dominant effect of transfusion on kidney graft survival. Transplantation 1980;29:153–158.

110. Opelz G. Improved kidney graft survival in nontransfused recipients. Transplant Proc 1987;19:149–152.

111. Groth CG. There is no need to give blood transfusions as pretreatment for renal transplantation in the cyclosporine era. Transplant Proc 1987;19:153–154.

112. Aldrete JA, Daniel W, O'Higgins JW, et al. Analysis of anesthetic-related morbidity in human recipients of renal homografts. Anesth Analg 1971;50:321–329.

113. Morgan M, Lumley J. Anaesthetic consideration in chronic renal failure. Anaesth Intensive Care 1975;3: 218–226.

114. Burke JF Jr., Francos GC. Surgery in the patient with acute or chronic renal failure. Med Clin North Am 1987;71:489–497.

115. Rabiner SF, Drake FR. Platelet function as an indicator of adequate dialysis. Kidney Int 1975;2–3:S144–146.

116. Reissell E, Taskinen MR, Orko R, Lindgren L. Increased volume of gastric contents in diabetic patients undergoing renal transplantation: lack of effect with cisapride. Acta Anaesthesiol Scand 1992:36;736–740.

117. Linke CL, Merin RG. A regional anesthetic approach for renal transplantation. Anesth Analg 1976;55:69–73.

118. Vandam LD, Harrison H, Murray JE, Merrill JP. Anesthetic aspects of renal homotransplantation in man. Anesthesiology 1962;23:783–792.

119. Wyant GM. The anaesthetist looks at tissue transplantation: three years' experience with kidney transplants. Can Anaesth Soc J 1967;14:255–275.

120. Estafanous FG, Porter JK, El Tawil MY, Popowniak KL. Anaesthetic management of anephric patients and patients in renal failure. Can Anaesth Soc J 1973;20:769–781.

121. Trudnowski RJ, Mostert JW, Hobika GH, Rico R. Neuroleptanalgesia for patients with kidney malfunction. Anesth Analg 1971;50:679–684.

122. Logan DA, Howie HB, Crawford J. Anaesthesia and renal transplantation: an analysis of fifty-six cases. Br J Anaesth 1974;46:69–72.

123. de-Temmerman P, Gribomont B. Enflurane in renal transplantation: report of 375 cases. Acta Anaesthesiol Scand 1979;71(Suppl):24–31.

124. Samuel JR, Powell D. Renal transplantation. Anaesthetic experience of 100 cases. Anaesthesia 1970;25:165–176.

125. Munda R, Alexander JW, First MR, et al. Pulmonary infections in renal transplant recipients. Ann Surg 1978;187:126–133.

126. Carlier M, Squifflet J, Pirson Y, et al. Maximal hydration during anesthesia increases pulmonary arterial pressures and improves early function of human renal transplants. Transplantation 1982;34:201–204.

127. Carlier M, Squifflet JP, Pirson Y, et al. Anesthetic protocol in human renal transplantation: twenty-two years of experience. Acta Anaesthesiol Belg 1986;37:89–94.

128. Davidson IJ, Sandor ZF, Coorpender L, et al. Intraoperative albumin administration affects the outcome of cadaver renal transplantation. Transplantation 1992;53:774–782.

129. Lauzurica R, Teixido J, Serra A, et al. Hydration and mannitol reduce the need for dialysis in cadaveric kidney transplant recipients treated with CyA. Transplant Proc 1992;24:46–47.

130. Hollenberg N, Birtch P, Rashid A, et al. The relationships between intra-renal perfusion and function serial hemodynamic studies in the transplanted human kidney. Medicine 1972;51:95.

131. Anderson C, Etheredge E. Human renal allograft blood flow and early renal function. Ann Surg 1977;186:564.

132. Luciani J, Frantz P, Thibault P, et al. Early anuria prevention in human kidney transplantation. Transplantation 1979;105:427.

133. Bloembergen W, Muirhead N, Moote C, et al. The effect of intraoperative mannitol on serum potassium in cadaveric renal transplantation. Transplantation 1991;2:792.

134. Bloembergen W, Muirhead N, Moote C, et al. Does intraoperative mannitol cause an increase in serum potassium in cadaveric renal transplantation? Clin Invest Med 1992;15:A149.

135. Grundmann R, Kammerer B, Franke E, et al. Effect of hypotension on the results of kidney storage and the use of dopamine under these conditions. Transplantation 32:184:1981.

136. Moreno M, Murphy C, Goldsmith C. Increase in serum potassium resulting from the administration of hypertonic mannitol and other solutions. J Lab Clin Med 1969;73:291–298.

137. Moote CA, Manninen PH. Mannitol administered during renal transplantation produces profound changes in fluid and electrolyte balance. Can Anaesth Soc J 1987;34:S120.

138. Hirshman CA, Edelstein G. Intraoperative hyperkalemia and cardiac arrests during renal transplantation in an insulin-dependent diabetic patient. Anesthesiology 1979;51:161–162.

139. Hirshman CA, Leon D, Edelstein G, et al. Risk of hyperkalemia in recipients of kidneys preserved with an intracellular electrolyte solution. Anesth Analg 1980;59:283–286.

140. Ghoneim MM, Pandya HB, Kelley SE, et al. Binding of thiopental to plasma proteins: effects on distribution in the brain and heart. Anesthesiology 1976;45:635–639.

141. Ghoneim MM, Pandya H. Plasma protein binding of thiopental in patients with impaired renal or hepatic function. Anesthesiology 1975;42:545–549.

142. Freeman FB, Sheff MF. The blood-cerebro-spinal fluid barrier in uremia. Ann Int Med 1962;56:233.

143. Dundee JW, Richards RK. Effect of azotemia upon the action of intravenous barbiturate anesthesia. Anesthesiology 1954;15:333.

144. Burch PG, Stanski DR. Decreased protein binding and thiopental kinetics. Clin Pharmacol Ther 1982;32:212–217.

145. Christensen JH, Andreasen F, Jansen J. Pharmacokinetics and pharmacodynamics of thiopental in patients undergoing renal transplantation. Acta Anaesthesiol Scand 1983;27:513–518.

146. Kirvela M, Olkkola RT, Rosenburg PH, et al. Pharmacokinetics of propofol and haemodynamic changes during induction of anaesthesia in uraemic patients. Br J Anaesth 1992;68:178–182.

147. Simons PJ, Cockshott ID, Douglas EJ, et al. Disposition in male volunteers of a subanaesthetic intravenous dose of an oil in water emulsion of 14C-propofol. Xenobiotica 1988;18:429–440.

148. Gepts E, Camu F, Cockshott ID, Douglas EJ. Disposition of propofol administered as constant rate intravenous infusion in humans. Anesth Analg 1987;66:887–891.

149. Servin F, Desmonts JM, Haberer JP, et al. Pharmacokinetics and protein binding of propofol in patients with cirrhosis. Anesthesiology 1988;69:887–891.

150. Gray PA, Park GR, Cockshott ID, et al. Propofol metabolism in man during the anhepatic and reperfusion phases of liver transplantation. Xenobiotica 1992;22:105–114.

151. Mather LE, Selby DG, Runciman WB, MacLean CF. Propofol: assay and regional mass balance in the sheep. Xenobiotica 1989;19:1337–1347.

152. Dogra S, Issac PA, Cockshott ID, Foy JM. Pulmonary extraction of propofol in post-cardiopulmonary bypass patients. J Drug Dev 1989;2:133.

153. Mulder GJ, Brouwer S, Scholtens E. High-rate intestinal conjugation of 4-methylumbellifoerone during intravenous infusion in the rat in vivo. Biochem Pharmacol 1984;33:2341–2344.

154. de Gasperi A, Mazza E, Noe L, et al. Pharmacokinetic profile of the induction dose of propofol in chronic renal failure patients undergoing renal transplantation. Minerva Anestesiol 1996;62:25–31.

155. Kirvela M, Yli-Hanakala A, Lindgren L. Comparison of propofol/alfentanil anaesthesia with isoflurane/N20 fentanyl anaesthesia for renal transplantation. Acta Anaesthesiol Scand 1994;38:662–664.

156. Monk PS, Lumley J. Anaesthetic aspects of renal transplantation. Ann Royal Coll Surg 1972;50:254.

157. Schleimer R, Benjamini E, Eisele J, Henderson G. Pharmacokinetics of fentanyl as determined by radioimmunoassay. Clin Pharmacol Ther 1978;23:188.

158. Bower S. Plasma protein binding of fentanyl: the effect of hyperlipoproteinaemia and chronic renal failure. J Pharmacy Pharmacology 1982;34:102–106.

159. Corrall IM, Moore AR, Strunin L. Br J Anaesth 1980; 52:101.

160. Don HF, Dieppa RA, Taylor P. Narcotic analgesics in anuric patients. Anesthesiology 1975;42:745–747.

161. Ball M, Moore RA, Fisher A, et al. Renal failure and the use of morphine in the intensive care. Lancet 1985; 1:784–786.

162. McQuay HJ, Moore RA. Be aware of renal function when prescribing morphine. Lancet 1984;2:284–285.

163. Osborne RJ, Joel SP, Slevin ML. Morphine intoxication in renal failure; the role of morphine-6-glucuronide. Br Med J Clin Res Ed 1986;292:1548–1549.

164. Mostert JW, Evers JL, Hobika GH, et al. Cardiorespiratory effects of anaesthesia with morphine or fentanyl in chronic renal failure and cerebral toxicity after morphine. Br J Anaesth 1971;43:1053–1060.

165. Rengard C, Twycross RG. Metabolism of narcotics. BMJ 1984;288:860.

166. Olsen GD. Morphine binding to human plasma proteins. Clin Pharm Ther 1975;17:31–35.

167. Moore A, Sear J, Baldwin D, et al. Morphine kinetics during and after renal transplantation. Clin Pharm Ther 1984;35:641–645.

168. Sear J, Moore A, Hunniset A, et al. Morphine kinetics and kidney transplantation: morphine removal is influenced by renal ischemia. Anesth Analg 1985;64: 1065–1070.

169. Aitkenhead AR, Vater M, Achola K, et al. Pharmacokinetics of single dose IV morphine in normal volunteers and patients with end-stage renal failure. Br J Anaesth 1984;56:813–819.

170. Woolner DF, Winter D, Frendin TJ, et al. Renal failure does not impair the metabolism of morphine. Br J Clin Pharm 1986;22:55–59.

171. Chauvin M, Sandouk P, Scherrmann JM, et al. Morphine pharmacokinetics in renal failure. Anesthesiology 1987;66:327–331.

172. Sawe J, Odar-Cederlof I. Kinetics of morphine in patients with renal failure. Eur J Clin Pharm 1987; 32:377–382.

173. Sear JW, Hand CW, Moore RA, McQuay HJ. Studies on morphine disposition: influence of renal failure on the kinetics of morphine and its metabolites. Br J Anaesth 1989;62:28–32.

174. Hanna MH, D'Costa F, Peat SJ, et al. Morphine-6-glucuronide disposition in renal impairment. Br J Anaesth 1993;70:511–514.

175. Armstrong PJ, Bersten A. Normeperidine toxicity. Anesth Analg 1986;65:536–538.

176. Szeto HH, Inturrisi CE, Houde R, et al. Accumulation of normeperidine, an active metabolite of meperidine, in patients with renal failure of cancer. Ann Intern Med 1977;86:738–741.

177. Chauvin M, Lebrault C, Levron JC, Duvaldestin P. Pharmacokinetics of alfentanil in chronic renal failure. Anesth Analg 1987;66:53–56.

178. Sear JW, Bower S, Potter D. Disposition of alfentanil in patients with chronic renal failure. Br J Anaesth 1986;58:812P.

179. Bower S. Plasma protein binding of fentanyl: the effect of hyperlipoproteinaemia and chronic renal failure. J Pharm Pharmacol 1982;34:102–106.

180. Schedewie HK, Lee LA, Cowan GS, et al. Hepatic clearance of sufentanil in humans. Anesthesiology 1985;63:708–710.

181. Davis PJ, Stiller RL, Cook DR, et al. Pharmacokinetics of sufentanil in adolescent patients with chronic renal failure. Anesth Analg 1988;67:268–271.

182. Fyman PN, Reynolds JR, Moser F, et al. Pharmacokinetics of sufentanil in patients undergoing renal transplantation [see comments]. Can J Anaesth 1988;35:312–315.

183. Sear JW. Sufentanil disposition in patients undergoing renal transplantation: influence of choice of kinetic model. Br J Anaesth 1989;63:60–67.

184. Wiggum DC, Cork RC, Weldon ST, et al. Postoperative respiratory depression and elevated sufentanil levels in a patient with chronic renal failure. Anesthesiology 1985;63:708–710.

185. Katz J, Kountz SL, Cohn R. Anesthetic considerations for renal transplant. Anesth Analg 1967;46:609–613.

186. Katz RL, Gissen AJ. Neuromuscular and electromyographic effects of halothane and its interaction with D-tubocurarine in man. Anesthesiology 1967;28:564.

187. Miller RD, Way LW, Dolan WM, et al. Comparative neuromuscular effect of pancuronium, gallamine and succinylcholine during Forane and halothane anesthesia in man. Anesthesiology 1971;35:509.

188. Bevan DR, Donati F, Gyasi H, Williams A. Vecuronium in renal failure. Can Anaesth Soc J 1984;31:491–496.

189. Fairley HB. Prolonged intercostal paralysis due to a relaxant. BMJ 190;2:986.

190. Rouse JM, Galley RLA, Bevan DR. Prolonged curarisation following renal transplantation. Anaesthesia 1977;32:247.

191. Jacobsen RH, Christiansen AH, Lunding M. The role of the anaesthetist in the management of acute renal failure. Br J Anaesth 1968;40:442–450.

192. Miller RD, Way WL, Hamilton WK, Layzer RB. Succinylcholine-induced hyperkalemia in patients with renal failure. Anesthesiology 1972;36:138–141.

193. Ryan DW. Preoperative serum cholinesterase concentration in chronic renal failure. Clinical experience of suxamethonium in 81 patients undergoing renal transplant. Br J Anaesth 1977;49:945–949.

194. Desmond JW, Gordon RA. The effect of haemodialysis on blood volume and plasma cholinesterase levels. Can Anaesth Soc J 1969;16:292–301.

195. Thomas JL, Holmes JH. Effect of hemodialysis on plasma cholinesterase. Anesth Analg 1970;49:323–325.

196. Koide M, Waud BE. Serum potassium concentrations after succinylcholine in patients with renal failure. Anesthesiology 1972;36:142–145.

197. Compamanes C, Bellville JE, Boyan CP, et al. Cardiac conduction disturbances during anesthesia in the uremic patient. Anesth Analg 1959;38:283–285.

198. Hampers CL, Bailey GL, Hager EB, et al. Major surgery in patients on maintenance hemodialysis. Am J Surg 1968;115:747–754.

199. Roth F, Wuthrich H. The clinical importance of hyperkalemia following suxamethonium administration. Br J Anaesth 1969;41:311–316.

200. Powell JN. Suxamethonium-induced hyperkalemia in a uremic patient. Br J Anaesth 1970;42:806–807.

201. Gronert GA, Theye RA. Pathophysiology of hyperkalemia induced by succinylcholine. Anesthesiology 1975;43:89–99.

202. Walton JD, Farman JV. Suxamethonium hyperkalemia in uraemic neuropathy. Anaesthesia 1973;28:66–68.

203. McLeod K, Watson MJ, Rawlins MD. Pharmacokinetics of pancuronium in patients with normal and impaired renal function. Br J Anaesth 1976;48:341–345.

204. Cohen EN, Brewer HW, Smith D. The metabolism and elimination of D-tubocurarine. Anesthesiology 1967;28:309–317.

205. Miller RD, Cullen DJ. Renal failure and postoperative respiratory failure: recurarization? Br J Anaesth 1976;48:253–256.

206. Riordon DD, Gilbertson AA. Prolonged curarisation in a patient with renal failure. Br J Anaesth 1971;43:506.

207. Abrams RE, Hornbein TF. Inability to reverse pancuronium blockade in a patient with renal failure and hepatic disease. Anesthesiology 1975;42:362.

208. Geha DG, Blitt CD, Moon BJ. Prolonged neuromuscular blockade with pancuronium in the presence of acute renal failure: a case report. Anesth Analg 1976;55:343.

209. Havill JM, Mee AD, Wallace MR, et al. Prolonged neuromuscular blockade with pancuronium in the presence of renal failure. Anaesth Intensive Care 1978;6:234.

210. Miller RD, Stevens WC, Way WL. The effect of renal failure and hyperkalemia on the duration of pancuronium neuromuscular blockade in man. Anesth Analg 1973;52:661.

211. d'Hollander A, Camu F, Sanders M. Comparative evaluation of neuro-muscular blockade after pancuronium administration in patients with and without renal failure. Acta Anaesthesiol Scand 1978;22:21.

212. Bevan DR, Smith CE, Donati F. Postoperative neuromuscular blockade: comparison between atracurium, vecuronium, and pancuronium. Anesthesiology 1988;69:272–276.

213. Beemer GH, Rozental P. Postoperative neuromuscular function. Anaesth Intensive Care 1986;14:41–45.

214. Howardy-Hansen P, Rasmussen JA, Jensen BN. Residual curarization in the recovery room: Atracurium versus Gallamine. Acta Anaesthesiol Scand 1989;33:167–169.

215. Viby-Mogensen J, Jorgensen BC, Ordin H. Residual curarization in the recovery room. Anesthesiology 1979;50:539–541.

216. Cody MW, Dorman FM. Recurarization after vecuronium in a patient with renal failure. Anaesthesia 1987;42:993–995.

217. Slater RM, Pollard BJ, Doran BRH. Prolonged neuromuscular blockade with vecuronium in renal failure. Anaesthesia 1988;43:250.

218. Agoston S, Seyr M, Khuenl-Brady KS, Henning RH. Use of neuromuscular blocking agents in the intensive care unit. Anesth Clin North Am 1993;22:345–359.

219. Orko R, Heino A, Rosenberg PH. Vecuronium inpatients with and without renal failure. Acta Anaesth Scand 1985;29:325–329.

220. Hunter JM, Jones RS, Utting JE. Comparison of vecuronium, atracurium and tubocurarine in normal patients and in patients with no renal function. Br J Anaesth 1984;56:941–951.

221. Fahey MR, Morris RB, Miller RD, et al. Pharmacokinetics of ORG NC 45 (Norcuron) in patients with and without renal failure. Br J Anaesth 1981;53:1049–1053.

222. Bevan DR, Donati F, Gyasi H, Williams A. Vecuronium in renal failure. Can Anaesth Soc J 1984;31:491–496.

223. Bencini AF, Scaf AHF, Sohn YJ, et al. Disposition and urinary excretion of vecuronium bromide in anesthetized patients with normal renal function or renal failure. Anesth Analg 1986;65:245–251.

224. Lepage JY, Malinge M, Cozian A, et al. Vecuronium and atracurium in patients with end-stage renal failure. Br J Anaesth 1987;59:1004–1010.

225. Peschaud JL, Kienlen J, Rey G, et al. Pharmacodynamics of vecuronium in patients with and without renal failure. Anesthesiology 1990;73:A916.

226. Beauvoir C, Peray P, Daures JP, et al. Pharmacodynamics of vecuronium in patients with and without renal failure: a meta-analysis. Can J Anaesth 1993;40(8):696–702.

227. Pollard BJ, Doran BR. Should vecuronium be used in renal failure? [letter; comment]. Can J Anaesth 1989;36:602–603.

228 Wierda JM, Proost JH, Schiere S, Hommes FD. Pharmacokinetics and pharmacokinetic dynamic relationship of rocuronium bromide in humans. Eur J Anaesthiol 1994;9(Suppl):66–74.

229. Fahey MR, Rupp SM, Fisher DM, et al. The pharmacokinetics and pharmacodynamics of atracurium in patients with and without renal failure. Anesthesiology 1984;61:699.

230. Hughes R, Chapple DJ. The pharmacology of atracurium: a new competitive neuromuscular blocking agent. Br J Anaesth 1981;53:31–44.

231. Mogan-Long D, Chabrol B, Baude C, et al. Atracurium in patients with renal failure. Clinical trial of a neuromuscular blocker. Br J Anaesth 1986;58:44S–48S.

232. de Bros FM, Lai A, Scott R, et al. Pharmacokinetics and pharmacodynamics of atracurium during isoflurane anaesthesia in normal and anephric patients. Anesth Analg 1986;65:743–746.

233. Fahey MR, Rupp SM, Canfell C, et al. Effect of renal failure on laudanosine excretion in man. Br J Anaesth 1985;57:1049–1051.

234. Vine P, Boheimer N, Ward S, et al. Laudanosine pharmacokinetics after bolus atracurium in acute hepatic failure (with acute renal failure). Br J Anaesth 1986;58:1327P.

235. Lien CA, Belmont MR, Abalos A, et al. The cardiovascular effects and histamine-releasing properties of 51W89 in patients receiving nitrous oxide-opioid-barbiturate anaesthesia. Anesthesiology 1995;82:1131–1138.

236. Belmont MR, Lien CA, Abalos A, et al. The clinical neuromuscular pharmacology of 51W89. Anesthesiology 1995;82:1139–1145.

237. Boyd AH, Eastwood NB, Parker CJR, Hunter JM. Pharmacodynamics of the 1R-cis 1'R-cis isomer of atracurium (51W89) in health and chronic renal failure. Br J Anaesth 1995;74:400–404.

238. De Wolf AM, Freeman JA, Scott VL, et al. Pharmacokinetics and pharmacodynamics of cisatracurium in patients with end-stage liver disease undergoing liver transplantation. Br J Anaesth 1996;76:624–628.

239. Smith CE, van Miert MM, Parker CJ, Hunter JM. A comparison of the infusion pharmacokinetics and pharmacodynamics of cisatracurium, the 1R-cis 1'R-cis isomer of atracurium, with atracurium besylate in healthy patients. Anaesthesia 1997;52:833–841.

240. Cook DR, Freeman JA, Lai AA, et al. Pharmacokinetics of mivacurium in normal patients and in those with hepatic or renal failure. Br J Anaesth 1992;69:580–585.

241. Blobner M, Jelen-Esselborn S, Schneider G, et al. Effect of renal function on neuromuscular block induced by continuous infusion of mivacurium. Br J Anaesth 1995;74:452–454.

242. Miller RD, Way LW, Dolan WM, et al. The dependence of pancuronium and D-tubocurarine induced neuromuscular blockades on alveolar concentrations of halothane and Forane. Anesthesiology 1972;37:573.

243. Rupp SM, Fahey MR, Miller RD. Neuromuscular and cardiovascular effects of atracurium during nitrous oxide-fentanyl-isoflurane anaesthesia. Br J Anaesth 1983;55:67S–70S.

244. Miller RD, Rupp SM, Fisher DM, et al. Clinical pharmacology of vecuronium and atracurium. Anesthesiology 1984;61:144.

245. Rupp SM, Miller RD, Gencarelle PJ. Vecuronium induced neuromuscular blockade during enflurane, isoflurane and halothane anesthesia in humans. Anesthesiology 1984;60:102.

246. Cronnelly R, Stanski DR, Miller RD, Sheiner LB. Pyridostigmine kinetics with and without renal function. Clin Pharmacol Ther 1980;28:78–81.

247. Morris RB, Cronnelly R, Miller RD, et al. Pharmacokinetics of edrophonium in anephric and renal transplant patients. Br J Anaesth 1981;53:1311–1313.

248. Cronnelly R, Stanski DR, Miller RD, et al. Renal function and the pharmacokinetics of neostigmine in anesthetized man. Anesthesiology 1979;51:222–226.

249. Mazze RI, Woodruff RE, Heerdt ME. Isoniazid-induced enflurane defluoridation in humans. Anesthesiology 1982;57:5–8.

250. Mazze RI, Calverley RK, Smith NT. Inorganic fluoridenephrotoxicity: prolonged enfluorane and halothane anesthesia in volunteers. Anesthesiology 1997;46:265–271.

251. Cousins MJ, Greenstein LR, Hitt BA, Mazze RI. Metabolism and renal effects of enflurane in man. Anesthesiology 1976;44:44–53.

252. Eichorn JH, Hedley-Whyte J. Renal failure following enflurane anesthesia. Anesthesiology 1976;45:557–560.

253. Hartnett MN, Lane W, Bennett WM. Non-oliguric renal failure and enflurane. Ann Int Med 1974;81:560.

254. Loehning RW, Mazze RI. Possible nephrotoxicity from enflurane in a patient with severe renal disease. Anesthesiology 1974;40:203–205.

255. Goldman E, Goldman MC, Sherill D, Aldrete JA. Enflurane and renal function after transplantation. Anesthesiology 1979;51:S24.

256. de-Temmerman P, Gribomont B. Enflurane in renal transplantation: report of 375 cases. Acta Anaesthesiol Scand 1979;71(Suppl):24–31.

257. Wickstrom I. Enflurane anesthesia in living donor renal transplantation. Acta Anaesthesiol Scand 1981;25:263–269.

258. Slayter KL, Sketris IS, Gulanikar A. Halothane hepatitis in a renal transplant patient previously exposed to isoflurane [letter]. Ann Pharmacother 1993;27:101.

259. Holaday DC, Rudofsky S, Truehaft PS. The metabolic degradation of methoxyflurane in man. Anesthesiology 1970;33:579.

260. Mazze RI, Cousins MJ, Barr GA. Renal effects and metabolism of isoflurane in man. Anesthesiology 1974;40:536–542.

261. Knill RL, Clement JL. Ventilatory responses to acute metabolic acidemia in humans awake, sedated and anesthetized with halothane. Anesthesiology 1985;62:745–753.

Chapter 12
Corneal Transplantation

Kathryn E. McGoldrick and Jonathan Mardirossian

Chapter Plan

The cornea, a clear, spheric tissue covering the iris and pupil, is the most anterior structure of the globe (Figure 12-1). Because light enters the eye through the cornea and because the cornea is responsible for approximately two-thirds of the refracting power of the eye, the cornea must remain transparent, smooth, and of relatively uniform curvature for maximal optical efficiency. Five layers constitute the cornea: the epithelium, Bowman's layer, the stroma, Descemet's membrane, and the endothelium. Although each layer plays a vital role in preserving the clarity of the cornea, the endothelium is paramount. The corneal stroma must be of uniform structure and devoid of opacity or vascularization.

Moreover, stromal deturgescence depends on endothelial function and is critical for corneal transparency. The endothelium is exquisitely vulnerable to mechanical or chemical trespass and has limited capacity for repair. By contrast, corneal epithelium possesses enviable powers of regeneration, and the intact epithelium provides a formidable barrier against most bacteria. If the cornea loses its structural integrity, the viability of the eye is threatened; if the cornea becomes opacified, vision is severely compromised.

Many disease processes can attack the cornea, including inflammation; bacterial, viral, and fungal infections; trauma; congenital or hereditary disorders; vitamin A deficiency; and a spectrum of metabolic diseases. Moreover, corneal edema resulting from endothelial dysfunction may be the legacy of previous intraocular surgery[1] or degenerative alterations. Corneal transplantation, or keratoplasty, can restore corneal function by substituting clear, smooth, healthy donor tissue for the diseased cornea.

History of Corneal Transplantation

Transplantation of human donor material to restore corneal transparency occupies a unique position in the history and science of tissue transplantation. Not only was the cornea the first solid tissue to be transplanted successfully from one individual to another, the cornea also has a degree of immunologic privilege not possessed by other tissues. Indeed, corneal

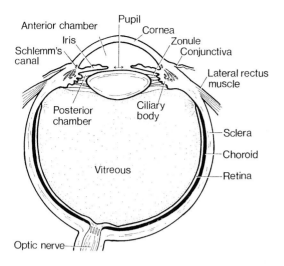

Anterior chamber
Pupil
Iris
Cornea
Schlemm's
canal
Zonule
Conjunctiva
Lateral rectus
muscle
Posterior
chamber
Ciliary
body
Sclera
Choroid
Vitreous
Retina
Optic nerve

Figure 12-1. Ocular anatomy.

transplantation is the most commonly performed transplant procedure. Its results are increasingly satisfying, except in eyes with chronic inflammation or severe exposure.

In 1824, Reisinger first performed full-thickness corneal transplantation, or penetrating keratoplasty, in rabbits.[2] Attempts to transplant corneas in humans met with failure throughout most of the nineteenth century owing to lack of appropriate suture material, suboptimal magnification, and ignorance of immunology. von Hippel,[3] who first performed successful lamellar grafting in humans in 1886, virtually revolutionized corneal transplantation research through the development of his trephine and other increasingly refined instruments. von Hippel's contribution, in conjunction with the development of Lister's theories of antisepsis and the discovery of anesthetic agents, eventually enabled the first successful penetrating corneal graft by Zirm in 1906.[4] Additional refinements in grafting technique can be credited to many people over the ensuing decades, including Paton and others who pioneered in the areas of donor procurement and tissue preservation.[5]

Gradually, the number of corneal transplantations increased during the twentieth century, with 2,000 being performed in 1963.[6] During the next three decades, major advances led to a dramatic increase in the number of successful corneal transplantations. These included the use of the operating

microscope; the availability of topical corticosteroids and other immunosuppressants; improved procurement, processing, and preservation of donor tissue; and appreciation that the corneal endothelium is critical for corneal hydration and clarity. However, the improvements in keratoplasty techniques and in training of corneal surgeons only partially explain the fact that more than 40,000 corneal transplants were performed in 1990 in the United States. Additionally, the indications for surgery have expanded. The increase in the incidence of corneal edema, largely because of the dramatic growth in the number of cataract operations being performed, has played a large part in the increase in keratoplasty.

Types of Keratoplasty

Keratoplasty involves the replacement of diseased cornea by a graft of homologous tissue or, occasionally, by a synthetic substitute. During the early era of corneal transplantation surgery, lamellar, or partial-thickness, keratoplasty was the procedure of choice. Later, penetrating, or full-thickness, keratoplasty became more common as surgical techniques improved and as realization of the importance of the endothelium in regulating corneal hydration became more widely disseminated. Today, lamellar keratoplasty is reserved for certain types of superficial opacity. Although this partial-thickness technique circumvents the risks of an intraocular procedure, the visual results are typically limited by eventual opacification at the interface between the host and donor.

Indications for Corneal Transplantation

The indications for corneal transplantation fall into two major categories. The first is *tectonic*, in which surgery is undertaken to restore the integrity of the cornea. Tectonic grafts may be necessary to eradicate disease processes that have not responded to medical treatment. Progressive ulceration or an infectious process refractory to medical therapy may require surgical intervention. Additionally, an acute corneal perforation may necessitate keratoplasty to restore the anterior chamber because a flat chamber may predispose to the eventual development of intractable glaucoma. The second major category involves *visual indications*, in which the altered state of the cornea prevents adequate vision. Only replacement of an optically inadequate cornea by optically satisfactory tissue can restore vision. Indeed, corneal transplantation is more commonly undertaken to restore optical clarity than to remove disease or to repair perforated or ectatic tissue.

From a pathophysiologic perspective, four major factors undermine the cornea's ability to refract light properly: grossly distorted corneal contour, microscopic irregularity of the corneal surface, increased stromal thickness, and stromal opacity. Diseases, such as keratoconus, marginal degenerations, and postinflammatory scarring, may produce deviations from sphericity and interfere with vision (Figure 12-2). Endothelial decompensation, often resulting in corneal edema, may trigger microscopic irregularity of the corneal surface and increased stromal thickness. Stromal opacity may be the result of postinfectious or posttraumatic scarring.

Although the most common indications for penetrating keratoplasty at the beginning of the twentieth century were corneal scars and later keratoconus, the most frequent indication in the United States at this time is corneal edema. Corneal clarity is inextricably linked to maintenance of a delicate balance of water movement. Water flows into the cornea from the anterior chamber. It must be pumped out by the endothelial monolayer, which is incapable of regeneration once damaged. With loss of endothelial cells, the stroma swells, the cornea becomes edematous and cloudy, and bullous keratopathy results. As the population becomes increasingly elderly, there is increased prevalence of degenerative endothelial disease, such as Fuchs' dystrophy.[7] But even more significant is the marked increase in corneal edema resulting from prior anterior segment surgery.[8] Indeed, most patients with bullous keratopathy have undergone cataract extraction. Pseudophakic bullous keratopathy describes the condition noted when a lens implant is present; aphakic bullous keratopathy describes the condition when no implant is present.

Table 12-1 summarizes data collected by the Eye Bank Association of America describing indications for corneal transplantation. (In Great Britain, keratoconus remains the most common indication for keratoplasty,[9] whereas in the United States today, the majority of patients with keratoconus can be successfully managed with contact lenses.[10, 11]) In

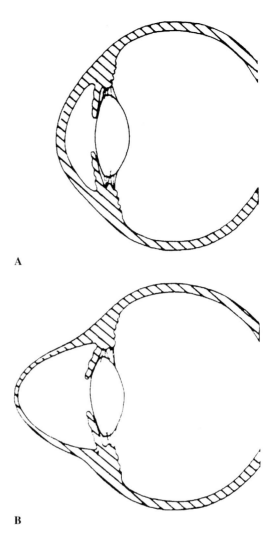

A

B

Figure 12-2. A. Sagittal view of normal cornea. **B.** The protruding, conical cornea characteristic of keratoconus.

the near future, it may be necessary to add another category as an indication for corneal transplantation: complications after such refractive surgical procedures as radial keratotomy, automated lamellar keratoplasty, or excimer laser photorefractive surgery.

Prognostic Factors

Multiple factors interact to determine the prognosis for obtaining a clear graft and for improving vision. In general, these factors pertain to the state of the

Table 12-1. Indications for Penetrating Keratoplasty in 1994

Indication	Percent of Patients
Pseudophakic bullous keratopathy	22.14
Aphakic bullous keratopathy	6.18
Fuchs' endothelial dystrophy	10.55
Corneal dystrophy (other than Fuchs')	3.75
Keratoconus	13.16
Congenital opacities	1.07
Viral or postviral keratitis	1.33
Microbial or postmicrobial keratitis	0.60
Syphilitic or postsyphilitic keratitis	0.32
Noninfectious ulcerative keratitis	0.96
Noninfectious ulcerative perforation	2.49
Corneal degeneration	3.56
Chemical injuries	0.42
Trauma	1.37
Regraft associated with allograft rejection	3.02
Regraft unrelated to allograft rejection	6.11
Unspecified causes of corneal scarring or edema	22.97

Source: Adapted from Eye Bank Association of America. Corneal Transplant Recipient Diagnosis Report. Washington, DC: Eye Bank Association of America, 1994;15.

recipient cornea and the pathologic condition necessitating the transplant, as well as the condition of the ocular adnexa and the presence of coexisting noncorneal ocular pathology. The likelihood of rejection is greater in the presence of intraocular inflammation with scarring, with corneal vascularization, with large grafts exceeding 8.5 mm in diameter, and in the pediatric population. In addition to their limited ability to cooperate, pediatric patients tend to have less successful results after penetrating keratoplasty than do adults, owing to the presence of other ocular malformations, amblyopia, glaucoma, and technical problems in manipulating the more malleable pediatric tissues.

Grafts can also fail in the absence of rejection. Tear function must be evaluated preoperatively because a dry eye or inadequate blinking can foster problems postoperatively. Intact functioning of cranial nerves V and VII is mandatory for surface protection of the graft. In the presence of corneal anesthesia or impaired facial nerve function, tarsorrhaphy may have to be performed to promote adequate healing. Glaucoma should be controlled before performing keratoplasty because pre-

existing glaucoma is often exacerbated by corneal surgery and borderline or latent glaucoma may be unmasked after keratoplasty. Hypotony, however, is associated with an even worse prognosis, and little can be done to correct low tension. Although a meticulous ophthalmic examination often detects other ocular pathology, corneal opacification can interfere with inspection of the retina and optic nerve. In these circumstances, techniques such as visual evoked potentials can be used to estimate visual prognosis.

Broadly speaking, transplants for corneal dystrophies, keratoconus, and small central scars have the best prognosis, with a 90–95% chance of success. This figure is reduced to approximately 85% with transplantation for chronic interstitial keratitis and bullous keratopathy. Transplants for acute corneal perforations and active herpes simplex or bacterial keratitis have only approximately a 50–60% chance of remaining clear. Indeed, herpes simplex infection and corneal dystrophies can recur in the donor graft. Moreover, patients with pemphigoid and, especially, those who sustained severe chemical burns, have an extremely discouraging prognosis for maintaining a clear graft.

Last, the skill and expertise of the surgeon in executing a technically exacting operation and his or her attention to the prevention and prompt management of postoperative complications contribute in no small way to a successful outcome. Similarly, the patient's willingness and ability to meticulously comply with perioperative instructions also influence the surgical result.

Associated Preoperative Considerations

A thorough medical and social history as well as physical and ocular examination must be undertaken before transplantation. The prognostic factors discussed previously must be meticulously evaluated and explained to the patient. Obviously, dry-eye syndrome must be addressed, and intraocular pressure must be controlled. The general physical condition of the patient may render him or her an unacceptable risk for surgery under either local or general anesthesia. If transplantation is being contemplated for a young child, the family's ability to observe the patient carefully and to be intimately involved in the demanding aspects of postoperative care must be assessed. Moreover, proximity to the surgeon and ability to visit the surgeon quickly if signs of graft failure develop should be considered.

Major considerations are whether the patient is disabled from corneal disease and the probability that surgery may actually improve vision. Clearly, the risk-benefit ratio is especially critical in a one-eyed patient. In patients with two eyes, the status of the other eye must be carefully assessed, and the likelihood of adequate binocular vision should be considered. In patients in whom funduscopic examination is inadequate owing to obscurement by the cornea or media, special testing, such as laser interferometry or other tests of macular function, should be performed to realistically assess the likelihood of visual improvement after transplantation.[10] In patients with pseudophakic bullous keratopathy, the type, stability, and position of an existing intraocular lens should be carefully noted. Some lenses, such as the closed-loop anterior chamber variety, are more likely than others to incite corneal damage. Consideration should be given to replacing the potentially hazardous lens with a safer type. In patients with a coexisting cataract, corneal transplantation combined with cataract extraction and intraocular lens implantation may be necessary.

Donor Material

Tissue selection and preservation depend on whether lamellar or penetrating keratoplasty is indicated. If disease is confined to the anterior portion of the cornea, a lamellar keratoplasty can be sufficient. With these partial-thickness transplants, the risk of rejection is low because donor corneal endothelium, which contains the cells most vulnerable to rejection, is not transplanted. Tissue used for lamellar keratoplasty need not contain viable cells. Thus, the donor material may be fresh, preserved by any of a variety of short-term methods, or kept in a dehydrated or frozen state and restored to normal hydration or temperature immediately before use as the lamellar donor graft.

Penetrating keratoplasty, however, mandates careful tissue selection and storage. It is widely accepted that endothelial viability is absolutely essential for successful outcome. Surgeons avoid tissue from eyes with a history of inflammatory conditions, trauma, or previous anterior segment surgery.

The Eye Bank Association of America establishes criteria for donor tissue selection and eye banking in the United States. The age of the donor per se is not a determining factor in graft survival.[12] It is acknowledged, however, that endothelial abnormalities become increasingly common as the eye ages. It is also recognized that donors less than 1 year of age often have a flaccid cornea that may cause extreme myopia in the recipient.

The blood of all potential donors is tested for human immunodeficiency virus, syphilis, and hepatitis A, B, and C. No tissue from donors testing positive for any of these conditions is accepted for transplantation. Other donor conditions that preclude transplantation include Creutzfeldt-Jakob disease; death from neurologic disease of unknown etiology; slowly debilitating neurologic disease; congenital rubella; rabies; septicemia; and known or suspected drug abuse. In addition to these absolute contraindications, other donor exclusion criteria can include patients with Parkinson's disease, multiple sclerosis, diabetes, jaundice, chronic lymphatic leukemia, chronic immunosuppression, and a history of prolonged mechanical life support. In these circumstances, a careful risk-benefit assessment must be undertaken.

Donor corneas are harvested as whole globes or as corneoscleral rims. The interval between donor death and enucleation ideally should be as brief as possible. Although some surgeons believe the interval should be less than 8 hours, some eye banks provide tissues that have been in situ for as long as 18 hours before enucleation, provided the corpse was properly refrigerated. Whole globes may be stored at 4°C in a sterile dry container[13] for 2 days or may be cryopreserved at –80°C for a virtually indefinite interval.[14] Alternatively, the cornea may be excised and placed in an appropriate tissue culture medium.[15] A variety of media, combining dextran, antibiotics, and assorted tissue culture factors and chemicals, allow a corneoscleral button to maintain excellent endothelial viability for approximately 1 week. Storage in artificial media is the most common preservation method used in the United States today.

In contrast to other organ transplants, donor-recipient antigen matching is usually not performed for corneal transplantation. In most circumstances, the likelihood of obtaining a clear graft approaches 90% without antigen matching or systemic immunosuppression. That corneal grafts are typically well tolerated can be attributed to the absence of blood vessels or lymphatics in the normal cornea, the lack of presensitization to tissue-specific antigens in most recipients, and anterior chamber–associated immune deviation. The latter is a series of unique immunologic properties of the anterior chamber, the most important of which is selective suppression of delayed hypersensitivity.[16] Reactions to corneal grafts do occur, however, especially in individuals whose own corneas were injured by previous inflammatory disease. Such corneas may have developed lymphatics and blood vessels, providing both afferent and efferent channels for immunologic reactions in the engrafted cornea.

Many foreign elements exist in corneal grafts that might stimulate the immune system of the host to reject the donor tissue. The corneal stroma is regularly perfused with immunoglobulin G and serum albumin from the donor, although only minimal, if any, other blood proteins are present. These serum proteins of donor origin quickly diffuse into the recipient stroma and are therefore removed from the graft site, but they are theoretically immunogenic. The histocompatibility HLA system may play an important role in graft rejections. Several investigators demonstrated that HLA incompatibility between donor and recipient is significant in determining graft survival, particularly when the corneal bed is vascularized. Most cells of the body possess these HLAs, including the endothelial cells of the corneal graft as well as certain stromal cells.

Despite several analytic studies supporting the role of HLA incompatibility in corneal graft rejection, one multicenter clinical trial found no significant benefit in HLA typing for high-risk grafts, such as patients with corneal vascularization or a history of previous graft rejection.[17] In this study, however, ABO blood typing did afford a modest protective effect in high-risk cases. These surprising findings are stimulating many investigators to restudy the role of major and minor antigens in corneal graft rejection.

Regardless of the method of preservation of donor tissue and of whether HLA matching or ABO blood typing is undertaken, the distribution of tissue is determined at the local level, often facilitated through computer-assisted distribution centers. These centers coordinate the functions of affiliated eye banks and allow efficient and effective distribution of tissue.

Surgical Procedure

Each patient must have appropriate medical and ophthalmic evaluation before surgery. As previously mentioned, the preoperative ophthalmic evaluation should identify conditions whose modification or correction may improve the prognosis for a successful graft. These factors include active anterior segment inflammation, lid margin irregularities, inadequate lid closure, and uncontrolled glaucoma.

The donor eye is prepared in one of two ways. For penetrating keratoplasty, the corneoscleral cap is placed endothelium up on a Teflon block. The trephine is pressed down into the cornea, and a full-thickness button is punched out. In lamellar keratoplasty, a partial-thickness trephine incision is made in the cornea of a whole globe and the lamellar button is dissected free. Occasionally, certain refinements in technique may be necessary.

A trephine is positioned on the central corneal mark and a partial-thickness cut (approximately 0.3 mm) is made to remove the recipient's corneal button. It is prudent not to enter the anterior chamber with a trephine; entrance to the anterior chamber is more safely accomplished with a sharp blade held at an angle. The incision is then extended around the circumference of the host's button with corneal scissors. Before introducing the scissors, it is often useful to insert a viscoelastic substance, such as sodium hyaluronate (Viscoat). This reforms the chamber to facilitate excision with the scissors and helps to prevent forward displacement of the lens-iris diaphragm, the vitreous, or the intraocular contents. After the recipient's button has been removed, it is stored in sterile saline. It is imperative to keep this tissue sterile so that it can be resutured into the patient if the donor tissue is damaged. After the host button has been excised, relevant concomitant procedures can be performed. An attempt is made to correct factors that contributed to the original problem. Synechiae may be lysed, colobomas may be corrected, bulging or adherent vitreous may be removed, intraocular lenses may be exchanged or stabilized, or cataract extraction may be performed.

After all concurrent procedures have been completed and appropriate anterior chamber depth reestablished, the donor button is transferred into the host bed. Throughout the procedure, it is mandatory to prevent direct trauma to the donor corneal endothelium.

Intraocular bleeding from the iris or wound edge usually is self-limited. If it persists, use of irrigating fluid with epinephrine or cautery may prove helpful. The graft is then sutured into place.

Although rare, one of the most devastating complications of any intraocular procedure is an expulsive choroidal hemorrhage, in which brisk bleeding between the choroid and sclera pushes the ocular contents out through the surgical incision. Although this serious complication may not be preventable, risk factors include a history of glaucoma, increased axial length, elevated intraocular pressure, arteriosclerosis, and tachycardia.[18] Intraoperative hypertension may also contribute to the problem.[19, 20] Rapid closure of the wound and drainage of the suprachoroidal hemorrhage are imperative to avoid this catastrophic complication. The visual prognosis is grim if eye contents are extruded. The incidence of suprachoroidal expulsive hemorrhage is 0.56% for keratoplasty, 0.41% for retinal and vitreous procedures, 0.16% for lens-related procedures, and 0.15% for glaucoma surgery.[18]

Suture knots are buried within the stroma of the cornea. Burying the knot enhances patient comfort and eliminates a nidus for irritation and infection. In cases in which the knots cannot be buried completely, applying a soft contact lens in the immediate postoperative period may be beneficial. After completion of the surgical closure, the wound is inspected and, if leakage is observed, additional sutures are placed. Subconjunctival and topical antibiotics are frequently applied, and the eye is then covered with a soft patch and a protective metal shield.

Anesthetic Techniques

Preoperative Assessment

In the United States today, the vast majority of corneal transplantations are scheduled, rather than truly emergent, procedures. Therefore, patients should be well evaluated and in optimal medical condition in terms of coexisting diseases. Furthermore, surgical candidates will have fasted the requisite number of hours. Because a significant percentage of keratoplasties are performed on an outpatient basis, the anesthesiologist's selection of anesthetic agents and techniques must permit a rapid emergence devoid of unpleasant, prolonged side effects. Many patients requiring corneal transplantation are elderly, and special age-related considerations apply, such as altered pharmacokinetics and pharmacodynamics. The margins of safety in fragile geriatric patients are narrowed, and it is important to administer drugs slowly with the minimal effective dose.

Clearly, inappropriate preoperative medical preparation can contribute to perioperative problems.[21] Eye surgery patients tend to be a high-risk group, often having such conditions as hypertension, diabetes or other endocrinopathies, pulmonary disease, or coronary artery disease. Eye surgery, however, tends to be relatively low-risk surgery owing to minimal blood loss, fluid shifts, and postoperative pain. Indeed, mortality associated with ophthalmic surgery[22, 23] is considerably more infrequent than mortality after general surgery.[24, 25]

How should the anesthesiologist and ophthalmologist prepare the high-risk patient having low-risk surgery? First, the high-risk patient's personal physician should be consulted. Patients seeing a physician for treatment of chronic medical problems should visit their physician before surgery. Second, medical history and physical examination should guide all preoperative testing if one is to take a rational approach in the current era of cost-containment. The patient should be deemed an unacceptable risk for elective surgery if he or she is currently medically unstable or has a reversible medical condition that is likely to produce a perioperative complication. Using the aforementioned principles, the following guidelines have been implemented in many institutions. Patients age 50 years and older or with hypertension (regardless of age) all have a preoperative electrocardiogram (ECG). Patients age 65 years and older, with diabetes, or on diuretic therapy have an ECG, serum electrolytes, glucose, and complete blood cell count. Obviously, patients with symptoms of coronary artery disease (regardless of age) would have, at a minimum, a preoperative ECG.

In 1996, the American College of Cardiology and the American Heart Association published guidelines for perioperative cardiovascular evaluation of patients having noncardiac surgery.[26] They consider the major clinical predictors of increased perioperative cardiovascular risk to be unstable coronary syndromes, such as recent myocardial infarction with evidence of important ischemic risk and unstable or severe angina; decompensated congestive heart failure; significant dysrhythmia (e.g., high-grade atrioventricular block or supraventricular dysrhythmias with uncontrolled ventricular rate); and severe valvular disease. The anesthesiologist must also consider the patient's functional capacity and the surgery-specific risk. Thus, a patient with stable angina occurring occasionally on exercise presenting for eye surgery is unlikely to require aggressive preoperative testing. However, the breathless patient on restricted activity with congested neck veins who is unable to lie flat should be studied more extensively and brought to optimal condition before being offered surgery.

The hypertensive patient also deserves mention. Hypertensive patients are at increased risk of left ventricular hypertrophy, congestive heart failure, dysrhythmias, ischemia, and stroke. Untreated hypertensive patients with a sustained systolic blood pressure above 200 mm Hg or a sustained diastolic pressure above 110 mm Hg should be referred to an appropriate physician for antihypertensive therapy before elective surgery. Patients with left ventricular hypertrophy should be assumed to have impaired autoregulation of coronary perfusion; they are vulnerable to ischemia with merely a moderate intraoperative reduction in blood pressure. Therefore, the anesthesiologist must reset the limits of acceptable blood pressure fluctuations perioperatively and attempt to maintain pressures within a 20% range from baseline.[27]

Patients with insulin-dependent diabetes mellitus require individualized treatment. Preoperatively, regardless of age, recommended evaluation includes ECG, electrolytes, glucose, and complete blood count. For patients with renal disease, a blood urea nitrogen and creatinine are indicated. History and physical examination provide information about autonomic dysfunction as well as any anticipated difficulty with intubation. Patients are instructed not to administer their usual insulin on the morning of surgery, and a blood sugar is obtained shortly after the patient's arrival at the surgical facility. Surgery should be postponed if fasting glucose is 400 mg/dl or greater or if any evidence of ketosis is present. If the glucose is 120 mg/dl or greater, one-half the usual subcutaneous dose of neutral protamine Hagedorn (NPH) and regular insulin is administered. An intravenous infusion containing 5% dextrose solution is started at a rate of 100–125 ml per hour. Solu-

tions containing lactate are generally avoided because lactate is gluconeogenic. The dextrose infusion is continued during the perioperative period until the patient can resume oral intake. The anesthesiologist continues to monitor the blood glucose well into the recovery period, usually targeting a level in the range of 120–180 mg/dl. Hyperglycemia in excess of 200 mg/dl can be treated with regular insulin according to a sliding scale. Before aggressively treating with regular insulin, however, the anesthesiologist must bear in mind that the peak effect from the preoperative NPH dose is 8–12 hours after its administration. Vigilance is necessary to protect against the potentially devastating complication of hypoglycemia.

Patients with chronic obstructive pulmonary disease, who have bronchospasm, coughing, copious sputum production, and hypoxemia or hypercarbia, present a challenge for the clinician, whether the surgery is performed under local or general anesthesia.[28] Under local anesthesia, the patient may be unable to lie flat, and paroxysms of coughing can jeopardize the eye. General anesthesia can result in postoperative sputum retention, bronchopneumonia, and respiratory failure. Moreover, an acute exacerbation of bronchospasm intraoperatively can render inflation of the lungs extremely difficult and precipitate serious barotrauma. The patient, therefore, should be questioned preoperatively about the effects of exercise and recumbency as guides to respiratory function. Peak flow is a reliable indicator of bronchospasm and the response to bronchodilators. Depending on the findings, arterial blood gases and other more sophisticated tests of pulmonary function may be indicated. Nebulized beta$_2$-adrenergic receptor agonists, steroid therapy, breathing exercises, and even postural drainage may be necessary to have the patient in peak condition for surgery.

A thorough history includes knowledge of all drugs—topical and systemic—the patient is taking. Patients should be asked explicitly about the use of eyedrops because these agents can have systemic effects and can interact with assorted anesthetic drugs (Table 12-2). If the patient is taking systemic anticoagulants, the patient's internist is consulted about stopping or lowering the dose of anticoagulation treatment. Discontinuing anticoagulation can have serious medical consequences. Several studies suggest that cataract surgery can be performed safely under regional anesthesia without discontinuing anti-

Table 12-2. Anesthetic Implications of Ocular Drugs

Drug	Potential Problems
Acetazolamide	Acidosis, hypokalemia, and hyponatremia with chronic use; allergic reactions associated with sulfonamide structure
Acetylcholine	Bradycardia, hypotension, increased salivation and bronchial secretions, bronchospasm
Atropine	Flushing, thirst, tachycardia, agitation, disorientation
Betaxolol (Betoptic)	Although typically has minimal effect on pulmonary and cardiovascular parameters, betaxolol considered contraindicated in patients with sinus bradycardia, > first-degree atrioventricular block, cardiogenic shock, or overt cardiac failure
Cocaine	Corneal toxicity, hypertension and hypertensive crises, dysrhythmias, agitation, hyperthermia, cardiorespiratory arrest; contraindicated in patients taking sympathomimetic agents
Cyclopentolate	CNS toxicity, dysarthria, disorientation, convulsions
Echothiophate iodide	Prolonged action of succinylcholine and ester-linked local anesthetics owing to long-acting anticholinesterase activity; cholinergic side effects, such as vomiting, hypotension, abdominal pain
Epinephrine	Nervousness, hypertension, dysrhythmias, headache, faintness
Mannitol	Renal failure, allergic reactions, electrolyte imbalance, congestive heart failure, hypotension, hypertension, myocardial ischemia
Phenylephrine	Hypertension, headache, tremulousness, cerebral hemorrhage, myocardial ischemia and infarction; dysrhythmias
Pilocarpine	Hypertension, tachycardia, bronchospasm, pulmonary edema, sweating, nausea, vomiting, diarrhea
Scopolamine	CNS excitation and disorientation
Timolol	Systemic nonselective beta-blockade; exacerbation of myasthenia gravis
Tropicamide	CNS aberrations; behavioral disturbances, psychotic reactions; vasomotor collapse (very rare)

CNS = central nervous system.
Source: Adapted from KE McGoldrick, J Mardirossian. Ophthalmic Surgery. In KE McGoldrick (ed), Ambulatory Anesthesiology: A Problem-Oriented Approach. Baltimore: Williams & Wilkins, 1995;507–535.

coagulants,[29–31] especially if the prothrombin time is approximately 1.5 times control.[32] Issues pertaining to donor tissue preservation often render it impractical to have patients avoid aspirin for 10 days before surgery. Moreover, platelet function is difficult to assess because Ivy bleeding time is often a poor predictor of perioperative hemostasis.[33] Nonetheless, if possible, many ophthalmologists prefer that patients avoid aspirin for at least 10 days before intraocular surgery under local or general anesthesia.

In some patients, acute reduction of intraocular pressure before surgery is indicated, particularly in those with elevated pressure or those undergoing cataract surgery and intraocular lens implantation in conjunction with penetrating keratoplasty. Intravenous mannitol (0.5–2.0 g/kg) administered over a 30- to 60-minute interval just before surgery reduces forward vitreous pressure as well as intraocular pressure, thereby facilitating cataract removal and intraocular lens implantation. However, serious systemic disturbances may result from rapid infusion of large doses of mannitol. These complications include congestive heart failure, pulmonary edema with hypoxia, electrolyte imbalance, hypertension or hypotension, myocardial ischemia, painful bladder distention, and, rarely, allergic reactions. Clearly, the patient's renal and cardiovascular status must be thoroughly evaluated before administration of mannitol. Intravenous acetazolamide may be an alternative therapy.

General versus Local Anesthesia Technique

Although no outcome studies are available to suggest the superiority of local over general anesthesia, penetrating keratoplasty is most frequently performed in the United States using local (retrobulbar or peribulbar block) anesthesia and intravenous conscious sedation. Many surgeons prefer general anesthesia for corneal transplantation, however, particularly if the patient is aphakic or other manipulations involving the vitreous are contemplated. Movement during certain critical manipulations could prove disastrous. Similarly, patients undergoing keratoplasty to repair a perforated cornea require general anesthesia because performance of a retrobulbar or peribulbar block could cause extrusion of intraocular contents through the corneal defect. Other relative surgical contraindications for local anesthesia include high myopia with an axial length greater than 26 mm or significant enophthalmos: Such conditions predispose to inadvertent globe perforation. Indeed, any patient who sustained a previous complication in association with ocular regional anesthesia may fare better under general anesthesia. Besides pediatric patients, individuals who are deaf or who speak a foreign language and those with claustrophobia or excessive anxiety are often poor candidates for local anesthesia. Other relative contraindications include tremors, chronic coughing, and inability to lie flat or hold still for the 1.5- to 2.0-hour surgical duration.

It cannot be overemphasized that penetrating keratoplasty is a delicate intraocular procedure that requires a motionless eye and stable intraocular pressure to protect against extrusion of intraocular contents. The devastating consequences of patient movement during intraocular surgery are graphically documented in the Closed Claims Analysis.[34]

Local Anesthesia

When corneal transplantation is planned under local anesthesia, usually either a retrobulbar or peribulbar block is performed. Occasionally, a sub-Tenon's injection is selected instead (see Sub-Tenon's Anesthesia).

Retrobulbar Block

Technique.   Retrobulbar injection of local anesthetic provides akinesia of the extraocular muscles by blocking cranial nerves III and VI within the muscle core. Blocking the ciliary nerve within the cone also affords analgesia for the conjunctiva, cornea, and uvea. A separate facial nerve block is then executed to anesthetize cranial nerve VII supplying the orbicularis oculi muscle; this prevents eyelid squeezing that could lead to increased intraocular pressure and extrusion of eye contents during delicate intraocular surgery.

Approximately 10–30 mg of intravenous methohexital or 0.3–0.5 mg/kg of propofol[35] is administered immediately before needle insertion (assuming no contraindications to either drug) to provide analgesia and amnesia. Intravenous midazolam, 1 mg, is another useful agent to provide amnesia. What must be assiduously avoided, however, is heavy sedation in the form of high doses of opioids, ben-

zodiazepines, and hypnotics. Such polypharmacy is extremely undesirable because of the pharmacologic vagaries observed in the geriatric population and the attendant hazards of respiratory depression, airway obstruction, hypotension, behavioral aberrations, and protracted recovery time. This unsatisfactory approach has all the disadvantages of an unintubated general anesthetic without the advantage of controllability usually associated with general anesthesia. By definition, patients under conscious sedation must be capable of cooperating, of responding rationally to instructions, and of maintaining airway patency. On the other hand, excessive anxiety should also be avoided because tachycardia and hypertension can have detrimental effects, particularly in patients with coronary artery disease. The goal should be a calm, cooperative, aware patient. Patients with orthopedic deformities or severe arthritis must be carefully positioned on the operating table with comfortable padding; a pillow under the knees may alleviate back pain. Supplemental oxygen should be delivered via a nasal cannula that can be fitted for end-tidal CO_2 sampling. The patient must be kept comfortably warm because of the risks of shivering in patients with coronary artery disease or, for that matter, in any patient having delicate eye surgery. Continuous ECG monitoring is crucial, lest performance of the retrobulbar block, pressure on the globe, or tugging on the extraocular muscles stimulate the oculocardiac reflex arc and produce dangerous dysrhythmias (Figure 12-3). Similarly, continuous oxygen saturation monitoring is essential.

Traditionally, patients were instructed to look upward and inward during the retrobulbar injection to remove the inferior oblique muscle from the trajectory of the retrobulbar needle. (An additional advantage of superonasal gaze is that the patient looks away from the needle as it is inserted inferotemporally.) In 1981, however, Unsöld and colleagues,[36] using computed tomography scanning of a cadaver orbit as the needle is inserted, exposed the risks of the traditional Atkinson position of superonasal gaze. They discovered that this position brings the optic nerve as well as the ophthalmic artery and the superior orbital vein into the path of the retrobulbar needle. The likelihood of perforating the optic nerve or penetrating the meningeal sheath surrounding the optic nerve, thereby allowing local anesthesia to spread throughout the cen-

Stimulation

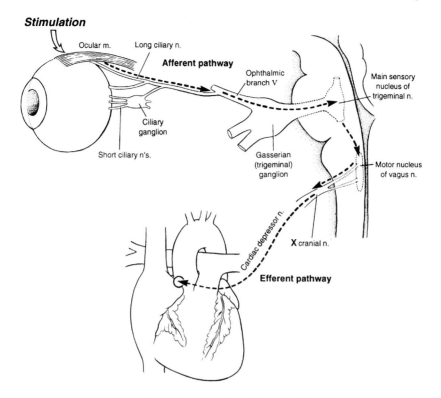

Figure 12-3. Traction on the extraocular muscles initiates the oculocardiac reflex. The afferent pathway consists of the long and short ciliary nerves, which meet in the ciliary ganglion. The ophthalmic division of the trigeminal nerve then transports the impulse to the gasserian ganglion, where the afferent arc continues to the main sensory nucleus of the trigeminal nerve in the brain stem. Fibers in the reticular formation synapse with the nucleus of the vagus nerve, just below the fourth ventricle. Efferent fibers from the vagus then travel to the heart, producing bradycardia or other dysrhythmias. (n. = nerve; m. = muscle.) (Reprinted with permission from SA Vassallo, LR Ferrari. Anesthesia for Ophthalmology. In CJ Cote, JF Ryan, ID Todres, NG Goudsouzian [eds], A Practice of Anesthesia for Infants and Children [2nd ed]. Philadelphia: Saunders, 1993;325.)

tral nervous system (CNS), is increased because the nerve is stretched in this position. Hence, the current recommendation is to have the patient look in primary gaze (Figure 12-4) or inferonasally.[37, 38]

Conventional ophthalmic wisdom had long maintained that the force necessary to perforate an eye during retrobulbar injection is noticeably greater with a blunt needle than with a standard hypodermic needle. In 1993, Waller and colleagues[39] measured scleral perforation pressure with specific needle tips in preserved and unpreserved human cadaver eyes. These investigators confirmed that the non–cutting-edge, blunt-tipped needles do in fact have higher scleral perforation pressures than do those with cutting edges. Grizzard et al., however, maintain that perforations produced by a blunt needle tip may cause more serious retinal damage

than its sharper counterpart would.[40] Waller's group also demonstrated that large-caliber (23-gauge) needles require more force to perforate the globe than do 25-gauge needles of the same tip design.[39]

Patient discomfort produced by the blunted needle may be minimized by first making an intradermal wheal of local anesthetic at the skin entry site with a sharp 25- or 27-gauge needle. The retrobulbar needle (no longer than 31 mm)[41] is then inserted through the lower lid in the inferotemporal quadrant, at the junction of the lateral and middle thirds of the margin (see Figure 12-4). (Alternatively, a transconjunctival approach can be used by pulling down the lower lid and inserting the needle through the inferior cul-de-sac.) The needle is then directed perpendicular to the skin surface, with the bevel facing the globe to reduce the risk of perforation.

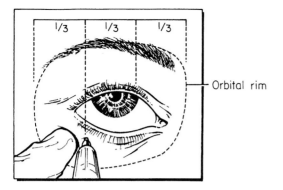

Figure 12-4. Retrobulbar injection is performed with the eye in primary gaze and the retrobulbar needle inserted either transconjunctivally or through the lower lid in the lateral one-third of the eye (inferotemporal quadrant).

After the needle passes the equator of the globe, it should be directed slightly lower than the orbital apex, toward the inferior part of the superior orbital fissure (Figure 12-5). The syringe should be aspirated before injection to ascertain that the needle is not inside a vessel. Although satisfactory retrobulbar block is achieved using injections of 2 ml of anesthetic solution in the muscle cone, many clini-

cians inject larger volumes (4–5 ml) and use hyaluronidase (75–150 units) to facilitate diffusion throughout the orbit. These larger volumes, however, may produce additional pressure on the globe and conjunctival chemosis. Combinations of 1% or 2% lidocaine mixed with 0.5% or 0.75% bupivacaine are popular choices for the local anesthetic solution. After completing the injection, the ophthalmologist typically applies firm, intermittent digital pressure to help distribute the anesthetic and lower intraocular pressure. If complete akinesia and adequate analgesia have not been achieved, it may be necessary to perform a supplemental retrobulbar injection or a transconjunctival quadrant block adjacent to the functioning extraocular muscle. The superior oblique muscle, located outside the muscle cone, will not be paralyzed by retrobulbar blockade. Therefore, the eye may intort when the patient is asked to look down.

Complications.   Retrobulbar injection is associated with both ocular and systemic complications (Table 12-3). Despite the use of specially designed blunt retrobulbar needles, perforation of the globe can occur. A published study from one retinal

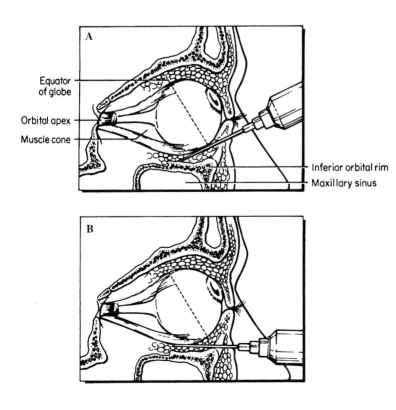

Figure 12-5. After the retrobulbar needle passes the equator of the globe (**A**), it should be directed slightly lower than the orbital apex, toward the inferior part of the superior orbital fissure inside the muscle cone (**B**).

Table 12-3. Complications of Retrobulbar Blockade

Ocular
    Retrobulbar hemorrhage
    Globe perforation
    Vascular occlusion
    Optic nerve injection
Systemic
    Cardiac dysrhythmias
    Respiratory depression or apnea
    Seizures
    Myocardial depression

Table 12-4. Risk Factors for Globe Perforation

Axial length >26 mm by ultrasound
Severe enophthalmos
Previous scleral buckle
Repeated surgeries
Posterior staphyloma
Repeated injections
Uncooperative patient who moves

surgery practice reports an approximate incidence of 1 in 1,000.[41] Waller and colleagues, however, discovered no instance of scleral perforation associated with more than 4,000 retrobulbar or peribulbar injections.[39] Risk factors for globe perforation are listed in Table 12-4. The patient often complains of intense, immediate ocular pain with sudden loss of vision after perforation of the globe.[42] Approximately half the time, the clinician does not recognize unintentional ocular perforation when it occurs because the scleral perforation pressure may be so low as to be imperceptible, especially with sharp needles. In 30% of cases, the eye may feel hypotonic, possibly owing to loss of vitreous. In 10% of cases, however, the eye may feel very hard because of elevated intraocular pressure after injection of local anesthetic into the globe. Clearly, when iatrogenic perforation of the eye occurs, the scheduled surgical procedure must be postponed and appropriate retinal consultation and treatment undertaken.

The most common complication is retrobulbar hemorrhage, occurring as often as 1–3% of the time after retrobulbar injection.[43] Vascular or hematologic disease may predispose a patient to develop a retrobulbar hemorrhage. In addition, aspirin and anticoagulant therapy may be associated with this complication. Signs and symptoms of retrobulbar hemorrhage include pain, increasing proptosis, and, frequently, subconjunctival or eyelid ecchymoses. The ophthalmologist should monitor the patient's intraocular pressure and central retinal artery pulsations carefully to detect impending retinal artery occlusion. Because the oculocardiac reflex may occur several hours after the initial hemorrhage if blood continues to extravasate from the cone and

intraocular pressure increases, ECG monitoring of the patient should be performed accordingly. If external pressure on the globe is sufficient to compress the retinal arterial circulation, a deep lateral canthotomy should be performed to decompress the orbit rapidly. If this maneuver fails to reestablish normal retinal blood flow, an anterior chamber paracentesis should be done to decompress the globe. Inadequate or delayed treatment of this complication may cause unilateral blindness. The planned surgical procedure should be postponed until all signs of the hemorrhage have resolved, and prudence suggests that the rescheduled surgery be performed under general anesthesia.

Optic atrophy and permanent loss of vision may occur, even in the absence of retrobulbar hemorrhage.[44, 45] Postulated mechanisms include direct injury to the nerve, injection into the nerve sheath producing compressive ischemia, and intraneural sheath hemorrhage.[44, 46] Retinal vascular occlusion has been observed after retrobulbar injection without evidence of a retrobulbar hemorrhage.[45, 47] Each patient who experienced vascular occlusion without concomitant hemorrhage had a severe coexisting hematologic or vascular disorder.

Systemic complications associated with retrobulbar block are rare but potentially lethal. A partial list of these sequelae includes stimulation of the oculocardiac reflex arc producing associated dysrhythmias, including asystole; intravascular injection of local anesthetic triggering initial CNS excitation,[48] which may be followed by obtundation and cardiovascular collapse; and unintentional injection of local anesthetics into the CNS, which can produce respiratory arrest.

Although the amount of local anesthetic agent administered with retrobulbar blockade usually is not sufficient to produce systemic toxicity if unintentionally injected into a vein, this is not the case

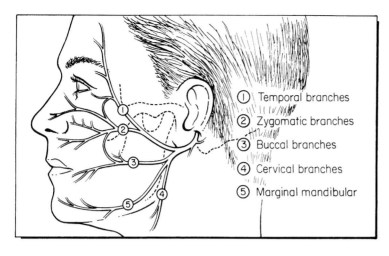

Figure 12-6. Anatomy of the facial nerve.

① Temporal branches
② Zygomatic branches
③ Buccal branches
④ Cervical branches
⑤ Marginal mandibular

with inadvertent intra-arterial injection. Indeed, only 1.8 ml of 2% lidocaine injected into an artery in the head and neck region can produce serious complications, including virtually instantaneous seizures secondary to ophthalmic artery injection, with retrograde flow into the cerebral circulation.[49]

Since 1980, several reports have appeared documenting serious CNS depression after retrobulbar block. Although one study reported an incidence of 0.79%,[50] other studies suggest that the occurrence is more unusual, typically appearing once in 350–500 cases.[51–54] There is a continuum of sequelae, depending on the amount of drug that gains entrance to the CNS and the specific area to which the drug spreads.[55] Onset of symptoms is variable, ranging from 2 to 40 minutes.[51] The protean CNS signs may include violent shivering,[56] contralateral amaurosis; eventual loss of consciousness; apnea; and hemiplegia, paraplegia, quadriplegia, or hyperreflexia. Blockade of the eighth to twelfth cranial nerves results in deafness, vertigo, vagolysis, dysphagia, aphasia, and loss of neck muscle power. Although these signs may be present in various combinations, once it is apparent that the local anesthetic has spread to the CNS, the anesthesiologist must be prepared to provide immediate cardiopulmonary resuscitation if necessary. When properly treated, these patients quickly recover completely. However, delay in diagnosing and treating respiratory arrest secondary to brain stem anesthesia can be fatal.

Various precautions can be taken to prevent brain stem anesthesia. As mentioned previously, the traditional Atkinson position of superonasal gaze during retrobulbar block places the optic nerve closer to the advancing needle. The needle tip can pierce the meningeal sheath surrounding the optic nerve, allowing local anesthesia to spread through the CNS. The optic nerve is less vulnerable with the globe in primary gaze or looking inferonasally.[37] Moreover, avoidance of deep penetration of the orbit is important to prevent this and other serious complications, including ocular perforation. Even without penetration of the optic nerve sheath, central spread of local anesthetic from deep orbital injection *may* be a rare possibility.[57] Therefore, the maximal needle length currently recommended for retrobulbar block is 31 mm (1.25 in.).[38]

Facial Nerve Blocks

A separate facial nerve block is necessary in conjunction with retrobulbar block to achieve akinesia of the eyelids (Figure 12-6). When hyaluronidase is mixed with larger volumes of local anesthetics and used in combination with an orbital decompression device, however, an effective spread from the orbit through the orbital septum occurs to produce eyelid akinesia.[58]

A variety of approaches can be used to block the facial nerve distal to its exit point from the skull through the stylomastoid foramen. Moving distally to proximally to the foramen, the techniques include the Van Lint, Atkinson's, O'Brien's, and Nadbath-Rehman methods.

The classic Van Lint technique involves inserting the needle at the lateral orbital rim and making a small intradermal wheal (Figure 12-7). The needle

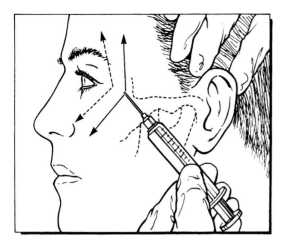

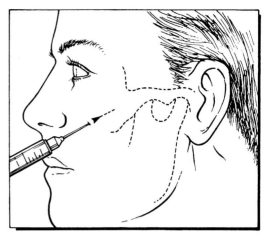

Figure 12-7. Classic Van Lint technique (*dashes*) blocks the facial nerve at the lateral orbital rim. The modified technique (*solid lines*) moves the injection more laterally to avoid eyelid edema.

Figure 12-8. Atkinson's block. The needle is inserted at the inferior aspect of the zygomatic arch, usually below the lateral margin of the orbital rim. Local anesthetic (5–10 ml) is injected along the zygomatic arch as the needle is advanced.

is then advanced into the deep tissues along the inferolateral orbital margin. As the needle is withdrawn, 2–4 ml of anesthetic is injected. The needle is then redirected along the superotemporal orbital margin. Again, anesthetic is injected as the needle is withdrawn. Pressure is then applied to the area to promote diffusion of the anesthetic. This method has the side effect of producing lid edema. Therefore, the technique has been modified by placing the injection more laterally to block the facial nerve as it traverses the periosteum of the orbital rim.

Initially described in 1953, the Atkinson's method involves blocking the branches of the facial nerve as they cross the zygomatic arch[59] (Figure 12-8). First, a skin wheal is made at the lower margin of the zygomatic arch just below the lateral orbital rim. The needle is directed superiorly and posteriorly along the zygoma (aimed just lateral to the midpoint between the tragus and lateral orbital rim). Five to 10 ml of anesthetic solution is injected as the needle is withdrawn.

In 1929, O'Brien described a facial nerve block over the mandibular condyle inferior to the posterior zygomatic process.[60] The needle is inserted to the level of the periosteum (Figure 12-9). Approximately 3 ml of anesthetic solution is injected as the needle is withdrawn. Because of the variable course of the facial nerve, especially in this area, the block may be inadequate. The following modifications,

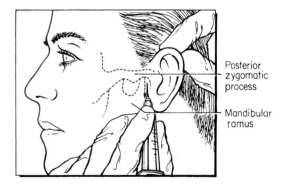

Figure 12-9. O'Brien's block. The injection is performed over the condyle of the mandible just inferior to the posterior zygomatic process. The condyle is located approximately 1 cm anterior to the tragus. Local anesthetic (2–3 ml) is injected as the needle is withdrawn. Care is taken to avoid direct injection into the temporomandibular joint.

therefore, have been recommended: After injecting over the condyle, the needle should be partially withdrawn and redirected inferiorly along the posterior edge of the ramus of the mandible. The anesthetic solution is injected while withdrawing the needle. The needle is repositioned anteriorly along the zygomatic arch, and the anesthetic is injected while withdrawing the needle.

Complete akinesia of all the muscles that are innervated by the facial nerve, not just the orbicu-

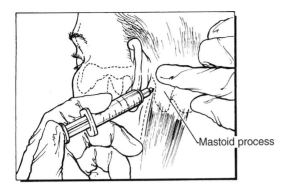

Figure 12-10. Nadbath-Rehman block. The anesthesiologist's index finger is placed on the mastoid process, and the needle is inserted between the mastoid process and the posterior border of the mandibular ramus. The needle is advanced anterocephalad to avoid the jugular foramen.

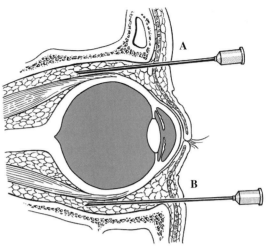

Figure 12-11. Sagittal view of the globe and adnexa. With peribulbar block, the superonasal (A) and the inferotemporal (B) needles do not enter the muscle cone, and the local anesthetic solution is deposited just beyond the equator of the globe.

laris oculi muscle, can be achieved with the Nadbath-Rehman block, first described in 1963.[61] The main trunk of the facial nerve is blocked at the concavity just below the external auditory meatus, between the anterosuperior border of the mastoid process and the posterior border of the mandibular ramus (Figure 12-10). A 25- or 27-gauge, 12-mm needle is inserted into the skin, and an intradermal wheal is made. The needle is then advanced its full length perpendicularly into the tissue. The plunger is withdrawn to ensure that the needle is not intravascular, and approximately 3 ml of anesthetic solution is injected as the needle is withdrawn. Gentle massage is applied to enhance diffusion of the local anesthetic. The major advantage of this technique is the consistent course of the facial nerve from the stylomastoid foramen to the posteromedial surface of the parotid gland, before the nerve divides into its five branches. Thus, complete facial nerve akinesia results, including the lower facial musculature. The patient must be informed of this effect during the preoperative interview and be reassured that the facial paralysis is transient. Patients may develop sudden dysphagia, hoarseness, respiratory distress, pooling of secretions, or laryngospasm.[62, 63] Presumably, these symptoms result from ipsilateral paralysis of the glossopharyngeal, vagus, and spinal accessory nerves that exit the skull via the jugular foramen, which is located only 10 mm medial to the stylomastoid foramen. Complete facial hemiparesis can be undesirable in the outpatient setting because family members may misinterpret its effects as a stroke. Moreover, profound facial hemiparesis interferes with liquid and solid intake.

Peribulbar Block

Technique.   Many consider peribulbar block easier, safer, and less painful than retrobulbar block because the muscle cone is not entered (Figure 12-11). In addition, separate facial nerve block is usually unnecessary because the relatively large volume (8–10 ml) of injected local anesthetic typically diffuses into the eyelids.

Patient preparation, including monitoring and sedation, is the same as that described for retrobulbar block. Davis and Mandel advocated a peribulbar or periconal technique in 1986,[64] and several modifications of their original protocol have since evolved. Two injections are required; these are placed inferotemporally, in the same entrance site as for retrobulbar block, and then superonasally, in the lid fold between the supraorbital notch and the trochlea. A 25-gauge, 1-in. needle is used and directed parallel to the floor and roof, respectively, of the orbit and just beyond the equator of the globe. After careful aspiration, 4–5 ml of anesthetic is injected in each site. Onset is slower than with retrobulbar blockade and may be delayed for as long as 15–20 minutes. Zahl and colleagues[65] reported that onset is accelerated by adding sodium

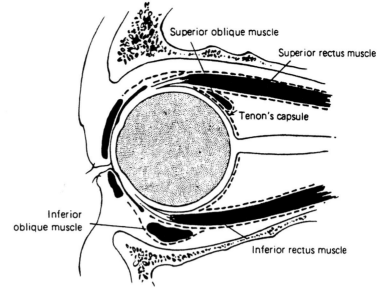

Figure 12-12. Tenon's capsule (*dashes*) envelops the eye and extraocular muscles as a continuous fibrous sheath.

bicarbonate to bupivacaine and hyaluronidase. Others believe that pH adjustment of local anesthetic bottled at pH 6.0 or above to reach pH 7.4 has minimal effect.[66] In a region of rapid blood flow, such as orbital connective tissue, transcapillary extraction is facilitated when the concentration of the base form of the local anesthetic predominates.

Complications.   Peribulbar block has a higher failure rate than retrobulbar block. Additionally, the larger volume of anesthetic solution deposited in the orbit produces increased forward pressure on the eyeball, which some surgeons find objectionable. This increased volume elevates orbital pressure, displaces the lids, and can increase vitreous pressure, all of which are undesirable. Moreover, anesthetic solution often moves forward around the eye, causing the conjunctiva to balloon and making proper fixation of the scleral support ring difficult. Therefore, retrobulbar anesthesia is more popular than peribulbar anesthesia for corneal transplant surgery. Other potential complications include eyelid ecchymoses, peribulbar hemorrhage, and perforation of the globe.

Sub-Tenon's Anesthesia

Tenon's capsule is the fascia that envelops the eye as a continuous fibrous sheath (Figure 12-12). Sub-Tenon's anesthesia involves an anterior approach that eliminates such risks of blind injection as optic nerve perforation and retrobulbar hemorrhage and

minimizes the risk of globe perforation. This form of periocular anesthesia is used for cataract extraction,[67] corneal transplantation, adult strabismus repair, pterygium excision, and retinal and glaucoma surgery. The degree of abolition of extraocular muscle movement is proportional to the volume and depth of injectate. The local anesthetic solution diffuses retrograde to anesthetize the long and short ciliary nerves and the ciliary ganglion, providing anesthesia to the cornea, iris, and ciliary body while preserving optic nerve function.

The clinician applies 1 drop of 0.5% topical tetracaine at the superotemporal and inferior fornices. Using a 30-gauge half-inch needle with the bevel up, tangential to the globe, he or she injects 4–5 ml of local anesthetic (mixture of 2% lidocaine and 0.75% bupivacaine) with hyaluronidase in the superotemporal quadrant of the globe, 5–15 mm from the limbal margin, into the sub-Tenon's space. An additional 2 ml of local anesthetic with hyaluronidase is then injected into sub-Tenon's space inferonasally. Although inexpensive, easy, and safe, sub-Tenon's anesthesia produces variable degrees of chemosis that may be surgically detrimental.

General Anesthesia

As previously mentioned, no outcome studies are available to indicate the preeminence of one type or form of anesthesia over another. Patients who require general anesthesia for corneal transplantation do well, provided hemodynamic stability is maintained and the eye is kept motionless, with a constant intraocular pressure to protect against extrusion of intraocular contents. Proper control of arterial blood pressure is always important, but it has special implications for retinal perfusion in the patient with glaucoma who is undergoing corneal transplantation. If the patient's mean arterial pressure is markedly reduced, the retinal perfusion pressure may be inadequate, and retinal ischemia and permanent retinal damage may ensue. On the other hand, marked elevation of retinal arteriole pressure can also be deleterious: When the intraocular pressure is suddenly lowered as the surgeon enters the globe and removes the central cornea, hemorrhage can occur. Therefore, it is imperative for the anesthesiologist to know the patient's normal blood pressure.

The exigencies of ophthalmic anesthesia mandate that the anesthesiologist be positioned remote from the patient's airway; this necessity can create certain logistic problems. Many anesthetic techniques can be used safely for elective intraocular surgery. Virtually any of the inhalation drugs can be given after intravenous induction of anesthesia with a barbiturate or propofol. Because postoperative vomiting is extremely undesirable owing to its dramatic effect of increasing intraocular pressure, propofol is an excellent induction agent that is consistently associated with less nausea and vomiting than other agents.[68, 69] In patients with advanced coronary artery disease, however, the cardiodepressant effects of barbiturates or propofol are unwelcome. Etomidate, therefore, may be kinder to the cardiovascular system but can trigger postoperative nausea and vomiting. The choice of muscle relaxant for intubation is made after considering the patient's airway, the presence of symptomatic reflux, and the hemodynamic consequences of the agent. Intravenous or topical lidocaine and small doses of fentanyl on induction may help to attenuate the hemodynamic effects of intubation. Owing to logistical problems, it is essential to secure the endotracheal tube meticulously. The nonoperative eye should be carefully taped shut to protect it from injury. It is prudent to administer a prophylactic antiemetic, such as 20 µg/kg of droperidol, or 4 mg of ondansetron intravenously. (These antiemetic drugs have not been studied in the specific context of corneal transplantation but have proved efficacious for other types of eye surgery.[70, 71])

Volatile agents are titrated. Because akinesia is important for delicate intraocular surgery, administration of a nondepolarizing muscle relaxant in conjunction with peripheral nerve monitoring is advocated to ensure a 90–95% twitch suppression level during surgery. Isoflurane, desflurane, or sevoflurane are appropriate choices for maintenance. Alternatively, a total intravenous anesthetic technique with propofol may be selected. Vecuronium is commonly administered for paralysis owing to its favorable hemodynamic profile and its intermediate duration of action. Ventilation is controlled and continuously monitored by end-tidal CO_2 measurement. This measure prevents hypercarbia and its ocular hypertensive effect and detects disconnection of the endotracheal tube from the anesthesia circuit, which is obscured by the logistical demands of draping in the ophthalmic patient. Continuous monitoring of arterial oxygen saturation by pulse oximetry is also important. A sufficiently deep level of anesthesia is mandatory until the wound has been sutured completely closed; coughing, for example, can increase intraocular pressure more than 40 mm Hg and result in extrusion of intraocular contents. After completion of surgery, any residual neuromuscular blockade is reversed, and intravenous lidocaine can be given a few minutes before extubation to prevent or attenuate periextubation coughing. Depending on such factors as the patient's airway anatomy, fasting status, or history of reflux, the anesthesiologist may select awake or deep extubation. In skilled hands, either technique is satisfactory. If postoperative nausea and vomiting occur, intravenous droperidol, 10 µg/kg, or ondansetron, 4 mg (or 50 µg/kg in the pediatric patient), is given.

Postoperative Management and Complications

The ophthalmologist should be notified immediately if a patient complains of severe periorbital or intraocular pain or develops nausea because these symptoms could signal increased intraocular pressure.

Most surgeons administer both topical antibiotics and steroids in the immediate postoperative period. The regimen varies depending on a variety of clinical factors. Typically, a broad-spectrum topical antibiotic, such as tobramycin, is administered several times a day for a few to several days. Systemic antibiotics are seldom necessary. Similarly, clinical response ultimately determines the frequency and duration of topical steroid use. If the eye is inflamed, sometimes up to 1 drop per hour of 0.1% dexamethasone or 1% prednisolone is necessary for several days. Because it has been suggested that steroids have a beneficial effect on endothelial function, long-term administration may be helpful in patients who had grafts performed to correct corneal edema. Prolonged steroid use not only increases the likelihood of local infection but also can increase the risk of glaucoma and posterior subcapsular cataracts. Therefore, patients must be monitored closely for signs of these complications. Significant elevations in intraocular pressure are treated with topical or systemic antiglaucoma medications. Systemic steroids are rarely indicated after corneal transplantation.

In addition to increased intraocular pressure and corneal infection, other early postoperative complications include primary graft failure, wound leakage, persistent epithelial defects, and intraocular infection or endophthalmitis (Table 12-5).

Late complications after corneal transplantation include glaucoma, astigmatism, wound dehiscence, and graft rejection. Early increases in intraocular pressure after penetrating keratoplasty may be caused by inflammation or obstruction of the trabecular meshwork due to intraoperative use of viscoelastic substances. Late increases in pressure may result from corneal-iris adhesions, chronic inflammation, or disruption of the anterior chamber angle by surgery. Topical and systemic antiglaucoma medications may be beneficial, but surgical correction may be necessary.

Although most graft rejections occur within the first few years after transplantation,[72] immunologically mediated rejection may happen at any time. Therefore, each patient should be warned of the possibility of this complication occurring several years after what appeared to be a successful transplant. Graft rejection may involve either the corneal epithelium or endothelium, and in each instance two phenomena are common.[73, 74] The first manifestation of epithelial rejection is a linear opacity that migrates across the surface of the graft. This phenomenon typically produces minimal, if any, symptoms and the prognosis is good even without treatment. The second major manifestation of epithelial rejection is the appearance of small,

Table 12-5. Postoperative Complications

Early
    Increased intraocular pressure (e.g., secondary to hemorrhage, inflammation, trabecular obstruction)
    Corneal infection
    Primary graft failure
    Wound leaks
    Persistent epithelial defects
    Intraocular infection and endophthalmitis
Late
    Glaucoma
    Astigmatism
    Wound dehiscence
    Graft rejection

round, patchy infiltrates in the subepithelial zone that may produce irritation and blurry vision. Topical steroids are effective in reversing this phenomenon. Epithelial rejection usually does not lead to graft failure. Endothelial rejection, however, is associated with the potential for irreversible permanent corneal edema. The first manifestation is the appearance of inflammation at the junction of the graft and host. This may be manifested by keratic precipitates, endothelial haze, localized edema, and occasionally flare and cells in the anterior chamber. Although pathognomonic, Khodadoust line is a late manifestation of the endothelial precipitates, as the line forms a linear pattern progressing across the endothelial surface of the graft. Indeed, the diagnosis of graft rejection should be made and the condition treated with topical steroids before the appearance of Khodadoust line because the ophthalmologist should document meticulously any keratic precipitates after a corneal graft and treat accordingly. The second major manifestation of endothelial graft rejection is extremely serious and involves generalized corneal edema in association with keratic precipitates, flare, or cells. Even with aggressive treatment, the prognosis is grim.

Clearly, the mainstay of therapy for graft rejection is topical steroids. Many ophthalmologists favor the use of 1% prednisolone every hour around the clock in all rejections until signs of improvement are observed; the medication is then tapered slowly. Because the earliest symptoms of graft rejection are rather nonspecific (e.g., discomfort, blurred vision, tearing, or redness of the eye), the surgeon must educate the patient and the patient's family about the absolute necessity to see an ophthalmologist immediately if such symptoms appear in a grafted eye. Graft rejection is truly an ophthalmic emergency, and the sooner patients are diagnosed and appropriately treated, the better the prognosis.

Surgery after Corneal Transplantation

The care of a corneal transplant recipient undergoing surgery is not dramatically different from that of patients who have not required lamellar or penetrating keratoplasty. Ocular medications, both topical and systemic, should be continued perioperatively. Intraoperatively, the eyelids should be taped closed to avoid exposure and ocular injury. Relative hypotension should be avoided to minimize the risk of retinal ischemia and optic nerve damage, and direct pressure on the eye, which can produce central retinal artery or vein occlusion or wound dehiscence, should be avoided.

If the patient requires reoperation on the eye for wound leakage or dehiscence after corneal transplantation, an open-globe situation prevails. The patient must be deeply anesthetized and completely paralyzed before laryngoscopy and intubation. Failure to take these precautions will produce a dramatic increase in intraocular pressure that could lead to extrusion of intraocular contents.

Conclusions

Impressive advances in materials and equipment, microsurgical techniques, donor tissue procurement and preservation, anesthetic techniques and agents, and the knowledge of pharmacology and immunology have resulted in the dramatic success of corneal transplantation. Indeed, penetrating keratoplasty is the most frequently performed transplant operation. The growing popularity of photorefractive surgery may lead to the eventual need for increasing numbers of corneal transplantations.[75]

Acknowledgments

The authors wish to express their gratitude to Marion Mangino and Jill Fuggi for typing the manuscript.

References

1. Breebart AC, Nuyts RMMA, Pels E, et al. Toxic endothelial cell destruction of the cornea after routine extracapsular cataract surgery. Arch Ophthalmol 1990; 108:1121–1125.
2. Reisinger F. Die Keratoplastik ein Versuch Zur Erweitering der Augenheilkunde. Baiersche. Ann Abhandl 1824;1:207.
3. von Hippel A. On transplantation of the cornea. Berichte Ophthalmol 1886;18:54.
4. Zirm E. Eine erfolgreiche totale keratoplastik. Graefes Arch Clin Exp Ophthalmol 1906;64:580–581.
5. Foster CS. Lamellar Keratoplasty. In FA Jakobiec, DM Albert (eds), Principles and Practice of Ophthalmology. Philadelphia: Saunders, 1994;319–325.
6. Eye Bank Association of America. News release, eye banking statistics, activity reports. Washington, DC: Eye Bank Association of America, 1990.
7. Adams AP, Filatov V, Tripathi BJ, et al. Fuchs' endothelial dystrophy of the cornea. Surv Ophthalmol 1993; 38:149–168.
8. Waring GO III. The 50-year epidemic of pseudophakic corneal edema [editorial]. Arch Ophthalmol 1989;107: 657–659.
9. Morris RJ, Bates AK. Changing indications for keratoplasty. Eye 1989;3:455–459.
10. Boruchoff SA. Penetrating Keratoplasty. In DM Albert, FA Jakobiec (eds), Principles and Practice of Ophthalmology. Philadelphia: Saunders, 1994;325–337.
11. Belin MW, Fowler WC, Chambers WA. Keratoconus: evaluation of recent trends in the surgical and nonsurgical correction of keratoconus. Ophthalmology 1988; 95:335–339.
12. Sharif KW, Casey TA. Penetrating keratoplasty for keratoconus: complications and long-term success. Br J Ophthalmol 1991;75:142–146.
13. Kaufman HE, Varnell ED, Kaufman S, et al. K-sol corneal preservation. Am J Ophthalmol 1985;100: 299–304.
14. Capella JA, Kaufman HE, Robbins JE. Preservation of viable corneal tissue. Arch Ophthalmol 1965;74:669–673.
15. McCarey B, Kaufman HE. Improved corneal storage. Invest Ophthalmol 1974;13:165–173.
16. Mizuno K, Clark AF, Streilein JW. Anterior chamber-associated immune deviation induced by soluble antigen. Invest Ophthalmol Vis Sci 1989;30:1112–1119.
17. The Collaborative Corneal Transplantation Studies Research Group. The Collaborative Corneal Transplantation Studies (CCTS): effectiveness of histocompatibility matching in high-risk corneal transplantation. Arch Ophthalmol 1992;110:1392–1403.
18. Speaker MD, Guerriero PN, Met JA, et al. A case-control study of risk factors for intraoperative suprachoroidal expulsive hemorrhage. Ophthalmology 1991;98:202–210.

19. Whitehouse GM, Filipic M, Francis IC. Expulsive choroidal hemorrhage: a clinical and pathological review. Aust N Z J Ophthalmol 1990;17:225–232.

20. McMeel JW. Uveal Tract Circulatory Problems. In DM Albert, FA Jakobiec (eds), Principles and Practice of Ophthalmology. Philadelphia: Saunders, 1994;389–396.

21. Kraushar MF, Turner MF. Medical malpractice litigation in cataract surgery. Arch Ophthalmol 1987;105: 1339–1343.

22. Petruscak J, Smith RB, Breslin PM. Mortality related to ophthalmological surgery. Arch Ophthalmol 1973; 89:106–109.

23. Quigley HA. Mortality associated with ophthalmic surgery: a twenty year experience. Am J Ophthalmol 1974;77:517–524.

24. Hovi-viander M. Death associated with anaesthesia in Finland. Br J Anaesth 1980;52:483–489.

25. Vacanti CJ, Van Houten RJ, Hill RC. A statistical analysis of the relationship of physical status to postoperative mortality in 68,388 cases. Anesth Analg 1970;49:564–566.

26. Report of the American College of Cardiology/American Heart Association Task Force on Practice Guidelines (Committee on Perioperative Cardiovascular Evaluation for Noncardiac Surgery). Executive summary of the ACC/AHA Task Force report: guidelines for perioperative cardiovascular evaluation for noncardiac surgery. Anesth Analg 1996;82:854–860.

27. Van Maren GA, Brown BR. Hypertensive Patients. In KE McGoldrick (ed), Ambulatory Anesthesiology: A Problem-Oriented Approach. Baltimore: Williams & Wilkins, 1995;127–136.

28. Nunn JF, Milledge JS, Chen D, Dore C. Respiratory criteria for surgery and anaesthesia. Anaesthesia 1988;43:543–551.

29. McMahan LB. Anticoagulants and cataract surgery. J Cataract Refract Surg 1988;14:569–571.

30. Hall DL, Steen WH, Drummond JW, et al. Anticoagulants and cataract surgery. Ophthalmic Surg 1988;19:221–222.

31. Robinson GA, Nylander A. Warfarin and cataract extraction. Br J Ophthalmol 1989;73:702–703.

32. Feitl ME, Krupin T. Retrobulbar anesthesia. Ophthalmol Clin North Am 1990;3(1):83–91.

33. Lind SE. The bleeding time does not predict surgical bleeding. Blood 1991;77:2547–2552.

34. Gild WM, Posner KL, Caplan RA, et al. Eye injuries associated with anesthesia: a closed claims analysis. Anesthesiology 1992;76:204–208.

35. Ferrari LR, Donlon JV. A comparison of propofol, midazolam, and methohexital for sedation during retrobulbar and peribulbar block. J Clin Anesth 1992;4:93–96.

36. Unsöld R, Stanley JA, DeGroot J. The CT-topography of retrobulbar anesthesia: Albrecht von Graefes. Arch Klin Exp Ophthalmol 1981;217:125–136.

37. Liu C, Youl B, Moseley I. Magnetic resonance imaging of the optic nerve in extremes of gaze: implications for the positioning of the globe for retrobulbar anaesthesia. Br J Ophthalmol 1992;76:728–733.

38. Katsev DA, Drews RC, Rose BT. An anatomic study of retrobulbar needle path length. Ophthalmology 1989; 96:1221–1224.

39. Waller SG, Taboada J, O'Connor P. Retrobulbar anesthesia risk: do sharp needles really perforate the eye more easily than blunt needles? Ophthalmology 1993; 100:506–510.

40. Grizzard WS, Kirk NM, Pavan PR, et al. Perforating ocular injuries caused by anesthesia personnel. Ophthalmology 1991;98:1011–1016.

41. Ramsay RC, Knobloch WH. Ocular perforation following retrobulbar anesthesia for retinal detachment surgery. Am J Ophthalmol 1978;86:61–64.

42. Duker JS, Belmont JB, Benson WE, et al. Inadvertent globe perforation during retrobulbar and peribulbar anesthesia: patient characteristics, surgical management, and visual outcome. Ophthalmology 1991;98:519–526.

43. Morgan CM, Schatz H, Vine AKM, et al. Ocular complications associated with retrobulbar injections. Ophthalmology 1988;95:660–665.

44. Ellis PP. Retrobulbar injections. Surv Ophthalmol 1974; 18:425–430.

45. Klein ML, Jampol LM, Condon PI, et al. Central retinal artery occlusion without retrobulbar hemorrhage after retrobulbar anesthesia. Am J Ophthalmol 1982;93: 573–577.

46. Sullivan KL, Brown GC, Forman AR, et al. Retrobulbar anesthesia and retinal vascular obstruction. Ophthalmology 1983;90:373–377.

47. Cowley M, Campochiaro PA, Newman SA, et al. Retinal vascular occlusion without retrobulbar or optic nerve sheath hemorrhage after retrobulbar injection of lidocaine. Ophthalmic Surg 1988;19:859–861.

48. Meyers EF, Ramirez RC, Boniuk I. Grand mal seizures after retrobulbar block. Arch Ophthalmol 1978;96: 847–848.

49. Aldrete JA, Roma-Salas F, Arora S, et al. Reverse arterial blood flow as a pathway for central nervous system toxic responses following injection of local anesthetics. Anesth Analg 1978;57:428–433.

50. Wittpen JR, Rapoza P, Sternberg P, et al. Respiratory arrest following retrobulbar anesthesia. Ophthalmology 1986;93:867–870.

51. Nicoll JMV, Acharya PA, Ahlen K, et al. Central nervous system complications after 6,000 retrobulbar blocks. Anesth Analg 1987;66:1298–1302.

52. Ahn JC, Stanley JA. Subarachnoid injection as a complication of retrobulbar anesthesia. Am J Ophthalmol 1987;103:225–230.

53. Stanley JA. Subarachnoid injection as a complication of retrobulbar block. Saudi Bull Ophthalmol 1987;2:13–15.

54. Hamilton RC, Gimbel HV, Strunin L. Regional anaesthesia for 12,000 cataract extraction and intraocular lens implantation procedures. Can J Anaesth 1988;35:615–623.

55. Hamilton RC. Brain stem anesthesia as a complication of regional anesthesia for ophthalmic surgery. Can J Ophthalmol 1992;27:323–325.

56. Nicoll JMV, Acharya PA, Edge KR, et al. Shivering following retrobulbar block [letter]. Can J Anaesth 1988;35:671.

57. Shantha TR. The relationship of retrobulbar local anesthetic spread to the neural membranes of the eyeball, optic nerve and arachnoid villi in the optic nerve [abstract]. Anesthesiology 1990;73:A850.

58. Martin SR, Baker SS, Muenzler WS. Retrobulbar anesthesia and orbicularis akinesia. Ophthalmic Surg 1986;17:232–233.

59. Atkinson WS. Akinesia of the orbicularis. Am J Ophthalmol 1953;36:1255–1258.

60. O'Brien CS. Akinesia during cataract extraction. Arch Ophthalmol 1929;1:447–449.

61. Nadbath RP, Rehman I. Facial nerve block. Am J Ophthalmol 1963;55:143–146.

62. Cofer HF. Cord paralysis after Nadbath facial nerve block. Arch Ophthalmol 1986;104:337.

63. Wilson CA, Ruiz RS. Respiratory obstruction following the Nadbath facial nerve block. Arch Ophthalmol 1985;103:1454–1456.

64. Davis DB, Mandel MR. Posterior peribulbar anesthesia: an alternative to retrobulbar anesthesia. J Cataract Refractive Surg 1986;12:182–184.

65. Zahl K, Jordan A, McGroarty J, et al. pH adjusted bupivacaine and hyaluronidase for peribulbar block. Anesthesiology 1990;72:230–232.

66. Hustead RF, Hamilton RC. Pharmacology. In JP Gills, RF Hustead, DR Sanders (eds), Ophthalmic Anesthesia. Thorofare, NJ: Slack, 1993;69–102.

67. Tsuneoka H, Ohki K, Taniuchi O, et al. Tenon's capsule anaesthesia for cataract surgery with intraocular lens implantation. Eur J Implant Refractive Surg 1993; 5:29–34.

68. Watcha MF, White PF. Postoperative nausea and vomiting: its etiology, treatment, and prevention. Anesthesiology 1992;77:162–184.

69. McCollum JSC, Milligan KR, Dundee JW. The antiemetic effect of propofol. Anaesthesia 1988;43:239–240.

70. Watcha MF, Bras PJ, Cieslak GD, Pennant JH. The dose-response relationship of ondansetron in preventing postoperative emesis in pediatric patients undergoing ambulatory surgery. Anesthesiology 1995;82: 47–52.

71. Brown RE, James DG, Weaver RG, et al. Low-dose droperidol versus standard-dose droperidol for prevention of postoperative vomiting after pediatric strabismus surgery. J Clin Anesth 1991;3:306–309.

72. Price FW Jr, Whitson WE, Collins KS, et al. Five-year corneal graft survival: a large, single-center patient cohort. Arch Ophthalmol 1993;111:799–805.

73. Aldredge OC, Krachmer JH. Clinical types of corneal transplant rejection: their manifestations, frequency, preoperative correlates and treatment. Arch Ophthalmol 1981;99:599–604.

74. Larkin DFP. Corneal allograft rejection. Br J Ophthalmol 1994;78:649–652.

75. O'Brart DPS, Lohmann CP, Fitzke FW, et al. Disturbances in night vision after excimer laser photorefractive keratectomy. Eye 1994;8:46–51.

Chapter 13

Intensive Care Unit Management of Transplantation-Related Problems

Michael R. Pinsky, Derek C. Angus, Arthur J. Boujoukos, and Edward Thomas

Chapter Plan

The number of critically ill patients who are candidates for organ transplantation, who actually receive a donor organ, or who have received an organ transplant in the past and now require intensive care has increased markedly since the mid-1980s. In the United States alone, almost 10,000 kidneys are transplanted each year. More than 2,000 livers and approximately 2,000 hearts are transplanted annually. Thus, it is highly likely that an intensivist will routinely care for such patients, even in the smallest of community hospitals.

Transplantation-related problems can occur throughout the lifetime of organ transplantation candidates and recipients. Generally, intensive care problems occur in three distinct phases of the process, starting with the preoperative phase when the patient is a transplantation candidate. In this phase, support of end-stage organ failure may exceed the bounds of conventional management. Caregivers know that if the patient is stable through the acute process and rendered ready for transplantation, no degree of single-organ failure would limit his or her candidacy for transplantation of that organ. The second time these patients are in the intensive care setting is the immediate postoperative period, when issues of surgery and homeostasis are considered within the limits of vascular patency, graft viability, and related surgical problems. These immunocompromised patients may have deterioration of the grafted organ or related immunologic sequelae. As such, they often require subsequent readmission remote to the transplantation procedure to treat recurrent infections, rejection, and unrelated issues. Their chronic care also requires consideration of complex interactions among antirejection therapy, immunologic status, graft function, and associated sequelae.

This chapter covers intensive care unit (ICU) care of patients who undergo transplantation procedures for solid organs, including kidney, heart, heart-lung, lung, liver, and multiple visceral organs. ICU-related

Table 13-1. Transplantation-Related Problems in the Intensive Care Unit

---

Preoperative support of unstable patients due to end-organ failure

Immediate postoperative technical problems related to the surgery and routine care of the postoperative patient

Recovery of the transplanted organ's function

Immunosuppression and organ rejection

Infection

---

management issues in these patients can be grouped into two broad categories: (1) the problems common to most organ-transplantation patients (Table 13-1) and (2) specific problems unique to each procedure and organ transplanted. Kidney and bone marrow transplant recipients generally do not require postoperative admission to the ICU unless they require intensive care management of conditions associated with their underlying disease process or problems occurring as a result of their organ transplant.

Support of Potential Organ Donors

Any patient younger than 60 years with no pre-existing malignancy or systemic infectious process is a potential organ donor. Although it may seem reprehensible to consider potentially viable patients potential donors, failure to consider them early enough to allow successful harvesting of viable organs is a major cause of organ wastage today.[1] Brain death criteria are discussed in Chapter 3.

Once a patient is defined as brain dead, or when withdrawal of therapy is being considered for ethical reasons or because of the patient's own wishes, issues of management shift from maintaining a viable brain to maintenance of visceral organ perfusion and integrity without damaging potentially transplantable organs. For example, use of a balloon counterpulsation device in a donor greatly increases the incidence of mediastinitis, thereby reducing the chances that either the heart or the lungs can be used to aid in another person's fight to live. Similarly, high-dose alpha-adrenergic vasopressor therapy, which is important in maintaining cerebral blood flow in profoundly hypotensive subjects, impairs renal and splanchnic blood flow, which may damage these visceral organs. Brain death is often

associated with markedly altered endocrinologic status as pituitary function is lost. Care of electrolyte, osmolality, thyroid hormone, and adrenocortical hormone replacement reflects additional concerns that the supporting intensivist should address in these donors.[2, 3] The reader is directed to Chapter 4 for a detailed description of these issues.

Preoperative Support of the Patient with End-Organ Failure Awaiting Transplantation

Organ transplantation candidates are usually ill. With the possible exception of renal transplantation candidates, whose internal milieu can be kept relatively stable by hemodialysis, and the liver transplantation candidate with isolated hepatic neoplasm, all transplantation candidates have the potential for severe decompensation and are terminally ill from their organ failure and related systemic complications. When a patient is being evaluated for organ transplantation, care must be made to sustain overall nutrition and bodily integrity to minimize risks of infections and promote recovery after transplantation. In this regard, the maintenance of overall homeostasis is performed in a fashion similar to other critically ill patients, with some important exceptions.

Because the patient may undergo organ transplantation, the caregiver may choose to use aggressive temporary artificial support modalities that may not otherwise be considered an option in patients with end-organ failure. Many examples of this divergence from normal standards of care can be given, but only a few are used here. First, mechanical ventricular assist devices (VADs) in patients with severe left ventricular (LV) or right ventricular (RV) failure may be used, even though the caregiver knows that these highly invasive devices do not improve deteriorating cardiac function on their own. In the pretransplantation setting, mechanical VADs are used as a bridge to transplantation. (See Chapter 5 for a detailed discussion of this subject.) Patients with end-stage liver failure may proceed to acute renal failure for a variety of reasons, including the development of the hepatorenal syndrome, prerenal (hypovolemic) failure, and renal (parenchymal) failure. In nontransplantation candidates, the development of renal failure in addition to pre-existing liver failure is an ominous sign and usually portends death. As such, it is usually not treated in these individuals because it does not change the outcome. In the liver transplantation candidate, however, renal failure may or may not be reversible but is not a contraindication to transplantation. Thus, these patients are routinely dialyzed, if necessary, before transplantation.

Because all patients undergoing organ transplantation receive massive amounts of immunocompromising agents to suppress the rejection process, they are at increased risk of developing serious systemic infections. Clearly, pre-existing infections become even more serious after transplantation; thus, the presence of an active infection is a major contraindication to organ transplantation. Therefore, the caregiver aggressively attempts to identify and eradicate all active sites of infection before surgery. The most common sites for infection include the kidneys and lungs in all patients and the abdomen in patients with liver failure.

Finally, because these patients will undergo major surgery, require immunosuppression, and risk organ rejection, the caregiver must also consider the impact of preoperative therapies on subsequent transplantation. For example, large-bore cannulation of central arteries to insert an extracorporeal membrane oxygenator (ECMO) device for support of the heart and lungs reduces the number of potential sites for subsequent vascular access and increases the risk of systemic infection and mediastinitis after lung or heart-lung transplantation. These important issues must be addressed by the entire health care team, including the transplant surgeon, the intensivist, the anesthesiologist, the primary referring specialist, the patient, and family.

Organ-Specific Postoperative Management

Liver Transplantation

Postoperative Problems

The liver transplantation patient is highly demanding in the technical aspects of surgery and the medical aspects of patient support before and after transplantation. The clinical course after orthotopic liver transplantation (OLT) is highly variable and is influenced by the recipient's preoperative status, the condition of the donor organ, and the intraoperative course of the recipient. A stable recipient with well-preserved extrahepatic end-organ function who undergoes an unremarkable liver transplantation procedure with good postoperative graft function may be extubated within 24 hours, transferred from the ICU within 2 days, and discharged from the hospital after 2–3 weeks. With the present shortage in organ availability, however, recipients often are severely compromised before liver transplantation. This may lead to a protracted postoperative course because preoperative organ dysfunction induced by persistent end-stage liver disease often persists and is aggravated by poor graft function.

Throughout the recent history of OLT, aggressive interventional diagnostic and therapeutic efforts are the hallmark of programs with the best long-term survival rates. To a large extent, the postoperative management of OLT recipients is similar to that after other major abdominal surgery, with the obvious additions of titrated immunosuppression and the pivotal role of graft function. This chapter addresses patient management issues (Table 13-2) specific to OLT by organ system.

Allograft Function.   Hepatic graft function is perhaps the most important element in determining the postoperative course of OLT patients. Early graft function is evaluated by serial determinations of glucose, lactate, bilirubin, prothrombin time, and bile production (if a choledochocholedochostomy with T-tube is present). The arterial ketone body ratio may also be used as an indicator of hepatic metabolism and has been shown to correlate with graft survival.[4] Subsequently, serum transaminases: (alanine aminotransferase, aspartate aminotransferase), canalicular enzymes (gamma-glutamyltransferase, alkaline phosphatase), prothrombin time, bilirubin levels, and bile production are followed as markers of hepatic function.

Knowing the condition of the organ donor and of procurement and implantation problems is essential for the accurate interpretation of laboratory findings. This is particularly true in the early postoperative period because initial elevation of bilirubin, transaminases, and canalicular enzymes is common. This rise may reflect the preoperative values of the recipient and injury to the donor organ during procurement (i.e., preservation injury). In the absence of problems, the bilirubin typically returns to normal levels in a few days. Mild organ harvesting and preservation injury sometimes results in

Table 13-2. Postoperative Complications after Orthotopic Liver Transplantation

Allograft dysfunction
Neurologic
    Encephalopathy
    Seizures
    Intracerebral hemorrhage
    Central nervous system infection
    Central pontine myelinolysis
    Progressive multifocal leukoencephalopathy
Cardiovascular
    Ongoing third-space fluid loss
    Hemorrhage
    Hypotension or hypertension
    Cardiac tamponade
Pulmonary
    Pulmonary edema (nonhydrostatic and hydrostatic)
    Aspiration
    Atelectasis
    Right phrenic nerve injury
    Pleural effusion
    Infection
    Hepatopulmonary syndrome
    Hypoxemia
    Pulmonary hypertension
Gastrointestinal
    Pancreatitis
    Gastrointestinal bleed
    Gastritis
    Fungal esophagitis
    Cytomegalovirus enteritis
    Vascular enteric fistulas
    Functional pyloric obstruction
    Delayed enteral feeding
Renal
    Hepatorenal syndrome
    Renal failure
Endocrine
    Hyperglycemia or hypoglycemia
    Hypothyroidism
    Adrenal insufficiency
Infections
    Postoperative bacterial surgical infections
    Opportunistic infections
    Posttransplantation lymphoproliferative disease

Table 13-3. Differential Diagnosis of Hepatic Graft Dysfunction

Preservation injury
Technical complications: hepatic artery or portal vein
    thrombosis, biliary obstruction
Rejection
    Hyperacute
    Acute
    Chronic
Sepsis
Hepatitis
    Viral (including cytomegalovirus, Epstein-Barr virus,
        adenovirus)
    Chemical
Posttransplantation lymphoproliferative disease
Cholestasis
Systemic hypoperfusion
Venous congestion
Medication side effects

transaminase elevation for several days after transplantation before slowly trending toward normal levels. Canalicular enzymes often show a marked rise before returning to normal levels over several weeks. The severity of these abnormalities and their duration reflect the degree of injury to the liver both before and during transplantation.

In the presence of marked, prolonged elevation of bilirubin, lactate, and liver enzymes due to serious graft injury, a return of synthetic function as reflected by normalization of the international normalized ratio and arterial ketone body ratio (acetoacetic acid to beta-hydroxybutyric acid) may be the most reliable indices of graft function. Rarely, laboratory values may return to near-normal levels despite severely impaired graft function. In such cases, the only signs of graft dysfunction may be impaired extrahepatic organ function, including encephalopathy, coagulopathy, renal insufficiency, mild hypotension due to vasodilation, ongoing third-space fluid losses, and impaired overall clinical recovery.

Allograft Dysfunction. The differential diagnosis of altered graft function is extensive (Table 13-3), and evaluation is complicated because the pattern of laboratory abnormalities is not a reliable indicator of the specific process involved. Although confounding factors (e.g., fluid overload, transfusion of red blood cells, and medication side effects) should be considered, technical problems and graft rejection should always be included in the differential diagnosis of graft dysfunction.

Prompt diagnosis of anatomic problems that induce these abnormalities is essential because delayed diagnosis can eliminate the opportunity for surgical correction and result in unnecessary secondary damage to the hepatic allograft. Furthermore, if anatomic problems are misdiagnosed as rejection and treated with increased immunosuppression, the patient may be unnecessarily exposed to increased risk of infection. Corticosteroids may also result in transient improvement of symptoms and laboratory abnormalities, thereby further delaying the correct diagnosis.

Hepatic artery thrombosis occurs in approximately 5% of patients in the early postoperative period and may present with sudden decompensation, marked elevation of all serologic markers, enteric bacteremia, and multiple-organ dysfunction syndrome. A hallmark of primary nonfunction of the liver is a failure to wake up within hours of surgery, assuming that a severe encephalopathy was not present preoperatively, and hypoglycemia. Furthermore, difficulty in warming the patient to 37°C may also indicate graft dysfunction. It is common for patients to arrive in the ICU hypothermic due to exposure of abdominal contents to ambient air temperature, the length of the surgical procedure, and a large amount of fluid resuscitation. Hepatic arterial occlusion in the late postoperative period typically presents with recurrent enteric bacteremia without an identifiable source, but it may also result in diffuse biliary strictures or progressive biliary ductopenia with formation of multiple intrahepatic bilomas or abscesses. In some patients, late arterial occlusion is well tolerated and produces no symptoms. Hepatic artery occlusion may also present as disruption of the bile duct because perfusion of the donor portion of the duct depends entirely on hepatic arterial flow. Conversely, the presentation may be subtler, manifesting as slowly evolving cholestatic jaundice. In either case, timely diagnosis is essential because prompt surgical intervention is effective in approximately one-half these cases.[5]

Portal venous thrombosis results in recurrent symptoms of portal hypertension, including ascites, splanchnic congestion, and gastrointestinal (GI) hemorrhage (variceal or hypertensive gastropathy). Stenosis of the superior caval anastomosis or suprahepatic caval thrombosis may mimic Budd-Chiari syndrome with hepatic congestion, lower-extremity edema, portal hypertension, and renal failure. Thrombotic or anatomic occlusion of the infrahepatic vena cava commonly results in edema of the lower extremities but may also result in renal dysfunction.

Initial evaluation of hepatic vessel patency can be made at the bedside by Doppler ultrasound imaging. If blood flow is not seen or if clinical suspicion of vascular occlusion is high and ultrasound findings are equivocal, selective angiography is indicated. Vascular stenosis or thrombosis may be addressed surgically or by balloon arterial dilation.

Biliary obstruction characteristically presents with signs and symptoms of cholestasis and may be due to anastomotic stenosis, kinking of a redundant duct, or bile sludging. If biliary obstruction is suspected, cholangiography should be performed either by T-tube or percutaneously. If a bile leak is demonstrated, hepatic arterial patency must be evaluated as previously discussed. Disruption of the bile duct in the absence of hepatic arterial thrombosis is uncommon but may present with periportal biloma, rising bilirubin, and sepsis. Cholestasis due to biliary sludging may respond to treatment with ursodeoxycholic acid (ursodiol).

Rejection must always be included in the differential diagnosis of graft dysfunction. Clinical presentation varies from explosive decompensation to gradually progressive hepatic failure. Despite a consistent clinical presentation and laboratory evidence of graft injury, the final diagnosis of rejection can only be made by liver biopsy. Biopsy may be performed percutaneously, under direct visualization, or via the transjugular approach. The transjugular approach to liver biopsy offers the obvious advantage in severely coagulopathic patients that all subsequent bleeding will be into the vascular tree. A disadvantage is that it requires a needle catheter to cross the upper caval anastomosis.

The existence of hyperacute rejection of hepatic allografts has been widely debated,[6–10] but catastrophic graft failure immediately after implantation has been reported.[11] It is characterized by sudden absence of bile production, fever, marked transaminasemia, coagulopathy, and graft necrosis. There is no proved mode of medical therapy. Although temporizing measures, such as plasmapheresis, have been tried, these patients should be listed for emergent retransplantation.

Acute cellular rejection typically occurs 5–14 days after OLT but should always be considered in the differential diagnosis of graft dysfunction at any time. The clinical presentation of acute cellular rejection is variable and may include fever, leukocytosis, thrombocytopenia, eosinophilia, and extrahepatic organ dysfunction. Elevated serum concentrations of bilirubin and hepatic enzymes are present, but the pattern of enzyme elevation is variable and the degree of elevation may not correlate with the histologic severity of rejection. Liver biopsy reveals inflammation and mononuclear infiltration of the portal triads. Treatment consists of intensification of the immunosuppressive regimen. Clearly, the presentation of acute cellular rejection resembles that of acute infection in several aspects, making the differential diagnosis difficult without a tissue diagnosis. Chronic rejection occurs later, typically after the fourth postoperative week. It is characterized by an indolent course of progressive graft dysfunction. Histologically, there is progressive loss of bile canaliculi from the portal triads, which has led some authors to use the term *ductopenic rejection* (see Figure 17-4). The mechanism of graft injury is thought to be due to antibody-mediated damage of the arteriolar epithelium. The clinical course is less severe than in acute cellular rejection, consistent with the lack of inflammation seen at pathology, and patients may be essentially asymptomatic until hepatic insufficiency develops. Chronic rejection is more difficult to treat, often being refractory to increased levels of immunosuppression. Once ductopenia develops, retransplantation may be the only recourse.

Neurologic Complications

Patients with good mental status before OLT and good graft function should awaken shortly after arrival in the ICU. Severe pretransplantation encephalopathy, hepatic dysfunction, side effects of immunosuppressant therapy, and medications that alter neurologic function may slow neurologic recovery. To the extent that other factors can be excluded, however, neurologic function is a sensitive marker of hepatic function.

Severe systemic insults, such as hypothermia, hyperthermia, malnutrition, infection, endocrine imbalances, electrolyte abnormalities, and dysfunction of multiple organ systems with potential neurologic effects may either precede or follow liver transplantation. These factors, combined with the use of multiple medications and the central role of the liver in drug metabolism, make metabolic encephalopathy a common etiology of altered mental status. Cyclosporine and tacrolimus may cause neurologic symptoms, ranging from mild psychomotor slowing to a condition resembling the "locked-in" syndrome.[12–14] Even if one or more of these etiologic factors is present, an aggressive diagnostic approach is required because altered mental status is also an early indicator of graft dysfunction or an intracranial process (hemorrhagic infection).

Although not common, seizures may be seen in patients after OLT. Several commonly used medications, including tacrolimus, cyclosporine, and OKT3, predispose to seizures.[13] Hyponatremia, hypomagnesemia,[15] and hypocholesterolemia[16] have been identified as comorbid factors. Nevertheless, focal neurologic deficits or seizures mandate emergent evaluation for cerebrovascular events, such as intracerebral hemorrhage as a result of an underlying coagulopathy, central nervous system (CNS) infection, or other intracranial process, because an erroneous diagnosis of metabolically induced seizures may delay appropriate treatment. Computed tomography (CT) or magnetic resonance imaging of the head, lumbar puncture, and blood culture analysis are all potential diagnostic tools in this setting. Akinetic seizures are a rare complication of OLT but must be included in the differential diagnosis of unresponsive patients.

Demyelination due to central pontine myelinolysis or progressive multifocal leukoencephalopathy[14] can cause decreased responsiveness and motor deficits. Steroid myopathy should also be considered, particularly in patients chronically treated with corticosteroids or prolonged courses of steroid-based muscle relaxants.[17–21] CNS infection is rare in the early postoperative period, but immunosuppression makes spinal fluid cultures essential in the presence of suggestive neurologic symptoms.

Cardiovascular Complications

The hyperdynamic, vasodilatative state often seen before OLT continues into the postoperative period. This hyperdynamic state gradually resolves but may be delayed by graft dysfunction or sepsis. Because peripheral vasomotor tone is low, these patients do not tolerate decreases in cardiac output, even to levels above "normal."

Ongoing third-space fluid loss is common in the initial perioperative interval. Vigorous intravascular volume resuscitation is often required. However, intravascular fluid administration should be carefully titrated once right atrial pressure exceeds 10 mm Hg because of the potential for hepatic congestion. Accordingly, to balance these conflicting factors, invasive hemodynamic monitoring is often required. In selected cases, echocardiography may be helpful in evaluating ventricular filling status and function. Systemic hypotension is treated in the usual fashion, with intravascular fluid replacement given to maintain right-sided filling pressures between 5 and 10 mm Hg and left-sided filling pressures between 10 and 16 mm Hg. Vasopressor therapy using dopamine or norepinephrine is indicated if hypotension persists despite adequate filling pressures and cardiac output, because hepatic artery graft perfusion is pressure limited.

Although uncommon, cardiac tamponade may occur in the immediate postoperative period because of many factors, including coagulopathy, atrial damage with high caval anastomosis, and inadvertent pericardial entry at the superior limit of the midline incision. Furthermore, because baseline vasodilatation may exist, the usual signs of tamponade may be masked, resulting in what appears to be normal cardiac output, right-sided filling pressures, and systemic vascular resistance despite inadequate systemic perfusion.

Because of the presence of residual coagulopathy and multiple vascular anastomoses, even brief hypertensive episodes can induce severe hemorrhage and hepatic graft dysfunction. Arterial pressures in excess of 160/95 mm Hg may induce anastomotic bleeding; thus, they should be reduced. Although pain and agitation are the most common signs of hypertension in the early postoperative period, hypertension can occur as a complication of both cyclosporine and tacrolimus.[22, 23] Hypertension due to cyclosporine or tacrolimus frequently responds to diuresis but may require routine antihypertensive medication.

Pulmonary Complications

Fluid shifts and humoral vasoactive factors present in patients with liver failure lead to variable degrees of pulmonary dysfunction due to decreases in lung compliance, alveolar diffusion, and increases in physiologic dead space. With two exceptions, management of mechanical ventilation and weaning are the same as in other patients. First, because elevated airway pressures are transmitted to the central venous system, hepatic congestion may occur. Thus, to avoid hepatic vascular congestion, airway pressures should not be allowed to remain elevated.

Second, because of the concern about aspiration in the immunosuppressed patient, clinically significant encephalopathy is a relative contraindication to extubation even if respiratory mechanics would suggest otherwise.

Atelectasis is very common after OLT due to the usual postoperative causes as well as two complications specific to this procedure. The engrafted liver may limit excursion of the right hemidiaphragm if it is significantly larger than the native liver, as is often the case in cirrhotic patients. Furthermore, right hemidiaphragm paresis can result from phrenic nerve damage during native hepatectomy if the dissection is complicated by extensive adhesions of the liver to the diaphragm. Phrenic nerve function usually recovers, but the time course is variable, and full recovery may take months.

Pleural effusions are also common, particularly in the presence of postoperative ascites and severe hypoalbuminemia. Drainage by thoracentesis or tube thoracostomy may be necessary if respiration is compromised. Effusions are typically right sided but may also be present bilaterally. Presence of an isolated left-sided effusion is uncommon and should prompt evaluation for pancreatitis or other subphrenic process.

In the immediate postoperative period, diffusely increased capillary permeability and hypoalbuminemia often result in pulmonary edema. This is usually transient and resolves with improving hepatic graft function and mobilization of third-space fluids, although poor graft function may result in more severe edema formation or delayed edema resolution. Gas exchange is usually better preserved than chest radiographs indicate. De novo formation of nonhydrostatic edema may result from the administration of OKT3 or severe hepatic graft injury. Even in the documented presence of these factors, new pulmonary infiltrates must be aggressively evaluated. Invasive hemodynamic assessment or bronchoalveolar lavage with or without protected tip brush specimens for quantitative bacterial and fungal cultures and opportunistic pathogens, such as *Pneumocystis carinii* and cytomegalovirus (CMV), are indicated in patients with new pulmonary infiltrates and fever.[24, 25]

Hepatopulmonary syndrome is a unique clinical entity characterized by hypoxemia and decreased alveolar arterial oxygen diffusion in the setting of chronic liver disease.[26] The diagnosis can be confirmed by demonstrating right-to-left intrapulmonary shunting on bubble contrast echocardiography.[27] Although the hypoxemia was originally thought to be due to anatomic intrapulmonary shunts, more recent work has shown severe ventilation-perfusion mismatch to be the mechanism of hypoxemia.[28, 29] Therefore, ventilatory support with enriched fraction of inspired oxygen usually improves arterial oxygenation. The syndrome typically resolves after successful transplantation,[30] but return to normal lung function may take several months. Early tracheostomy should be considered when prolonged (more than 2 weeks) gas exchange abnormalities preclude effective weaning from ventilatory support.

Pulmonary hypertension may also be associated with end-stage liver disease,[31–33] but this is a diagnosis of exclusion. Pulmonary vasodilator therapy may be attempted in hemodynamically impaired subjects but is not reliably effective. Pharmacologic manipulation of pulmonary artery pressures is problematic because systemic hypotension often results. Patients with systolic pulmonary artery pressures greater than 45 mm Hg (or mean pulmonary artery pressure greater than 35 mm Hg) and those with lower pulmonary artery pressures and evidence of RV failure are considered poor candidates for OLT. Post-OLT survival of patients with pre-existent pulmonary hypertension is 10–40%. Improvement of pulmonary hypertension does occur after transplantation but,[34–36] as in the case of the hepatopulmonary syndrome, may take months.

Gastrointestinal Complications

Elevations of serum amylase and lipase occur in approximately 20% of patients after OLT. However, only 5% develop clinical pancreatitis.[37] Evaluation and management are straightforward. Mild cases respond well to the usual supportive measures. Severe pancreatitis, however, frequently leads to hepatic graft dysfunction and has a grim prognosis in this population.

Upper GI bleeding requires immediate evaluation for recurrence of portal hypertension. Stress gastritis is a common finding in the early postoperative period, but later in the course, CMV enteritis,[38] fungal esophagitis, and gastric invasion due to post-transplantation lymphoproliferative disease[39] must be considered. Lower GI bleeding may be due to hemobilia, bleeding at the afferent limb of the Roux-en-Y jejunojejunostomy, or infectious enteritis, but more problematic lesions, such as vascular enteric fistulas from the hepatic or splenic arteries, must be considered. Evaluation must be rapid and may entail endoscopy, selective arteriography, and radionuclide bleeding scans. If the patient becomes unstable and a primary vascular lesion is suspected, immediate surgical re-exploration should be considered.

Renal Complications

Hepatorenal syndrome is a well-described cause of renal failure in patients with end-stage liver disease; it usually resolves after OLT.[40–44] Recovery of renal function may vary considerably and depends on the postoperative course. However, the presence of renal insufficiency before OLT increases the chance for a negative outcome from OLT.

Postoperative factors that may further compromise renal function include the almost universal administration of nephrotoxic medications (including tacrolimus[2] and cyclosporine[45, 46]), pronounced third-space fluid losses (functional hypovolemia), and the usual metabolic and hemodynamic insults experienced by critically ill patients.

Hepatic graft dysfunction may result in clinical deterioration of extrahepatic organ function. This is particularly true of renal function, but the actual relationship of renal function to graft injury or dysfunction is difficult to define because of the multiple coincident factors associated with graft dysfunction. These include changes in immunosuppressive drugs, intravascular volume status, and the humoral effects of infection or rejection on hepatic dysfunction.

Evaluation and management of renal failure are straightforward. Use of continuous ultrafiltration in selected patients requiring extracorporeal support (J. A. Kellum, personal communication, January 8, 1995) and prophylactic administration of a diuretic agent[47] are presently under study and may prove beneficial in these patients.

Endocrine Complications

Hyperglycemia is a common problem after OLT. Glucose intolerance is a recognized side effect of tacrolimus,[14] cyclosporine,[48] and corticosteroid therapies. This is particularly true when relatively high doses of corticosteroids are used to treat hepatic graft rejection. Hyperglycemia due to the initial stages of a high-dose corticosteroid taper may be difficult to control even with high dosages of insulin. New-onset hyperglycemia may also be an early sign of infection or acute rejection.

Hypoglycemia is much less common due to early institution of nutritional support. Adrenal insufficiency due to chronic corticosteroid administration may result in hypoglycemia if corticosteroids are abruptly discontinued. Hypoglycemia due to hepatic graft dysfunction is an ominous sign suggesting severe graft injury.

Both autoimmune hepatitis and primary biliary cirrhosis are associated with an increased incidence of thyroid insufficiency. A high index of suspicion should be maintained in patients with these primary disorders who manifest mental status changes, decreased myocardial contractility, or failure to wean from mechanical ventilation due to muscular weakness or decreased respiratory drive.

Corticosteroids are routinely used in the immunosuppressive regimen. Sudden discontinuation or decrease in steroid dosage may result in adrenal insufficiency and should be considered in patients with the usual signs and symptoms as well as unexplained pressor requirement and failure to wean from mechanical ventilation. The Cortrosyn Stimulation Test (Organon Canada, Ltd., Scarborough, Ontario, Canada) may be useful in evaluation of such patients. In practice, however, steroids are usually given in high enough doses to preclude adrenal crises.

Infectious Complications

Universal use of immunosuppressive agents makes infection an omnipresent risk in these patients. If severe infection or sepsis occurs, immunosuppression should be decreased or discontinued if possible. The situation is particularly difficult when graft rejection makes this option impossible.

Early postoperative infections result from infectious agents similar to those found in the general surgical population. Commonly isolated organisms are staphylococci, the enteric bacteria, and *Candida* species. After several weeks, increased vigilance for viral and opportunistic infections is necessary as the effects of T-cell suppression become more pronounced.[49] Prophylactic coverage with broad-spectrum antibiotics for 24–72 hours after surgery

is routine. The specific antibiotics used vary. Colonization with *Candida* is common in these patients,[44, 50] and prophylactic coverage with low-dose (10–20 mg/day) amphotericin B may be indicated after OLT if the procedure lasts more than 12 hours, if the transfusion requirement is large, or if there is peritoneal soiling. Re-exploration and retransplantation may also be indications for amphotericin B prophylaxis, although the efficacy of such treatment is currently unproved. Patients routinely receive prophylaxis for *P. carinii* either with trimethoprim-sulfamethoxazole or inhaled pentamidine.

CMV is also a common pathogen in these patients.[51, 52] Clinical expression of the infection varies from asymptomatic seroconversion to disseminated disease resulting in multisystem organ failure and death. Seronegative patients receiving seropositive organs are at the highest risk of infection. Disease in seropositive recipients is less frequent and may represent either reactivation of latent virus or superinfection by an immunologically distinct strain. Primary infection carries a significantly worse prognosis.[53] It is routine practice at our institution to perform weekly CMV antigenemia[54–56] determinations in the early postoperative period. Prophylaxis with specific antiviral agents, such as ganciclovir and acyclovir[57] or CMV hyperimmune globulin,[58] should be considered. (See Chapter 18 for a more detailed discussion of transplantation-related infections.)

Posttransplantation lymphoproliferative disease is caused by Epstein-Barr virus (EBV) infection. It can present with mild constitutional symptoms or a rapidly progressive disseminated lymphomatosis. Treatment consists of reducing immunosuppression and antiviral agents (acyclovir). Surgical excision of tumor masses may also be beneficial.[10] Because lymphoproliferative disease resembles lymphoma, however, it may require chemotherapy and is difficult to contain while the patient is receiving immunosuppressive therapy.

Several studies have shown that selective decontamination of the digestive tract (SDD) significantly decreases pharyngeal and GI colonization with aerobic gram-negative bacteria and fungi.[59–61] SDD has also been shown to reduce clinically significant infections with gram-negative organisms after OLT.[54, 62] However, corresponding decreases in postoperative mortality and ICU length of stay have not been demonstrated. Nevertheless, because infection with gram-negative organisms is a significant cause of morbidity and mortality in these patients, SDD may be appropriate.

Cardiac Transplantation

Pulmonary Hypertension

Pre-existing pulmonary hypertension (pulmonary vascular resistance in excess of 5 Wood units) is a major contraindication to heart transplantation. Pulmonary hypertension can be due to passive congestion of the pulmonary vasculature from the failing left ventricle. In these cases, calculated pulmonary vascular resistance is not increased because the increase in pulmonary artery pressure is matched by an increase in left atrial pressure. Usually, such patients' pulmonary arterial pressures decrease after successful cardiac transplantation. Pulmonary hypertension may also be due to increased pulmonary vascular resistance from multiple recurrent pulmonary emboli, vascular obliteration, or pulmonary arterial medial hypertrophy. In these cases, whether a subject is still a candidate for cardiac transplantation is related to the vasodilative potential of the pulmonary vasculature. These issues are usually addressed in the preoperative cardiac evaluation; they rarely present as unexpected postoperative problems. One notable exception is the subject with apparent passive pulmonary congestion in whom pulmonary arterial pressures do not decline after transplantation with the resultant decrease in pulmonary outflow pressure or pulmonary artery occlusion pressure (P_{PAO}). In such patients, P_{PAO} was not the downstream pressure to pulmonary blood flow; improving LV function only unmasked the diseased pulmonary vasculature, which, when presented with the increase in cardiac output after surgery, increased its inflow pressures. However, because the newly transplanted right ventricle is neither hypertrophied nor prepared to handle the markedly increased right-sided ejection pressures, the management of these patients is problematic. Often, the pulmonary vascular resistance decreases if the patient is supported long enough. The degree of vasoreactivity of the pulmonary vasculature after cardiac transplantation is highly variable, however, and the use of selective pulmonary vasodilator agents, such as intravenous prostaglandin E (PGE), prostacyclin, and inhaled nitric oxide, may not produce measurable hemody-

namic effects. If these patients do not respond to pharmacologic agents, consideration must be given to emergent mechanical RV assist device (RVAD) insertion or reinstitution of cardiopulmonary bypass (peripheral) until such time as the pulmonary vasculature relaxes or the right ventricle hypertrophies. Neither of these adaptive processes occurs quickly. Thus, this is a condition better avoided by proper patient selection than treated.

Finally, as with all forms of transplantation, it is important to diagnose pre-existent infection because the postoperative response of an infected, immunocompromised patient to antibiotics is suboptimal at best. Because most heart transplantation candidates have severe LV dysfunction and cardiac enlargement, some pulmonary congestion, atelectasis, and effusions are common. Furthermore, left lower-lobe collapse is uniformly seen as the enlarged left ventricle compresses and collapses this region of the lung. Thus, the diagnosis of pneumonia requires special attention to history, associated physical findings, and confirmatory laboratory results. The final arbitrator of the presence or absence of a pneumonic process is increasingly becoming quantitative cultures from bronchoalveolar lavage. More than 10^5 colony-forming units of a single organism in a patient with fever, pulmonary infiltrates, and elevated white cell count are definitive criteria for pneumonia. Surgery must be postponed until the infection resolves. The clearance of pulmonary infiltrates may lag behind resolution of active infection by many weeks; operational resolution of fever, leukocytosis, purulent sputum, and positive sputum cultures for the same organism is taken as evidence of no active pulmonary infection. These criteria are also used as a determinant for listing a subject as a transplantation candidate.

Ventricular Assist Devices

The use of mechanical VADs is seen in the management of heart transplant recipients at two potential phases of their illness. The first is the pretransplantation setting (bridge-to-transplantation VAD), and the second is after transplantation. Transplantation candidates who deteriorate clinically may require intravenous inotropic support or, ultimately, an intra-aortic balloon counterpulsation pump, which confines them to bed rest until transplantation. The survival of these patients to transplantation is in the range of 40% after 6 months; it can improve significantly with "bridge" VAD support until a donor heart is available.[63] An LV assist device may even allow status I transplant candidates to be discharged from the hospital while awaiting an organ. The challenge has been to select patients at imminent risk of ischemic organ injury without intervening too late.

In the posttransplantation setting, temporary VADs have been used to aid recovery from LV or RV failure (due to hyperacute rejection, preservation injury, or air embolism) and later episodes of acute cellular rejection. The success of temporary VADs is obviously determined by the reversibility of the myocardial pathology. In a subgroup of 125 heart transplant patients who required a VAD for posttransplantation shock, 38% were weaned and 22% survived to hospital discharge.[64] (See Chapter 5 for more detailed discussion of the mechanical devices available and anesthetic considerations.)

Surgical Considerations

As with any surgery, it is important for the intensivist to understand the surgical procedure and any unusual aspects of the intraoperative or preoperative care that may affect the postoperative course. (See Chapter 6 for details.)

Technically, several problems can arise in the immediate postoperative period. Surgical bleeding is common. A common site is not the mediastinum but the intra-atrial septum (due to torsion during insertion) and the great vessel anastomoses. Furthermore, torsion of pulmonary artery outflow tract can occur, especially with change in body position. Other postoperative complications include coronary artery–RV fistula after endomyocardial biopsy (8%) and mediastinitis. Mediastinitis is rare except in patients requiring preoperative support with an intra-aortic balloon counterpulsation pump. Risk with use of implantable VADs is known.

Posttransplantation Heart Physiology

Because parts of the donor atria are retained, there are two P waves, one from the native heart and one from the donor heart. However, the electrical activity from the native atrial tissue does not cross the suture line and therefore does not influence cardiac electrical activity. The transplanted heart is denervated (parasympathetic and sympathetic demonstration). As such, it demonstrates far fewer

Table 13-4. Postoperative Complications after Orthotopic Heart Transplantation

Arrhythmias
Sinus bradyarrhythmias
Cardiovascular insufficiency
    Acute rejection
    "Stunned myocardium"
    Right heart failure (due to pulmonary hypertension, prolonged ischemia time)
Pulmonary
    Atelectasis
    Infection
    Respiratory alkalosis
Renal or electrolyte disturbances
    Hypomagnesemia
    Hypophosphatemia
    Metabolic alkalosis
    Hypochloremia

respiratory sinus arrhythmias and no response to vagus-mediated manipulations in atrioventricular (AV) nodal conduction.[65] Thus, digitalis does not block AV nodal conduction and atropine does not increase heart rate in a bradycardic state. Furthermore, heart rate and inotropic changes induced by varying metabolic demands are delayed, making rapid changes in physiologic stresses more dangerous because hypotension may develop despite adequate blood volume, peripheral vasomotor tone, and even adequate intrinsic cardiac contractility.

Postoperative Problems

Routine postoperative problems common to all cardiovascular surgery patients also occur in cardiac transplant patients. Problems unique to cardiac transplant patients include arrhythmias, cardiovascular insufficiency, specific pulmonary problems, and renal or electrolyte disturbances (Table 13-4).

In the immediate postoperative period, marked sinus bradycardia may occur due to intraoperative cardiac cooling. In general, some degree of chronotropic support is indicated to maintain cardiac output if the heart rate is less than 90 beats per minute (bpm). In practice, either isoproterenol or dobutamine infusions are used and titrated to effect. The dosage needed is usually very small and rarely needed for more than 24 hours. Finally, once stable, the heart rate of the denervated heart is a sinus tachycardia in the range of 90–110 bpm as a result of the denervated parasympathetic tone. This represents the normal rhythm of a cardiac transplant patient; it need not be treated as abnormal.

Severe ventricular failure in the immediate postoperative period usually represents hyperacute rejection and is uniformly fatal unless the patient is placed on artificial cardiac support. It is manifest by a generalized hypokinetic myocardium by echocardiographic examination and reduced responsiveness to inotropic support. Postoperative myocardial depression lasting more than 24 hours due to ischemia, reperfusion, or "stunned myocardium" also occurs in cardiac transplantation. In this setting, progressive myocardial dysfunction, characterized by increased filling pressure requirements to maintain a reasonable cardiac output, appears between 6 and 8 hours after surgery and continues for another 6 hours. Stunned myocardium rarely is a cause of myocardial depression more than 24 hours after surgery. In general, inotropic support with dobutamine (5–10 m/kg/minute) should be considered if the cardiac index exceeds 2.5 liters per minute per m^2. Similarly, recalcitrant pulmonary hypertension should be treated aggressively with intravenous PGE$_1$ (20–80 µg/kg/minute). The dose of PGE$_1$ may be limited due to hypotension and may worsen gas exchange due to its negating effect on hypoxic pulmonary vasoconstriction. If it will resolve, meaning that it is not due to primary pulmonary hypertension, it usually does so within 24 hours. As described previously, persistent pulmonary hypertension associated with cor pulmonale often requires mechanical RVAD support if it does not respond to pulmonary vasodilator therapy. Inhalational nitric oxide may become the selective pulmonary vasodilator of choice. It has been shown to reduce pulmonary vascular resistance with no effect on systemic blood pressure, and its efficacy is currently under investigation.

Left lower-lobe atelectasis is common immediately after surgery because of the pre-existent cardiomegaly compressing this portion of the lungs. It is treated conservatively with recruitment maneuvers and supplemental positive end-expiratory pressure (PEEP) until it resolves, and then the PEEP can be lowered to minimal levels. However, persistent atelectasis or new pulmonary infiltrates on daily chest roentgenogram should be aggressively evaluated. One must consider infection rather than volume overload. Early fiberoptic bronchoscopy with appropriate cultures from bronchoalveolar lavage and bronchial brushings should be considered if infiltrate does not clear with routine maneuvers. Gram-negative bacilli are the most common pathogen in the immediate postoperative period because all patients are on perioperative antibiotic prophylaxis with either a first- or second-generation cephalosporin that covers gram-positive organisms. Chronic infiltrates or those not responsive to antibiotic therapy raise the diagnostic possibility of fungal, *P. carinii*, *Nocardia*, and viral infections. These can usually be diagnosed by bronchial biopsy and cultures as well as immunologic studies in established chronic infections. These infectious complications are treated with the usual antibiotic and chemotherapeutic agents but for extended periods.

Electrolyte imbalances due to chronic diuretic use are also common in this patient group. Hypomagnesemia presents as tachycardia, depressed ventricular function, low systemic vascular resistance, and an increased risk of coronary spasm. It mimics hypokalemia on electrocardiogram. The diagnosis is made by measuring serum Mg^{+2}; treatment is with intravenous MgSO$_4$. Hypophosphatemia may also occur, characterized by decreased muscle strength and failure to wean from mechanical ventilatory support; treatment is with intravenous NaPO$_4$ or KPO$_4$. Finally, respiratory alkalosis is commonly seen in the immediate postoperative period and is often artificial. It is due to hypothermia and resolves within 8–12 hours. If metabolic alkalosis is seen, as it often is later in the postoperative course, it is usually due to chloride loss. If urinary chloride is less than 10 mEq/liter, intravenous KCl or saline infusions may be needed to correct pH.

Acute rejection is characterized by acute heart failure; it is a medical emergency. It is usually treated with high-dose steroids or antithymocyte globulin. The complications of antithymocyte immunosuppression can range from mild influenza-like syndrome to full-blown septic shock with hypotension and adult respiratory distress syndrome (ARDS). It may also cause fever, chills, thrombocytopenia, and inflammation at the site of intramuscular injection. Whereas OKT3 produces a more generalized influenza-like syndrome, hypotension and acute pulmonary infiltrates with hypoxemia may occur as a result of the induced inflammatory mediators released from T cells after its administration.

Heart-Lung or Isolated Lung Transplantation

Heart-lung transplantation is usually performed to treat end-stage pulmonary disease because it is technically easier to perform than lung transplantation and it simultaneously treats cor pulmonale. Advances in surgical technique have made unilateral lung transplantation a more attractive option for many patients with end-stage lung disease, thereby making heart-lung transplantation less attractive.

Surgical Considerations

Unilateral lung transplantation requires three anastomoses: main stem bronchus, pulmonary artery, and pulmonary vein. In general, it is preferable to transplant the left lung because it allows easier access to vessels from posterior lateral thoracotomy. This form of transplantation does not require cardiopulmonary bypass unless cor pulmonale occurs at the time of cross-clamping the left pulmonary artery. Double-lung transplantation is performed from a standard median sternotomy, and cardiopulmonary bypass is usually used with both lungs removed from the patient's chest via mediastinal incisions that avoid damaging the phrenic nerves. Thus, there are three anastomoses: the trachea, atrial cuff, and pulmonary artery. Finally, heart-lung transplantation is performed with a standard median sternotomy and cardiopulmonary bypass. Both lungs are removed from the patient's chest via mediastinal incisions that avoid damaging the phrenic nerves. The heart is then removed, sparing the right atrial cuff. The lungs are inserted through the mediastinal incisions in an effort to prevent damage to the phrenic nerves. Three anastomoses here include the trachea, aorta, and right atrium. The cough reflex cannot be elicited by stimuli distal to the anastomosis due to denervation. After heart-lung transplantation, the carina has lost its sensory innervation, and these patients are at particular risk for silent aspiration.

Postoperative Problems

The primary concern in the immediate postoperative period after any form of lung transplantation is pulmonary insufficiency; noncardiogenic pulmonary edema (NCPE), rejection, and infection are the major contributors encountered in the first postoperative week.

Table 13-5. Management of Postoperative Complications of Lung Transplantation

Noncardiogenic pulmonary edema
Fluid restriction
Diuresis, prn
Inotropic support, prn
Maintain adequate hemoglobin level
FiO_2 to maintain adequate arterial saturations (>92%); using PEEP $\leq$10 mm Hg
Minimize peak airway pressures and use inverse ratio ventilation, if necessary
Physiotherapy, tracheal toilet
Promote frequent coughing, deep breathing
Nitric oxide, prn
ECMO, prn
Rejection
Confirm by transbronchial biopsy
Acute rejection immunosuppression protocol
Infection
Confirm microbe identity with culture, transbronchial washings, or biopsy, prn

prn = as needed; FiO_2 = fraction of inspired oxygen; PEEP = positive end-expiratory pressure; ECMO = extracorporeal membrane oxygenation.

Pulmonary Problems

All patients demonstrate some degree of NCPE, as shown by increased pulmonary markings on chest radiograph, increased intrapulmonary shunt, decreased lung compliance, increased work of breathing, and impaired gas exchange. Several factors contribute to NCPE and include reperfusion injury secondary to graft ischemia, inadequate graft preservation, lymphatic interruption, and inappropriate fluid resuscitation. Management consists of ventilatory support aimed at achieving appropriate gas exchange with minimal peak airway pressures. If necessary, increased inspired oxygen concentrations with concomitant inotropic support and diuresis are used to maintain adequate perfusion pressure and oxygen delivery (Table 13-5). In the most severe cases, acute pulmonary infiltrates manifesting as acute hypoxemic respiratory failure may need to be treated with ECMO while the underlying cause, such as acute reperfusion injury or graft rejection, resolves.

NCPE presents most often as a massive pulmonary capillary leak, hypoxemia, decreased compliance, and respiratory failure consistent with ARDS. Supportive and respiratory management is identical to that for

ARDS, although the acuity is often such that refractory hypoxemia and acidosis precipitate management with ECMO. Cannulation is generally peripheral, and venovenous ECMO is preferred over venoarterial ECMO because cardiac function is generally preserved. Furthermore, venovenous ECMO does not predispose the transplanted lungs, which are devoid of bronchial circulation, to the additional ischemic insult posed by bypassing the pulmonary circulation with a venoarterial circuit. Management is often complicated by bleeding into the chest. Nonetheless, in our experience, survival to hospital discharge is approximately 70%, with 1–9 days of support. In six patients in whom ECMO was instituted more than 7 days after transplant, none survived.[66]

Early postoperative bleeding may come from numerous intrathoracic sites. Tradition has it that adequate pleural suction reduces bleeding. Clearly, replacing clotting factors documented to be deficient is important.

Airway problems represent unique aspects of the care of heart-lung or lung transplantation patients. Airway anastomotic failure can occur. Dehiscence of the tracheal anastomosis presents as either air leaks or infection into the thorax and mediastinum. The risk factors for dehiscence include anastomosis ischemia due to inadequate revascularization techniques (omental wrap failure) and failure of wound healing due to excess corticosteroid use. Airway stricture can develop at the anastomotic site. It is difficult to correct using dilation techniques and silicone (Silastic) stents. Recurrent infections are only worsened by the insertion of the stent, and dilation techniques provide only temporary relief and are associated with risk of rupture.

Immunosuppression and Rejection

Immunosuppression therapies are similar to those for cardiac transplantation, with varying doses of tacrolimus, rabbit antithymocyte globulin, and OKT3 used. Acute cellular rejection is very common within the first 2 months and may result in ICU admission. The usual presentation is fever, dyspnea, and signs of pulmonary insufficiency described previously. The diagnosis is often made on clinical grounds once infection has been excluded. Bronchoalveolar lavage is useful in excluding infection but has not proved useful in staging acute cellular rejection. Occasionally, transbronchial biopsy or open-lung biopsy is necessary to confirm diagnosis if the risk of increased immunosuppression is high. Treatment is merely to increase standard immunosuppression therapy; the response is usually good.

Chronic rejection may also occur and require readmission to the ICU. The onset is usually insidious, presenting with dyspnea, cough, and a normal chest roentgenogram but worsening of the restrictive pattern on pulmonary function testing. Diagnosis requires tissue, and the preferred route is transbronchial biopsy. Long-term outcome is usually good. The major morbidity from chronic rejection is due to bronchiolitis obliterans. Isolated cardiac rejection in heart-lung transplant patients can occur, but it is diagnosed less often than is lung rejection. It is not clear, however, how often heart rejection occurs without lung rejection, whereas lung rejection without heart rejection is common. Presumably, lung rejection presents earlier because of the air-fluid interface, allowing diagnosis before respiratory failure, whereas cardiac rejection must induce functional problems before it is recognized.

Infections

Heart-lung and lung transplant recipients are at increased risk of respiratory infection for reasons beyond immunosuppression. These include denervation of the airways abolishing the cough reflex, ischemic dysfunction of airway mucosa impairing mucociliary clearance, the airway anastomosis forming a barrier to movement of secretions, and disruption of lymphatics preventing normal circulation of immune effector cells. Bacterial pneumonia is the most common cause of infection, with CMV infection being next most common. Before the routine use of antibiotic prophylaxis, *P. carinii* infections were common. Depending on the clinical situation, bronchoalveolar lavage with or without a transbronchial biopsy may be required to confirm the identity of the invading microbe. For example, a negative bronchoalveolar lavage in a patient who is suspected of infection with *P. carinii* mandates a transbronchial biopsy to confirm or exclude the diagnosis.

Renal Transplantation

Most patients do not require routine postoperative intensive care after renal transplantation, and thus do

Table 13-6. Common Causes for Intensive Care Unit Admission of Renal Allograft Recipient

Cardiac dysfunction: cardiac history with left ventricle ejection fraction <30%

Continued ventilatory support: pre-existent pulmonary disease and poor nutrition

Hypertension: (systolic BP >200 mm Hg or diastolic BP >120 mm Hg) treatment with nitroprusside, labetalol, or esmolol intravenously

Pulmonary edema: after OKT3 therapy for rejection, hypervolemia

Hyperkalemia: requires emergent hemodialysis to prevent arrhythmias

Gastrointestinal complications
  Massive upper gastrointestinal bleeding requires routine stress ulcer prophylaxis (e.g., sucralfate or H$_2$-receptor blocker)
  Ogilvie's syndrome: colonic pseudo-obstruction; requires aggressive attempts at decompression, including colonoscopy

Neurologic complications
  Cerebrovascular events (9%)
  Infections (4%)
  Peripheral neuropathy (4%)
  Hypertensive encephalopathy (6%)

Infectious complications

BP = blood pressure.

Table 13-7. Potential Causes for Delayed Allograft Dysfunction

Medical
  Preservation injury, acute tubular necrosis
  Rejection
  Nephrotoxicity of immunosuppressive therapy
Surgical
  Vascular
    Renal artery thrombosis
    Renal vein thrombosis
    Postoperative hemorrhage
  Urologic
    Ureter or bladder leakage
    Ureteral obstruction
  Renal biopsy complications
    Hematoma
    Renal rupture
    Arteriovenous fistula
    Urine leaks
    Vascular thrombosis

not come to the attention of the intensivist until some untoward event occurs. Occasionally, patients require postoperative ICU care, but these indications usually reflect non–transplant-related issues. Indications for perioperative ICU care relate to other organ-system dysfunction, renal failure–related problems, graft rejection, and infection rather than renal transplantation per se. Related organ-system dysfunction often occurs in this patient population due to the precipitants of chronic renal failure, such as diabetes and hypertension. Table 13-6 lists some common indications for admission of the renal transplant recipient to the ICU.

The most common reason for admission of a kidney transplant recipient is a history of coronary artery disease or evidence of myocardial ischemia.[67] The patient is aggressively hydrated with intravenous fluids to ensure adequate renal perfusion in the immediate postoperative period (to maintain central venous pressure at 10–15 mm Hg); this may predispose patients with compromised LV function to pulmonary edema. Diabetic renal transplantation candidates have an exceptionally high incidence of coronary artery disease, with 25–40% of asymptomatic patients having significant (50–70%) stenosis of one or more coronary arteries.[68–70] After transplantation, standard measures to reduce the incidence of ischemia should be used, including careful attention to pain and anxiety, good pulmonary toilet, and careful blood pressure control. Blood pressure control measures include continuation of agents associated with withdrawal problems, such as beta blockers and clonidine, and close monitoring of volume status with pulmonary artery catheters.

Allograft Dysfunction

Physicians caring for renal transplant recipients should be knowledgeable about the assessment of delayed return to function. Most transplanted kidneys are functional by 2 weeks after transplantation, but a delay of 4–6 weeks is possible before adequate function is restored. Delayed return of function, as determined by the need for dialysis at 1 week post transplantation, is associated with a 15–20% lower graft survival rate at 1 year. It may be due to many causes.[71] Although preservation injury, rejection, and nephrotoxicity of immunosuppressant medications account for the majority of cases of delayed return to function, up to 5% of graft dysfunction is related to surgical complications (Table 13-7). Because these complications may be treatable if identified early, failure to diagnose the cause can result in loss of the graft and significant patient morbidity and mortality.

Hyperkalemia and pulmonary edema secondary to a delayed return of allograft function are the most common reasons for ICU admission in the initial postoperative period. Hyperkalemia can be treated with standard measures, such as glucose and insulin, loop diuretics, and intravenous bicarbonate. Several case reports indicate that potassium exchange resins should not be used because they may cause intestinal perforation.[72] Many physicians are also hesitant to begin dialysis in the early postoperative period, but it may be necessary for hyperkalemia and pulmonary edema unresponsive to more conservative measures.

High cyclosporine or tacrolimus levels indicate the possibility of renal insufficiency secondary to the nephrotoxicity of these agents. Renal function may improve promptly after reduction of the dosage of these agents, but the correlation between nephrotoxicity and drug levels is inconsistent. If technical problems have been excluded, and renal allograft dysfunction does not appear to be due to nephrotoxic agents or does not improve with reducing the dose of the nephrotoxic agent, rejection must be considered. The clinical signs of rejection are also nonspecific and may consist of allograft swelling and tenderness, fever, malaise, and leukocytosis. A renal biopsy is required to differentiate between acute rejection and acute tubular necrosis. Complications of renal biopsy include hematoma, renal rupture, AV fistulas, urine leaks, and vascular thrombosis; they can result in graft loss.

Acute rejection is characterized by a mononuclear interstitial infiltrate and occurs in up to 55% of all recipients.[73] It is usually treated with methylprednisolone bolus therapy, which is effective approximately 85% of the time.[74] Chronic rejection is the most frequent cause of late graft loss, but other causes of graft dysfunction must be excluded. In the initial evaluation of declining function, cyclosporine or tacrolimus levels should be determined. If elevated, the dosage of these drugs should be reduced; if no improvement in function is seen, other causes should be considered. The possibility of renal artery stenosis should be assessed when progressive hypertension or a renal bruit accompanies a loss in function. Recurrence of the disease that originally caused the renal failure can also cause decline in renal function. All diseases that cause renal failure can recur in the transplanted kidney, with the exception of Alport's syndrome. The diseases that most commonly recur in the allograft include diabetic nephropathy, type II membranoproliferative nephritis, immunoglobulin A nephropathy, and focal or segmental glomerular sclerosis.[75] Overall graft loss due to recurrent disease is only 5%. Renal biopsy is the best way to determine if chronic, acute, or recurrent rejection is the cause.

Surgical Complications

Surgical complications can be separated into two groups: vascular and urologic (see Table 13-7).

Hemorrhage from unligated small vessels, arterial lacerations, and disrupted ligatures is occasionally seen early post-transplantation. Repair of anastomotic suture-line bleeding is rarely indicated because of the high recurrence rate of rebleeding. A mortality rate as high as 33–50% has been reported with massive operative bleeding.[76] Low-grade nonanastomotic bleeding occurs after kidney transplantation because of the uremic coagulopathy that is often present. Uremic coagulopathy can be treated with desmopressin (DDAVP; 0.03 µg/kg), conjugated estrogens (0.7 mg/kg daily for 5 days), transfusion to a hematocrit of 30, and fibrinogen given as cryoprecipitate.[77–80] Large hematomas should be evacuated before they compress and occlude the renal vascular supply or ureter. Any undrained hematoma presents an infectious risk.

Renal artery thrombosis occurs in slightly more than 1% of kidney transplants.[81] Technical problems that can cause renal artery thrombosis include presence of an intimal flap, malanastomosis, and kinking of the artery; other causes include hyperacute rejection and hypercoagulable states. The hallmark of the condition is a sudden cessation of urine output; allograft loss occurs if not treated within 12 hours. Failure to diagnose can result in sepsis and is associated with a patient mortality rate as high as 50–60%.[82] This complication can occur late after transplantation, but 80% of cases occur in the first month.[83] Immediate exploration and reanastomosis are indicated, but in most cases salvage attempts fail and nephrectomy is required. Renal vein thrombosis occurs in 0.3–4.2% of patients and tends to occur shortly after transplantation.[84–86] It may be caused by kinking of the vein, compression of the vein by an adjacent hematoma or lymphocele, stenosis of the venous anastomosis, or ascending thrombophlebitis. Clinically, it is characterized by a painful swelling of the allograft with hematuria, proteinuria, and oliguria. Thrombectomy may save the kidney, but usually the thrombus has propagated into smaller vessels and the kidney cannot be salvaged.

Urologic complications are more common than vascular complications and may occur in up to 10% of transplants.[87] Leakage can occur from either the ureter or the bladder. The bladder usually leaks at the anterior edge of the cystotomy closure. Leakage usually presents before the fifth month after transplantation and is characterized by fever, increased creatinine, oliguria, and a painful mass in the area of the leak. Radiologic imaging techniques or the demonstration of a high creatinine level in fluid draining from a surgical wound or in percutaneously aspirated fluid can be used to make the diagnosis. Surgical repair is the treatment of choice. Ureteral obstruction can occur any time after transplantation. When it occurs early, it may be due to edema of the ureter, blood clots, compression by adjacent hematoma, or kinking of the ureter. Clinical signs are similar to those of rejection and include oliguria or anuria, pain over the allograft site, and increasing creatinine. Sepsis may develop. Traditionally, surgery has been the treatment of choice, but more recently, percutaneous or transurethral balloon dilation with or without stenting has shown value. Percutaneous transurethral nephrostomy tube placement may be performed to temporarily improve renal function before a more definitive procedure is attempted. Overall, the symptoms associated with surgical complications of renal transplantation are well recognized but not very specific.

Imaging techniques, including CT scans, angiograms, magnetic resonance angiograms, pyelography, cystography, and cystoscopy, have value in the diagnosis of posttransplantation technical complications, but the most useful tool in the initial evaluation for these conditions is color flow Doppler ultrasound. Radionuclide renal scintigraphy can also be easily performed at bedside and has supplemental value in the initial evaluation of graft dysfunction. There are many reports of the value of Doppler examination of the hemodynamics of allograft blood flow in differentiating rejection from ischemic injury and drug toxicity. In particular, the role of the resistive index has been touted, but clinical experience has shown the value of such techniques to be disappointing.[88]

Table 13-8. Infectious Complications after Renal Transplantation

Viral infections
Cytomegalovirus presenting as pneumonitis, gastritis, or colitis with hemorrhage (gastrointestinal bleeding may be severe)
Treatment: ganciclovir
Protozoal infections
Pneumocystis carinii less common since use of prophylactic trimethoprim-sulfamethoxazole
Treatment: trimethoprim-sulfamethoxazole
Fungal infections
Numerous types, many trivial, some serious, especially candidal esophagitis; systemic *Candida* and *Aspergillus* seen in patients with prolonged illnesses; consider *Nocardia*, *Cryptococcus*, and *Mucor* with pulmonary or cerebral infections
Treatment: amphotericin B, fluconazole

Infectious Complications

The primary reason for admission to the ICU after the initial postoperative period is infection. Infectious complications seen with kidney transplants are similar to those seen with other solid-organ transplants (Table 13-8). Almost 70% of all severe infections occur within the first 3 months of transplantation.[89] In the first month, the infectious complications are similar to those seen in nonimmunosuppressed postoperative patients. Infections of the lung, bladder, wounds, and catheter site with common bacteria or *Candida* occur, but the clinical consequences of such infections may be much more severe. Opportunistic infections occur most frequently 1–6 months post transplantation.[90] The etiology of infections must be aggressively pursued because of the high morbidity and mortality associated with them. Protective brush or bronchoscopic alveolar lavage should be performed promptly on patients with pneumonia, particularly when a nonlobar pneumonia and a nonproductive cough are present. In patients with unexplained abdominal pain, GI bleeding, and diarrhea, early endoscopy should be performed to establish whether fungal or viral infections are the cause. CMV is the most important pathogen during this period and can involve any organ system. Three patterns of infection are seen: Primary infections due to transplantation of a CMV-infected kidney or transfusions of CMV-carrying blood products into a CMV-seronegative patient are the most severe. Reactivation of endogenous latent virus is the least severe, and superinfection of CMV-seropositive patients causes illness intermediate in severity.[91] Because of the immune-modulating properties of CMV, superinfection with other opportunistic pathogens commonly complicates CMV infection.[92] Antithymocyte and antilymphocyte globulin appear to increase the risk for infections due to CMV. Additional opportunistic viral infections seen include other herpesviruses (herpes simplex, varicella-zoster, EBV) and hepatitis B and C.

Fungal infections with *Candida* species occur primarily in the urinary tract. *Aspergillus* colonizes the respiratory tract and CNS; *Cryptococcus* in the CNS is the most common infection.[93] In most fungal infections, amphotericin B remains the preferred therapy because the role of fluconazole has yet to be well established in immunosuppressed solid-organ recipients. Other notable pathogens include mycobacteria, both tuberculous and nontuberculous,[94] and parasites such as *P. carinii*. In all severe infections, a reduction or a discontinuation of immunosuppression is indicated. Beyond 6 months, infectious agents tend to be the pathogens found in the general population, with the exception that atypical infections still occur in some recipients, particularly those requiring high doses of immunosuppression. Chronic viral infections occur in 10–15% of renal transplant recipients, who are at risk for virus-related diseases, such as chronic hepatitis, hepatocellular carcinoma, and EBV-associated posttransplantation lymphoproliferative disorder. (For a more detailed discussion of diagnosis and management of infectious complications, see Chapter 18.)

Cardiovascular Complications

Cardiovascular disease ranks with sepsis as the major cause of death after renal transplantation. In one survey, the incidence of coronary artery disease was 15.1%—fourfold higher than predicted.[95] Diabetic patients are at particularly high risk, with up to 60% of their deaths due to cardiovascular complications.[96] Significant cardiac risk factors develop after renal transplantation, including hypertension and hyperlipidemia. Hyperlipidemia is believed to be caused by immunosuppressive medications, loop diuretics, and beta blockers.[97–99] Because of the high incidence of cardiac disease, it should not be assumed that pulmonary edema is solely due to volume overload secondary to renal insufficiency. Myocardial ischemia

should be excluded because hemodialysis of patients with myocardial ischemia can be disastrous.

At least half of all renal transplant recipients develop hypertension. In a small fraction of these patients, it may be severe enough to warrant ICU admission. Stenosis of the allograft renal artery, renin release from the native kidneys, rejection, cyclosporine, and tacrolimus can each be implicated in the pathogenesis of posttransplantation hypertension. Progressive hypertension that is refractory to therapy or that is accompanied by a renal bruit or decreased renal function without evidence of rejection suggests renal artery stenosis. Duplex sonography and captopril radionuclide scans are the most reliable noninvasive tests for this condition.[100] Angiotensin-converting enzyme (ACE) inhibitors can precipitate renal failure in patients with renal artery stenosis and should be avoided.[101] Surgery is the treatment of choice, with an 80% long-term success rate; balloon angioplasty is half as effective.[102] Native kidneys can also cause hypertension through renin release. In this situation, angiotensin inhibitors are of value. Nephrectomy is an option if ACE inhibitors are ineffective or cause renal insufficiency.[103] Hyperkalemia may be caused by ACE inhibitors and can be treated with diuretics. Hypertension due to cyclosporine and tacrolimus does not appear to be due to the renin-angiotensin system but to renal vasoconstriction and sodium retention. Diuretics or calcium channel blockers are most useful in this situation, as with hypertension associated with rejection.[104] Diuretics must be cautiously used so that prerenal azotemia does not develop. Cyclosporine levels should be closely monitored if either diltiazem or verapamil is begun because both medications can increase the blood levels of cyclosporine.[105, 106] Because of their adverse effect on lipid profiles, beta blockers and loop diuretics may be poor choices for long-term management of hypertension in these patients. Pulmonary edema, electrolyte disturbances, and complications of uremia may occur with declining renal function and necessitate ICU admission.

Gastrointestinal Complications

Significant GI complications have been reported in one-third or more of all renal transplant recipients, but these complications are probably less common today. Still, significant morbidity and mortality can occur when these conditions develop. Esophagitis due to fungal and viral infections and peptic ulcer disease sometimes occur in renal allograft recipients. Pancreatitis, possibly caused by high-dose corticosteroid or azathioprine administration, is also a relatively common problem, occurring in 2–7% of these patients.[107] In this situation, pseudocysts and pancreatic abscesses often develop and are accompanied by a mortality rate that has been reported in excess of 50%.[108] Colonic complications have been reported in 1–2% of renal allograft recipients, including colonic perforation, of which 50% occur in the cecum. Early series reported mortality rates in excess of 80%, and even today mortality rates exceed 30%.[109–111] CMV is a major contributor to GI disease in transplant recipients. Infections can occur on all levels of the GI tract, but CMV predominantly involves the colon and small bowel of transplant recipients. CMV infection can cause pain, diarrhea, severe GI hemorrhage, and perforation.[112] The introduction of anti-CMV treatment with ganciclovir has improved the prognosis of renal transplant recipients with GI and other CMV infections. If a CMV infection is suspected, the level of immunosuppression should be reduced. Hospitalized renal allograft recipients are frequently on antibiotics and at risk for *Clostridium difficile* colitis. *C. difficile* colitis does not always present as diarrhea but may present with acute abdominal pain and intestinal distention, and it should be considered in this setting.

Multivisceral Organ Transplantation

Although multivisceral transplantations (MVTs) have been documented in animals since 1964, the first successful MVT was reported in 1987.[113] Today, there are still only a handful of humans surviving with MVTs, and this procedure remains experimental.

The usual indications are upper abdominal malignancy or prior extensive resection after trauma or Crohn's disease.[114] Patients are considered candidates only when conventional therapy has failed and severe disability or life-threatening complications have developed. This changes the risk-benefit ratio in favor of these experimental procedures. As such, postoperative care of these patients is complicated by their markedly debilitated state. The long-term parenteral nutrition that these patients usually require leaves them at risk for intravenous catheter infection, multiple venous thromboses, and liver failure. This latter complication is an indication for combined OLT and small bowel transplantation.

Surgical Considerations

Patients undergoing MVT often have had multiple prior operations, making any intra-abdominal transplantation procedure hazardous. Furthermore, the abdominal cavity has usually shrunk secondary to scarring. Thus, procured organs must be smaller than expected for the recipient's size to allow abdominal wall closure.

The site and anastomoses in MVT depend on which organs are removed and which are replaced. The procedures performed at one site (University of Pittsburgh Medical Center) have included resection and transplantation of the liver, pancreas, spleen, some or all of the stomach, duodenum, jejunum, ileum, and, in some, partial colon.

Postoperative Problems

The principles of postoperative management include routine ICU care, nutrition, strict glucose control, immunosuppression with careful monitoring for rejection, and organ-specific support. This includes careful attention to nosocomial infection, multisystem organ function, and provision of supportive therapy as indicated (e.g., blood and blood products for bleeding complications) while the patient is weaned from the ventilator and rehabilitated.

Fluid and Electrolyte Balance

All MVT surgery involves significant manipulation, many hours of anesthesia, and extensive fluid losses. Postoperative third-space fluid requirements can be massive, and inadequate replacement leads to end-organ dysfunction, particularly renal failure. Consequently, central venous pressure monitoring, preferably with pulmonary arterial catheterization, is essential. Several liters of fluid may be required in the initial 24–48 hours postoperatively simply to maintain central pressures adequate to provide a satisfactory urine output of 0.5 ml/kg per hour. During this time, the patient may develop extensive peripheral edema, which dissipates over the next few days as the patient mobilizes fluids. It is important to appreciate that, although this phenomenon occurs after all abdominal surgery, these patients have significantly greater fluid shifts than do patients undergoing major nontransplantation abdominal surgery. Serum electrolytes should be checked every 6 hours initially. The patient often requires supplemental magnesium and phosphate. After the first few days, fluid requirements stabilize. Continued increases in fluid requirements herald infection or rejection.

Antimicrobial Prophylaxis

Infection is always a significant risk in transplant recipients. Initially, this often results from leaking from anastomoses from previous surgeries or the presence of fistulas and abscesses in the operative field. Anastomoses may be fashioned with bowel that sustains some unquantified injury during preservation. These anastomoses are technically difficult and may be in sites that cannot be seen well postoperatively. These patients require aggressive immunosuppression to prevent rejection. Furthermore, rejection results in compromised graft integrity; therefore, bacterial and fungal infection may occur concurrently with rejection. Surveillance cultures from drains and ostomies as well as catheter sites have particular value when sepsis develops and empiric antibiotics are required. Prophylaxis is directed at common bacterial, fungal, and viral pathogens.

Antibacterial. Contamination of the operative site with gram-negative (enterobacteriaceae) and gram-positive (*Staphylococcus* and *Enterococcus*) organisms requires broad-spectrum antibiotic coverage. Typically, we use ampicillin and cefotaxime for 48 hours, commencing on call to the operating room. The choice of agents varies, depending on the spectrum of resistance in a particular hospital. SDD is also added to those receiving an intestine graft.

Antiviral. Viruses of the herpes family commonly cause illness in solid-organ transplant recipients. Both primary infection (from the donor) and reactivation of latent recipient infection cause significant morbidity and require treatment. Primary infections that occur in a seronegative recipient who receives a graft from a seropositive donor often result in multiple organ involvement with high mor-

bidity and mortality. The likelihood of infection correlates with the intensity of immunosuppression. Recipients of multiple viscera are heavily immunosuppressed. The most common offending viruses are CMV and herpes simplex virus. Prophylaxis for both infections is currently provided with full-dose ganciclovir for at least 2 weeks and often longer, until oral acyclovir is tolerated.

Experience in bone marrow transplant recipients has demonstrated that prophylaxis directed specifically at very high-risk patients (those actively infected) is particularly effective without incurring the risk of supplying prophylaxis to low-risk patients. In a similar fashion, MVT patients with evidence of CMV infection (biopsy-proved) and those with colonization and high clinical suspicion or significant risk are all treated with high-dose ganciclovir. Ganciclovir-resistant organisms have been described. Patients with persistent infection or with intolerable side effects are treated with foscarnet. The most significant side effect of ganciclovir is bone marrow suppression, particularly neutropenia. If continued therapy is required, Filgrastim (Neupogen) may be administered. The major toxicity of foscarnet is renal failure, a common problem in these patients.

Antipneumocystic. All OLT, small bowel transplantation, and MVT patients are commenced on *P. carinii* pneumonia prophylaxis. This consists of trimethoprim-sulfamethoxazole every other day. In the event of suspect GI absorption, the drug is administered intravenously. If sulfa allergy is present, patients can be switched to pentamidine inhalations monthly. Therapy is continued for life.

Antifungal. Fungal infection is common in MVT patients. They are immunocompromised, have multiple intravascular catheters, receive parenteral nutrition, and require multiple antibiotics. No data currently define the roles of amphotericin B and the imidazoles, such as fluconazole, for prophylaxis. Patients at particularly high risk, including those with anastomotic leaks, particularly heavy immunosuppression, multiple sites colonized, and unremitting fever, are treated with full-dose amphotericin B.

Nutrition

Patients who have undergone abdominal exenteration have understandable digestive difficulties, and transfer to a normal diet is difficult. Almost all have lost significant body weight in the first 3 months post transplantation despite vigorous attempts to maintain adequate nutrition.

Many patients are already considerably debilitated, and many are malnourished. Although attempts are made to optimize the patient's condition before transplantation, the natural history of the underlying illness may thwart efforts to improve the patient's nutritional status. Furthermore, the extensive surgery and the postoperative course, which may include systemic infection and graft rejection, combine to produce an extremely severe catabolic stress. Although debate continues about the optimal feeding method during such stress, the experience at our institution is that significant weight loss and failure to thrive are very common. Accordingly, without direct evidence to the contrary, we favor early introduction of aggressive feeding regimens.

Enteral Nutrition.   Although donor intestine function is difficult to assess in the initial postoperative period, we use small amounts of isotonic tube feeding into the small bowel because it may be of benefit in preserving villous architecture. This is insufficient to meet the daily caloric requirements of the host. As bowel sounds develop and ileostomy output occurs, the tube feeding rate can be advanced. Eventually, all caloric requirements are met via enteral means. An important point is that, if the donor intestine appears to be functioning, it should be used.

Parenteral Nutrition.   Most patients receiving a multivisceral transplant require parenteral nutrition. Indeed, many may already have a dedicated total parenteral nutrition silicone catheter in place preoperatively. If the site is clean and there is no history of recent infection attributable to the catheter, it should be used as the dedicated parenteral nutrition catheter postoperatively. Otherwise, a port on a triple-lumen or pulmonary artery catheter should be dedicated to parenteral nutrition to minimize the risk of infection. Total parenteral nutrition should begin within the first 2–3 postoperative days and continued as long as there is any suspicion that caloric requirements are not being met by enteral feeding.

Exocrine Pancreatic Replacement.   Depending on the configuration of the multivisceral transplant, many patients do not have exocrine pancreatic function. Enteral feeding mandates exocrine pancreatic enzyme supplements to maximize absorption and minimize ileostomy output. These supplements are dissolved in the tube feedings or sprinkled on the food during preparation. Once the patient is stable, tablet supplements may be taken before each meal.

Blood Glucose Control

Hyperglycemia is common and multifactorial in etiology in patients after visceral organ transplantation. Pancreatectomy, high caloric load for parenteral nutrition therapy, corticosteroids, tacrolimus, cyclosporine, sepsis, and surgical stress often contribute. Glucose control is best effected by continuous insulin infusion in the initial postoperative period. The goal for most recipients is a blood glucose concentration less than 200 g/dl. However, pancreas transplant and intestine transplant recipients require tighter control. It is believed that donor islet cell viability may depend on the minimization of stress to produce insulin (i.e., elevated blood glucose level) during the engraftment phase over the first few days.[115] Consequently, all these patients are maintained on a continuous intravenous insulin infusion with hourly blood glucose analysis and adjustment to maintain blood sugar between 70 and 150 g/dl.

Small Bowel and Colon Transplantation

The freshly transplanted bowel is deemed at increased risk of translocation due to impaired mucosa-associated lymphoid tissue function, ischemic gut wall, and, when combined with an OLT, impaired Kupffer cell function. Consequently, we recommend early institution of a selective bowel decontamination regimen targeted at gram-negative bacilli and, depending on the microbiological environment of the hospital, gram-positive cocci. This promotes overgrowth of a protective layer of anaerobic bacteria with a consequent theoretical decrease of translocation of bacterial wall components and sepsis.

Similarly, to promote early recovery of bowel wall integrity, we recommend low-dose tube feeding as early as possible to reduce further villous atrophy and promote recovery of the existing villous architecture.

Daily history and examination of the GI system is the first step in monitoring bowel transplant function.

Attention to nausea, abdominal pain, bowel sounds, and abdominal tenderness and distention often provides early signs of problems. Additionally, the macroscopic appearance of the ileostomy provides clues as to the integrity of the bowel mucosa. The volume and character of the ileostomy drainage provides information about the absorptive capacity of the bowel—a sensitive marker of rejection. Culture of the ileostomy output aids in assessing the effectiveness of selective decontamination regimens. In contrast to other solid-organ recipients, small and large intestine recipients require routine (protocol) endoscopic biopsies even in the absence of potential problems. Finally, more exact studies of bowel function, such as D-xylose absorption tests and stool fat assays, are performed routinely to monitor ongoing bowel function. Again, as experience grows, the frequency of these tests may drop.

Postoperative Complications

Technical

The principal technical complication of bowel transplantation is an anastomotic leak. This is potentially devastating because leakage of bowel contents into the peritoneum of an immunocompromised host carries a high mortality. Consequently, signs of sepsis or peritonitis must be investigated immediately with a high index of suspicion for a bowel leak. Treatment is virtually always surgical (either a primary repair of the anastomosis or a defunctionalizing ostomy followed by late reanastomosis) with aggressive intra- and postoperative systemic and intraperitoneal antibiotics. There is little evidence yet as to the incidence of late stricture formation in small bowel transplant recipients, but this is certainly possible.

Rejection

Detection of early rejection of the transplanted intestines is often difficult. The clinical heralds of increased ostomy output, fever, and abdominal tenderness are nonspecific and may occur in both infectious and rejection episodes. We have found that routine and frequent biopsies are essential. As noted with other solid organs, resistant, cellular rejection is treated with increased dosage of tacrolimus and

corticosteroids. Resistant episodes may require treatment with OKT3. Rejection may be associated with compromise in bowel integrity and subsequent bacteremia and sepsis syndrome. Consequently, concomitant treatment of rejection and infection may be necessary. Ultimately, if severe rejection persists, surgical removal is indicated.

Infection

Bacterial

Small bowel transplant patients are at particularly high risk for intra-abdominal infection. Despite antimicrobial prophylaxis, bacterial infection may result from disruption of biliary and enteral anastomoses with resultant peritonitis. Early, aggressive surgical management combined with appropriate antibiotics and antifungal agents are essential. Despite these efforts, infection-related death remains quite common.

Other sites of infection include the lungs and the invasive catheter site. The usual diagnostic evaluation for these patients may not reveal the etiology. We favor bronchial lavage and protected brush specimen sampling with quantitative cultures to determine the offending organism. Clinical diagnosis of pneumonia is difficult and erroneous. Patients may present with clinical, radiographic, and laboratory signs consistent with a pulmonary infection, and yet it may have an intra-abdominal source. Furthermore, patients with allograft rejection may present with signs of respiratory embarrassment, which proceeds to frank ARDS; in fact, it may be difficult to distinguish from pneumonia.

Fungal

Fungal infection is common and may occur concomitantly with bacterial infection. The usual organisms are *Candida* and *Aspergillus*. As in other solid-organ transplant recipients, the finding of invasive aspergillosis is very grave. Currently, we approach basic fungal infections with full-dose amphotericin B therapy. Adjunctive therapy is flucytosine for *Candida*. The newer imidazoles, such as itraconazole for *Aspergillus*, are used when indicated. Other fungal infections, such as *Cryptococcus*, are reported in immunocompromised patients, such as solid-organ transplant recipients. The diagnosis must be considered in the patient with unexplained neurologic dysfunction and persistent headache.

Viral

Viral infection can also occur simultaneously with bacterial and fungal infection. In multivisceral transplant recipients, this viral infection may lead to graft dysfunction or failure. Intestinal infection is common, and an increase may herald the presence of CMV enteritis. Treatment is with ganciclovir and foscarnet, as described previously.

Conclusions

Intensive care management of the transplant population may involve support of end-stage organ failure patients who are awaiting transplantation, perioperative care of the transplant recipient, or care of the transplanted patient who requires ICU admission to manage postoperative complications, usually consisting of episodes of infection or rejection. Knowledge regarding the diagnosis and management of end-stage organ failure and its effects on other organ systems, allograft dysfunction, and rejection, as well as the infectious complications associated with the immunocompromised host, are germane to this patient population.

References

1. Mackersie RC, Bronsther OL, Shackford SR. Organ procurement in patients with fatal head injuries. Ann Surg 1991;213:43–50.
2. Davis CF. Coordination of cardiac transplantation: patient processing and donor organ procurement. Circulation 1987;75:29.
3. Slapak M. The immediate care of potential donors for cadaveric organ transplantation. Anesthesia 1978;33: 700–709.
4. Yamamoto Y, Ozawa K, Okamoto R, et al. Prognostic implications of postoperative suppression of arterial ketone body ratio: time factor involved in the suppression of hepatic mitochondrial oxidation reduction state. Surgery 1990;107:289–294.
5. Yanaga K, Le Beau G, Marsh JW, et al. Hepatic artery reconstruction for hepatic artery thrombosis after orthotopic liver transplantation. Arch Surg 1990;125: 628–631.
6. Ratner LE, Phelan D, Brunt EM, et al. Probable antibody-mediated failure of two sequential ABO-compatible hepatic allografts in a single recipient. Transplantation 1993;55:814–819.
7. Bird G, Friend P, Donaldson P, et al. Hyperacute rejection in liver transplantation: a case report. Transplant Proc 1989;21:3742–3744.
8. Starzl TE, Demetris AJ, Todo S, Kang Y. Evidence for hyperacute rejection of human liver grafts: the case of the canary kidney. Clin Transplant 1989;3:37–45.
9. Iwatsuki S, Rabin BS, Shaw BW Jr, Starzl TE. Liver transplantation against T-cell positive warm cross-matches. Transplant Proc 1984;16:1427–1429.
10. Gordon R, Funf J, Markus B, Fox I. The antibody cross-match in liver transplantation. Surgery 1986;100:705–715.
11. Cienfuegos JA, Pardo F, Hernandez JL, et al. Hyperacute rejection in liver transplantation: morphologic and clinical characteristics. Transplant Proc 1992;24:141–142.
12. de Groen PC, Aksamit AJ, Rakala J, et al. Central nervous system toxicity after liver transplantation: the role of cyclosporine and cholesterol. N Engl J Med 1987;317:861–866.
13. Lorber MI. Cyclosporine: lesson learned—future strategies. Clin Transplant 1991;5(Special Issue):505–516.
14. Fung JJ, Abu-Elmagd K, Todo S, et al. FK 506 in clinical organ transplantation. Clin Transplant 1991;5 (Special Issue):517–522.
15. Thompson CB, June CH, Sullivan KM, Thomas ED. Association between cyclosporine neurotoxicity and hypomagnesemia. Lancet 1984;2:1116–1120.
16. deGroen PC. Cyclosporine, low density lipoprotein and cholesterol. Mayo Clin Proc 1988;63:1012.
17. Op de Coul AAW, Lambregts PCLA, Koeman J, et al. Neuromuscular complications in patients given Pavulon (pancuronium bromide) during artificial ventilation. Clin Neurosurg 1985;87:17–22.
18. Ramsay DA, Zochodone DW, Robertson DM, et al. A syndrome of acute severe muscular necrosis in intensive care unit patients. J Neuropathol Exp Neurol 1993;52:387–388.
19. Danon MJ, Carpenter S. Myopathy with thick filament (myosin loss following prolonged paralysis with vecuronium during steroid treatment). Muscle Nerve 1991;14:1131–1139.
20. Waclawik AJ, Sufit RL, Beinlich BR, et al. Acute myopathy with selective degeneration of myosin filaments following status asthmaticus treated with methylprednisolone and vecuronium. Neuromuscul Disord 1992;2:119–126.
21. Griffin D, Fairman N, Coursin D, et al. Acute myopathy during treatment of status asthmaticus with corticosteroids and steroidal muscle relaxants. Chest 1992;102: 510–514.
22. Curtis JJ, Luke RG, Jones P, Diethelm AG. Hypertension in cyclosporine-treated renal transplant recipients is sodium dependent. Am J Med 1988;85:134–138.
23. Bennet W, Porter GA. Cyclosporine-associated hypertension [editorial]. Am J Med 1988;85:131.

24. Chaparala R, Kramer DJ, Miro A, et al. Comparison of clinical score, bronchoalveolar lavage, and protected brush specimen for the diagnosis of bacterial pneumonia in critically ill patients with liver disease. Am Rev Respir Dis 1993;147(Suppl):A38.

25. Chaparala R, Kramer DJ, Miro A, et al. Patient outcome after bronchoscopic evaluation of pulmonary infiltrates in liver transplant candidates. Am J Respir Crit Care Med 1994;149(4):A843.

26. Matuschak GM, Rinaldo JE, Pinsky MR, et al. Effect of endstage liver failure on the incidence and resolution of the adult respiratory distress syndrome. J Crit Care 1987;2:162.

27. Dansky HM, Schwinger ME, Cohen MV. Using contrast enhanced echocardiography to identify normal pulmonary arteriovenous connections in patients with hypoxemia. Chest 1992;102:1690–1692.

28. Rodriguez-Roisin R, Roca J, August AGN, et al. Gas exchange and pulmonary vascular reactivity in patients with liver cirrhosis. Am Rev Respir Dis 1987;135: 1085–1092.

29. Davis HH, Schwartz DJ, Letrak SS, et al. Alveolar capillary oxygen disequilibrium in hepatic cirrhosis. Chest 1978;73:507–511.

30. Scott V, Miro A, Kang Y, et al. Reversibility of the hepatopulmonary syndrome by orthotopic liver transplantation. Transplant Proc 1993;25:1878–1888.

31. Lebrec D, Capron JB, Dhumeux D, Benhamou JP. Pulmonary hypertension complicating portal hypertension. Am Rev Respir Dis 1979;120:849–856.

32. Morrison EB, Gaffney FA, Eignebrodt EH, et al. Severe pulmonary hypertension associated with macronodular cirrhosis and autoimmune phenomena. Am J Med 1980;69:513–549.

33. McDonnell PJ, Tove PA, Hutchins GM. Primary pulmonary hypertension and cirrhosis: are they related? Am Rev Respir Dis 1983;127:437–441.

34. Koneru B, Ahmed S, Weisse AB, et al. Resolution of pulmonary hypertension of cirrhosis after liver transplantation. Transplantation 1994;58:1133–1135.

35. Plevak D, Krowka M, Rettke S, et al. Successful liver transplantation in patients with mild to moderate pulmonary hypertension. Transplant Proc 1993;25:1840.

36. Scott V, DeWolf A, Kang Y, et al. Reversibility of pulmonary hypertension after liver transplantation: a case report. Transplant Proc 1993;25:1789–1790.

37. Alexander JA, Demetrius AJ, Gavaler JS, et al. Pancreatitis following liver transplantation. Transplantation 1988;45:1062–1065.

38. Jacobs F, Van de Stadt J, Bourgeois N, et al. Severe infections early after liver transplantation. Transplant Proc 1989;21:2271–2273.

39. Nalesnik MA, Makowka L, Starzl TE. Diagnosis and treatment of post-transplant lymphoproliferative disorders. Curr Prob Surg 1988;5:367–472.

40. Distant DA, Gonwa TA. The kidney in liver transplantation. J Am Soc Nephrol 1993;4:129–136.

41. Haller M, Schonfelder R, Briegel J, et al. Renal function in the postoperative period after orthotopic liver transplantation. Transplant Proc 1992;24:2704–2706.

42. Detroz B, Honore P, Monami B, et al. Combined treatment of liver failure and hepatorenal syndrome with orthotopic liver transplantation. Acta Gastroenterol Belg 1992;55:350–357.

43. Seu P, Wilinson AH, Shaked A, Busuttil RW. The hepatorenal syndrome in liver transplant recipients. Am Surgeon 1991;57:806–809.

44. Gonwa TA, Morris CA, Goldstein RM, et al. Long-term survival and renal function following liver transplantation in patients with and without hepatorenal syndrome—experience in 300 patients. Transplantation 1991;51:428–430.

45. Myers BD. Cyclosporine nephrotoxicity. Kidney Int 1986;30:964–974.

46. Kahan BD. Cyclosporine nephrotoxicity: pathogenesis, prophylaxis, therapy, and prognosis. Am J Kidney Dis 1986;8:323–331.

47. Driscoll DF, Wright-Pinson C, Jenkins RL, Bistram BR. Potential protective effects of furosemide against early renal injury in liver transplant recipients receiving cyclosporine-A. Crit Care Med 1989;17:1341–1343.

48. Basadonna G, Montorsi F, Kakizak K, Merrel R. Cyclosporine A and islet function. Am J Surg 1988; 156:191–193.

49. Kusne S, Dummer JS, Singh N, et al. Infection after liver transplantation: an analysis of 101 consecutive cases. Medicine 1988;67:132–143.

50. Kusne S, Dummer JS, Singh N, et al. Fungal infections in liver transplantation recipients. Transplantation 1985;40:347.

51. Balfour HH, Chace BA, Stapleton JA, et al. A randomized, placebo-controlled trial of oral acyclovir for the prevention of cytomegalovirus disease in recipients of renal allografts. N Engl J Med 1989;320:1381–1387.

52. Pomeroy C, Englund JA. Cytomegalovirus: epidemiology and infection control. Am J Infect Control 1987;15:107–119.

53. Gottesdiener KM. Transplanted infections: donor-to-host transmission with the allograft. Ann Intern Med 1989;101:1001–1016.

54. Le Goff C, Huralt de Ligny B, Freymuth F, et al. Comparison of quantitative cytomegalovirus leukocyte antigenemia with conventional diagnostic methods of cytomegalovirus detection in renal transplantation. Transplant Proc 1995;27:2452–2453.

55. Lamy ME, Mulongo NK, Vargas M, et al. Early diagnosis of CMV infection by detection of PP65 antigen in 91 renal transplant recipients. Transplant Int 1994;7: 237–242.

56. Lautenschlager I, Hockerstedt K, Salmela K. Quantitative CMV–antigenemia test in the diagnosis of CMV infection and in the monitoring of response to antiviral treatment in liver transplant recipients. Transplant Proc 1994;26:1719–1720.

57. Martin M, Manez R, Linden P, et al. A prospective, randomized trial comparing sequential ganciclovir-high dose acyclovir to high dose ganciclovir for prevention of cytomegalovirus disease in adult liver transplant recipients. Transplantation 1994;58:779–785.

58. Syndman DR, Werner BG, Heinze-Lacey B, et al. Use of cytomegalovirus immunoglobulin to prevent cytomegalovirus disease in renal transplant recipients. N Engl J Med 1987;317:1049.

59. Smith SD, Jackson RJ, Hannakan CJ, et al. Selective decontamination in pediatric liver transplants: a randomized prospective study. Transplantation 1993;55:1306–1309.

60. Badger IL, Crosby HA, Kong KL, et al. Is selective decontamination of the digestive tract beneficial in liver transplant patients? Interim results of a prospective, randomized trial. Transplant Proc 1991;23:1460–1461.

61. Wiesner RH, Hermans PE, Rakela J, et al. Selective bowel decontamination to decrease gram negative aerobic bacterial and candida colonization and prevent infection after orthotopic liver transplantation. Transplantation 1988;45:570–574.

62. van Zeijl JH, Kroes ACM, Metselaar HJ, et al. Infections after auxiliary partial liver transplantation. Experiences in the first ten patients. Infection 1990;18:146–151.

63. Frazier OH, Macris MP, Myers TJ, et al. Improved survival after extended bridge to cardiac transplantation. Ann Thorac Surg 1994;57:1416–1422.

64. Aufiero T. Combined registry for the clinical use of mechanical ventricular assist pumps and the total artificial heart [abstract]. Presented at the American Society for Artificial Internal Organs 1994 annual meeting. San Francisco, April, 1994.

65. Bernardi L, Keller F, Sanders M, et al. Respiratory sinus arrhythmia in the denervated human heart. J Appl Physiol 1989;67:1447–1455.

66. Glassman LR, Keenan RJ, Fabrizio MC, et al. Extracorporeal membrane oxygenation as an adjunct treatment for primary graft failure in adult lung transplant patients. J Thorac Cardiovasc Surg 1995;110:723–726.

67. Sadaghdar H, Chelluri L, Bowles SA, Shapiro R. Outcome of renal transplant recipients in the ICU. Chest 1995;107:1402–1405.

68. Weinrauch L, E'Elia EA, Healy RW, et al. Asymptomatic coronary artery disease: angiographic assessment of diabetes evaluated for renal transplantation. Circulation 1978;58:1184–1190.

69. Braun WE, Philips PF, Vidt DG, et al. Coronary artery disease in 100 diabetics with end stage renal failure. Transplant Proc 1984;10:603–607.

70. Lorber MF, Van Buren CT. Pre-transplant coronary arteriography for diabetic renal transplant recipients. Transplant Proc 1987;19:1539–1541.

71. Sanfilippo F, Vaughn WK, Spees EK, Lucas BA. The detrimental effects of delayed graft function in cadaver donor renal transplantation. Transplantation 1984;38:643–648.

72. Scott TR, Graham SM, Schwietzer EJ, Bartlett ST. Colonic necrosis following sodium polystyrene sulfonate (Kayexalate)-sorbitol enema in a renal transplant patient. Dis Colon Rectum 1993;36:607–609.

73. Solez K, Axelsen RA, Benediktsson H, et al. International standardization of criteria of the histologic diagnosis of renal allograft rejection. The Banff working classification of kidney transplant pathology. Kidney Int 1993;44:411–422.

74. Bell PR, Briggs JD, Calman KC, et al. Reversal of acute clinical and experimental organ rejection using large doses of intravenous prednisolone. Lancet 1971;1(7705):876–880.

75. Ramos EL, Tishor CC. Recurrent diseases in the kidney transplant. Am J Kidney Dis 1994;24:142–154.

76. Vidne BA, Leapman SB, Butt KM, et al. Vascular complications in human transplantation. Surgery 1976;79:77–81.

77. Mannucci PM, Remuzzi G, Pusineri F, et al. Deamino-8-D-arginine vasopressin shortens the bleeding time in uremia. N Engl J Med 1983;308:8–12.

78. Remuzzi G. Bleeding disorders in uremia: pathophysiology and treatment. Adv Nephrol Necker Hosp 1989;18:171–186.

79. Shemin D, Elnour M, Amarantes B, et al. Oral estrogens decrease bleeding time and improve clinical bleeding in patients with renal failure. Am J Med 1990;89:436–440.

80. Greger B, Bockhorn H, Reeb A, et al. Treatment of perioperative bleeding after kidney transplantation by conjugated estrogen. Transplant Proc 1987;19:3704–3706.

81. Goldman MH, Tilney NL, Vineyard GC, et al. A twenty-year survey of arterial complications of renal transplantation. Surg Gynecol Obstet 1975;141:758–760.

82. Louridas G, Botha JR, Meyers AM, et al. Vascular complications of renal transplantation: the Johannesburg experience. Clin Transpl 1987;1:240–245.

83. Groggel GC. Acute thrombosis of the renal transplant artery: a case report and review of the literature. Clin Nephrol 1991;36:42–45.

84. Debleke D, Sacks GA, Sandler M. Diagnosis of allograft renal vein thrombosis. Clin Nucl Med 1989;14:415–419.

85. Duckett T, Bretan P Jr, Cochran ST, et al. Noninvasive radiological diagnosis of renal vein thrombosis in renal transplantation. J Urol 1991;146:403–406.

86. Merion RM, Calne RY. Allograft renal vein thrombosis. Transplant Proc 1985;17:1746–1750.

87. Amante AJ, Kahan BD. Technical complications of renal transplantation. Surg Clin North Am 1994;74:1117–1131.

88. Pozniak MA, Dodd GD, Kelez F. Ultrasonographic evaluation of renal transplantation. Radiologic Clin North Am 1992;30:1053–1066.

89. Peterson PK, Balfour JJ, Fryd DS, et al. Fever in renal transplant recipients: causes, prognostic significance and changing patterns at the University of Minnesota Hospital. Am J Med 1981;71:345–351.

90. Hibberd PL, Rubin RH. Renal transplantation and

related infections. Semin Respir Infect 1993;8: 216–224.

91. Syndman DR, Rubin RH, Werner BG. New developments in cytomegalovirus prevention and management. Am J Kidney Dis 1993;21:217–218.

92. Rubin RH. The indirect effects of cytomegalovirus on the outcome of organ transplantation. JAMA 1989;261: 3607–3609.

93. Paya CV. Fungal infections in solid organ transplantation. Clin Infect Dis 1993;16:677–688.

94. Patel R, Roberts GD, Keating MR, Paya CV. Infections due to nontuberculous mycobacteria in kidney, heart and liver transplant recipients. Clin Infect Dis 1994;19:263–273.

95. Kasiske BL. Risk factors for accelerated atherosclerosis in renal transplant recipients. Am J Med 1988;84:985–992.

96. Fabrega AJ, Matas AJ, Payne ED, et al. Ten to 20 year follow-up of 123 consecutive HLA identical living related transplants from the pre-cyclosporine era. Clin Transpl 1990;4:145.

97. Drueke TB, Abdulmassih Z, Lacour B, et al. Atherosclerosis and lipid disorders after renal transplantation. Kidney Int 1991;31:S24–S28.

98. Pirsch JP, D'Alessandro AM, Jollinger W, et al. Hyperlipidemia and transplantation: etiologic factors and therapy. J Am Soc Nephrol 1992;2:S238–S242.

99. Kasiske BL, Tortorice KL, Heim-Duthoy KL, et al. The adverse impact of cyclosporine on serum lipids in renal transplant recipients. Am J Kidney Dis 1991;17:700–707.

100. Glicklich D, Jellis VA, Quinn J, et al. Comparison of captopril scan and Doppler ultrasonography as screening tests for transplant renal artery stenosis. Transplantation 1990;49:217–219.

101. Curtis JJ, Luke RG, Whelchel JD, et al. Inhibition of angiotensin converting enzymes in renal transplant recipients with hypertension. N Engl J Med 1983; 308:377–381.

102. Benoit G, Moukarzel M, Hiesse C, et al. Stenosis de l'artere du rein transplante: place des dilatations endoluminules. Presse Med 1991;20:2045–2047.

103. Laskow DA, Curtis JJ. Post-transplant hypertension. Am J Hypertens 1990;3:721–725.

104. Curtis JJ. Hypertension following kidney transplantation. Am J Kidney Dis 1994;23:471–475.

105. McCauley J, Ptachcinski R, Shapiro R. The cyclosporine sparing effects of diltiazem in renal transplantation. Transplant Proc 1989;21:3955–3957.

106. Maggio TG, Buitels DW. Increased cyclosporine blood concentrations due to verapamil administration. Drugs Intell Clin Pharm 1988;22:705–707.

107. Fernandez JA, Rosenberg JC. Post transplantation pancreatitis. Surg Gynecol Obstet 1976;143:795–798.

108. Renning JA, Waiden GD, Stevens LE, et al. Pancreatitis after renal transplantation. Am J Surg 1972;123:293–296.

109. Guice K, Rattazzi LC, Marchioro TL. Colon perforation in renal transplant patients. Am J Surg 1979;138: 43–48.

110. Stylianos S, Forde KA, Benvenisty AT, et al. Lower gastrointestinal hemorrhage in renal transplant recipients. Arch Surg 1988;123:739–744.

111. Yoshimura N, Oka T. Medical and surgical complications of renal transplantation: diagnosis and management. Med Clin North Am 1990;74:1025–1037.

112. Buckiner FS, Pomeroy C. Cytomegalovirus of the gastrointestinal tract in patients without AIDS. Clin Infect Dis 1993;17:644–656.

113. Starzl TE, Rowe M, Todo S, et al. Transplantation of multiple abdominal viscera. JAMA 1989;261:1449–1457.

114. Tzakis AG, Ricordi C, Alejandro R, et al. Pancreatic islet transplantation after upper abdominal exenteration and liver replacement. Lancet 1990;336:402–405.

115. Doyle H, Kramer DJ, Marino I, et al. Advances in Transplantation. In NR Webser, A Bodenham (eds), Clinical Anaesthesiology. London: Saunders, 1992;307–326.

Chapter 14

Anesthesia for the Previously Transplanted Patient

Jamal A. Alhashemi, Adrian W. Gelb, and Michael D. Sharpe

Chapter Plan

Better immunosuppressive therapy regimens, surgical techniques, and perioperative care have resulted in increased survival of patients who undergo organ transplantation. The number of organs transplanted per year continues to grow due to various initiatives to increase the donor pool (see Chapter 2). Because of these changes in transplantation surgery, anesthesiologists will encounter an increasing number of previously transplanted patients who present for nontransplantation surgery. The challenges posed by these patients are related to (1) altered organ function or physiology related to the transplanted organ, (2) altered organ function secondary to immunosuppressive therapy, (3) the potential for rejection of the transplanted organ, (4) increased risk of infection, and (5) the potential interaction of immunosuppressive agents with anesthetic drugs. First, we discuss the preoperative evaluation of the patient with a transplanted organ, with most of the remaining chapter devoted to the anesthetic management of patients with different organ transplants.

Preoperative Assessment

The primary objectives of preoperative evaluation of the transplant patient are (1) to exclude the presence of infection, (2) to evaluate the transplanted organ function, (3) to rule out allograft rejection, and (4) to determine the functional adequacy of other organ systems.

Although infectious mortality after organ transplantation has declined, infections remain a major cause of morbidity and mortality in transplant recipients. Most infections are bacterial, especially in the early posttransplantation period, but cytomegalovirus, the most common viral pathogen, is associated with the highest morbidity and mortality among transplant recipients.[1] During the preoperative visit, it is of paramount importance that infection be sought aggressively and ruled out before proceeding with elective surgery. This is particularly true in the early posttransplantation period, when the intensity of immunosuppression is highest and the presentation of infection may be atypical. Fever should be specifically asked about because it could be a marker of infection or an underlying graft rejection. Although fever is relatively common in solid-organ transplant

Table 14-1. Preoperative Investigations

Complete blood count
Serum electrolytes, calcium, magnesium
Serum urea, creatinine, glucose
Liver function tests: aspartate aminotransferase, alanine
    aminotransferase, alkaline phosphatase, bilirubin,
    gamma-glutamyl transferase
Serum amylase and lipase
Urinalysis
International normalized ratio (prothrombin time), partial
    thromboplastin time
Blood gases (lung transplants)
Electrocardiogram
Pulmonary function tests (lung transplants)
Echocardiogram (heart transplants)

recipients, its presence should not be attributed to noninfectious causes (e.g., rejection) until a thorough search for infection has been completed.[2]

Table 14-1 lists the minimum preoperative laboratory tests to evaluate the function of different organ systems. Additional test results of allograft function are usually available in the medical record. Alternatively, they can be obtained from the transplant service that is following the patient. Further laboratory tests may be necessary, in liaison with the appropriate specialty, when there is evidence of an organ system malfunction. The latter may occur as a manifestation of allograft dysfunction (e.g., renal dysfunction secondary to low output state in a heart transplant patient) or as an adverse effect of immunosuppressant therapy. Elective surgery should be postponed if infection or rejection is suspected until the diagnosis is made. The transplant team's advice on the perioperative management of immunosuppressive therapy should also be sought, especially if dose adjustment is necessary due to change in the route of drug administration. In general, however, immunosuppressive drugs should be continued in the perioperative period and the dosage adjusted according to serum drug levels.

Anesthetic Considerations Related to the Transplanted Organ

Heart

The Denervated Heart

The inevitable interruption of cardiac autonomic innervation during orthotopic heart transplantation results in a unique physiologic state. This state is characterized by a relatively stable resting heart rate of 90–100 beats per minute and absence of neural-mediated cardiac reflexes (i.e., baroreceptor-mediated changes in heart rate and cardiac responses to airway instrumentation, carotid sinus massage, and Valsalva maneuver). Due to lack of sympathetic neural input to the heart, demands for increased cardiac output (as occurs during exercise) are met by increases in stroke volume rather than heart rate.[3] With sustained demand, however, the heart rate does increase (albeit slowly over 4–5 minutes); this corresponds to the time required for the adrenal medulla to secrete endogenous catecholamines.[4] Accordingly, the denervated heart retains the ability to respond to endogenous catecholamines and other direct-acting drugs, such as isoproterenol. In contrast, drugs that alter heart rate through modulation of parasympathetic or sympathetic output (e.g., atropine and pancuronium) have little to no effect on the denervated heart. Compared to its effects on sinoatrial node function, denervation does not influence arterioventricular node function or ventricular conduction times.[5] As a result, resting stroke volume and indices of myocardial function are also little changed in the absence of allograft rejection or pulmonary hypertension.[6, 7] In addition, the pressure-volume relationship is maintained, and it constitutes an important compensatory determinant of cardiac output. Traditionally, it was believed that autonomic efferent denervation is permanent in human recipients of orthotopic heart transplants.[8, 9] However, some reports suggest that at least partial reinnervation may occur as early as 1 year after transplantation.[10–16] The changes in pulmonary function tests (PFTs) that occur secondary to long-standing heart failure do not improve after heart transplantation and resolution of the cardiac failure.[17]

Arrhythmias after orthotopic heart transplantation are a common complication, with a reported incidence of up to 50%.[18] Conventional antiarrhythmic agents are usually effective in treating the dysrhythmia, but caution must be exercised because many of these drugs have inherent negative inotropic properties. Permanent pacing may be required in 11% of patients to treat significant bradyarrhythmias resulting from postoperative sinus node dysfunction or atrioventricular block.[19, 20] In some cases, however, the need for pacing has also been the result of severe graft rejection.[21, 22] Mortality rates were very high in those patients. In the absence of rejection, long-term pacing may not be required in most patients beyond 3 months post transplantation.[19, 23] In summary, posttransplantation arrhythmias are frequently encountered, but they decrease over time. An increase in their frequency or severity should alert to the possibility of underlying rejection.[21, 24]

Perioperative Anesthetic Management

Noncardiac surgical intervention is required in approximately 15–30% of heart transplant recipients at various times after transplantation.[25, 26] During the preoperative visit, these patients should be assessed for the presence of rejection and infection. In addition, secondary organ dysfunction due to adverse effects of immunosuppressive drugs or in association with rejection and low cardiac output should be sought. Rejection episodes are observed most frequently in the first 3 months post transplantation, with a peak incidence at 1 month.[27] They are a major cause of morbidity and mortality after heart transplantation, and they significantly increase the intraoperative mortality of noncardiac surgery. The anesthesiologist should specifically seek symptoms of altered exercise tolerance, shortness of breath, and fatigue because they usually precede other symptoms of heart failure. Clinical evidence of early failure is an indication to delay elective surgery to allow further investigation of the patient for graft rejection. Graft failure can also be caused by accelerated graft atherosclerosis, which is thought to be a form of chronic rejection and occurs in up to 50% of patients at 5 years post transplantation.[28] Clinical distinction between graft rejection and accelerated coronary artery disease is often difficult because angina is usually not perceived in the presence of cardiac denervation. Under these circumstances, endomyocardial biopsy remains the gold standard for diagnosing graft rejection and should be considered before elective surgery. Echocardiography is of limited value. Plasma interleukin-6 and tumor necrosis factor have been reported to be elevated in patients with graft rejection and may thus be of value as noninvasive tests in the future.[29]

Laboratory evaluation of the heart transplant recipient should include 12-lead electrocardiogram (ECG), complete blood cell count (CBC), blood urea nitrogen (BUN), serum electrolytes, and creatinine. In addition, the results of a recent echocar-diogram and endomyocardial biopsy should be reviewed with the transplant team. The patient's ECG may demonstrate two P waves: one originating from the native atrium and the other from the donor sinoatrial node. The native atrial rhythm is physiologically inconsequential because the generated action potentials do not cross the anastomotic suture line. Atrial dysrhythmia may be observed on the 12-lead ECG, but it is usually benign.[30] Previous ECGs, however, should always be reviewed because recent increases in frequency or severity of dysrhythmias may be a marker for rejection and warrant further investigation. Eleven percent of heart transplant recipients have a permanent pacemaker.[19] Dizziness, syncope, and other symptoms of pacemaker malfunction should be sought in these patients. The absence of paced beats on the ECG should prompt a cardiology consultation to interrogate the pacemaker and determine its functional integrity before proceeding with surgery.

The anesthetic management of patients with a transplanted heart poses challenges. An intra-arterial catheter for blood pressure monitoring is recommended for major operative procedures. The use of central venous and pulmonary artery catheters is guided by the complexity of the surgical procedure and the anticipated intraoperative and postoperative blood loss and fluid shifts. Maintenance of adequate preload is mandatory before and after induction of either general or regional anesthesia because these patients are preload dependent for maintenance of adequate cardiac output. Blood loss should be rapidly corrected and peripheral vasodilation avoided. Many patients have impaired but stable renal function because of cyclosporine immunosuppression.[31] Therefore, it may be necessary to avoid drugs that are secreted or excreted by the kidneys (i.e., muscle relaxants). Anesthesia induction can be achieved with a variety of anesthetic agents. Ketamine should probably be avoided in patients who are hypertensive, either chronically or secondary to cyclosporine therapy, because it may elicit an exaggerated hypertensive response. Tachycardia should not be relied on as an early manifestation of light anesthesia and the depth of anesthesia. Drugs that are known to be myocardial depressants (e.g., halothane) should be administered with caution in patients receiving antidysrhythmic medications because of the latter's negative inotropic properties. Intraoperative bradycardia is best treated with drugs, such as isoproterenol, epinephrine, or ephedrine, which increase heart rate directly by stimulating beta-adrenergic receptors. The administration of an anticholinesterase (e.g., neostigmine and edrophonium) has been shown to provoke a bradycardic response, which is smaller in magnitude than that observed in patients with normal autonomic innervation.[32, 33] The potential remains for severe bradycardia after administration of an anticholinesterase without a muscarinic antagonist, however, and antimuscarinic drugs should always be administered to counteract this side effect in patients with a transplanted heart.

Regional anesthesia is not contraindicated in heart transplant recipients. In fact, peripheral nerve blockade is probably advantageous because it avoids the hemodynamic perturbation that is sometimes seen with general anesthesia. On the other hand, central neuraxial blockade carries the risk of profound hypotension due to decreased preload and lack of compensatory tachycardia in the face of severe vasodilatation. The risk of hypotension in association with major conduction block should not constitute a contraindication to its performance in the heart transplant patient. Instead, adequate patient hydration and judicious use of vasopressors should make this block a useful addendum to the anesthesiologist's armamentarium.

Lung

The Denervated Lung

Based on the indication for lung transplantation, patients may undergo single-lung (SLT), double-lung (DLT), or heart-lung transplantation (HLT). The transplanted lung is denervated distal to the surgical anastomosis. Therefore, in SLT (or DLT performed as a sequential SLT), carinal innervation is spared, and patients have an intact cough reflex in response to carinal stimulation. In contrast, tracheal resection during en bloc DLT or HLT results in disruption of distal tracheal and carinal innervation with consequent loss of the carinal cough reflex.[34] This places the patient at risk for silent aspiration, retention of secretions, and development of infection. The concomitant impairment of mucociliary clearance in the transplanted lung further increases the risk of pneumonia.[35] Postural drainage and chest physiotherapy should therefore be encouraged, particularly in the postoperative period. Although ani-

mal studies suggest that reinnervation takes place after canine lung transplantation, there is no evidence of reinnervation in humans.[36, 37]

Airway tone and function are little affected by the loss of parasympathetic efferent innervation of the bronchial smooth muscles. There is no evidence to suggest that pulmonary transplantation has any effect on respiratory rate or rhythm or sleep respiratory patterns.[38] SLT results in preferential perfusion of the denervated lung, which also receives 60–70% of ventilation.[39] This increase in perfusion has been attributed to decreased pulmonary vascular resistance in the denervated lung. The concomitant increase in ventilation together with an intact hypoxic pulmonary vasoconstriction results in maintenance of ventilation-perfusion matching in the transplanted lung.[40] In patients with CO_2 retention, preoperative hypercapnia and the blunted ventilatory response to CO_2 return to normal by the end of the first month after transplantation.[41] The ventilatory response to exercise is substantially preserved in the lung transplant recipient, and arterial CO_2 response to exercise is normal.[42, 43] In addition, ventilatory responses to hypoxia and hypercapnia in heart-lung transplant patients are comparable to those in normal patients.[44]

A significant decline in lung volumes is frequently observed in the immediate posttransplantation period. This can be explained by changes in thoracic mechanics that are associated with transplant surgery. After the first month of transplantation, there is a gradual improvement in total lung capacity, forced vital capacity, forced expiratory volume in 1 second, and diffusion capacity for carbon monoxide. Most patients are symptom-free with good exercise tolerance within 3 months of the transplantation. Double-lung transplant patients exhibit near-normal PFTs within 6 months of transplantation, whereas single-lung transplant patients continue to have impaired though improved PFTs due to the presence of a diseased native lung.[45, 46]

Perioperative Anesthetic Management

Long-term survival of lung transplant patients is lower than that of heart allograft recipients; thus, fewer lung transplant patients present for elective surgery. The most common indication for general anesthesia in this patient population is bronchoscopy, lung biopsy, and bronchoalveolar lavage. Gastrointestinal disorders, such as pancreatitis and cholecystitis, and posttransplantation lymphoproliferative disease are also common indications for surgical intervention in lung transplant patients. The incidence of posttransplantation lymphoproliferative disease is fairly high among lung transplant recipients, which may reflect the more intense immunosuppression protocol necessary in this group of patients compared to other transplanted organ recipients.[47]

Preoperative evaluation of the lung transplant patient is centered on (1) determining the presence of rejection or infection, (2) evaluation of the extent of disease in the native lung in patients with single-lung transplant, and (3) evaluation of the effects of immunosuppressive drugs on other organ functions. Graft rejection and infection are major threats to patient survival and therefore must be carefully excluded before proceeding with elective surgery. They both occur most frequently in the first 3 months after surgery, but rejection or infection may develop at any time after transplantation.[48] During the preoperative visit, patients should be asked about shortness of breath, fatigue, cough, fever, sputum production, need for home oxygen, and changes in exercise tolerance. The development of dry cough and dyspnea 8–12 months after transplantation should alert to the possibility of obliterative bronchiolitis (OB). OB is usually a manifestation of chronic rejection, but it may be related to acute rejection or repeated viral infections (cytomegalovirus). The typical presentation is that of minimally productive cough followed in months by dyspnea. Thereafter, the disease takes the form of accelerated chronic obstructive pulmonary disease, with wheezing and crackles on clinical examination and severe airway obstruction with a restrictive element on PFTs. Arterial blood gases show decreased Po_2 and widened alveolar-arterial oxygen gradient, whereas elevated Pco_2 is not observed until late in the disease.

Routine laboratory workup of the lung transplant patient should include CBC, serum electrolytes, BUN, creatinine, blood glucose, arterial blood gases, PFTs, ECG, and chest radiograph. Abnormal PFTs are frequently observed in single-lung transplant patients who have no evidence of rejection due to the effects of the diseased native lung on global pulmonary function. Therefore, changes in PFTs over time are more important than absolute values in determining the presence of rejection or infection.[49] Any deterioration in PFTs should prompt a search for rejection and infection in collaboration with the trans-plant team, and elective surgery should be delayed.[50] The distinction between rejection and infection is of paramount importance because treatment of rejection involves additional immunosuppression that could make an underlying infection worse. Chest radiograph and bronchoalveolar lavage are of limited value in distinguishing between these two conditions, and transbronchial lung biopsy is often required to establish the diagnosis of rejection.[51, 52] High-resolution computed tomography has been suggested as a useful aid in determining the need for transbronchial biopsy in lung transplant patients with suspected rejection.[53] The test has limited sensitivity, however, and together with the high morbidity and mortality associated with misdiagnosing pulmonary graft rejection, it is likely that the real value of this test is in deciding where, rather than when, to perform the biopsy. Other abnormalities that may be encountered during preoperative laboratory testing include elevated serum creatinine concentration and increased blood glucose levels. In the absence of primary organ dysfunction, these abnormalities are usually secondary to cyclosporine and corticosteroid immunosuppression, respectively. Corrective measures and consultation with appropriate services should be done before proceeding with elective surgery.

Lung transplant recipients present a unique case because the anesthesiologist frequently instruments the patient's airway. This has led some to recommend strict asepsis when handling the airway as well as air filters, sterile laryngoscopes, and breathing circuits. Although this practice is theoretically plausible, there is no evidence to support its widespread adoption over standard practice.

Intraoperative monitoring is dictated by the planned surgical procedure and the general status of the patient. Routine invasive monitoring to measure intraoperative arterial blood gases should be discouraged because of the added risk of line infection in a population that is already at increased risk. If direct arterial pressure monitoring is justifiable, radial lines are better than femoral lines because of the femoral lines' higher risk of infection. There is no contraindication to central venous and pulmonary artery catheterization in the lung transplant patient, provided there are appropriate indications for their use. Although it may be tempting to choose the side of the native lung for central line insertion, there is no evidence to suggest that one side is better or safer than the other.

The choice between general and regional anesthesia rests on patient's preference, the expertise of the anesthesiologist, and the planned surgical procedure. If general endotracheal anesthesia is chosen, nasotracheal intubation should be avoided because of the increased risk of bacteremia; otherwise, appropriate prophylactic antibiotics must be administered before intubation. Simple mask and laryngeal mask airway are not contraindicated, but the main concern is the possibility of an unrecognized aspiration in patients who have no carinal cough reflex.

Another important consideration during airway management in the lung transplant recipient is airway anastomotic complications. These occur in approximately 15% of patients and include stenosis, granulation tissue formation, and bronchomalacia.[54] Significant airway stricture results in characteristic changes in PFTs and can be seen on computed tomography.[55] Therefore, whenever possible, the cuff of the endotracheal tube should be placed just beyond the vocal cords to avoid unnecessary trauma to the airway in patients with a tracheal anastomosis. If it is required, a double-lumen tube should be positioned under direct vision using fiberoptic bronchoscopy.

All anesthetic drugs and inhalational agents, including nitrous oxide, can be safely administered to lung transplant patients. The trachea should be extubated only when the patient is fully awake and able to cough in response to verbal commands. Postural drainage, chest physiotherapy, and incentive spirometry are crucial adjuncts to the postoperative care of these patients.

Major conduction anesthesia can be safely performed in the lung transplant patient. However, excessive fluid preloading should be avoided because it may increase the risk of pulmonary edema due to lymphatic disruption. Furthermore, the lung allograft is particularly prone to pulmonary edema due to the presence of a vascular permeability defect, which is always present to some extent in the acute postoperative period (see Chapter 7). On the other hand, adequate hydration is essential in patients with heart-lung transplant because of the associated cardiac denervation and preload dependence for maintaining adequate cardiac output. Accordingly, the balance between adequate and excessive fluid administration may be a fine one, and judicious fluid preloading is the rule.

Liver

Graft Function

Animal data suggest that denervation of the liver, in contrast to the heart, does not affect its hemodynamics. Therefore, in the absence of such complications as hepatic artery thrombosis, hepatic blood flow after liver transplantation should be normal if cardiac output is adequate. The liver's synthetic ability usually normalizes within 2 weeks after transplantation, but liver enzymes and serum bilirubin may take longer to reach normal values. Serum bilirubin rises slightly in the immediate posttransplantation period due to the inevitable ischemic insult of the allograft, but there is a steady decline thereafter. Abnormal elevation of bilirubin levels more than 3 months after transplantation suggests rejection, biliary obstruction, or hepatitis C infection.[28] In contrast, serum aspartate aminotransferase (AST) levels continue to be above normal limits in up to 50% of patients by 12 months post transplantation, and normal values are observed in only 80% of subjects by the fourth postoperative year. Alkaline phosphatase and gamma-glutamyl transferase (GGT) are the least likely of all liver enzymes to normalize after transplantation, with approximately 30% of patients exhibiting normal values within 4 years.[56]

By the third postoperative day, all procoagulant factors achieve normal activity. In contrast, the anticoagulant proteins (proteins C and S, antithrombin III, and heparin cofactor II) show delayed recovery, with more than one-half of patients exhibiting decreased antithrombin III activity on day 5 postoperatively.[57] This imbalance between procoagulants and coagulation inhibitors usually resolves by the end of the second postoperative week; the patient's coagulation profile is then expected to be normal.[58] Other hematologic aberrations that are typical in the immediate postoperative period include low hemoglobin and low leukocyte and platelet counts. The observed hematologic changes are partly due to intraoperative hemodilution from blood products, but the observed decline in platelets may also be attributed to intraoperative vascular endothelial injury at the time of allograft anastomosis. Thrombocytopenia usually continues into the fifth postoperative day before it starts to improve, but clinical bleeding solely due to deficient platelets is seldom seen. On the other hand, platelet transfusion may at times be required for very low levels (less than 20,000 µl) to avoid spontaneous hemorrhage, especially intracerebral hemorrhage.

Perioperative Anesthetic Management

Surgery in the early posttransplantation period is usually required for complications related to the transplant surgery (e.g., biliary leak or intra-abdominal abscess). Anesthetic management of such cases could present a formidable challenge because many patients might still have the cardiovascular, renal, and electrolyte derangements that existed before the initial surgery with or without concurrent sepsis. The preoperative evaluation of such patients should therefore be geared to optimizing the various physiologic abnormalities as well as ruling out the presence of graft rejection. The latter is of paramount importance in the preanesthetic assessment of patients with liver allograft, whether they present early or late after transplantation, because elective surgery should be postponed in the presence of rejection. Accordingly, anesthetic history should include specific inquiry about fever, malaise, new onset of jaundice, changes in urine or stool color, pruritus, abrupt weight gain, and ankle edema.[56] The patient should be examined for signs of liver dysfunction (e.g., edema, ascites, asterixis) and for side effects of immunosuppressive therapy (e.g., hypertension, Cushing's syndrome, fungal skin infection).

Laboratory evaluation of graft function is initially based on standard liver function tests; serum bilirubin, AST, alanine aminotransferase, alkaline phosphatase, GGT, albumin, and international normalized ratio (INR). Because these markers decline at variable rates among different patients after transplantation, changes in trend over time are more important than absolute values. Among all enzymes, serum AST is the most reliable indicator of the adequacy of immunosuppression, and a continuous rise of this enzyme post transplantation suggests rejection and the need for more immunosuppression. Also, elevated serum bilirubin and prothrombin time (PT) or INR, and low albumin levels more than 3 months after transplantation provide evidence of ongoing rejection. Alternatively, continuous deterioration in liver function tests may represent the presence of allograft infection. Hepatitis C has been observed to recur in more than one-half of cases in which liver transplantation was performed for hepatitis C.[59]

Cytomegalovirus infection and primary viral hepatitis are some other etiologic factors implicated in the pathogenesis of allograft infection.[60, 61] In contrast to other enzymes, serum alkaline phosphatase and GGT are markers of cholestasis, and their elevation usually indicates biliary tract obstruction, which is a known complication of the transplant procedure. Accordingly, significant changes in any liver function tests should prompt detailed investigation of graft function by the transplant team before proceeding with elective surgery. A tissue biopsy is usually needed for definitive diagnosis when allograft rejection is suspected.[62, 63]

In the presence of normal allograft function, choice of anesthetic technique (general, regional, or combined regional-general) is guided by the nature of the surgical procedure and the patient's preference. Volatile anesthetics and drugs that are metabolized in the liver can be safely administered to the liver transplant patient.[64–66] On the other hand, one may elect to avoid drugs that are known to decrease hepatic blood flow, such as propranolol and cimetidine, but there is no evidence to support this practice.[67]

Kidney

Graft Function

Despite complete denervation of the kidney after renal transplantation, animal data suggest that renal plasma flow and urinary potassium excretion remain intact in the denervated kidney, whereas urinary sodium and bicarbonate excretion are elevated.[68] Serum erythropoietin levels increase markedly in the immediate posttransplantation period, and then they return toward normal values over time.[69] The rise in erythropoietin levels results in resumption of normal erythropoietic activity, with subsequent resolution of anemia of chronic renal failure. This process could be hampered by delayed graft function and by onset of rejection, but erythropoiesis is usually restored on recovery of graft function.[70, 71]

Perioperative Anesthetic Management

Among all allograft recipients, anesthesiologists are most likely to encounter kidney transplant patients because kidney transplantation remains the most commonly performed transplant procedure worldwide. In addition to assessment of renal function, preoperative evaluation of these patients should also involve careful assessment of the cardiovascular system because cardiovascular disease remains the leading cause of death in this population. Although hypertension is commonly observed in patients with end-stage renal disease, up to 50% of renal transplant recipients develop hypertension postoperatively due to such factors as allograft rejection, cyclosporine therapy, steroids, and vascular stenosis of the renal graft.[72] Hypertension together with pre-existing risk factors (e.g., diabetes, atherosclerosis, hyperlipidemia) account for the increased cardiovascular morbidity and mortality in this population.

Laboratory investigations should include CBC, serum creatinine, BUN, urinalysis, liver enzymes, blood glucose, serum electrolytes (including calcium and magnesium), and an ECG. Serum creatinine is likely to be chronically elevated yet stable in patients receiving cyclosporine immunosuppression.[45, 73, 74] This is in part due to cyclosporine-induced nephropathy, but it may also reflect chronic rejection. The distinction between these two conditions is almost impossible to ascertain on clinical grounds, but it is crucial in cases in which there is markedly elevated or progressively rising creatinine levels because treatment of the two conditions is vastly different. Ultrasound of the kidney has been suggested as a noninvasive test in the investigation of these patients, but needle biopsy of the allograft remains the diagnostic modality of choice.[75] Immunosuppression with cyclosporine, tacrolimus, and steroids has also been associated with the development of posttransplantation hyperlipidemia and impaired glucose tolerance.[76, 77] The former is observed in nearly half of renal allograft recipients and has necessitated treatment with lipid-lowering agents in many patients. Assessment of liver function is required in patients receiving lipid-lowering agents because these drugs have been implicated as causes of drug-induced hepatitis. In addition, glucose levels should be monitored perioperatively, and insulin therapy may be required for hyperglycemia. Specialized tests of cardiovascular function (e.g., echocardiography) are not routinely performed and should be guided by findings in the patient's history and physical examination.

The choice between general and regional anesthesia is generally guided by the nature of the planned surgical procedure and the patient's preference. The presence of renal allograft per se is not a contraindication to major conduction blockade, even in the presence of mild renal dysfunction. Spinal anesthesia has indeed been used for renal transplantation surgery in patients with end-stage renal disease without adverse effects.[78] On the other hand, central neuraxial blockade is not recommended if there is clinical evidence of platelet dysfunction as a result of uremia. If general anesthesia is chosen, ketamine induction is best avoided because many renal transplant patients are hypertensive and may exhibit exaggerated hemodynamic response to ketamine administration. Propofol is probably the induction agent of choice, although thiopental is still widely used despite its prolonged duration of action in patients with renal impairment. Morphine remains the most commonly used opioid in the postoperative period, but its repeated administration may result in prolonged respiratory depression in patients with chronic renal failure due to accumulation of its active metabolite, morphine-6-glucuronide.[79] Similarly, meperidine must be used with caution in patients with impaired renal function due to accumulation of normeperidine, a metabolite that has convulsant activity.[80]

Most renal transplant patients have at least a 20% reduction in graft function secondary to cyclosporine-induced nephropathy or chronic rejection. Therefore, caution must be exercised when administering drugs that are excreted by the kidney because their duration of action may be prolonged.[74] The underlying principle is that drugs handled by the kidney are not absolutely contraindicated in the presence of renal impairment; nonetheless, it is common sense to avoid long-acting drugs for short surgical procedures.

Small Bowel

Graft Function

Intestinal motility returns 7–15 days after small bowel transplantation, but gastric emptying may continue to be delayed for a prolonged period. The ability of the transplanted bowel to resume normal absorption varies according to dietary constituents.

Dietary sugars are well absorbed shortly after motility has been established. Fat absorption may be abnormal for a more prolonged period. Diarrhea and dehydration are frequent problems after bowel transplantation and usually result from a short native or transplanted colon. Other causes include fat malabsorption, rejection, and infection. Treatment with antidiarrheal drugs should be considered only after rejection and infection are excluded.

Perioperative Anesthetic Management

Preoperative assessment of patients with a small bowel transplant does not differ from that of other organ transplant recipients; rejection and infection should be ruled out before proceeding with elective surgery. During history taking, patients should be asked about fatigue, fever, diarrhea, blood in the stool, nausea and vomiting, and abdominal pain. Physical examination should determine the patient's state of hydration because many may have chronic diarrhea and dehydration. It is important to realize that rejection in these patients leads not only to loss of graft function but also to bacterial translocation and increased risk for systemic infection. The latter is further increased by the intense immunosuppression regime that is frequently used in the treatment of rejection. Although there are several clinical indicators of failing graft function, the diagnosis of rejection should always be confirmed by endoscopy and biopsy.[81–83] Among vascularized solid-organ grafts, the transplanted small bowel is unique in its ability to elicit graft-versus-host disease (GVHD). This may be due to the large number of lymphocytes in the graft, which migrate extensively between the graft and the host even in the absence of rejection. GVHD should be suspected if there is unexplained hemolysis, pancytopenia, pneumonitis, diarrhea, altered mental status, and skin rash. GVHD has been less of a clinical problem than was initially feared.[84]

Preoperative laboratory investigations should include an assessment of liver function tests (see Table 14-1). Disturbed liver function is common in patients with a history of prolonged total parenteral nutrition before transplantation. Serum creatinine concentration may be elevated as a result of the increased immunosuppression requirement in this patient population. Anesthetic management

is similar to that of patients with a liver transplant. Strict aseptic technique and avoidance of unnecessary invasive monitors are of paramount importance in the management of the patient with a small bowel transplant.

Pancreas

Patients with a pancreatic transplant have undergone either simultaneous pancreas-kidney transplantation, pancreas after kidney transplantation, or pancreas transplantation alone. Pancreatic transplantation is usually reserved for patients with type 1 diabetes with severe complications. This is because pancreatic transplantation is associated with the highest surgical complication rate of all solid-organ transplantations. In one review, surgical complications, including intra-abdominal infection and abscess formation, anastomotic leak, and vascular graft thrombosis, occurred in 35% of pancreatic transplant recipients.[85] The anesthetic management of such patients is complicated by increased risk for major bleeding and postoperative sepsis.

Pancreatic control of blood glucose is seen as early as immediately after reperfusion during the transplantation procedure. However, insulin may be required in the immediate postoperative period to control the rise in blood sugar that may occur secondary to steroid immunosuppression and the stress of surgery. Subsequently, treatment with insulin is usually unnecessary unless graft function is compromised. The preoperative assessment of pancreas transplant patients scheduled for elective surgery should include careful examination of the abdomen for tenderness over the pancreas. Other biochemical features of graft rejection that should be elucidated during preoperative testing include increased serum amylase concentration, elevated serum lipase, and a fall in urinary amylase in patients with bladder-drained pancreatic transplant.[86] Serum amyloid A and pancreatic-specific proteins have been suggested as noninvasive markers for graft rejection.[87] Whenever graft rejection is suspected clinically or on simple laboratory tests, however, the transplant team should be consulted for guidance on further diagnostic workup. Definitive diagnosis of pancreatic graft rejection is usually obtained by tissue biopsy.

Immunosuppressive Agents

Immunosuppressive drugs are a cornerstone in the posttransplantation management of allograft recipients. They have contributed tremendously to improved patient survival, but at the same time, they are responsible for significant posttransplantation morbidity. During the preoperative visit, it is important to determine the presence or absence of any side effects related to the immunosuppressive therapy (Table 14-2) and whether the observed adverse effects require corrective measures preoperatively. Treatment of immunosuppressant-induced side effects should be done in collaboration with the transplant team and the appropriate consulting service. Preoperatively, immunosuppressive drugs should be continued up to the time of surgery. If changes are required in their route of administration, they should be made in consultation with the transplant team responsible for patient follow-up. Appropriate serum levels should be drawn after the planned changes to confirm the maintenance of adequate immunosuppression throughout the perioperative period.

Steroid Supplementation

Most, if not all, allograft recipients receive corticosteroid immunosuppression and are therefore at risk for adrenal insufficiency when exposed to the perioperative stress of surgery. For this reason, it has been customary to administer supraphysiologic doses of supplemental steroids to all patients in the perioperative period. This practice has been challenged, however, and maintenance doses of corticosteroids have been recommended without perioperative supplementation.[88, 89] This recommendation is supported in part by the poor correlation between adrenal cortisol secretion in corticosteroid-treated patients and the dose and duration of glucocorticoid therapy.[90] Spontaneous recovery of the hypothalamic-pituitary-adrenal axis has been observed in patients receiving daily low-dose steroid therapy.[91] In summary, current evidence suggests that the traditional amount of perioperative steroid supplementation is excessive and unwarranted. The "no-supplement" recommendation cannot be generalized until its safety and efficacy is confirmed in carefully conducted, randomized, controlled clinical trials. Until the final

Table 14-2. Side Effects of Immunosuppressive Agents

Agent	Side Effects
Cyclosporine	Nephrotoxicity
	Hypertension
	Gingival hyperplasia
	Hyperkalemia
	Central nervous system: paresthesia, seizures, coma
	Hypomagnesemia
	Hepatotoxicity
Steroids	Infection
	Hyperglycemia
	Hypertension
	Hepatitis
	Peptic ulceration
	Myopathy
	Hyperlipidemia
	Mood changes
	Adrenal suppression
Azathioprine	Infection
	Hepatic dysfunction
	Bone marrow suppression; anemia, thrombocytopenia, leukopenia
	Pancreatitis
	Nausea, vomiting, diarrhea
Antilymphocyte globulin	Fever, chills
	Anaphylaxis
	Leukopenia, thrombocytopenia
	Serum sickness
	Renal dysfunction
	Phlebitis, erythema
OKT3	Fever, chills
	Infection
	Nausea and vomiting
	Aseptic meningitis, seizures
	Pulmonary edema
	Encephalopathy
	Anaphylaxis
	Bronchospasm
	Chest pain
Tacrolimus (FK506)	Nephrotoxicity
	Headache
	Nausea and vomiting
	Flushing
	Tremor
	Hyperglycemia
	Psychological disturbances
Mycophenolate	Nephrotoxicity
	Headache
	Nausea and vomiting
	Flushing
	Tremor
	Hyperglycemia
	Psychological disturbances

verdict is reached, the low-dose supplementation recommended by Symreng et al. appears to be a reasonable approach to perioperative steroid coverage in the transplanted patient.[92]

Interaction of Cyclosporine and Anesthetic Agents

Few studies have focused on the interaction of cyclosporine and anesthetic agents, and most of these involve animal models. Brown et al. demonstrated in humans that oral cyclosporine administered less than 4 hours preoperatively results in subtherapeutic levels.[93] Isoflurane anesthesia has been implicated as the cause of this effect because decreased gastric emptying and reduced small bowel absorption has been shown to occur in the rat during isoflurane anesthesia.[94] Once steady-state therapeutic levels have been reached, however, a 3-hour isoflurane anesthetic (in animals) does not alter cyclosporine pharmacokinetics.[95]

A number of case reports have implicated cyclosporine as potentiating or prolonging neuromuscular block during vecuronium[96, 97] and pancuronium[98] administration, although the mechanism is unclear. Gramstad et al. demonstrated in cats a potentiation of neuromuscular block by cyclosporine during vecuronium and atracurium administration.[99] It is therefore reasonable to assume that patients receiving cyclosporine may be more sensitive to nondepolarizing muscle relaxants, and their recovery times may be prolonged.

Conclusions

Patients with a transplanted organ presenting for nontransplant surgery are becoming more common in our anesthetic practice. Successful anesthetic management of these patients includes assessment of the transplanted organ and of other organs that may be affected by either transplant organ dysfunction or chronic immunosuppressive therapy. Fever or acute deterioration in the transplanted organ may represent rejection or infection, and these entities must be ruled out before elective surgery. Contact with the patient's transplant center is helpful in determining the function of the transplanted organ and recommendations for perioperative immunosuppressant therapy.

Acknowledgements

The authors thank Lynn Hinchcliffe and Linda Hunte for their assistance in preparation of this chapter.

References

1. Boden MD, Dummer JS. Infections after organ transplantation. J Intensive Care Med 1997;12:166–186.
2. Fischer SA, Trenholme GM, Levin S. Fever in the solid organ transplant patient. Infect Dis Clin North Am 1996;10:167–184.
3. Kent KM, Cooper T. The denervated heart. A model for studying autonomic control of the heart. N Engl J Med 1974;291:1017–1021.
4. Stinson EB, Griepp RB, Schroeder JS, et al. Hemodynamic observations one and two years after cardiac transplantation in man. Circulation 1972;45:1183–1194.
5. Firestone LL. General anesthetics. Int Anesthesiol Clin 1988;26:248–253.
6. Verani MS, George SE, Leon CA, et al. Systolic and diastolic ventricular performance at rest and during exercise in heart transplant recipients. J Heart Transplant 1988;7:145–151.
7. Frist WH, Stinson EB, Oyer PE, et al. Long-term hemodynamic results after cardiac transplantation. J Thorac Cardiovasc Surg 1987;94:685–693.
8. Pope SE, Stinson EB, Daughters GT, et al. Exercise response of the denervated heart in long-term cardiac transplant recipients. Am J Cardiol 1980;46:213–218.
9. Kavanagh T, Yacoub MH, Mertens DJ, et al. Cardiorespiratory responses to exercise training after orthotopic cardiac transplantation. Circulation 1988;77:162–171.
10. Stark RP, McGinn AL, Wilson RF. Chest pain in cardiac-transplant recipients. Evidence of sensory reinnervation after cardiac transplantation [see comments]. N Engl J Med 1991;324:1791–1794.
11. Rudas L, Pflugfelder PW, Kostuk WJ. Vasodepressor syncope in a cardiac transplant recipient: a case of vagal re-innervation? Can J Cardiol 1992;8:403–405.
12. Rudas L, Pflugfelder PW, Menkis AH, et al. Evolution of heart rate responsiveness after orthotopic cardiac transplantation. Am J Cardiol 1991;68:232–236.
13. Wilson RF, Laxson DD, Christensen BV, et al. Regional differences in sympathetic reinnervation after human orthotopic cardiac transplantation. Circulation 1993;88:165–171.
14. Bracht C, Hoerauf K, Vassalli G, et al. Circadian variations of blood pressure and heart rate early and late after heart transplantation. Transplantation 1996;62:1187–1190.
15. Fagard R, Macor F, Vanhaecke J. Signs of functional efferent reinnervation of the heart in patients after cardiac transplantation. Acta Cardiol 1995;50:369–380.
16. Bernardi L, Bianchini B, Spadacini G, et al. Demon-

strable cardiac reinnervation after human heart transplantation by carotid baroreflex modulation of RR interval. Circulation 1995;92:2895–2903.

17. Ohar J, Osterloh J, Ahmed N, Miller L. Diffusing capacity decreases after heart transplantation. Chest 1993;103:857–861.

18. Pavri BB, O'Nunain SS, Newell JB, et al. Prevalence and prognostic significance of atrial arrhythmias after orthotopic cardiac transplantation. J Am Coll Cardiol 1995;25:1673–1680.

19. Scott CD, McComb JM, Dark JH, Bexton RS. Permanent pacing after cardiac transplantation [see comments]. Br Heart J 1993;69:399–403.

20. Markewitz A, Schmoeckel M, Nollert G, et al. Long-term results of pacemaker therapy after orthotopic heart transplantation. J Card Surg 1993;8:411–416.

21. Blanche C, Czer LS, Fishbein MC, et al. Permanent pacemaker for rejection episodes after heart transplantation: a poor prognostic sign. Ann Thorac Surg 1995;60:1263–1266.

22. Cooper MM, Smith CR, Rose EA, et al. Permanent pacing following cardiac transplantation. J Thorac Cardiovasc Surg 1992;104:812–816.

23. Raghavan C, Maloney JD, Nitta J, et al. Long-term follow-up of heart transplant recipients requiring permanent pacemakers. J Heart Lung Transplant 1995;14:1081–1089.

24. Blanche C, Czer LS, Trento A, et al. Bradyarrhythmias requiring pacemaker implantation after orthotopic heart transplantation: association with rejection [see comments]. J Heart Lung Transplant 1992;11:446–452.

25. Augustine SM, Yeo CJ, Buchman TG, et al. Gastrointestinal complications in heart and in heart-lung transplant patients. J Heart Lung Transplant 1991;10:547–555.

26. Bhatia DS, Bowen JC, Money SR, et al. The incidence, morbidity, and mortality of surgical procedures after orthotopic heart transplantation. Ann Surg 1997;225:686–693.

27. Kirklin JK, Naftel DC, Bourge RC, et al. Rejection after cardiac transplantation. A time-related risk factor analysis. Circulation 1992;86:II236–II241.

28. Sharpe MD. Anaesthesia and the transplanted patient. Can J Anaesth 1996;43:R89–R98.

29. Abdallah AN, Billes MA, Attia Y, et al. Evaluation of plasma levels of tumour necrosis factor alpha and interleukin-6 as rejection markers in a cohort of 142 heart-grafted patients followed by endomyocardial biopsy [see comments]. Eur Heart J 1997;18:1024–1029.

30. Liem LB, DiBiase A, Schroeder JS. Arrhythmias and clinical electrophysiology of the transplanted human heart. Semin Thorac Cardiovasc Surg 1990;2:271–278.

31. Lewis RM, Van BC, Radovancevic B, et al. Impact of long-term cyclosporine immunosuppressive therapy on native kidneys versus renal allografts: serial renal function in heart and kidney transplant recipients. J Heart Lung Transplant 1991;10:63–70.

32. Backman SB, Fox GS, Stein RD, Ralley FE. Neostigmine decreases heart rate in heart transplant patients. Can J Anaesth 1996;43:373–378.

33. Backman SB, Stein RD, Fox GS, Polosa C. Heart rate changes in cardiac transplant patients and in the denervated cat heart after edrophonium. Can J Anaesth 1997;44:247–254.

34. Hathaway T, Higenbottam T, Lowry R, Wallwork J. Pulmonary reflexes after human heart-lung transplantation. Respir Med 1991;85(Suppl A):17–21.

35. Herve P, Silbert D, Cerrian J, et al. Impairment of bronchial mucociliary clearance in long-term survivors of heart/lung and double-lung transplantation. Chest 1993;103:59–63.

36. Stretton CD, Mak JC, Belvisi MG, et al. Cholinergic control of human airways in vitro following extrinsic denervation of the human respiratory tract by heart-lung transplantation. Am Rev Respir Dis 1990;142:1030–1033.

37. Higenbottam T, Jackson M, Woolman P, et al. The cough response to ultrasonically nebulized distilled water in heart-lung transplantation patients. Am Rev Respir Dis 1989;140:58–61.

38. Sanders MH, Costantino JP, Owens GR, et al. Breathing during wakefulness and sleep after human heart-lung transplantation. Am Rev Respir Dis 1989;140:45–51.

39. The Toronto Lung Transplant Group. Experience with single-lung transplantation for pulmonary fibrosis. JAMA 1988;259:2258–2262.

40. Robin E, Theodore J, Burke CM, et al. Hypoxic pulmonary vasoconstriction persists in the human transplanted lung. Clin Sci 1987;72:283–287.

41. Trachiotis G, Knight S, Hann M, et al. Respiratory responses to CO_2 rebreathing in lung transplant recipients. Ann Thorac Surg 1994;58:1709–1717.

42. Grassi B, Ferretti G, Xi L, et al. Ventilatory response to exercise after heart and lung denervation in humans. Respir Physiol 1993;92:289–304.

43. Duncan S, Kagawa F, Starnes V, Theodore J. Hypercarbic ventilatory responses of human heart-lung transplant recipients. Am Rev Respir Dis 1991;144:126–130.

44. Sanders MH, Owens GR, Sciurba FC, et al. Ventilation and breathing pattern during progressive hypercapnia and hypoxia after human heart-lung transplantation. Am Rev Respir Dis 1989;140:38–44.

45. Williams TJ, Snell GI. Early and long-term functional outcomes in unilateral, bilateral, and living-related transplant recipients. Clin Chest Med 1997;18:245–257.

46. Bando K, Paradis IL, Keena RJ, et al. Comparison of outcomes after single and bilateral lung transplantation for obstructive lung disease. J Heart Lung Transplant 1995;14:692–698.

47. Penn I. Incidence and treatment of neoplasia after transplantation. J Heart Lung Transplant 1993;12:S328–S336.

48. Bando K, Paradis IL, Komatsu K, et al. Analysis of time-dependent risks for infection, rejection, and death after pulmonary transplantation. J Thorac Cardiovasc Surg 1995;109:49–57.

49. Becker FS, Martinez FJ, Brunsting LA, et al. Limitations of spirometry in detecting rejection after single-

lung transplantation. Am J Respir Crit Care Med 1994; 150:159–166.

50. Van MA, Melot C, Antoine M, et al. Role of pulmonary function in the detection of allograft dysfunction after heart-lung transplantation. Thorax 1997;52:643–647.

51. Gryzan S, Paradis IL, Hardesty RL, et al. Bronchoalveolar lavage in heart-lung transplantation. J Heart Transplant 1985;4:414–416.

52. Millet B, Higenbottam TW, Flower CD, et al. The radiographic appearances of infection and acute rejection of the lung after heart-lung transplantation. Am Rev Respir Dis 1989;140:62–67.

53. Loubeyre P, Revel D, Delignette A, et al. High-resolution computed tomographic findings associated with histologically diagnosed acute lung rejection in heart-lung transplant recipients. Chest 1995;107:132–138.

54. Kshettry VR, Kroshus TJ, Hertz MI, et al. Early and late airway complications after lung transplantation: incidence and management. Ann Thorac Surg 1997;63:1576–1583.

55. Anzueto A, Levine SM, Tillis WP, et al. Use of the flow-volume loop in the diagnosis of bronchial stenosis after single lung transplantation. Chest 1994;105:934–936.

56. O'Grady J, Williams R. Long-term Management, Complications, and Disease Recurrence. In WC Maddrey (ed), Transplantation of the Liver. New York: Elsevier, 1988;143–165.

57. Stahl RL, Duncan A, Hooks MA, et al. A hypercoagulable state follows orthotopic liver transplantation. Hepatology 1990;12:553–558.

58. Velasco F, Villalba R, Fernandez M, et al. Diminished anticoagulant and fibrinolytic activity following liver transplantation. Transplantation 1992;53:1256–1261.

59. Shuhart MC, Bronner MP, Gretch DR, et al. Histological and clinical outcome after liver transplantation for hepatitis C. Hepatology 1997;26:1646–1652.

60. Sido B, Hofmann WJ, Otto G, et al. Cytomegalovirus infection in liver transplantation: graft infection and clinical relevance. Transplant Proc 1992;24:2641–2642.

61. Singh N, Gayowski T, Ndimbie OK, et al. Recurrent hepatitis C virus hepatitis in liver transplant recipients receiving tacrolimus: association with rejection and increased immunosuppression after transplantation. Surgery 1996;119:452–456.

62. Baumgartner U, Scholmerich J, Kremer B, et al. Early detection of graft dysfunction after orthotopic liver transplantation in man by serum and biliary bile acid analysis. Hepatogastroenterology 1995;42:950–960.

63. Hayry P, Lautenschlager I. Transplant aspiration cytology: applications to kidney and liver transplantations. Transplant Proc 1991;23:1760–1761.

64. Essen P, Eleborg L, Blomqvist B, et al. Fluoride plasma concentration after isoflurane anesthesia during and after liver transplantation. Transplant Proc 1989;21:3530.

65. Fisher DM, Ramsay MA, Hein HA, et al. Pharmacokinetics of rocuronium during the three stages of liver transplantation. Anesthesiology 1997;86:1306–1316.

66. Marcel RJ, Ramsay MA, Hein HA, et al. Duration of rocuronium-induced neuromuscular block during liver transplantation: a predictor of primary allograft function. Anesth Analg 1997;84:870–874.

67. Puff MR, Carey WD. The effect of cimetidine on cyclosporine A levels in liver transplant recipients: a preliminary report. Am J Gastroenterol 1992;87:287–291.

68. Zincke H, Ott NT, Woods JE, Wilson DM. The role of denervation in renal transplantation on renal function in the dog. Invest Urol 1976;14:210–212.

69. Sun CH, Ward HJ, Paul WL, et al. Serum erythropoietin levels after renal transplantation. N Engl J Med 1989;321:151–157.

70. Besarab A, Caro J, Jarrell BE, et al. Dynamics of erythropoiesis following renal transplantation. Kidney Int 1987;32:526–536.

71. Besarab A, Caro J, Jarrell BE, et al. Effect of cyclosporine and delayed graft function on posttransplantation erythropoiesis. Transplantation 1985;40:624–431.

72. Sear JW. Kidney Transplants: Induction and Analgesic Agents. In D Royston, TW Feeley (eds), Anesthesia for the Patient with a Transplanted Organ. Boston: Little, Brown, 1995;45–68.

73. Salas M, Loertscher R, Caro JJ. Effect of cyclosporin weaning on glomerular filtration rate in renal transplantation. Nephron 1996;74:309–312.

74. Linder R, Lindholm A, Restifo A, et al. Long-term renal allograft function under maintenance immunosuppression with cyclosporin A or azathioprine. A single center, five-year follow-up study. Transpl Int 1991;4:166–172.

75. Linkowski GD, Warvariv V, Filly RA, Vincenti F. Sonography in the diagnosis of acute renal allograft rejection and cyclosporine nephrotoxicity. AJR Am J Roentgenol 1987;148:291–295.

76. Krentz AJ, Dousset B, Mayer D, et al. Metabolic effects of cyclosporin A and FK506 in liver transplant recipients. Diabetes 1993;42:1753–1759.

77. Canzanello VJ, Schwartz L, Taler SJ, et al. Evolution of cardiovascular risk after liver transplantation: a comparison of cyclosporine A and tacrolimus (FK506). Liver Transpl Surg 1997;3:1–9.

78. Linke CL, Merin RG. A regional anesthetic approach for renal transplantation. Anesth Analg 1976;55:69–73.

79. Chauvin M, Sandouk P, Scherrmann JM. Morphine pharmacokinetics in renal failure. Anesthesiology 1987;66:327–331.

80. Armstrong PJ, Bersten A. Normeperidine toxicity. Anesth Analg 1986;65:536–538.

81. Tabasco-Minguillan J, Hutson W, Weber K, et al. Prospective evaluation of endoscopy in acute cellular rejection and cytomegalovirus infection. Transplant Proc 1996;28:2778–2779.

82. Hassanein T, Schade RR, Soldevilla-Pico C, et al. Endoscopy is essential for early detection of rejection in small bowel transplant recipients. Transplant Proc 1994;26:1414–1415.

83. Kuusanmaki P, Halttunen J, Paavonen T, et al. Value of

mucosal biopsies in the monitoring of acute small bowel rejection. Transpl Int 1997;10:192–196.

84. Abu-Elmagd K, Todo S, Tzakis A, et al. Rejection of human intestinal allografts: alone or in combination with the liver. Transplant Proc 1994;26:1430–1431.

85. Gruessner RW, Sutherland DE, Troppmann C, et al. The surgical risk of pancreas transplantation in the cyclosporine era: an overview. J Am Coll Surg 1997; 185:128–144.

86. Benedetti E, Najarian JS, Gruessner AC, et al. Correlation between cystoscopic biopsy results and hypoamylasuria in bladder-drained pancreas transplants. Surgery 1995;118:864–872.

87. Muller TF, Trosch F, Ebel H, et al. Pancreas-specific protein (PASP), serum amyloid A (SAA), and neopterin (NEOP) in the diagnosis of rejection after simultaneous pancreas and kidney transplantation. Transpl Int 1997;10:185–191.

88. Bromberg JS, Baliga P, Cofer JB, et al. Stress steroids are not required for patients receiving a renal allograft and undergoing operation. J Am Coll Surg 1995;180: 532–536.

89. Friedman RJ, Schiff CF, Bromberg JS. Use of supplemental steroids in patients having orthopaedic operations. J Bone Joint Surg Am 1995;77:1801–1806.

90. Schlaghecke R, Kornely E, Santen RT, Ridderskamp P. The effect of long-term glucocorticoid therapy on pituitary-adrenal responses to exogenous corticotropin-releasing hormone [see comments]. N Engl J Med 1992;326:226–230.

91. LaRochelle GE Jr, LaRochelle AG, Ratner RE, Borenstein DG. Recovery of the hypothalamic-pituitary-adrenal (HPA) axis in patients with rheumatic diseases receiving low-dose prednisone. Am J Med 1993;95:258–264.

92. Symreng T, Karlberg BE, Kagedal B, Schildt B. Physiological cortisol substitution of long-term steroid-treated patients undergoing major surgery. Br J Anaesth 1981;53:949–954.

93. Brown MR, Brajtbord D, Johnson DW, et al. Efficacy of oral cyclosporine given prior to liver transplantation. Anesth Analg 1989;69:773–775.

94. Gelb AW, Freeman D, Robertson KM, et al. Isoflurane alters the kinetics of oral cyclosporine. Anesth Analg 1991;72:801–804.

95. Freeman DJ, Sharpe MD, Gelb AW. Effects of nitrous oxide/oxygen-isoflurane anesthesia on blood cyclosporine concentrations in the rabbit. Transplantation 1994;58: 640–642.

96. Sidi A, Kaplan RF, Davis RF. Prolonged neuromuscular blockade and ventilatory failure after renal transplantation and cyclosporine. Can J Anaesth 1990;37: 543–548.

97. Wood GG. Cyclosporine-vecuronium interaction [letter]. Can J Anaesth 1989;36:358.

98. Crosby E, Robblee JA. Cyclosporine-pancuronium interaction in a patient with a renal allograft. Can J Anaesth 1988;35:300–302.

99. Gramstad L, Gjerlow JA, Hysing ES, et al. Interaction of cyclosporine and its solvent, Cremophor, with atracurium and vecuronium. Br J Anaesth 1986;58:1149–1155.

Chapter 15

Role of Nutrition in the Care of the Transplant Patient

Adam E. Levy and J. Wesley Alexander

Chapter Plan

Throughout history, physicians have recognized an association between nutrition and disease. The Edwin Smith papyrus, dating from 1600 BC, is perhaps the first written record of the use of dietary intervention to treat specific maladies.[1] Yet it was well into the middle of the twentieth century before the means and ability to analyze and manipulate this relationship came of age. Studley's landmark study in 1936 was the first to objectively document a 20-fold increase in postoperative mortality in surgical patients who had lost more than 20% of their total body weight preoperatively.[2] Since the 1950s, the significance of hypoproteinemia was first appreciated as a cause of prolonged ileus, wound dehiscence, and poor bone callus formation.[3] The use of accurate instruments to measure in vivo metabolic rate has demonstrated that injury and organ failure can profoundly alter regulation of the body's nutritional economy. More recently, the advent of efficient means to deliver specific enteral and parenteral nutrition has provided physicians an opportunity to treat nutritional derangements at a time when intervention can have a significant impact.

Perhaps nowhere are the principles and challenges of scientific nutritional management better highlighted than the solid-organ transplant recipient. These patients, by virtue of their end-stage organ failure, often have profound nutritional and metabolic derangements, which can have a striking effect on perioperative outcome. This, coupled with the consequences of postoperative immunosuppression and allograft-specific idiosyncrasies, demands a thorough understanding of the distinctive metabolic and physiologic changes that occur when delivering a patient from end-stage organ failure to organ replacement and a return to health.

Table 15-1. Estimating Energy Expenditures

Basal energy expenditure (men) = 66.473 + 13.7516 (weight in kg) + 5.0033 (height in cm) − 6.7550 (age in years)	
Basal energy expenditure (women) = 655.095 + 9.563 (weight in kg) + 1.8496 (height in cm) − 4.6756 (age in years)	
Estimating stress factor for basal energy requirements	

Patient status	Stress factor
Mild starvation	0.85–1.00
Postsurgical intervention	1.00–1.05
Severe infection	1.30–1.55
Cancer	1.10–1.45

Activity factor = 1.25 for ambulatory patients
Total energy expenditure = (basal energy expenditure) × (stress factor) × (activity factor)

Since the first successful solid-organ allograft in 1954, care of the transplant patient has rapidly evolved into a separate medical entity involving members from all major specialties. As the number of transplant recipients continues to rise (more than 18,000 per year in North America), an ever-widening circle of clinicians have some contact with these patients.[4] This necessitates an understanding of their unique demands and requirements.[4] The goal of this chapter is to introduce the general principles of pre- and postoperative nutritional assessment common to all surgical patients. We also highlight the most recent literature on the particular needs of the transplant recipient and organ-specific requirements. Related topics are the types of diets available, advantages of enteral versus parenteral nutrition, monitoring of nutritional support, complications of nutritional therapy, and research on the role of specific macronutrients, immunomodulatory diets, and the effect of diet on bacterial translocation.

General Preoperative Assessment

Numerous studies have demonstrated that an inordinate number of deaths and complications occur in malnourished surgical patients. Yet, despite intensive clinical and experimental research, no single test or procedure can accurately predict postoperative outcome in the malnourished surgical candidate. Consequently, various multimodal nutritional indices and procedures based on a thorough history and physical examination were developed to determine which patients are at risk for postoperative complications.

The preoperative evaluation of nutritional status begins with a consideration of four basic categories that define nutritional health: (1) basal energy expenditure, (2) fat and protein reserves, (3) level of metabolic stress, and (4) degree of physiologic impairment attributed to malnutrition. Much information can be gained about energy and protein balance by assessing the frequency and size of a patient's meals and comparing these results with an estimate of the rate of weight loss. A more comprehensive survey can be accomplished by including a 24-hour food recall or analysis of a food diary coupled with a calorie count. The presence of nausea, vomiting, fever, and intestinal, renal, or other chronic diseases are all clues to increased energy losses. Based on this information, one can calculate approximate values for basal energy expenditure, thermal effect of food, physical activity, and metabolic stress. With these values, an approximation of total body energy expenditure can be generated according to a modification of the Harris-Benedict equation (Table 15-1).[5]

For more sophisticated measurement, indirect calorimetry can be used to determine basal metabolic rate, but energy expenditure due to physical activity is difficult to measure by this method.

Assessment of body composition begins with a baseline measurement of height and weight. If a patient has sustained a weight loss before evaluation, determination of original weight is a necessary but difficult task. Although there are many tables for approximating ideal weight, studies suggest that a patient's recall of prior weight appears to be most accurate.[6] The rapidity and extent of preoperative weight loss is often used as an index of malnutrition and is based on the percentage of weight loss that has occurred over the previous 6 months (Table 15-2).[7] In general, patients with severe weight loss exceeding 10% more typically have marasmic malnutrition, whereas patients with features consistent

Table 15-2. Evaluation of Weight Loss

Evaluation of weight change over time

$$\% \text{ weight change} = \frac{\text{usual weight} - \text{actual weight}}{\text{usual weight}} \times 100$$

Definition of moderate and severe weight loss over time*

Time	Moderate weight loss (%)	Severe weight loss (%)
1 week	1–2	>2
1 month	5	>5
3 months	7.5	>7.5
6 months	10	>10

*GL Blackburn, BR Bistran, BS Maini, et al. Nutritional and metabolic assessment of the hospitalized patient. JPEN J Parenter Enteral Nutr 1977;1:11–22.

with kwashiorkor may exhibit more moderate changes over time.

Physical examination continues to be an important and relevant assessment technique. A 20% loss of body weight is associated with a marked decrease in muscle mass and subcutaneous fat, giving the patient an emaciated and haggard appearance.[8] This is most prominent about the malar eminence, supraclavicular fossa, and buttocks. In contrast, physical evaluation of hypermetabolic patients, such as those having liver failure, can be misleading due to a relative conservation of fat stores and an expansion of total body water, leading to a preservation of normal body contour. Despite these limitations, however, gross loss of fat stores can also be determined readily by palpation of a number of skinfolds. It has been demonstrated that if the dermis can be palpated between the fingers on examining the patient's triceps or biceps skinfolds, the patient's total body fat is generally less than 10%.[9]

Body fat and fat-free mass can be further assessed by anthropometric techniques. Because approximately 50% of total body fat is stored in the subcutaneous space, serial measurements of skinfold thickness can provide an accurate indication of fat stores compared to reference standards. Two types of measurements are normally recorded: skinfold thickness and limb circumference. Although a measurement of a specific skinfold thickness may be useful over time, measurements over several areas of the body, including triceps, biceps, and subscapular areas, are more useful.[10] This strategy, combined with limb circumference, provides the most accurate measurement. Once total body fat is calculated, fat-free body mass can also be derived. It is important to

note that anthropometric measurements are most sensitive when used to observe patients over the long term, and single measurements can often result in misleading conclusions. Furthermore, these tests are subject to high interobserver variability due to changes in skin turgor, total body water, and skin elasticity, making them less sensitive for patients with chronic disease.[11]

Given the relative inaccuracy of anthropometric measures, several laboratory tests can provide a more reliable indication of energy stores. Creatinine is a by-product of protein metabolism, and because the vast majority of protein is deposited in skeletal muscle tissue, it can furnish an accurate index of protein stores. A 24-hour urine creatinine excretion indexed by height can be compared to standard reference tables of creatinine excretion of adults of similar height, thereby generating a rough estimate of skeletal muscle mass. Calculation of the creatinine height index (CHI) is illustrated in the following equation.[12]

$$\text{CHI} = \frac{\text{measured urinary creatinine (mg/day)}}{\text{ideal urinary creatinine (mg/day)}*} \times 100$$

A patient whose CHI is less than 25% of normal is considered nutritionally challenged.[13] By definition, this test is limited by the requirement for normal renal function, which can be altered by a variety of pathophysiologic states, including renal, hepatic, and diabetic disease. More elaborate methods, generally not available to the clinician, include determination of the ratio of exchangeable sodium

*Estimated from height in centimeters.

to exchangeable potassium by isotope dilution techniques, measurement of potassium 40 by whole-body gamma camera imaging, and gamma neutron activation.[14–16]

Protein depletion can also be estimated by assaying various blood components, including retinol binding protein, prealbumin, transferrin, and albumin. The relatively long half-life of albumin compared to other circulating proteins makes its measurement a more reliable index of chronic protein malnutrition.[17] In a large retrospective study of patients undergoing colorectal surgery, Hickman et al. measured preoperative albumin levels and correlated them to postoperative morbidity and mortality.[18] They found that if the albumin level was 3.5 g/dl or lower, the postoperative mortality rate was 28% and the overall complication rate was 61%. In contrast, patients with a serum albumin greater than 3.5 g/dl had a mortality of 4.1% and a morbidity of 28%.[18] Transferrin is an intravascular iron-transport protein with a half-life of 8–10 days; it has also been proposed as a measure of protein stores. Transferrin levels below 200 mg/dl are considered indicative of malnourishment.[19] However, some studies suggest that this index has a relatively high false-positive prediction of malnutrition and may not provide meaningful clinical information.[20] Other measurements, such as prealbumin and retinol binding protein, are relatively less well defined. (The reader is directed to an excellent discussion of these topics by Church et al.[21]) As with anthropometric measurements, changes in total body water may affect accuracy of serum protein measurement through concentration or dilution of the index protein.

Due to the rapid turnover of cells within the lymphoid compartment, cell-mediated immunity, as measured by total lymphoid count (TLC) or skin anergy test batteries, is highly sensitive to protein depletion and can provide a rough estimate of protein reserves. Its calculation is demonstrated by:

$$TLC = \frac{\% \text{ lymphocytes} \times \text{white blood cells (cells/}\mu l)}{100}$$

Generally, weight loss must exceed 10% of well weight before suppression of immunocompetence.[17] TLC values below 1,200 cells/μl are considered consistent with moderate malnutrition; values less than 800 indicate severe nutritional depletion.[7] Studies by Seltzer et al. demonstrated that TLC below 1,500 cells/μl was associated with a fourfold increase in mortality in a series of 500 consecutive medical and surgical admissions.[22] Skin anergy testing is another measure of cell-mediated immunity used to assess malnutrition. When multiple antigens are placed intradermally, patients may be classified into three groups depending on their response: normal immunocompetence (two or more positive reactions), relative anergy (one positive reaction), or complete anergy (all negative reactions). Several studies have attempted to correlate these responses to nutritional status and postoperative outcome, but this test appears to be only moderately predictive and can be influenced by an assortment of non–nutrition-related disease states.[23, 24]

Loss of physiologic function remains one of the most important and clinically relevant measurements of malnutrition. Grip strength and respiratory function are two tests that have proved to be highly predictive of severe nutritional compromise. In a study by Pettigrew et al., grip pressure of less than 64 kPa in men and 47 kPa in women was up to 87% specific for clinically significant malnutrition.[25] Respiratory function, as measured by vital capacity and peak expiratory flow rate, is also a sensitive predictor of surgical risk.[26] Both tests can be rapidly assessed by asking the patient to grip the examiner's index and middle fingers and squeeze for 10 seconds or by measuring the volume of forced expiratory reserve with a simple bedside spirometer.

Assessment of metabolic stress allows the clinician to determine how efficiently the patient is using current energy stores. An individual with prolonged simple starvation often has a metabolic rate substantially below that of normal controls. When nutritional supplementation can be accomplished, it results in a preferential replenishment of vital protein reserves. In contrast, infection, liver failure, or recent trauma elevates metabolic rate, and replenishment of energy stores is confounded by a conversion of whole-body energy metabolism toward glycogen and fat formation. Thus, determination of metabolic stress can allow the clinician to establish how quickly and efficiently the malnourished patient will respond to aggressive therapy.

Preoperative Nutritional Assessment in the Transplant Patient

The pretransplant patient with a long history of chronic disease is particularly likely to be malnourished. These patients require a heightened awareness and demand a detailed knowledge of their unique organ-specific requirements and limitations.

Kidney Transplant Patient

Chronic renal failure necessitating hemodialysis has been demonstrated to affect nutritional status adversely, with up to 50% of patients exhibiting moderate-to-severe protein calorie depletion.[27] Such patients lose protein through frequent dialysis and also have inadequate oral nutritional intake. These losses are even more exaggerated among patients undergoing peritoneal dialysis.[28] A study of the nutritional intake of dialysis patients demonstrated that, despite aggressive nutritional counseling, the vast majority of end-stage renal disease (ESRD) patients fell short of their desired target nutritional goals of 35 kcal/kg per day and 0.8–1.4 g of protein/kg per day while attempting to maintain dietary restrictions on sodium, potassium, phosphorus, calcium, and protein intake.[29] Studies have also documented that the malnutrition in ESRD is not exacerbated by an elevated basal metabolic rate, as is common with end-stage liver failure.[30] Despite this reduced nutritional intake, ESRD patients paradoxically have hypertriglyceridemia and hypercholesterolemia. This may be due to enhanced production of very low-density lipoproteins and reduced secretion of lipoprotein lipase.[31] In summary, the poor nutritional status associated with ESRD seems to be related to an inability to maintain adequate oral intake against mounting protein and calorie losses.

Heart Transplant Patient

The heart transplant candidate may have a specific form of protein calorie malnutrition, termed *cardiac cachexia*. This chronic wasting, often seen in individuals with long-standing rheumatic or valvular disease, is often the most dramatic manifestation of this syndrome. Although its etiology is not well understood, this form of malnutrition often heralds increased morbidity and mortality after transplant.[32] It is theorized that chronic tissue hypoxia due to poor perfusion brings about intestinal malabsorption and gut atrophy as well as impaired nutrient delivery, leading to a self-perpetuating form of mal-

nutrition.[33] Once heart transplantation is achieved, however, nutritional supplementation can rapidly reverse this otherwise downward spiral.

Liver Transplant Patient

In contrast to terminal heart or kidney disease, end-stage liver failure engenders both a disruption of normal metabolic synthetic function and depletion of protein reserves, reduced oral intake, and malabsorption.[34] Loss of hepatic reserve is most prominently demonstrated by increased protein catabolism to maintain the gluconeogenesis required by glucose-oxidizing tissues, such as the brain and blood. In a healthy adult, glycogen reserves can meet whole-body glucose requirements for approximately 36 hours after cessation of oral intake. Beyond that time, extensive fat stores can be used for the production of ketoacids, thereby greatly reducing but not eliminating the need for protein catabolism. In a patient with end-stage liver failure and impaired gluconeogenesis, this interval may be reduced to as little as 6–10 hours. In addition, the loss of hepatocellular ketosynthetic function forces the body to rely increasingly on vital protein stores for metabolic substrate.[35] Inadequate oral intake also plagues these patients due to nausea, vomiting, malabsorption, and the administration of drugs such as lactulose and neomycin. Finally, increased losses can also occur due to frequent diarrhea, as well as iatrogenic attempts to remove accumulated ascites. Despite this discouraging outlook, aggressive nutritional support and counseling can help prevent or slow further losses before organ replacement.

Lung Transplant Patient

Patients with end-stage lung disease present with a more varied spectrum of nutritional compromise. Madill et al. demonstrated that pretransplant evaluation of patients with idiopathic pulmonary fibrosis and primary pulmonary hypertension reveal normal or near-normal nutritional indices.[36] In contrast, those with emphysema, cystic fibrosis, or bronchiectasis more often present with severe protein-calorie malnutrition despite normal or supranormal caloric intake. It is hypothesized that chronic infection in these individuals results in increased energy requirements and development of malnutrition.

Conclusions about Nutritional Assessment in the Pretransplant Patient

As noted in the previous sections, some manifestations of end-stage organ failure can interfere with the evaluation of nutritional status using traditional objective parameters. For example, body weight may not be a valid index due to ascites or edema masking the loss of lean muscle mass. Administration of diuretics can lead to exaggerated fluctuations in the extracellular fluid compartment and thus to inaccurate conclusions. Anthropometric measurements have been proposed as a more accurate yardstick of nutritional status. Variations in hydration and skin compressibility and elasticity are not accounted for by available standards of anthropometric measurement, and spurious results can occur even with experienced operators. Biochemical indices of nutritional health may also be severely affected by chronic renal and hepatic failure altering CHI, nitrogen balance studies, 3-methylhistidine excretion, skin antigen testing, and various serum protein levels, making their interpretation problematic.[37–40]

In an attempt to improve the predictive power of individual observations and measurements, various multiparameter indexes were developed. The two most commonly used in clinical practice include the prognostic nutritional index (PNI) and the subjective global nutritional assessment (SGNA) combined with selected serum protein measurements.[41, 42] The PNI is based on four measures selected by regression analysis, generating a percent risk assessment:

$$PNI (\% \text{ risk}) = 158 - 16 \text{ (serum albumin [g])} - \\ 0.78 \text{ (triceps skinfold [mm])} - \\ 0.2 \text{ (serum transferrin [mg/dl])} - \\ 5.8 \text{ (skin test reactivity [0–2])}$$

Although the PNI has been validated in a variety of surgical populations, it has not been predictive in transplant recipients. In one study, nearly all patients receiving a liver transplant had PNI scores that suggested high postoperative risk, yet very few actually manifested complications.[38] It has been suggested that this poor correlation may be due to the unusually rapid reversal of many of the adverse

Table 15-3. Subjective Global Nutritional Assessment (SGNA)

History
Weight loss in last 6 months
Dietary intake
Gastrointestinal symptoms
Functional capacity
Physical effects (e.g., muscle wasting, edema, ascites)
SGNA rating
A = well nourished
B = moderately malnourished
C = severely malnourished

metabolic abnormalities by liver transplantation. It may be that the serum protein levels used in the calculation of the index may not indicate malnutrition in the liver failure patient.

The SGNA is an index that surveys a patient's historic and physical findings, ultimately generating a rating of well nourished, moderately malnourished, or severely malnourished (Table 15-3).[43] Five features in the history are elicited. The first is overall weight loss in the past 6 months, with specific emphasis on weight gain or loss during the past 2 weeks. This allows discrimination of patients who may have sustained a significant weight loss but have plateaued or rebounded from those with ongoing weight loss. Patients are then classified as having normal or abnormal oral intake. If intake is abnormal, the duration and degree of intake are measured as suboptimal solid diet, hypocaloric diet, full liquid diet, or starvation. The third feature is the presence of gastrointestinal (GI) symptoms such as nausea, vomiting, anorexia, or diarrhea. These symptoms are considered significant if persistent beyond 2 weeks. The fourth category is functional capacity or energy level and includes duration and type of physical exertion, ranging from active to bedridden. The last feature gives some indication of the metabolic demands of a patient's underlying disease and is rated as high, medium, or low stress (e.g., a patient with ongoing sepsis has high stress).

Five features of the physical examination are weighted from normal (0) to mild (+1), moderate (+2), or severe (+3). The first is loss of subcutaneous fat measured in the patient's triceps region and the midaxillary line at the level of the lower ribs. The second measurement is loss of muscle mass and tone as determined by palpation. Finally, the presence of

Table 15-4. Effects of the Hypermetabolic Response

Clinical Response	Endocrine Response	Mediator Response
Increased cardiac output	Increased cortisol	Increased interleukin-1, interleukin-6
Increased temperature	Increased norepinephrine	Increased tissue necrosis factor
Redistribution of blood flow	Increased epinephrine	Increased eicosanoids
Increased metabolic rate	Increased insulin	
Increased heart rate	Increased glucagon	
Increased respiration		

sacral or ankle edema as well as the presence or absence of ascites is noted. Based on this directed history and physical examination, the clinician may determine an SGNA rank that best characterizes the patient's nutritional status. In contrast to the PNI, a rank is assigned based on subjective weighting of individual parameters rather than a fixed, numeric weighting scheme. Thus, a patient with ascites and weight gain but poor intake and muscle wasting can still be found severely malnourished based on the clinician's subjective rating. Despite concerns of interobserver variability, the SGNA has been found to be highly reproducible and reliable. It has also demonstrated excellent preoperative predictive capacity in liver transplant and dialysis patients.[44, 45] Thus, a comprehensive history and physical examination, coupled with the use of selected laboratory measurements in combination with an SGNA, appear to generate a reliable and reproducible approach to evaluating the nutritional status of the pretransplant patient.

Postoperative Considerations

Metabolic Changes in the Postoperative Patient

As with all surgical patients, operative intervention triggers significant alterations in metabolism, energy expenditure, and nitrogen balance. The changes in whole-body metabolism associated with surgical and traumatic injuries were first appreciated in the 1970s. In a study examining the metabolic requirements of burn victims, it was demonstrated that the metabolic rate increases proportionately to the percentage of total burned body surface area up to 50–60%.[46] In large burns, a patient's energy requirements are essentially double that of his or her normal basal metabolic rate. Subsequent studies examining the changes in metabolism associated with surgical

injury have documented a similar, albeit less dramatic, rise in basal metabolism of 5–20%, depending on the extent of iatrogenic tissue injury.[47] Table 15-4 lists the effects of the hypermetabolic response.

With all substantial tissue injury the cardiovascular system functions at an accelerated pace.[48] Cardiac output is enhanced, predominantly through an increase in heart rate, leading to augmented blood flow. However, the majority of this output is preferentially shunted to the area of tissue injury, supporting increased cellular activity; to the kidney, leading to an elevated glomerular filtration rate (GFR); and to the splanchnic viscera.[49, 50] Through the release of a variety of endogenous mediators, including interleukin-1 and tumor necrosis factor, the thermoregulatory centers in the hypothalamus are reset upward to a new reference point.[51] This leads to additional metabolic stress to maintain an elevated core body temperature through shivering and glucose use for heat production. Both protein and carbohydrate metabolism are altered with injury. Studies by Cuthberson first documented accelerated protein loss from the skeletal muscle compartment in association with long bone fractures.[52] Subsequent studies using 3-methylhistidine and creatinine kinase excretion, both markers of skeletal protein catabolism, have substantially confirmed these findings in a variety of injured states.[53, 54] Further studies of the time course of this response suggest that this protein catabolism peaks several days after injury and slowly declines over a period of several weeks.[52] Analysis of this skeletal protein catabolism by Garber et al. also revealed a preferential release of alanine and glutamine from the muscle compartment during this catabolic phase.[55] These two amino acids may constitute up to 70% of net peripheral amino acid release.[55] This appears to be due to alanine's dominant role as a precursor for gluconeogenesis in the liver and glutamine's function as an important respiratory fuel for gut entero-cytes. In response to the release of a variety of counterregulatory hormones, including epinephrine, cortisol, glucagon, interleukin-1 and -6, and a variety of prostaglandins, glucose production is greatly increased. These hormones also negatively affect both insulin release and peripheral glucose uptake by postreceptor inhibition, however, leading to the so-called diabetes of injury.

The body's use of nutrients is also modified by injury. In a series of experiments by Wolfe et al., the limits of efficient glucose oxidation were examined during injury.[56] These studies have demonstrated that recovering trauma and burn patients have an upper limit to the use of exogenously administered glucose of approximately 5–6 mg/kg per minute. Long et al. found that increasing carbohydrate intake up to 60–70% of total caloric needs slowed nitrogen loss.[57] Above this level, net nitrogen loss was not substantially affected. In fact, elevated glucose load above this critical level can be detrimental by shunting excess glucose through the fructose 1,6-diphosphate pathway; this leads to excess heat generation and acceleration of an already heightened metabolic response.[58] In addition, this excess glucose can substantially increase the risks and complications associated with hyperglycemia, including inappropriate osmotic diuresis, impaired wound healing, and altered lymphocyte and macrophage function.[59] In light of these discoveries, nutritional support of the injured patient, specifically total parenteral nutrition (TPN), most often includes a mixture of carbohydrate and fat to meet energy requirements. The administration of exogenous glucose is thus used to meet the energy requirements of the tissues that require it (e.g., central nervous system, renal medulla, and cellular blood elements). This reduces protein wasting for the substrate of gluconeogenesis, and fat can be used to replenish diminished lipid stores.

Metabolic Concerns Unique to the Transplant Patient

In addition to the changes in body metabolism associated with tissue injury, metabolic side effects unique to the transplant patient are related to the administration of immunosuppressive drugs, which may further alter the response to injury in the post-transplant patient (Table 15-5). After an uncompli-

Table 15-5. Metabolic Concerns Unique to the Transplant Patient

Increased catabolism related to high-dose steroids
Glucose intolerance from steroids, cyclosporine, and tacrolimus (FK506)
Electrolyte abnormalities: hyperkalemia, hypomagnesemia, polyuria
Hypertension
Hyperlipidemia with hypertriglyceridemia, especially prevalent with sirolimus

cated allograft placement, energy expenditure rises proportionately to the degree of injury and has been shown to be analogous to other surgeries of similar scope.[60] In contrast, protein catabolism after renal and hepatic transplantation has been observed to be significantly greater than that of comparable surgical procedures.[61, 62] This is due in large measure to the administration of high-dose corticosteroids used in the induction of immunosuppression. The use of steroids has been shown to increase the protein catabolic rate in a dose-dependent fashion. For example, in the weeks after kidney transplantation, the protein catabolic rate can range from 1.3 to 2.2 g/kg per day on immunosuppressive regimens using 60–200 mg/kg of prednisone.[63] It can increase up to 1.9–2.4 g/kg per day after treatment for acute rejection episodes with higher pulse steroid doses.[63] If left uncountered, this accelerated protein catabolism would rapidly lead to severe muscle wasting, pulmonary insufficiency, and infectious complications. These problems can be readily prevented by supplying a diet high in both fat and protein calories.

The transplant patient has a higher incidence of postoperative glucose intolerance than do other postsurgical populations. In addition to its strong protein catabolic effects, steroid therapy also exerts significant influence over glucose production and use, which can lead to transient or prolonged carbohydrate dysregulation. Such glucose intolerance has been observed in up to 16–47% of renal transplant patients in the first few months after surgery.[64–66] Both cyclosporine and newer agents, such as tacrolimus (FK506), may further exacerbate this dysregulation by their direct effects on insulin release by pancreatic islet cells.[67] Thus, although the postoperative transplant patient may have high energy and carbohydrate requirements, these must be carefully monitored to ensure adequate use and prevention of hyperglycemia.

Electrolyte abnormalities are common in the posttransplant period and are due, in part, to cyclosporine's influence on the renal cortical collecting ducts and their regulation of the extracellular fluid compartment.[68] Hyperkalemia may occur in conjunction with cyclosporine administration and is often exacerbated by delayed return of renal graft function.[69] This disturbance can in turn lead to impaired ammonium excretion and renal tubular acidosis. Hypomagnesemia is also seen in cyclosporine-treated patients and can rapidly lead to life-threatening complications, such as cardiac dysrhythmias.[70] Hypertension also is associated with cyclosporine use. It is thought to be related to sodium retention through an altered renal response to volume changes brought about by this drug.[68] It is important to consider these potential electrolyte abnormalities when planning dietary interventions in this critical postoperative period.

Hyperlipidemia and hypertriglyceridemia can affect both the early and late postoperative nutritional management of the transplant patient. Hyperlipidemia has been demonstrated to occur in up to 40–55% of transplant recipients.[71] Serum cholesterol often begins to rise in the first 90 days after transplant, and it appears to be circumstantially associated with the initiation of steroid immunosuppression. Although the etiology of this effect may be related to a number of contributing factors, steroids are known to enhance lipoprotein production as well as stimulate lipoprotein lipase, leading to enhanced release of triglycerides and free fatty acids.[72] Cyclosporine appears to exacerbate this effect. It is hypothesized that cyclosporine may disrupt the normal interaction between low-density lipoprotein receptors and ligands in addition to inhibiting secretion of cholesterol through the bile. These effects cannot be reversed unless immunosuppressive medication is discontinued; thus, the clinician must monitor serum lipids closely.

In summary, the immediate postoperative period is marked by substantial alterations in whole-body metabolism that follow a characteristic course common to the general surgical patient and the transplant patient. Administration of immunosuppressive drugs, however, particularly steroids and cyclosporine, can amplify this response, and these changes must be considered when planning nutritional intervention in the postoperative transplant patient.

Enteral versus Parenteral Nutrition

Despite the hypermetabolism identified in the early postoperative period, healthy, well-nourished individuals undergoing an uncomplicated elective surgery can usually tolerate 5–7 days of starvation without significant disability if small amounts of glucose are added to their intravenous fluids.[73] This usually amounts to approximately 500 calories per day from the administration of 2 liters of a 5% dextrose solution. It has been advocated that if oral intake is inadequate beyond this period, supplemental enteral nutrition, such as nasogastric feedings, should be initiated promptly. If the GI tract is not working, parenteral nutrition may be required.[73] It is important to note that during starvation and moderate stress, daily nitrogen losses commonly approach 10–15 g per day, whereas optimal nutritional support can at best be expected to achieve a positive nitrogen balance of 3–5 g per day.[74] Thus, for each 24 hours where adequate nutritional support is delayed, it may take 3–5 additional days just to recoup a single day's loss.

In the case of the malnourished postoperative patient, nutritional compromise is more rapidly associated with untoward outcome. Several studies have documented that major abdominal surgeries can worsen the malnourished state identified preoperatively. Herberer et al. demonstrated that the mean period of inadequate dietary intake in patients after GI surgery was 10 days.[75] Although most patients in this study began eating by 7 days, they were unable to consume enough to prevent a negative nitrogen balance for several more days. In an earlier study, Meguid and Meguid examined the inadequate oral nutrition period in a large series of patients undergoing resection of a GI malignancy. They found that malnourished patients began oral intake at an interval similar to well-nourished controls but did not achieve adequate intake before 10 days post procedure.[76] Thus, both these studies suggest that the malnourished state in the postoperative patient can be severely exacerbated by waiting for return of normal oral caloric intake, implying that more aggressive measures are needed. This has led to the call to limit this period of starvation to 5 days or less in malnourished individuals before starting more aggressive measures.[73] Indeed, immediate enteral feeding has been shown to significantly reduce postoperative complications and length of hospitalization. The magnitude of benefit is great, with overall infection being reduced by 50–70%. The vast majority of patients can start enteral nutrition within 6–8 hours of injury or operation, but enteral feedings should be delayed in unstable patients.

Enteral nutrition implies the use of the GI tract as the site of nutrient absorption. If a patient cannot tolerate oral nutrition but retains a functional GI tract, there are numerous routes of administration, including nasoenteric, esophagoenteric, and gastroenteric intubation, as well as needle catheter jejunostomy. With the advent of thin silicone (Silastic) tubing, nasoenteric intubation has now become the most common route of supplemental short-term nutrition therapy, given the ease of placement and prevention of complications.[77] Nasoenteric feeding also allows feeding continuously during anesthesia. In the patient for whom passing a tube past the pylorus is difficult, metoclopramide may be helpful.

The number of commercial enteral formulas available to the clinician has grown exponentially since the late 1980s. They include a variety of defined formula diets, which can be categorized into five distinct groups:

1. Mixtures of natural food that may or may not include more purified ingredients
2. Mixtures of protein isolates, such as soybean, egg white, or casein, and more highly purified sources of carbohydrates and lipids
3. Mixtures of hydrolyzed proteins with more highly purified sources of carbohydrates and lipids (so-called chemically defined elemental diets)
4. Mixtures of crystalline amino acids and purified sources of carbohydrates and lipids (i.e., elemental diets)
5. Formulations designed for specific disease states, such as renal, hepatic, or pulmonary failure or trauma

Considerations in selecting the most appropriate enteral formula are many. In general, because a large portion of the adult population has some degree of lactose insufficiency, formulas based on milk products should be avoided and are mostly limited to those found in the first category described above.[78]

The optimal form of amino acid preparation for nutrient absorption, intact protein, hydrolyzed protein, or free amino acids has been debated.

Although evidence is conflicting, some metabolic studies in both humans and animals suggests that, in general, free amino acids may have less biological availability than peptides or whole proteins and are more expensive to produce.[79] One notable exception is cases of malabsorption, such as chronic pancreatitis or celiac disease, where free amino acids have demonstrated some added usefulness.[80]

A variety of carbohydrates, including fructose and longer-chain sugars, have been advocated as more efficient energy sources. All are eventually digested to glucose, however, and these advantages appear to be minor. More significantly, the form of carbohydrate affects the osmolarity of the solution, which may range between 150 and 800 mOsm in commercially produced diets and can have important effects on transit time, absorption, intestinal discomfort, and diarrhea.[81] As a general rule, isotonic solutions are best tolerated.

The composition of lipids also varies considerably between proprietary formulations, but it is usually based on corn, safflower, or soybean oil. Some manufacturers have introduced formulas based on medium-chain triglycerides, which do not require pancreatic lipases for absorption and do not enter the eicosanoid pathway. All commercial formulations include at least 3–5% of polyunsaturated fat, such as linoleic and linolenic acid, to prevent essential fatty acid deficiency, but most have much higher levels—up to 50% of total fat. At this high concentration, omega-6 fatty acids were demonstrated to be immunosuppressive in some patients.[82] All complete defined formulas also contain a full range of vitamins, except vitamin K, that meet the recommended daily allowances for adults. With the interest in antioxidant vitamins, these compounds have been added to various formulas above physiologic needs, but their actual role is less well defined.[83] Finally, all nutritional support provides some form of electrolytes and trace elements. Again, there is substantial variation between formulations in the total concentration of sodium, potassium, chloride, calcium, phosphate, and magnesium. Choice of a particular diet should consider these differences in light of clinical needs.

Parenteral nutrition means the administration of nutrients directly into the circulation, bypassing intestinal absorption. By definition, its route of administration is through some form of intravenous cannula, which may be placed peripherally or centrally. Although peripheral administration has demonstrated usefulness in certain patient populations requiring short-term treatment, this discussion is limited to TPN through central venous access. The reader is referred elsewhere for further information on the topic.[84]

As with enteral nutrition, parenteral nutrient solutions have been developed to provide adequate calories, protein, vitamins, and electrolytes to achieve positive energy-nitrogen balance. Glucose is generally the source of carbohydrate calories in the form of dextrose monohydrate. In this form, it yields approximately 3.4 kcal/g. The majority of solutions available are 25–35% glucose by weight, with an osmolarity of 1,200–1,700 mOsm/liter. It is because of this hypertonicity that these solutions require administration through a large central vein with high flow to prevent endothelial damage and rapid thrombosis.

Lipid emulsions are used in conjunction with glucose to prevent essential fatty acid deficiency and provide supplemental calories. These solutions have a caloric density of 9 kcal/ml and are isotonic in relation to blood. In general, the lipid component of TPN should supply no more than 30% of nonprotein calories because beyond that level it may saturate the body's ability to use this fuel and may interfere with neutrophil and lymphocyte function. Standard lipid solutions normally contain a mixture of safflower and soybean oil; they are emulsified by the addition of egg phospholipids to homogeneous droplets that are similar in size to chylomicrons.

Crystalline amino acids in the levo form are provided in solution as a nitrogen source. Commercial solutions are formulated to consist of 40–50% essential amino acids and 50–60% nonessential amino acids. Although there are slight differences between various mixtures, they are not thought to be of clinical significance. Fluids, electrolytes, vitamins, and trace minerals are adjusted to meet specific patient needs.

Complications of Enteral and Parenteral Nutritional Therapy

Although both enteral and parenteral nutrition have been shown to be safe and effective, several complications related to each form of supplementation must be appreciated to ensure proper administration

Table 15-6. Complications of Enteral versus Parenteral Nutrition

Enteral route
  Tube displacement
  Tube malposition or pneumothorax
  Epistaxis
  Sinusitis
  Tube blockage
  Mucosal erosion
  Aspiration
  Diarrhea
Parenteral route
  Catheter-related sepsis
  Metabolic and electrolyte disturbance
  Depressed immune responses
  Intestinal atrophy
  Pneumothorax
  Thrombosis central vein
  Carotid artery injury
  Hematoma
  Pericardial tamponade
  Brachial plexus injury
  Hemothorax or hydrothorax

(Table 15-6). These risks can be divided into two basic categories: those related to tube or cannula placement and those specifically related to the administration of enteral or parenteral nutrition. Enteral nutrition most commonly requires the blind intubation of the GI tract, after which tube location is confirmed by radiograph. The importance of confirming tube position was highlighted in a study by Benya et al., who examined a series of 100 consecutive nasoenteric tube placements. They found that nearly one-fourth of all tubes were malpositioned, with the majority of these involving esophageal placement.[85] More important, they found a 1% incidence of pulmonary or pleural intubation, which is potentially disastrous if subsequent feeding is initiated. This is of particular importance when dealing with obtunded, intubated, or comatose patients. Other complications include sinusitis due to blockage of adequate drainage from the maxillary ostia and hemorrhage from mucosal erosion. These issues can usually be minimized by using newer silicone catheters, which are much smaller and more pliable than the older generations of vinyl or latex tubing.[77]

Clogging of feeding tubes with inspissated protein or pill fragments also complicates enteral supplementation, leading to intermittent administration and often mandating tube replacement. Mancuard et al. found that some formulas, including Osmolite (Ross Products Division, Abbott Laboratories, Columbus, OH) and Ensure (Ross Products Division, Abbott Laboratories), had significantly higher rates of formula-related tube occlusion than did Vivonex (Novartis Nutrition, Minneapolis, MN), Vital (Ross Products Division, Abbott Laboratories), and Citrotein (Novartis Nutrition).[86] Clogging also correlated with lowering the pH of formulas to below 5.0 by the addition of acidic medications and use of smaller-bore tubing (below 8 French). In light of these findings, routine flushing of the feeding tube is recommended after each use to reduce the number of these episodes.

Aspiration of tube feeding or bacteria by contaminated gastric contents is associated with significant morbidity and mortality related to chemical pneumonitis and pneumonia. Intragastric tube feedings are associated with an elevation of the gastric pH, leading to a less hostile environment for gram-negative bacterial colonization.[87] Strong et al. demonstrated that there may be equal risk of aspiration in gastric and postpyloric feedings.[88] Others, such as Montecalvo et al., suggest that postpyloric position may have significant advantages.[89] Ibanez et al. examined the effects of patient positioning in regard to gastroesophageal reflux and aspiration; they concluded that semirecumbency is associated with a small decrease in reflux over the supine position.[90] Based on these and other studies, it can be suggested that to reduce the risks of aspiration, patients should be fed postpylorically in a semirecumbent position. If this is not feasible, feedings should be administered into the stomach and titrated to a pH of 3.5–4.0 to decrease the incidence of nosocomial pneumonia from gastric colonization.[91]

Complications associated with the administration of enteral feedings are generally minor. They were reviewed extensively in an excellent monograph by Cataldi-Betcher et al.[81] This group examined 253 consecutive medical and surgical patients treated with enteral nutritional supplementation. Enteral feedings, excluding mechanical difficulties, had an overall complication rate of 8.2%, including 6.2% GI problems, such as diarrhea or poor gastric emptying, and metabolic complications of 2.0% (e.g., hyper- or hypokalemia and azotemia). Diarrhea is the most commonly reported complication of tube feeding and is associated with multiple etiologies, including rate

of delivery, osmolarity, additional medications, fat content, and bacterial infection.[92, 93] Edes et al. studied 29 episodes of diarrhea in hospitalized patients receiving enteral nutrition.[94] They found that the vast majority were osmotic complications related to the administration of various medications, such as antacids or elixirs containing sorbitol. Very few were directly related to the enteral feeding itself. He further observed that obtaining a stool osmotic gap (see following equation) was very helpful in rapidly differentiating possible etiologies of diarrheal complications associated with enteral feedings.

Stool osmotic gap = (stool osmolarity) − [2 × the sum
  of the concentrations of stool sodium and potassium]

In general, diarrhea is considered osmotic in origin if the stool osmotic gap is greater than 100 mmol/liter.

The process of initiating parenteral nutrition begins with the placement of a cannula in a large central vein. The subclavian or jugular vein is most commonly used, and the clinician should be comfortable with both sites of placement. In a prospective study of 200 consecutive central-line placements, Ryan et al. found an overall complication rate of 7%, including pneumothorax (3%), thrombophlebitis (1.5%), and carotid artery injury, mediastinal hematoma, hydrothorax, and brachial plexus injury (each 0.5%).[95] In the largest study to date, Wolfe et al. found a 1.3% incidence of major complications requiring invasive treatment.[96]

Catheter-related sepsis is perhaps the most common complication related to an indwelling central venous cannula. It has been reported to occur with an incidence of 7% in a multicenter study of patients undergoing parenteral nutritional therapy.[97] With the advent of multilumen catheters, there has been a dramatic increase in the number of catheter-related sepsis cases. Thus, if possible, a single-lumen line dedicated to TPN administration is advocated and is associated with significantly fewer line infections.[98] Although many fungal and bacterial pathogens have been implicated in line sepsis, the most common organisms are those typically found on the skin of patients and the personnel who care for them. These include the gram-positive organisms *Staphylococcus aureus*, *S. epidermidis*, and *Streptococcus viridans*; the gram-negative bacteria *Klebsiella*, *Pseudomonas*, *Serratia*, and *Escherichia coli*; and the fungus *Candida albicans*.[99] Treatment generally includes catheter removal, culture of the intracutaneous portion of the cannula, and replacement at a new site if necessary. Intravenous antibiotics may be required if fever and leukocytosis do not promptly subside with catheter removal. These should be directed by blood and line cultures.

Metabolic and electrolyte complications of parenteral therapy are more common than with enteral therapy because direct delivery of nutrients into the bloodstream bypasses the regulatory mechanisms inherent to intestinal absorption. It is estimated that up to 10% of adult patients on TPN have at least one metabolic complication related to therapy.[96] Long-term TPN is associated with various complications, including linoleic acid and trace metal deficiencies and hepatic and biliary abnormalities. Short-term treatment is most commonly associated with blood glucose regulatory dysfunction, which may occur in up to 25% of postoperative patients.[100–102] It is thus incumbent on the clinician to carefully monitor blood glucose every 4–6 hours initially and to administer insulin as needed to prevent hyperglycemia. Hyperglycemia may lead to further problems, such as impaired immune function and inappropriate osmotic diuresis. Increasing the percentage of calories derived from lipids may help to relieve this problem but is itself associated with immunosuppression in high concentrations. In summary, then, although enteral feeding may be more difficult to administer than TPN in seriously ill patients, it may provide better nutritional support, is less costly, and is associated with fewer complications than intravenous nutrition.

Role of Early Enteral Nutritional Supplementation in the Postoperative Patient

As noted earlier, nitrogen losses during moderately stressed starvation can be 10–15 g per day and may require several additional days of nutritional supplementation to make up for a single day's loss. During this period of starvation, the malnourished postoperative patient can fall even further behind, thereby exacerbating nutrition-related complications. In an attempt to prevent this mounting deficit, some clinicians have advocated initiation of enteral or parenteral nutrition at the earliest possible time. The role of early administration of postoperative TPN was addressed by Preshaw et al., who randomized postoperative patients undergoing bowel resection to an early 5-day course of TPN or no supplemental nutrition.[103] He found that

the number of anastomotic leaks in the nutritionally supplemented population was 50% less than in the unfed group. Collins et al. also demonstrated the benefits of aggressive early postoperative TPN.[104] He compared a group of postoperative cancer resection patients receiving TPN to those receiving amino acid solution and intravenous fluids alone. The TPN group had significantly fewer complications than did the two control arms in the study. Finally, Yamada et al. prospectively analyzed the effects of aggressive early TPN on a series of patients receiving chemotherapy and gastrectomy for a gastric malignancy.[105] The TPN-treated group not only had improved weight gain, serum proteins, and immunocompetence but also tolerated higher doses of chemotherapy and had improved disease-free survival.

Despite the improvements demonstrated by early initiation of parenteral nutrition, a growing body of evidence suggests that enteral nutrition is much more efficacious. In a study by Hoover et al. of 51 patients undergoing abdominal surgery, patients were randomized to groups receiving standard intravenous saline solutions or an enteral diet initiated immediately after surgery. The enterally fed patients required nearly 6 days less intravenous therapy than did controls.[106] In another study, Sagar et al. found that initiation of early enteral feedings versus standard intravenous therapy followed by an oral diet beginning on postoperative day 6 led to improved weight gain and nitrogen balance and a shorter hospital stay than controls.[107] More recently, Kudsk et al. randomized a series of 67 patients with matched abdominal trauma indexes to enteral or parenteral nutrition. They demonstrated that patients treated with a balanced enteral formula had significantly fewer septic episodes than did parenteral controls, including pneumonia (5 versus 14 episodes; $p = .03$) and line sepsis (0 versus 6 episodes; $p = .03$).[108] In perhaps the largest meta-analysis of perioperative nutrition to date, Moore et al. combined eight randomized prospective trials designed to compare the nutritional efficacy of early enteral versus TPN in high-risk trauma patients. Comparison of enteral ($n = 118$) to parenteral ($n = 112$) nutrition groups revealed that significantly fewer enterally fed patients experienced septic complications (18% versus 35%; $p = .01$).[109] Thus, although studies comparing early-initiation enteral with parenteral diet have demonstrated that both forms of therapy can improve weight gain and nitrogen balance over

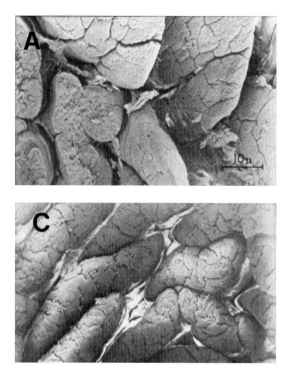

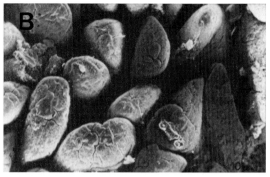

Figure 15-1. Electron micrograph scans of jejunal mucosa of guinea pigs after 30% total body surface area burn. **A.** The jejunal villi of the preburn group were tongue shaped and separated by narrow spaces. **B.** On postburn day 1, villous width was reduced, with wider spaces between villi in animals fed lactated Ringer's solution. **C.** Villi of animals that received enteral feeds were similar to those of the preburn group.

intravenous saline alone, multiple studies suggest that early enteral feeding in particular may be more cost-effective, reduce subjective postoperative stress, lower the prevalence of glucose intolerance, and reduce septic complications. On the whole, aggressive, early postoperative nutrition may be beneficial to the malnourished postoperative patient. Enteral nutrition may be the preferable route of feeding unless the GI tract cannot be otherwise used.

In animal studies, early enteral feeding prevents loss of villous height and mucosal mass (Figure 15-1). It also prevents translocation of microbes across the intestinal barrier and is associated with reduced hypermetabolic and stress responses (dampens increase in cortisol, norepinephrine, and glucagon).[110]

Role of Early Nutritional Supplementation in the Transplant Patient

Given that a large majority of transplant recipients have some form of malnutrition preoperatively, it is somewhat surprising that few studies are available to guide the clinician on the impact of early postoperative nutritional supplementation in this patient population. In particular, the postoperative liver transplant recipient almost universally exhibits protein-calorie malnutrition in addition to the stresses of catabolism induced by surgery and the initiation of immunosuppression. To date, only one controlled study has evaluated the benefits of nutritional support in this critical period. Reilly et al. randomized 28 liver transplant recipients to one of three treatment groups during the first 7 postoperative days.[111] These groups received either (1) isotonic glucose solution, (2) TPN providing 35 kcal/kg and 1.5 g/kg of protein per day, or (3) a similar TPN solution with protein enrichment for branched-chain amino acids. They found that both standard and branched chain–enriched TPN groups had significantly improved nitrogen balance over standard intravenous fluids alone. They also tended to have shorter lengths of stay in the intensive care unit (ICU), which translates to lower total hospital cost; but these trends did not reach statistical significance. The TPN formulation enriched with branched-chain amino acids did not appear to confer an advantage over standard TPN. Taken as a whole, this study suggests that early patient recovery from the ICU leads to significant cost savings and would justify aggressive early nutritional supplementation. Table 15-7 provides guidelines for the formulation of such aggressive parenteral nutrition from a review by Porayko et al.[34]

Although no studies have specifically addressed the administration of early enteral nutrition in this patient population, one could speculate that such nutrition, if permitted by gut function, may confer many of the same benefits but at a substantially lower cost. Recent experience at our own institution suggests that tube feedings can be initiated by the second postoperative day without complications.

In renal transplant recipients, some evidence suggests that early initiation of an enteral diet high in nitrogen and low in carbohydrate and continued through the first postoperative month can promote positive nitrogen balance and reduce the manifestations of cushingoid side effects induced by steroid immunosuppressive therapy. Whittier et al. randomized 12 consecutive renal transplant recipients to receive the experimental diet described above or an isocaloric control diet high in carbohydrate and low in protein.[112] Patients were begun on these oral diets by postoperative day 4. Positive nitrogen balance was achieved in six of six individuals ingesting the experimental diet. In contrast, five of six patients receiving the control diet did not achieve a nitrogen surplus. In addition, no patients who received the experimental diet developed a cushingoid appearance, whereas four of six control patients had severe cushingoid appearance; the remainder had moderate cushingoid side effects. Furthermore, the control group had a mean net loss of 47 oz of lean muscle mass, whereas the experimental group had a mean net gain of 114 oz. The mean number of rejection episodes was similar between the two groups. Thus, this study suggests that early initiation of this specific enteral diet can positively affect post–renal transplant morbidity. Our own experience at the University of Cincinnati Medical Center has been that uncomplicated renal transplant recipients usually receive a normal diet by the first postoperative day and almost never require intravenous hyperalimentation.

The role of early administration of supplemental nutrition in malnourished patients receiving combined kidney-pancreas transplantation has also been debated due to concerns that early nitrogen and carbohydrate administration could interfere with graft recovery. This issue was addressed in a study by Braga et al.[60] They randomized 26 consecutive diabetic uremic patients receiving kidney-pancreas

Table 15-7. Suggested Guidelines for Early Postoperative Total Parenteral Nutrition in Liver Transplantation

Content	Amount
Calories	Moderate calories (basal requirements + 15–20%)
Protein	High protein content (1.20–1.75 g/kg/day)
Fat	Accounts for 20–30% calories
Carbohydrate	Accounts for 70–80% calories
Sodium	90–180 mEq (2–4 g)
Fluid	As needed
Calcium	800–100 mg
Vitamins	Multivitamin or mineral supplementation (recommended daily allowance)

Source: Adapted from MK Porayko, S Dicecco, SJ O'Keefe. Impact of malnutrition and its therapy on liver transplantation. Semin Liver Dis 1991;4:305–314.

transplantation to one of three groups: (1) parenteral nutrition consisting of 0.15 g/kg per day of nitrogen and 30 kcal/kg per day of energy consisting of a 70% glucose solution and 30% lipids, (2) similar nitrogen and energy intake, with the nonnitrogen calories exclusively consisting of a glucose solution, and (3) a control group receiving standard intravenous fluids. All parenteral nutrition was initiated 24 hours after surgery and was continued for a mean of 6.8 days until the patient could resume oral intake. Parenteral nutrition did not alter insulin requirements or C-peptide levels compared to standard intravenous therapy, and early parenteral nutrition did not interfere with the recovery of kidney or pancreas graft function. However, the mean number of hyperglycemic episodes did vary according to the type of parenteral nutrition: 6.6 episodes for the glucose support group versus 1.5 episodes for the mixed-regimen group. The authors suggested that given the high proportion of malnourished kidney-pancreas transplant recipients and poor prognosis associated with septic complications, early parenteral nutrition may have a role in their treatment. In our transplant unit, an oral diet is usually initiated by the third postoperative day, and intravenous hyperalimentation is avoided unless ileus persists past the fifth postoperative day.

To date, no controlled studies have directly examined the impact of early nutritional support on lung transplantation. However, Holcombe and

Resler retrospectively reviewed the nutritional support records of 52 adult patients who had undergone lung transplantation at the University of North Carolina.[113] All patients in this study were initially begun on parenteral nutrition at a mean of 48 hours after surgery and were continued on this therapy to a mean of postoperative day 7. They found that preoperative malnutrition was most commonly identified in patients with cystic fibrosis compared with patients with other diagnoses. This supports the findings of Madill et al. discussed previously in this chapter.[36] It was also noted that omentopexy used to bolster the bronchial anastomosis at the time of surgery commonly leads to postoperative ileus, often preventing early initiation of enteral nutrition. Because preoperative malnutrition was not identified in a large number of the lung transplant recipients and most were able to resume oral intake after extubation, they suggested that the use of routine early parenteral nutrition should be examined more closely. They suggest that early parenteral nutrition might be restricted to patients in greatest need, such as the cystic fibrosis patient undergoing lung transplantation with omentopexy.

The use of nutritional support in the perioperative heart transplant recipient is not well defined, and protocols appear to vary from one institution to another. There is evidence to suggest, however, that the administration of intravenous fat emulsion used in parenteral nutrition should be monitored carefully. In an animal study, Grimes and Abel demonstrated that rapid infusion of fat emulsions significantly decreases force-velocity and length-tension relationships of the left ventricle.[114] In a follow-up study in humans recovering from coronary bypass procedures, Abel et al. observed no adverse hemodynamic changes when lipids were infused at less than 1.7 mg per minute.[115] If infusion rates climbed to 5.25 mg/kg per minute, however, significant myocardial depression was noted. Clearly, future research is needed to better define the role of postoperative nutrition in this growing transplant population.

Small bowel transplantation is now being performed in several centers in North America and Europe. These patients are routinely malnourished by virtue of their long-standing end-organ dysfunction and cannot be fed enterally after surgery due to prolonged ileus of the transplanted organ. Thus, they are begun on parenteral nutrition immediately after transplant and continue with this form of nutri-tion until the return of ileostomy output. Initial aversion to oral intake is usually the practice with these patients, but the avoidance of early enteral feeding may prove incorrect. Children undergoing this procedure may often require significant retraining to recover their desire to take food orally.[116]

Taken together, these studies suggest that patients undergoing solid-organ transplantation who are malnourished preoperatively may benefit from early aggressive enteral or parenteral nutritional support. In addition, for liver transplant recipients, at least one controlled study found that early parenteral nutrition may lead to shorter stays in the ICU, thereby providing significant cost savings over later initiation.[111] Our experience suggests that, in general, aggressive enteral feeding should be initiated as early as possible postoperatively and that intravenous hyperalimentation should be restricted to enteral failures.

Monitoring of Nutritional Support

Once the decision has been made to place a patient on nutritional support, some provision must be made to monitor and gauge the adequacy of this treatment. Traditionally, clinicians have relied on several parameters, including urine urea nitrogen (UUN) measurements and several selected visceral protein levels.

When protein is used for fuel by the body, nitrogenous wastes are produced and excreted mainly in the urine. This occurs in conjunction with obligatory nitrogen losses from skin, feces, GI tract, and bodily secretions that approximate 2 g per day. When anabolism has been achieved, protein is no longer used for fuel, and it becomes a substrate for cell growth. Thus, simply stated, nitrogen balance is the difference between nitrogen input and output, and it provides a rough approximation of the usage of protein stores. Most clinicians rely on an approximation of total urinary nitrogen (TUN), using a measurement of UUN obtained from a 24-hour urine collection. In general, there is a good correlation between the two measurements (80% ± 12%). However, several studies have called into question the validity of this estimate in certain stressed patients, such as the ICU patient.[117, 118] These studies have found that UUN can vary between 12% and 112% of actual TUN. These researchers suggest that direct TUN measurement or the sensitive pyrochemiluminescence technique be used in this population.

An alternative to nitrogen balance studies as an index of dynamic nutritional assessment is the measurement of albumin, prealbumin, transferrin, or retinol binding protein. Church and Hill examined the usefulness of these proteins as a marker of anabolism in 54 general surgical patients treated with parenteral nutritional therapy. Using TUN as a reference standard of nitrogen balance, they found that prealbumin had a sensitivity of 88%, a specificity of 70%, a positive predictive value of 93%, and a negative predictive value of 56% in detecting positive nitrogen balance.[21] In contrast, none of the other plasma proteins achieved more than 50% accuracy in estimating nitrogen balance. Such measurements have not been directly assessed in transplant patients, however, and we conclude that none of the available tests is worth the expenditure.

Introduction to Nutritional Immunomodulation

Throughout this chapter, evidence is presented to suggest that nutritional supplementation can have a positive impact on the malnourished transplant patient by improving such variables as nitrogen balance, requirement for mechanical ventilation, and complications of steroid immunosuppression. However, there is increasing evidence that particular components of this nutritional supplementation, such as specific amino acids, lipids, or vitamins, may have a role beyond their usefulness as metabolic substrate. These effects have spawned a new line of inquiry, termed *nutritional pharmacology*. Some experimental research now points to dietary intervention as a potential route for manipulation of the immune system and the rejection response to solid-organ allografts.

Among the amino acids, glutamine and arginine have been demonstrated to possess potent immunoregulatory properties. Arginine is a nonessential amino acid but may become essential during periods of stress and immune activation.[119] It has been demonstrated in rodents that arginine is beneficial for weight gain and wound healing in injured rats.[120] Arginine supplementation has also been shown to increase thymic weight, lymphoid count,

and mitogen-induced proliferation of lymphocytes in animals.[121] In vivo studies reflect these effects by demonstrating that a diet fortified with 2% arginine can improve survival in a third-degree burn affecting 30% of total body surface area in guinea pigs[122] or that arginine supplementation can improve resistance to transplantable solid-tumor models, such as Moloney sarcoma virus.[123] Although the specific mechanism of the immunomodulatory actions of arginine has yet to be defined, it may be multifactorial. Mechanisms may include an increase in cellular ornithine levels, alteration in nitric oxide metabolites, or modulation of membrane receptor signaling.[124] Furthermore, studies in a transfused mouse burn model at our own institution have demonstrated that enteral supplementation with arginine can improve gut barrier function and enhance survival over a balanced standard laboratory diet. These effects appear to be mediated by the arginine–nitric oxide pathway.[125]

The mucosa of the intestine consists primarily of enterocytes whose function is to digest and absorb nutrients and to form a physical barrier to keep unwanted pathogens from entering the body. Normally, this barrier function is highly efficient, but it can break down during periods of exceptional stress, leading to bacterial translocation.[126] Under these conditions, whole, viable microbes can pass through this epithelial layer, entering the blood or lymph and providing a potential source of systemic infection (Figure 15-2). During these periods of stress, skeletal muscle protein is degraded and preferentially aminated to form the branched-chain amino acids, alanine and glutamine. Although alanine is preferentially used by the liver as a substrate for gluconeogenesis, glutamine is metabolized by intestinal enterocytes and serves as their principal oxidizable fuel.[127] During times of injury, however, enteric glutamine consumption by visceral organs can exceed production in peripheral tissues, leading to gut atrophy. Currently, glutamine is not supplied in standard enteral or parenteral nutrient solutions due to concerns about potential stability and toxicity when stored in solution. However, some evidence from animal and human studies suggests that glutamine supplementation may help to protect mucosal integrity and limit the severity of multisystem organ failure in addition to sparing muscle catabolism and improving nitrogen balance.[128, 129]

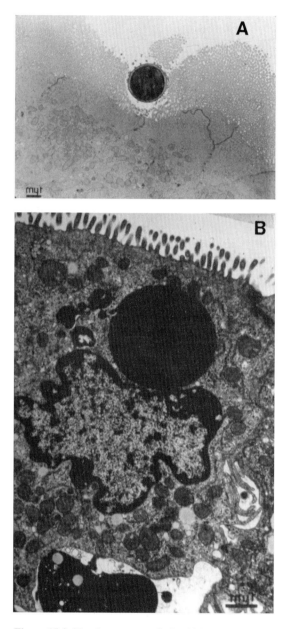

Figure 15-2. The phenomenon of microbial translocation is demonstrated after the introduction of *Candida albicans* into the ileum of a burned guinea pig. The *Candida* organism passes across the microvillus layer (**A**) and descends into the enterocyte (**B**).

Among the lipids, omega-3 fatty acids have demonstrated potent immunomodulatory properties. Dietary supplementation with such lipids leads to their incorporation into the cell membranes of lymphocytes and macrophages. This can result in three very important consequences. The first is a change in

the ratio of polyunsaturated to saturated fatty acids in the cell membrane, leading to enhanced fluidity, which may alter receptor signaling or function.[130] Supplementation with the omega-3 fatty acids can also result in a reduction of available arachidonic acid, which is the substrate necessary for the production of a number of important immune regulators, such as prostaglandins, thromboxanes, and leukotrienes via the cyclo-oxygenase pathway.[131] Finally, they may lead to enhanced production of prostaglandin E_3 and thromboxane A_3 (TXA_3) through the same pathway, both of which have less biological potency than do the prostaglandins of the series 2 subtype, such as TXA_2.[132]

Fish oil has several properties that suggest that it plays a key role in immunomodulation. It has been demonstrated to reduce blood pressure and decrease serum cholesterol as well as increase renal cortical blood flow and GFR.[133, 134] It is also a potent inhibitor of platelet aggregation and thrombus formation, and it appears to reduce small vessel arteriosclerosis.[135, 136] These effects are presumed to occur through fish oil's down regulation of TXA_2 production. In experimental transplant models, Perez et al. demonstrated that the administration of lipids can significantly reduce host responsiveness to solid-organ allografts, thereby leading to improved allograft survival.[137]

Just as glutamine is the preferential respiratory fuel of small bowel enterocytes, colonic enterocytes favor butyric acid as a primary source of energy.[138] The supplementation of diets with dietary fibers, such as pectin (a fermentable fiber polysaccharide), leads to degradation of this compound by enteric bacteria and thus to the release of butyric and other short-chain fatty acids.[139, 140] In studies examining intestinal adaptation to massive small bowel resection, the addition of pectins leads to improved mucosal growth and function.[141] Dietary supplementation with pectin has also demonstrated reduced colonic injury and improved recovery from experimentally induced colitis.[142]

Dietary nucleotides have been demonstrated to have immunoregulatory function. Mice that received H_2-incompatible heterotopic cardiac transplants and nucleotide-free diets had delayed rejection of their grafts compared to nucleotide-treated controls.[143, 144] This effect has been shown to be synergistic with cyclosporine in enhancing allograft survival.[145] It has also been demonstrated that nucleotide-free diets suppress lymphocyte responsiveness both in vivo and in vitro, reduce delayed hypersensitivity responses, and adversely affect resistance to opportunistic pathogens, such as *Candida albicans*.[146] To date, however, the clinical significance of these findings remains to be proved.

Several vitamins and trace minerals have received increasing attention as antioxidant agents. Vitamin E, in particular, may help to prevent lipid peroxidation of long-chain fatty acids within cell membranes. It is known that vitamin E has some influence on prostaglandin synthesis and appears to inhibit equally the cyclo-oxygenase and lipoxygenase pathways.[147] In vivo studies in rodent burn models suggest that vitamin E can improve outcome if administered before injury.[148] Vitamin C has been heralded as a powerful antioxidant and immunostimulatory agent, but substantial evidence to support these claims is lacking. The trace metal selenium, as an integral component of the enzyme glutathione peroxidase, is thought to be an essential nutrient in some species and possibly in humans.[149] Epidemiologic studies show a correlation between cancer rates and selenium blood levels.[150] Despite these promising implications, very little is known about the actual role or significance of these findings.

Many of the experimental findings described above are now finding applications in clinical practice. Alexander and Gottschlich examined 60 pediatric patients with more than 10% total body surface area burns; the children received either standard enteral tube feedings without fish oil or a diet containing 7.5% of the nonprotein calories derived from fish oil.[151] The group that received the fish oil–supplemented diet had a significantly lower incidence of wound infection and pneumonia as well as reduced hospital stay. Dietary supplementation with arginine has also demonstrated usefulness in immunosuppressed surgical patients. In a randomized prospective study of 30 cancer patients undergoing major operative procedures, those receiving enteral feedings supplemented with arginine experienced significant enhancement in T-cell activation as a result of concanavalin A and phytohemagglutinin stimulation compared to standard enteral feeding.[152]

The identification of the significant benefits of both fish oil and arginine has helped to spawn the creation of immune-enhancing diets that offer clinical benefits to stressed surgical patients. One such diet is Impact (Sandoz Nutrition, Minneapolis, MN). This commercially available enteral immunomodulatory diet has been studied extensively in animal models, including a variety of immunocompromised states.[153–155] Impact is specifically formulated to enhance immune function through supplementation with arginine, RNA, and fish oil containing omega-3 fatty acids. These supplements are thought to decrease the damage caused by the inflammatory response through multiple pathways.[123, 156] Several clinical studies highlight the effectiveness of Impact. Bower et al. compared Impact to a balanced enteral control diet in a prospective randomized, blinded, multicenter trial.[157] They found that Impact reduced length of stay in the ICU by 27% (22 days versus 30 days for control diet, $p = .05$). A trend in reduction of infectious complications among the Impact-fed group reached statistical significance only with urinary tract infections. Daly et al. randomized 85 patients undergoing surgery for GI malignancy to receive either Impact or a balanced enteral control diet.[158] Patients receiving Impact had significantly improved nitrogen balance and in vitro lymphocyte responsiveness compared to control diet. Mean length of hospital stay was significantly shorter for the Impact-fed group (15.8 versus 20.2 days, $p = .01$).

Moore et al. compared a similar immunomodulatory diet to a standard enteral formula in a group of 98 randomized patients with major torso trauma.[159] After 7 days of feeding, the group on the immunomodulatory diet had significantly greater increases in lymphocyte count and significantly fewer intraabdominal abscesses (0% versus 11% for control, $p = .02$). Kemen et al. compared the effect of postoperative enteral support with Impact to a control enteral diet in a series of 77 randomized surgical patients.[160] Infectious complications were reduced by 33% with Impact compared to standard enteral support, if the immunomodulatory diet was administered over 5 days. In another randomized prospective study of surgical patients, Daly et al. showed that patients fed Impact had an infection and wound complication rate of only 10% compared to 43% in patients receiving a standard enteral formula. In addition, hospital stay was reduced from 22 to 16 days in the Impact-fed group ($p = .05$).[161]

Future Applications and Trends in Nutritional Research in Transplantation

One of the greatest challenges facing transplantation science today is the discovery of new treatments that can achieve lasting organ survival without the risks inherent to general immunosuppression. The induction of donor-specific tolerance in the transplant recipient is a strategy that may soon provide a viable solution to this complex issue. Among the benefits of tolerance induction are donor-specific hyporesponsiveness, which allows otherwise normal immune function; a short treatment interval, eliminating the requirement for lifelong therapy; significant potential cost savings over present multidrug regimens; and improved use of scarce donor organs.

Transplantation scientists have noticed the potential of certain dietary supplements to profoundly influence immune regulation as well as organ-specific function. Some discoveries about the immunoreactive effects of specific fatty acids and amino acids (described previously) have led to the formulation of immunostimulatory diets, which have helped to ameliorate the immunocompromised state associated with sepsis, burn injury, or tumor burden.[123, 158, 162] Such diets have led to accelerated wound healing, decreased infection, and enhanced survival. At first glance, however, the use of such diets in the immunocompromised state associated with transplant recipients appears paradoxical. On one hand, it may relieve many potential complications, yet it could simultaneously risk reducing the effectiveness of immunosuppressive therapy, leading to allograft dysfunction or even accelerated rejection. Given this dilemma, the future application of such diets in allograft recipients could be problematic. Some evidence suggests that at least one method of immunosuppression could benefit from nutritional immunomodulation without loss of efficacy and may point toward the future role of diet as an adjunctive therapy for prolonging allograft survival.

Donor-specific blood transfusion (DST) with concurrent cyclosporine has been studied extensively since the discovery of this combination in 1982.[163] The versatility of DST with cyclosporine is suggested by its demonstrated effectiveness in a number of experimental transplant models. It continues to be used clinically at a number of institutions. Although the mechanism of this synergistic interaction has yet to be fully defined, it seems to require an intact immune system to generate an active immune response necessary for the production of donor-specific elements to sustain allografts.[164] Because this response is thought to be active rather than passive, it is hypothesized that dietary immunostimulation could improve the effectiveness of such a reaction, leading to enhanced allograft survival. Furthermore, its long-term use might reduce some of the significant risks associated with impaired nonspecific cellular immunosuppression, including surveillance against opportunistic infections and tumors.

To better define the potential of dietary immunomodulation in transplantation, Levy et al. examined whether allograft survival could be improved by the immunostimulatory diet of Impact in combination with DST and cyclosporine in a complete major histocompatibility complex (MHC)-mismatched rat heterotopic cardiac transplant model.[165] They found that control animals receiving a heart transplant without additional immunosuppressive treatment rejected briskly at 7.0 ± 0 days. Transplanted animals treated with a single DST and a 15-day course of cyclosporine, after which they received no supplemental immunosuppression, rejected at a mean of 72 ± 12 days. When animals had a diet of Impact substituted for standard rodent chow on the day before transplantation, mean survival was dramatically increased to 275 ± 53 days, with five of eight animals demonstrating functioning allograft beyond 300 days (Table 15-8).

Prior investigators from our own and other institutions have contended that the mechanism of DST-cyclosporine treatment is not merely a passive response but is generated by proliferation of suppressive elements, leading to an active reduction of alloreactive cells. Assuming such a mechanism, it may be that the addition of the immunostimulatory agents arginine, omega-3 fatty acids, and RNA catalyzes this dynamic reaction, leading to the substantial survival enhancement. Based partially on these findings, we have used Impact in several transplant recipients whose course was complicated by infection and have found it safe and effective for nutritional support.

Our laboratory study is the first report of synergy between a complete enteral immunomodulatory diet and an immunosuppressive therapy for the treatment of allografts. The mechanisms of this combi-

Table 15-8. Summary of Rat Cardiac Allograft Survival among Animals Treated with Impact versus Standard Enteral Laboratory Diet[a]

Group	Survival (Days)	Mean ± SEM	$p \leq .05$ Compared to Group No.
1. Untreated/standard diet	7, 7, 7, 7, 7, 7, 7, 8	7.0 ± 0.0	2, 3, 4, 5, 6
2. Untreated/Impact diet	7, 7, 7, 8, 9, 17, 19, 19, 22	12.8 ± 2.1	1, 3, 4, 5, 6
3. CsA/standard diet	9, 18, 18, 20, 32, 40, 44, 45, 47	30.3 ± 4.8	1, 2, 5, 6
4. CsA/Impact diet	15, 18, 18, 19, 25, 52, 115	33.0 ± 9.5	1, 2, 5, 6
5. DST/CsA/standard diet	47, 61, 66, 69, 71, 92, 99	72.1 ± 6.8	1, 2, 3, 4, 6
6. DST/CsA/Impact diet	40, 84, 179, 335, 389[b] × 3, 395	275 ± 53	1, 2, 3, 4, 5

DST = donor-specific blood transfusion at day 1; CsA = cyclosporine A, 10 mg/kg 24 hours preoperation; 2.5 mg/kg per day from day of operation to postoperation day 13.
[a]Impact (Sandoz Nutrition, Minneapolis, MN) diet begun at day 1 until rejection or death.
[b]Living animals.

nation therapy are speculative, and it is unknown whether other immunosuppressive regimens may be augmented by enteral immunomodulation. Future refinement of this diet may ultimately pave the way for an adjunctive therapy that generates consistent donor-specific tolerance without the risks of permanent systemic immunosuppression. Some studies have shown that arginine, fish oil, and oils high in omega-9 fatty acids independently prolong allograft survival when given with a short course of low-dose cyclosporine.[166, 167]

One study supports the efficacy of fish oil supplementation in allograft protection. Homan van der Heide et al. administered 6 g of fish oil daily to a cohort of renal transplant recipients for the first 3 months after transplant.[134] They demonstrated that fish oil supplementation to renal allograft recipients decreased the cumulative number of rejection episodes by 60% and improved 1-year graft survival from 87% to 96% compared to a population of coconut oil–treated renal transplant controls. GFR and renal plasma flow also improved. Thus, although the clinical application of immunomodulatory diets to transplantation is still in its infancy, this study highlights its potential.

Conclusions

For the majority of liver, renal, cardiac, and small bowel transplant recipients, the preoperative period is often complicated by malnutrition, which is a challenge to monitor and treat due to these patients' limited reserve. Given the difficulty in predicting the availability of a particular organ, pretransplant nutritional therapy most frequently relies on outpatient treatment and must not delay organ replacement. Such therapy most often consists of nutritional counseling and education during recurrent visits before transplantation.

The immediate posttransplant period is strongly influenced by high-dose, triple-drug immunosuppression, the impact of which is shown in many facets of a patient's metabolism. This includes a propensity for high rates of protein catabolism and frequent episodes of blood glucose dysregulation. Given the limited reserves of these patients, several days of little or no nutritional supplementation can put them further into nutritional debt and may translate into weeks of nutritional recovery and more complications. Definitive evidence is sparse, but several clinical studies suggest that initiation of nutritional supplementation, preferably enteral, as early as medically possible may help to prevent postoperative complications.

New discoveries in the field of nutritional pharmacology are rapidly transforming the subordinate role of nutritional management in the transplant patient. Only recently have compounds such as arginine, glutamine, and omega-3 fatty acids been appreciated for their far-ranging immunologic effects. Their dietary supplementation has demonstrated clinical usefulness. As this field continues to advance, the traditional role of nutritional management may soon include a provision for dietary immunomodulation that eventually may augment or even displace more conventional, long-term, drug-based immunosuppressive strategies.

References

1. Breasted J. The Edwin Smith Papyrus. Chicago: University of Chicago Press, 1984.

2. Studley HO. Percentage of weight loss: a basic indicator of surgical risk in patients with chronic peptic ulcer. JAMA 1936;106:458–460.

3. Rhoads JE, Fliegelman MT, Penzer LM. The mechanism of delayed wound healing in the presence of hypoproteinemia. Ann N Y Acad Sci 1955;63:268.

4. United Network for Organ Sharing. Transplant Registry, 1994.

5. Shanbhogue RLK, Chwals WJ, Weintraub M, et al. Parenteral nutrition in the surgical patient. Br J Surg 1987;74:172–180.

6. Metropolitan Life Foundation. Statistical Bulletin 1983;64:2–9.

7. Blackburn GL, Bistran BR, Maini BS, et al. Nutritional and metabolic assessment of the hospitalized patient. JPEN J Parenter Enteral Nutr 1977;1:11–22.

8. Keys A, Brozek J, Henshel A, et al. The Biology of Human Starvation. Minneapolis: University of Minnesota Press, 1950.

9. Hill GL. Nutritional assessment. In JF Fischer (ed). Total Parenteral Nutrition. Boston: Little, Brown, 1993; 139–152.

10. Darwin J, Womersley J. Body fat assessed from total body density and its estimation from skinfold thickness: measurements in 481 men and women aged 16 to 72 years. Br J Nutrition 1974;37:77.

11. Collins J, McCarty I, Hill G. Assessment of protein nutrition in surgical patients: the value of anthropometrics. Am J Clin Nutr 1979;32:1527.

12. Jeejeebhoy KN. Bulk or bounce: the object of nutritional support. JPEN J Parenter Enteral Nutr 1988; 12:539–549.

13. Bozzetti F, Migliavacca S, Gallus G, et al. "Nutritional" markers as prognostic indicators of postoperative sepsis in cancer patients. JPEN J Parenter Enteral Nutr 1985;9:464.

14. Shizgal HM, Spanier AH, Kurtz RS. Effect of parenteral nutrition on body composition in the critically ill patient. Am J Surg 1976;131:156.

15. Tellado-Dodriguez JM, Garcia-Sabrido JL, Shizgal HM, et al. NA_e/K_e ratio is a better index of nutritional status than standard anthropomorphic and biochemical indices. Surg Forum 1987;38:56.

16. Hill GL, Beddoe AH. In vivo neutron activation in metabolic and nutritional indices. J Clin Surg 1982;1:270.

17. Daly J. Malnutrition. In DW Wilmore, MF Brennen, AH Harken, et al. (eds), Care of the Surgical Patient. New York: Scientific America, 1988.

18. Hickman DM, Miller RA, Rombeau JL, et al. Serum albumin and body weight as predictors of postoperative course in colorectal cancer. JPEN J Parenter Enteral Nutr 1980;4:314.

19. Fletcher JP, Little JM, Guest PK. A comparison of serum transferrin and serum prealbumin as nutritional parameters. JPEN J Parenter Enteral Nutr 1987;11:144.

20. Rosa AM, Tuitt D, Shizgal HM. Transferrin: a poor measure of nutritional status. JPEN J Parenter Enteral Nutr 1984;8:523.

21. Church JM, Hill GL. Assessing the efficacy of intravenous nutrition in general surgical patients: dynamic nutritional assessment with plasma proteins. JPEN J Parenter Enteral Nutr 1987;11:135–139.

22. Seltzer MH, Bastidas JA, Cooper DM, et al. Instant nutritional assessment. JPEN J Parenter Enteral Nutr 1979;3:157.

23. Twomey P, Zeigler D, Rombeau J. Utility of skin testing in nutritional assessment: a critical review. JPEN J Parenter Enteral Nutr 1982;6:50.

24. Forse RA, Christou N, Meakins JL, et al. Reliability of skin testing as a measure of nutritional status. Arch Surg 1981;116:1284.

25. Pettigrew RA, Hill GL. Indicators of surgical risk and clinical judgment: a prospective comparative study. Br J Surg 1986;73:47.

26. Windsor JA, Hill GL. Weight loss with physiologic impairment: a basic indicator of surgical risk. Ann Surg 1988;207:290.

27. Compher C. Nutrition assessment in chronic renal failure. Nutr Supp Serv 1985;6:18–25.

28. Blumenkranz MJ, Gahl GM, Kopple JD, et al. Protein losses during peritoneal dialysis. Kidney Int 1981;19: 593–602.

29. Schoenfeld PY, Henry RR, Laird NM, et al. Assessment of nutritional status of the National Cooperative Dialysis Study population. Kidney Int 1983;23:S80–S88.

30. Moore L, Acchiardo S. Aggressive nutritional supplementation in chronic hemodialysis patients. Consult Renal Nutr Q 1987;11:14.

31. Manske CL. Lipid abnormalities and renal disease. Kidney 1988;20:25.

32. Abel RM. Nutritional support and the cardiac patient. In MD Caldwell (ed), Clinical Nutrition. Philadelphia: Saunders, 1986.

33. Pittman JG, Cohen P. The pathogenesis of cardiac cachexia. N Engl J Med 1964;271:403.

34. Porayko MK, Dicecco S, O'Keefe SJ. Impact of malnutrition and its therapy on liver transplantation. Semin Liver Dis 1991;4:305–314.

35. Silk DB. Parenteral nutrition in liver disease. J Hepatol 1988;7:277.

36. Madill J, Maurer JR, de Hoyos A. A comparison of preoperative and postoperative nutritional states of lung transplant recipients. Transplantation 1993;56:347–350.

37. Hehir DJ, Jenkins RL, Bistran BR. Nutrition in patients undergoing orthotopic liver transplantation. JPEN J Parenter Enteral Nutr 1985;9:695.

38. Dicecco SR, Wieners FI, Weisner RH, et al. Assessment of nutritional status of patients with endstage liver disease undergoing liver transplantation. Mayo Clin Proc 1989;64:89.

39. Hasse JM. Nutritional considerations in liver transplantation. Top Clin Nutr 1992;7:24.

40. Shronts EP, Teasley KM, Thoele SL, et al. Nutritional support in the adult liver transplant candidate. J Am Diet Assoc 1987;87:441.

41. Buzby G, Mullen J, Mathews P, et al. Prognostic nutritional index in gastrointestinal surgery. Am J Surg 1980;139:160–166.

42. Baker JP, Detsky AS, Wesson DE, et al. Nutritional assessment: a comparison of clinical judgment and objective parameters. N Engl J Med 1982;306:969.

43. Detsky AS, McLaughlin JR, Baker JP. JPEN J Parenter Enteral Nutr 1987;11:8–13.

44. Hasse J, Strong S, Gorman M, et al. Subjective global assessment: alternative nutrition-assessment technique for liver-transplant candidates. Nutrition 1993;9:339–343.

45. Enia G, Sicuso C, Alati G, et al. Subjective global nutritional assessment of nutrition in dialysis patients. Nephrol Dial Transplant 1993;8:1094–1098.

46. Wilmore DW, Long JM, Mason AD, et al. Catecholamine mediator of the hypermetabolic response to thermal injury. Ann Surg 1974;180:653.

47. Wilmore DW. Metabolic Management of the Critically Ill. New York: Plenum, 1977.

48. Wilmore DW, Aulick LH, Mason AD, et al. Influence of the burn wound on local and systemic responses to injury. Ann Surg 1977;186:444.

49. Aulick LH, Wilmore DW, Mason AD, et al. Muscle blood flow following thermal injury. Ann Surg 1978;188:778.

50. Aulick LH, Goodwin CW, Becker RA, et al. Visceral blood flow following thermal injury. Ann Surg 1981;193:112.

51. Breder CD, Dinardello CA, Saper CB. Interleukin-1 immunoreactive innervation of the human hypothalamus. Science 1988;240:321.

52. Cuthberson DP. The disturbance of metabolism produced by bony and non-bony injury, with notes on certain abnormal conditions of bone. Biochem J 1930;24:1244.

53. Threlfall CJ, Stoner HB, Glasko CB. Patterns in the excretion of muscle markers after trauma and orthopedic surgery. J Trauma 1981;21:140.

54. Young VR, Munro HN. Ntau-methylhistidine (3-methylhistidine) and muscle protein turnover: an overview. Fed Proc 1978;37:2291.

55. Garber AJ, Karl IE, Kipnis DM. Alanine and glutamine synthesis and release from skeletal muscle. J Biol Chem 1976;251:826.

56. Wolfe RR, O'Donnell TF, Stone MD, et al. Investigation of factors determining optimal glucose infusion rate in total parenteral nutrition. Ann Surg 1980;190:274.

57. Long JM, Wilmore DW, Mason, et al. Effect of carbohydrates and fat intake on nitrogen excretion during total intravenous feeding. Ann Surg 1977;185:417.

58. Wolfe RR, Herndon DN, Jahoor F, et al. Effect of severe burn injury on substrate cycling by glucose and fatty acids. N Engl J Med 1987;317:403.

59. Schumann D. Postoperative hyperglycemia: clinical benefits of insulin therapy. Heart Lung 1990;19:165–173.

60. Braga M, Castoldi R, Cristallo M, et al. Catabolic response and parenteral nutrition after simultaneous kidney-pancreas transplantation. Nutrition 1992;8:232–236.

61. Hay WE, Sargent JA, Freeman RB, et al. A computer-aided prospective study of protein catabolic rate and nitrogen balance after renal transplantation. Kidney Int 1984;25:343.

62. O'Keefe SJ, Williams R, Calne RY. Catabolic loss of body protein after human liver transplantation. BMJ 1980:1107–1108.

63. Manger P, Homan van der Heide J, Leendert CP. Are dietary interventions justified for recipients of organ transplants? In L Paul, K Solez (eds), Organ Transplantation. New York: Marcel Dekker, 1992.

64. Gunnarsson R, Lungrin G, Magnusson G, et al. Steroid diabetes: a sign of overtreatment with steroids in renal graft recipients? Scand J Urol Nephrol 1980;54:135.

65. Ruiz JO, Simmons RL, Callender CO, et al. Steroid diabetes in renal transplant recipients: pathogenic factors and prognosis. Surgery 1973;73:759.

66. Hill CM, Douglas JF, Rajkumar KV, et al. Glycosuria and hyperglycemia after kidney transplantation. Lancet 1974;2:490.

67. Yale JF, Chameluan M, Courchesnes S, et al. Peripheral insulin resistance and decreased serum insulin secretion after cyclosporine treatment. Transplant Proc 1988;20:985–988.

68. Laskow DA, Curtis JJ, Luke RG, et al. Cyclosporine-induced changes in glomerular filtration rate and urea excretion. Am J Med 1990;888:497–501.

69. Kamel K, Quaggins S, Ethier J, et al. Post-transplant hyperkalemia in patients on cyclosporine A. Kidney Int 1990;37:266.

70. June CH, Thompson CB, Kennedy MS, et al. Profound hypomagnesemia and renal magnesium wasting associated with the use of cyclosporine for marrow transplantation. Transplantation 1985;39:621–625.

71. Ghosh P, Evans D, Tomilson A, et al. Plasma lipids following renal transplantation. Transplantation 1973;15:521–523.

72. Perez R. Managing nutrition problems in transplant patients. Nutrition Clin Prac 1993;8:28–32.

73. ASPEN Board of Directors. Guidelines for the use of parenteral and enteral nutrition in adult and pediatric patients. JPEN J Parenter Enteral Nutr 1993;17:S1–S52.

74. ASPEN Board of Directors. Guidelines for the use of enteral nutrition in adult patients. JPEN J Parenter Enteral Nutr 1987;11:435–439.

75. Herberer M, Bodaky A, Iwatsohenko P, et al. Indications for needle catheter jejunostomy in elective abdominal surgery. Am J Surg 1987;153:545–552.

76. Meguid MM, Meguid D. Preoperative identification of the surgical cancer patient in need of postoperative supportive total parenteral nutrition. Cancer 1985;55:258–262.

77. Boyes RJ, Kruse JA. Nasogastric and nasoenteric intubation. Crit Care Med 1992;8:865–878.

78. Rao DR, Bello H, Warren AP, et al. Prevalence of lactase maldigestion: influence and interaction of age race and sex. Dig Dis Sci 1994;39:1519–1524.

79. Sarwer G, Pease RW. The protein quality of some enteral products is inferior to that of casein as assessed by rat growth methods and digestibility-corrected amino acid scores. J Nutrition 1994;124:2223–2232.

80. Silk DB, Kumar PJ, Perrett D, et al. Amino acid and peptide absorption in patients with coeliac disease and dermatitis herpetiformis. Gut 1984;15:1–8.

81. Cataldi-Betcher EL, Seltzer MH, Slocum BA, et al. Complications occurring during enteral nutritional support: a prospective study. JPEN J Parenter Enteral Nutr 1983;7:546–552.

82. Taraszewski R, Jensen GL. N-6 Fatty Acids. In S Bell, G Blackburn, G Kabbash (eds), Diet, Nutrition and Immunity. Boca Raton, FL: CRC Press, 1994;165–177.

83. Barber DA, Harris SR. Oxygen free radicals and antioxidants: a review. Am Pharm 1994;24:26–35.

84. Payne-James JJ, Khawaja HT. First choice for total parenteral nutrition: the peripheral route. JPEN J Parenter Enteral Nutr 1993;17:468–478.

85. Benya R, Langer S, Mobarhan S. Flexible nasogastric feeding tube tip malposition immediately after placement. JPEN J Parenter Enteral Nutr 1990;14:104–109.

86. Mancuard RP, Perkins AM. Clogging of feeding tubes. JPEN J Parenter Enteral Nutr 1988;12:403–405.

87. Driks MR, Craven DE, Celli BR, et al. Nosocomial pneumonia in intubated patients given sucralfate as compared with antacids or histamine type-2 blockers. N Engl J Med 1987;317:1376–1382.

88. Strong RM, Condon SC, Solinger MR, et al. Equal aspiration rates from postpylorus and intragastric-placed small-bore nasoenteric feeding tubes: a randomized prospective study. JPEN J Parenter Enteral Nutr 1992;16:59–62.

89. Montecalvo MA, Steger KA, Farber HW, et al. Nutritional outcome and pneumonias in critical care patients randomized to gastric versus jejunal tube feedings. Crit Care Med 1992;20:1377–1386.

90. Ibanez C, Penafiel A, Raurich JM. Gastroesophageal reflux in intubated patients receiving enteral nutrition: effect of supine and semirecumbent positions. JPEN J Parenter Enteral Nutr 1992;16:419–422.

91. Heyland D, Bradley C, Mandell LA. Effect of acidified enteral feedings on gastric colonization in the critically ill patient. Crit Care Med 1992;20:1388–1393.

92. Rolfe RD, Holebrain S, Finegold SM. Bacterial interference. Difficile and normal fecal flora. J Infect Dis 1981;143:470.

93. Keohane PP, Altrill H, Love M, et al. Relation between osmolarity of diet and gastrointestinal side effects in enteral nutrition. BMJ 1984;283:678.

94. Edes TE, Walk BE, Austin JL. Diarrhea in tube-fed patients: feeding formula not necessarily the cause. Am J Med 1990;83:91–93.

95. Ryan JA, Abel RM, Abbott WM, et al. Catheter complications in total parenteral nutrition: a prospective study of 200 consecutive patients. N Engl J Med 1974;290:757.

96. Wolfe BM, Ryder MA, Nishikawa RA, et al. Complications of parenteral nutrition. Am J Surg 1986;152:93.

97. Goldman DA, Maki DG. Infection control in total parenteral nutrition. JAMA 1973;223:1360.

98. Pemperton LB, Lyman B, Lander V, et al. Sepsis from triple-lumen versus single-lumen catheters during total parenteral nutrition in surgical or critically ill patients. Arch Surg 1986;121:591.

99. Sitzmann JV, Townsend TR, Siler MC, et al. Septic and technical complications of central venous catheterization: a prospective study of 200 consecutive patients. Ann Surg 1985;202:766.

100. Collins FD, Sinclair AJ, Royale JP, et al. Plasma lipids in linolenic acid deficiency. Nutr Metab 1971;13:150.

101. Jeejeebhoy KN, Chu RC, Marliss EB, et al. Chromium deficiency, glucose intolerance, and neuropathy reversed by chromium supplementation in a patient receiving long-term parenteral nutrition. Am J Clin Nutr 1977;30:531.

102. Klein S, Nealon WH. Hepatobiliary abnormalities associated with total parenteral nutrition. Semin Liver Dis 1988;8:237.

103. Preshaw RM, Attisha RR, Hollingsworth WJ, et al. Randomized sequential trial of parenteral nutrition in healing of colonic anastomosis in man. Can J Surg 1979;22:437–439.

104. Collins JP, Oxby CB, Hill GL. Intravenous amino acids and intravenous hyperalimentation as protein sparing therapy after major surgery: a controlled clinical trial. Lancet 1978:788–791.

105. Yamada N, Koyama H, Hioki K, et al. Effect of post-operative total parenteral nutrition (TPN) as an adjunct to gastrectomy for advanced gastric carcinoma. Br J Surg 1983;70:267.

106. Hoover AC, Ryan JA, Anderson EJ, et al. The nutritional benefits of immediate post-operative feeding of an elemental diet. Am J Surg 1980;139:153–159.

107. Sagar S, Harland P, Shields R. Early post-operative feeding with elemental diet. BMJ 1979;1:293–295.

108. Kudsk KA, Minard G, Wojtysiak SL, et al. Visceral protein response to enteral versus parenteral nutrition and sepsis in patients with trauma. Surgery 1994;116:516–523.

109. Moore FA, Feliciano DV, Andrassy RJ, et al. Early enteral feeding, compared with parenteral, reduces postoperative septic complications. The results of a meta-analysis. Ann Surg 1992;216:172–183.

110. Mochizuki H, Trocki O, Dominioni L, et al. Mechanism of prevention of postburn hypermetabolism and catabolism by early enteral feeding. Ann Surg 1984; 200:297–310.

111. Reilly J, Mehta R, Teperman L, et al. Nutritional support after liver transplantation: a randomized study. JPEN J Parenter Enteral Nutr 1990;14:384–391.

112. Whittier FC, Evans DH, Dultton S, et al. Nutrition in

renal transplantation. Am J Kidney Dis 1985;6: 405–411.

113. Holcombe BJ, Resler R. Nutrition support for lung transplant patients. Nutr Clin Prac 1994;9:235–239.

114. Grimes TB, Abel RM. Acute hemodynamic effects of intravenous fat emulsions in dogs. JPEN J Parenter Enteral Nutr 1979;3:40–44.

115. Abel RM, Fisch D, Grossman ML. Hemodynamic effects of intravenous 20% soy oil emulsion following coronary artery bypass. JPEN J Parenter Enteral Nutr 1983;7:534–540.

116. Reyes J, Tzakis AG, Todo S, et al. Small bowel and liver/small bowel transplantation in children. Semin Pediatr Surg 1993;2:289–300.

117. Konstantinides FN, Konstantinides NN, Li JC, et al. Urinary urea nitrogen: too insensitive for calculating nitrogen balance studies. JPEN J Parenter Enteral Nutr 1991;15:189–193.

118. Loder PB, Kee AJ, Horsburgh R, et al. Validity of urine urea nitrogen as a measure of total urinary nitrogen in adult patients requiring parenteral nutrition. Crit Care Med 1989;17:309–312.

119. Daly JM, Reynolds J, Sigal RK, et al. Effect of dietary protein and amino acids on immune function. Crit Care Med 1990;18:586–593.

120. Seifer E, Rettura G, Barbul A, et al. Arginine: an essential amino acid for injured rats. Surgery 1978;84(2):224–230.

121. Barbul A. Arginine and immune function. Nutrition 1990;6:53.

122. Saito H, Trocki O, Wang SL, et al. Metabolic and immune effects of dietary arginine supplementation after burn. Arch Surg 1987;122:784–789.

123. Rettura G, Padawer J, Barbul A, et al. Supplemental arginine increases thymic cellularity in normal and murine sarcoma virus-inoculated mice and increases the resistance to murine sarcoma virus. JPEN J Parenter Enteral Nutr 1979;3:409.

124. Hacker-Shahin B, Drogee W. Putrescine and its biosynthetic precursor L-ornithine augment the in vivo immunization against minor histocompatibility antigens and syngeneic tumor cells. Cell Immunol 1986;20:434.

125. Gianotti L, Alexander JW, Pyles T, et al. Arginine-supplemented dirt improves survival in gut-derived sepsis and peritonitis by modulating bacterial clearance. The role of nitric oxide. Ann Surg 1993;217:644–653.

126. Wolochow H, Hildebrand GJ, Lamanna C. Translocation of microorganisms across the intestinal wall of the rat. J Infect Dis 1966;116:523–528.

127. Windmueller HG. Glutamine utilization by the small intestine. Adv Enzymol Relat Areas Mol Biol 1982; 53:201.

128. Burke DJ, Alverdy JC, Aoys E, et al. Glutamine-supplemented total parenteral nutrition improves gut immune function. Arch Surg 1989;124:1396.

129. Fox AD, Kripke SA, Del'aula JA, et al. The effect of glutamine-supplemented enteral diet on methotrexate induced enterocolitis. JPEN J Parenter Enteral Nutr 1988;12:325.

130. Farias R, Nioji B, Moreno R, et al. Regulation of allosteric membrane bound enzymes through changes in membrane fluidity. Biochem Biophys Acta 1975;415:231.

131. Chavali SR, Forse RA. The Role of N-3 Polyunsaturated Fatty Acids in Immune Response during Infection and Inflammation. In S Bell, G Blackburn, G Kabbash (eds), Diet, Nutrition and Immunity. Boca Raton, FL: CRC Press, 1994.

132. Endres S, Ghorbani R, Kelly VE, et al. The effect of dietary supplementation with n-3 polyunsaturated fatty acids on the synthesis of interleukin-1 and tumor necrosis factor by mononuclear cells. N Engl J Med 1989;320:265.

133. Shimamura T, Wilson A. Influence of dietary fish oil on aortic, myocardial, and renal lesions of SHR. J Nutr Sci Vitaminol (Tokyo) 1991;37:581–590.

134. Homan van der Heide JJ, Bilo HJG, Tegzess AM, et al. The effects of dietary supplementation with fish oil on renal function in cyclosporine-treated renal transplant recipients. Transplantation 1990;49:523–527.

135. Goodnight S, Harris W, Connor W. The effect of dietary omega-3 fatty acids on platelet composition and function in man. Blood 1981;58:880.

136. Sarris G, Mitchell S, Billingham M, et al. Inhibition of accelerated cardiac graft arteriosclerosis by fish oil. J Cardiovasc Surg 1989;97:841–855.

137. Perez RV, Munda R, Alexander LW. Dietary immunoregulation of transfusion-induced immunosuppression. Transplantation 1988;45:614–617.

138. Roediger WE. Utilization of nutrients by isolated epithelial cells of the rat colon. Gastroenterology 1982;83:424.

139. Soergel KH. Absorption of Fermentation Products from the Colon. In W Kasper, H Goebel (eds), Colon and Nutrition: Proceedings of the 32nd Falk Symposium held during intestinal week, Titisee, May 29–31,1981. Lancaster, UK: MTP Press, 1982;27.

140. Ruppin H, Bar-Meir S, Soergel KH, et al. Absorption of Short Chain Fatty Acids by the Colon. Lancaster, UK: MTP Press, 1980;78:1500.

141. Elsen RJ, Bistrian BR. Recent developments in short chain fatty acid metabolism. Nutrition 1991;7:7–10.

142. Rolandelli RH, Saul SH, Settle RG, et al. Comparison of parenteral nutrition and enteral feeding with pectin in experimental colitis in the rat. Am J Clin Nutr 1988; 47:715.

143. Van Buren CT, Kullarni AD, Schandle, et al. The influence of dietary nucleotides on cell mediated immunity. Transplantation 1983;36:350.

144. Van Buren CT, Kim E, Kullarni AD, et al. Nucleotide-free diet and suppression of the immune response. Transplant Proc 1987;4(Suppl 5):57.

145. Van Buren CT, Kullarni AD, Rudolph F. Synergistic effect of nucleotide-free diet and cyclosporine on allograft survival. Transplant Proc 1983;12:296–297.

146. Rudolph FB, Kulkarni AD, Fandslow WC. Role of RNA as a dietary source of pyrimidines and urines in immune function. Nutrition 1990;6:45–52.

147. Meydani SN, Meydani M, Verdon CP, et al. Vitamin E

supplementation suppresses prostaglandin E_2 synthesis and enhances the immune response of aged mice. Mech Ageing Dev 1986;34:191.

148. Fang CH, Peck MD, Alexander JW, et al. The effect of free radical scavengers on outcome after infection in burned mice. J Trauma 1990;30:453–456.

149. Neve J, Vertongen F, Molle L. Selenium deficiency. Clin Endocrin Metab 1985;14:629.

150. Clark LC. The epidemiology of selenium and cancer. Fed Proc 1985;44:2584.

151. Alexander JW, Gottschlich MM. Nutritional immunomodulation in burn patients. J Crit Care Med 1989;18:S149.

152. Daly JM, Reynolds JV, Thom A, et al. Immune and metabolic effects of arginine in the surgical patient. Ann Surg 1988;208:512.

153. Chandra R, Baker M, Whang S, et al. Effects of two feeding formulas on immune responsiveness and mortality in mice challenged with *Listeria monocytogenes*. Immunol Lett 1991;27:45–48.

154. Kulkarni A, Kumar S, Pizzini R, et al. Influence of dietary glutamine and impact on in vivo cell-mediated immune response in mice. Nutrition 1990;6:66–69.

155. Leiberman M, Shou J, Torres A, et al. Effect of nutrient substrates on immune function. Nutrition 1990;6:88–91.

156. Katz D, Kvetan V, Askanazi J. Enteral nutrition: potential role in regulating immune function. Curr Opin Gastroenterol 1990;6:199–203.

157. Bower RH, Lavin PT, LiCari JJ, et al. A modified enteral formula reduces hospital length of stay in patients in intensive care units. Crit Care Med 1993;42:219.

158. Daly JM, Lieberman MD, Goldfine J, et al. Enteral nutrition with supplemental arginine, RNA, and omega-3 fatty acids in patients after operation: immunologic, metabolic, and clinical outcome. Surgery 1992;112:56–67.

159. Moore FA, Moore EE, Kudsk KA, et al. Clinical benefits of an immune-enhancing diet for early postinjury enteral feeding. J Trauma 1994;37:607.

160. Senkel M, Mumme A, Eickhoff U, et al. Early postoperative enteral immunonutrition: clinical outcome and cost-comparison analysis in surgical patients. Crit Care Med 1997;25:1489–1496.

161. Daly JM, Weintraub FN, Shou J, et al. Enteral nutrition during multimodality therapy in upper gastrointestinal cancer patients. Ann Surg 1995;221:327–338.

162. Gottschlich M, Jenkins M, Warden G, et al. Differential effects of three enteral dietary regimes on selected variables in burn patients. JPEN J Parenter Enteral Nutr 1990;14:225–236.

163. Miller C, Martinelli G, Racelis D, et al. Prolongation of rat cardiac allografts by pretransplant administration of blood transfusions and cyclosporine A. Transplantation 1982;33:335–337.

164. Levy A, Alexander JW. The significance of timing of additional short-term immunosuppression in the donor-specific transfusion/cyclosporine treated rat. Transplantation 1996;62:262–266.

165. Levy A, Alexander JW. Nutritional immunomodulation enhances cardiac allograft survival in rats treated with donor specific transfusion and cyclosporine. Transplantation 1995;60:812–815.

166. Alexander JW, Valente JF, Greenberg NA, et al. Dietary amino acids as new and novel agents to enhance allograft survival. (Submitted).

167. Alexander JW, Valente JF, Greenberg NA, et al. Dietary ω-3 and ω-9 fatty acids uniquely enhance allograft. Survival in cyclosporine-treated and donor-specific transfusion-treated rats. Transplantation 1998;65:1304–1309.

Chapter 16

Hematologic Considerations in the Transplant Patient

Yoogoo Kang and Thomas A. Gaisor

Chapter Plan

Organ transplantation is frequently complicated by hemostatic and hematopoietic defects resulting from systemic effects of end-stage organ disease, surgical bleeding, donor organs with hypothermia, ischemic preservation, and grafted organs recovering from ischemia and reperfusion injury. In this chapter, pathophysiology and perioperative management of coagulation and the erythropoietic system of patients undergoing organ transplantation are described.

Heart and Lung Transplantation

Preoperative Considerations

The frequency and severity of perioperative bleeding during heart, combined heart and lung, or isolated lung transplantation depend on a combination of the following factors: (1) type of intrathoracic transplantation, (2) underlying disease state, (3) requirement for cardiopulmonary bypass, (4) preoperative medications, (5) preoperative hepatic and renal function, and (6) previous intrathoracic surgery.

Heart Transplantation

Patients undergoing heart transplantation with end-stage heart failure typically have cardiac dilation.[1] Thus, they are prone to formation of mural thrombi and potential embolization, especially with atrial fibrillation. These patients often receive either heparin or warfarin therapy. Chronic preoperative heparin administration can produce a relative antithrombin III (AT-III) deficiency with subsequent difficulty in maintaining an adequate activated clotting time (ACT) during cardiopulmonary bypass. Additional heparin, fresh frozen plasma (FFP), or AT-III concentrate may be indicated to prevent activation of coagulation and thrombin formation[2] with possible increased postoperative bleeding.[3] Chronic heparin therapy can also produce thrombocytopenia and platelet dysfunction.[4, 5] Chronic warfarin therapy may require the administration of FFP and vitamin K for reversal of its effects but does not appear to increase perioperative bleeding or the incidence of complications during heart transplantation.[3] Although hepatic cirrhosis is typically a contraindication to heart transplantation, right atrial hypertension can cause passive hepatic congestion, leading to diminished hepatic synthetic function and decreased coagulant levels. Coagulopathy associated with hepatic dysfunction, demonstrated by an elevation of the prothrombin time (PT), may exacerbate the effects of cardiopulmonary bypass and concomitant warfarin therapy.

Heart and Lung Transplantation

Patients with complex congenital heart disease and Eisenmenger's syndrome and those with primary pulmonary hypertension with right heart failure typically require combined heart and lung transplantation. Intra- and postoperative bleeding during combined heart and lung transplantation complicates the perioperative course. In the early series, it was a major cause of early postoperative morbidity and mortality.[6-8] The scenario of extensive perioperative bleeding, multiple blood product transfusion, compromised function of the transplanted lung, development of multiorgan failure, and ultimate death was a common one.[9] Bleeding accounted for 36% of intraoperative deaths and for 8% of total deaths in one series.[10] Postoperative blood loss greater than 2 liters was a significant prognostic indicator of early death in another.[11]

Bleeding during combined heart and lung transplantation is multifactorial. In these patients, who are prone to pulmonary thromboembolic events, preoperative medications might include aspirin, dipyridamole, and oral anticoagulants, such as warfarin. Because of the emergent nature of the transplantation procedure, these drugs were often ingested the day of the operation. Presently, anticoagulants are more selectively administered to patients with atrial fibrillation, ventricular thrombus, and embolic phenomena of unclear etiology. Long-standing pulmonary arterial hypertension often results in an element of right ventricular dysfunction, which causes hepatic congestion leading to diminished hepatic synthetic function, decreased coagulant levels, and prolonged PT. Because of

chronic hypoxemia there can be large posterior mediastinal and pleural collateral blood vessels. Prolonged cardiopulmonary bypass was therefore required for surgical dissection and hemostasis.

Modifications of the surgical technique used during combined heart and lung transplantation include limited dissection of the posterior mediastinum, increased surgical stapling, use of the argon beam coagulator, and use of various topical coagulants and fibrin glue. These have led to better posterior mediastinal hemostasis as well as a significant reduction in bleeding and subsequent transfusion requirements.[12] Introduction of the bilateral thoracosternotomy or clamshell incision further facilitates exposure and takedown of adhesions.[13] With improved surgical technique and pharmacologic drugs, exsanguinating hemorrhage during combined heart and lung transplantation has become less of a problem.[14]

Lung Transplantation

Patients with septic pulmonary disease, such as cystic fibrosis or bronchiectasis, undergo bilateral sequential lung transplantations, in most cases without the need for cardiopulmonary bypass. Perioperative bleeding can be excessive in these patients; causes include vascular pleural adhesions, enlarged mediastinal lymph nodes, and cachexia and sepsis, with their effects on coagulation.[15]

Patients with either primary pulmonary hypertension or Eisenmenger's syndrome with a correctable intracardiac defect, such as an atrial septal defect or patent ductus arteriosus, can be successfully treated with a single-lung transplantation. These patients require cardiopulmonary bypass for correction of the intracardiac defect and subsequent lung transplantation. They resemble combined heart and lung transplantation candidates but typically have less severe right heart dysfunction that could contribute to a perioperative coagulopathy.

Most patients awaiting lung transplantation have chronic obstructive pulmonary disease and are likely to need only single-lung transplantation. Cardiopulmonary bypass is not necessary in the majority of these patients. Bleeding is not often an issue, but repeated chest tube insertions for pneumothorax and the introduction of thorascopic pulmonary reduction procedures for bullous disease can lead to pleural adhesions, which can result in significant bleeding. Despite multiple thoracic procedures, lung transplantation is not contraindicated.[16]

Previous thoracotomy and sternotomy were once absolute contraindications to lung transplantation due to increased bleeding and subsequent morbidity and mortality, but now lung transplantation candidates with previous intrathoracic procedures are considered on an individual basis. These patients have increased perioperative bleeding, requiring a greater number of transfused blood products, but they do not appear to have a significantly increased morbidity or mortality over patients with no previous intrathoracic procedure unless cardiopulmonary bypass is used.[17]

For these reasons, the degree of bleeding is greatest in combined heart and lung transplantation, next in single-lung transplantation and double-lung transplantation requiring cardiopulmonary bypass, and least in single-lung transplantation performed without cardiopulmonary bypass.

Preoperative Evaluation

Preoperative evaluation of patients undergoing intrathoracic transplantation is extensive and includes evaluation of right heart function; assessment of potential hepatic congestion and renal dysfunction, both of which could compromise hemostatic mechanisms[18]; and a baseline coagulation profile consisting of platelet count, PT, and activated partial thromboplastin time (aPTT). Bleeding time, thrombin time, fibrinogen, and fibrin degradation products are not routinely obtained. The use of these coagulation tests in predicting postoperative mediastinal drainage in 897 patients undergoing cardiac surgical procedures (coronary operations, valve replacement, and reoperative procedures) requiring cardiopulmonary bypass was not shown to be of any value.[19] The value of these tests in predicting perioperative hemorrhage during heart or lung transplantation remains unstudied.

In the early heart and lung transplantation experiences, the primary focus was on organ preservation, surgical technique, and perioperative management. With progress in all aspects of cardiothoracic transplantation and longer recipient waiting times, autologous predonation can be considered. Factors influencing the safety and usefulness of predonation are the patients' underlying disease and their physio-

logic dependence on intravascular volume, baseline hemoglobin levels, and the ultimate need for blood transfusion. Combined heart and lung transplantation recipients appear to be good candidates for predonation in that they are typically polycythemic, although they may require volume replacement during phlebotomy. Patients with chronic obstructive pulmonary disease as single-lung transplantation candidates typically have a slightly elevated hemoglobin level and would tolerate predonation. However, transfusion during an uncomplicated single-lung transplantation is unusual. Septic patients (i.e., those with cystic fibrosis and bronchiectasis) are often chronically anemic; predonation is inappropriate for them. Autologous predonation with frozen storage and subsequent thawing and reinfusion was reported in a heart transplant patient.[20] The feasibility of autologous predonation has been demonstrated in a small series of heart and lung transplantation candidates.[21] The cost-effectiveness, safety, and efficacy of preoperative autologous donation requires further study.[22–24]

Autologous blood can be collected in the immediate preoperative period in heart transplantation candidates who start with a normal hematocrit. The immediate preoperative collection of autologous blood is more appealing in the patients with complex congenital heart disease who are undergoing combined heart and lung or lung transplantation. Several units of blood can be collected with normovolemic hemodilution before cardiopulmonary bypass, or blood can be sequestered during cardiopulmonary bypass. In either case, the autologous blood is reinfused after heparin neutralization with protamine. The intraoperative collection of autologous blood is often not possible in the chronically anemic patient and has limited value in uncomplicated single-lung transplantations in which bleeding is not an issue.

The efficacy of autologous platelet-rich plasmapheresis during routine cardiac surgical procedures has yet to be established, likely due to the inability to obtain large platelet volumes in a timely fashion.[25, 26] Therefore, this technique is not typically used during cardiothoracic transplantation. One of the mainstays of blood conservation methods is the use of intraoperative salvage by means of a cell-saving device, with reinfusion of washed red blood cells (RBCs).

Although erythropoietin has been used safely in other cardiac patients,[27] its use in patients undergoing heart and lung transplantation has yet to be tested other than in a small series of infants awaiting heart transplantation, in whom daily erythropoietin appeared to be effective in maintaining a stable hematocrit in the face of iatrogenic blood loss.[28] The benefit of increasing the hematocrit must be weighed against the development of possible increased blood viscosity and thrombotic events in these patients with low-flow states.

The complications and risks of blood product transfusion are well known and include fluid overload, nonallergic reactions, hemolytic transfusion reactions, transmission of infectious agents (e.g., viral hepatitis, human immunodeficiency virus, and cytomegalovirus [CMV]), production of HLA alloantibodies, and graft-versus-host disease. These are concerns in any patient, but the perioperative management of lung transplantation patients requires judicious fluid administration and the avoidance of CMV infection.[29]

Prophylactic Pharmacologic Therapy

Pharmacologic agents are sometimes used as prophylaxis to reduce perioperative bleeding and subsequent transfusion requirements during heart and lung transplantation. These include the antifibrinolytics (epsilon-aminocaproic acid [EACA], aprotinin, and tranexamic acid) and platelet agents, such as dipyridamole and 1-(3-mercaptopropionic acid)-8-D-arginine vasopressin (desmopressin [DDAVP]). Most studies of these agents were performed on patients who were at increased risk for bleeding and undergoing more routine cardiac procedures, including patients undergoing redo cardiac procedures, patients with pre-existing coagulopathy, and patients on antiplatelet or anticoagulant drugs. The relative efficacy of agents is controversial. Patient populations are often dissimilar between studies, and no consensus exists on a uniform method of assessing efficacy and outcome between these agents in relatively routine cardiothoracic procedures,[30] let alone heart and lung transplantation. The antifibrinolytic drugs, EACA and tranexamic acid, clearly influence coagulation and the hemostatic mechanisms during cardiac procedures using cardiopulmonary bypass, typically by decreasing postoperative chest-tube drainage and, sometimes, transfusion requirements.[31, 32] Aprotinin has been shown to be efficacious in decreasing chest-

tube drainage and transfused blood products.[33, 34] A meta-analysis of prophylactic drug treatment in the prevention of postoperative bleeding found that desmopressin, antifibrinolytic drugs, and aprotinin were all effective in decreasing postoperative chest-tube drainage.[35] Aprotinin and the antifibrinolytics were effective in decreasing the amount of transfused blood products, but only aprotinin was effective in increasing the percentage of patients who receive no transfused blood products. None of the prophylactic drug therapies had a direct effect on mortality.[35]

A small series of patients undergoing combined heart and lung transplantation and double-lung transplantation appeared to benefit from the administration of aprotinin by decreased transfused blood products and decreased chest-tube drainage.[36] One case report demonstrated a marked decrease in bleeding and transfusion requirements in a cystic fibrosis patient undergoing combined heart and lung transplantation compared to historic controls.[15] In a retrospective analysis, aprotinin was found to decrease postoperative blood loss and blood product replacement (packed RBCs [pRBCs] and platelets, but not FFP) in patients undergoing sequential single-lung transplantations under cardiopulmonary bypass.[37] A large, randomized, placebo-controlled prospective study is necessary to confirm these results, but this is unlikely given the perceived benefit of aprotinin in these cases.

Cardiopulmonary Bypass

The effects of cardiopulmonary bypass on hemostatic mechanisms are numerous and complicated. They include, but are not limited to, contact activation through factor XII, activation of the complement cascade, leukocyte activation, quantitative and qualitative platelet defects, fibrinolysis, hemodilution, hypothermia, the effects of heparin, and the reversal of heparin with protamine.[38–40]

The effects of cardiopulmonary bypass on pulmonary function after any cardiothoracic procedure remains unclear, but clinically, they range from frank pulmonary edema or "pump lung" to pulmonary infiltrates and experimentally measured increased interstitial lung water. The incidence of severe pulmonary dysfunction has decreased, likely due to better perioperative management and improvements in cardiopulmonary bypass materials and techniques, but subtle changes in the microvascular permeability of the pulmonary endothelium still occur. Proposed mechanisms have included complement activation with subsequent leukocyte and platelet activation.[41] Ischemia and subsequent reperfusion are known to damage the endothelium of all organs. Pulmonary endothelial permeability in several transplanted lungs was demonstrated to be greater than that of healthy volunteers, but it was not uniformly greater.[42] A large series reported the effects of cardiopulmonary bypass on early allograft dysfunction: Patients undergoing lung transplantation requiring cardiopulmonary bypass had lower arterial to alveolar oxygen tension ratios, more severe pulmonary infiltrates on chest roentgenograms, prolonged intubation, and a slightly worse graft survival and patient survival compared to patients who did not require cardiopulmonary bypass for their lung transplantation.[43] The two groups required significantly different amounts of transfused blood products. The use of a heparin-coated cardiopulmonary bypass circuit combined with reduced systemic heparinization did not improve early graft function in a canine model of single-lung transplantation.[44]

After discontinuation of cardiopulmonary bypass, protamine is administered to neutralize heparin. Various methods to determine the protamine dosage are used, including a dose matched to the total heparin administered or a dose determined by a measurement of residual heparin concentration. Whatever method is used, a return to baseline ACT is the goal. Surgical hemostasis should be meticulous, using additional suture and electrocautery. If bleeding persists, clotting tests, including platelet count, PT, aPTT, fibrinogen, and fibrin(ogen) degradation products (FDPs), can be obtained to help guide blood product therapy. The use of thromboelastography (TEG) with algorithms for interpretation has been effective in guiding therapy during liver transplantation[45] and has been advocated to guide replacement therapy during cardiac procedures,[46] but it is not uniformly accepted.[47, 48]

Management of Coagulation

Management of coagulation during heart, combined heart and lung, or isolated lung transplantation, especially when cardiopulmonary bypass is used, represents another challenge in these already demanding procedures. Replacement therapy is usually with blood components. Modified whole blood is sometimes available and is indicated when transfusion of pRBCs and FFP is expected. Transfusion of pRBCs is indicated to maintain the hemoglobin level between 7 and 10 g/dl in the lung transplantation patient. The lowest acceptable hemoglobin is determined by the patient's needs and the operative team. Heart and lung transplantation patients receive CMV-seronegative blood to minimize the occurrence of CMV infection. The use of leukocyte-depleted blood to attenuate HLA alloimmunization and possible leukocyte-mediated lung injury is not routine practice, but it is an option if retransplantation is an issue. Platelets are administered for persistent bleeding, typically after a prolonged cardiopulmonary bypass with a normal or near-normal ACT. A measured platelet count may not indicate a qualitative platelet defect. Platelets can be administered as pooled random-donor platelets or as a single-donor apheresis product. Transfusion of FFP is ideally dictated by a prolonged PT (greater than 1.5 international normalized ratio [INR]) in the presence of clinical bleeding. In the case of massive bleeding with quick response laboratory data unavailable, FFP is sometimes transfused in combination with pRBCs. Transfusion of cryoprecipitate is limited to patients with massive bleeding and is governed by fibrinogen concentration, typically less than 100 mg/dl.

Liver Transplantation

Coagulation in Patients with End-Stage Liver Disease

Bleeding tendency and coagulopathy are well described in patients with end-stage liver disease, given that the liver plays the central role in the production of most clotting factors and inhibitors as well as the clearance of their activated forms. Furthermore, liver disease affects all phases of coagulation, namely, the vascular phase, platelet phase, coagulation cascade, fibrin polymerization phase, and fibrinolysis phase.

The vascular phase of coagulation appears to be impaired in patients with liver disease because the disease is associated with peripheral vasodilation, reduced elasticity and contraction of vessels, and decreased interaction between the vessel walls and platelets.[49]

A significant alteration is seen in the platelet phase. Thrombocytopenia is observed in up to 70% of patients,[45] although production of platelets is normal or increased.[50] Thrombocytopenia is induced by splenomegaly, shortened platelet survival time, platelet consumption, sequestration of platelets in the regenerating liver, folic acid deficiency in alcoholic liver disease, and toxic effects of ethanol on megakaryocytes.[51–54] Platelet dysfunction is a common occurrence and appears to be associated with decreased content of arachidonic acid and adenine nucleotides in platelets.[55] The impaired aggregation of platelets appears to be related to an increase in small, hypofunctional platelets.[56] Platelet dysfunction is observed with no correlation between platelet count and bleeding time[50] and diminished clot retraction.[53, 54] Also, abnormal platelet function in patients with hepatorenal syndrome is caused by dialyzable or nondialyzable plasma factors.

The coagulation cascade is adversely affected by low levels of procoagulants and inhibitors produced by the liver, including coagulation factors (I, II, V, VII, VIII, IX, X, XI, XII, XIII, Fletcher, Fitzgerald, prekallikrein, plasminogen, and high–molecular-weight kininogen), inhibitors (AT-III and alpha$_1$-antitrypsin), and regulatory proteins (C$_1$ inhibitor and alpha$_2$-macroglobulin). The fibrinogen level is generally normal or increased, but excessive sialic acid content in the fibrinogen molecule results in dysfibrinogenemia.[57] Dysfibrinogenemia affects the polymerization of fibrin[58] and is demonstrated by prolonged thrombin time. The level of factor VIII is frequently increased because of increased level of von Willebrand's factor (vWF) antigen and its activity.[59] A generalized deficiency in coagulation factors prolongs PT, and decreases in levels of factors IX and XII prolong aPTT. In addition, the low level of proteinases with antithrombin activity (AT-III and alpha$_1$-antitrypsin) and regulatory proteins (C$_1$ inhibitor and alpha$_2$-macroglobulin) may theoretically result in thrombosis.[60] Fibrin polymerization is impaired by the low level of factor XIII and dysfibrinogenemia.

The fibrinolytic system is also affected by liver disease because the levels of several proteins involved in fibrinolysis (plasminogen, protein C, protein S, and alpha$_2$-antiplasmin) can be low, and a large endothelial area increases the level of tissue plasminogen activator (tPA).

More important, the imbalance between coagulation and its inhibition and fibrinolysis and its inhibition results in all forms of coagulopathy. The hypocoagulable state is caused by impaired hepatic synthesis of clotting factors and quantitative and qualitative defects of platelets. Excessive activation of coagulation may occur when the hepatic clearance of activated clotting factors is decreased. Fibrinolysis develops when levels of fibrinolysis inhibitors (alpha$_2$-antiplasmin and histidine glycoprotein) are low,[61, 62] or the hepatic clearance of tPA is decreased.[63, 64] A hypercoagulable state may be seen in patients with Budd-Chiari syndrome or with protein C or protein S deficiency.

Impaired coagulation of patients with end-stage liver disease is shown in Tables 16-1 and 16-2.[65] As expected, patients with hepatocellular disease develop more significant abnormalities. The levels of factors I, II, V, VII, IX, and XI are less than 50% of normal, and the test results of thrombin time, AT-III level, platelet count, and PT are abnormal in more than 80% of the population. Furthermore, in more than 20% of patients, FDPs are present, and fibrinolytic activity is detected. Derangement of coagulation in patients with cholestatic disease is less pronounced: All clotting factor levels are greater than 70% of normal, and fewer than half of patients show abnormal results of various tests. On the other hand, the majority of patients with uncomplicated hepatic malignancies have relatively normal coagulation profiles, although tumor necrosis may trigger activation of coagulation. Patients with congenital metabolic disorders, such as Dubin-Johnson, Gilbert, or Rotor's syndrome, have low titers of factor VII,[66, 67] and patients with familial antithrombin deficiency, an autosomal dominant genetic disease, are prone to developing thromboembolism.

Perioperative Changes in Coagulation

The abnormal coagulation system undergoes complex changes during liver transplantation (Table 16-3). This is well summarized in the early clinical experience of liver transplantation[68–70]:

> There was an intraoperative bleeding diathesis at the same time as fibrinolysis and hypofibrinogenemia developed. In four of the cases, the hemorrhage was eventually controlled after the administration of EACA, fibrinogen, and fresh blood. Subsequently, three of four

Table 16-1. Mean Values of Coagulation Tests of Patients Undergoing Liver Transplantation*

Group	No.	PT	aPTT	TT	Platelet	AT-III	Fibrinogen	FDP	Lysis
Normal	—	≤13.5 secs	≤36 secs	≤20 secs	≥150 × 10³/μl	≤7 U/ml	≥150 dl	0	0
PNC	20	16.8 (95)	40.9 (79)	30.3 (85)	92 (90)	0.36 (95)	182 (40)	+ (25)	+ (20)
Misc.	10	28.9 (80)	48.3 (80)	29.2 (80)	199 (70)	0.49 (90)	183 (50)	+ (11)	+ (33)
SC	8	13.0 (25)	39.8 (75)	21.2 (63)	189 (63)	0.82 (50)	473 (0)	0 (0)	0 (0)
PBC	16	12.3 (25)	35.7 (38)	21.7 (56)	249 (38)	0.94 (25)	389 (0)	+ (13)	0 (0)
Ca	10	11.9 (0)	30.9 (10)	20.1 (55)	308 (0)	0.97 (22)	455 (0)	0 (0)	0 (0)
All	4	16.3 (52)	39.0 (59)	25.3 (67)	188 (55)	0.67 (60)	313 (20)	+ (13)	+ (11)

*Percentage of patients with abnormal values is shown in parentheses.
PT = prothrombin time; aPTT = activated partial thromboplastin time; TT = thrombin time; AT-III = antithrombin III; FDP = fibrinogen degradation products; PNC = postnecrotic cirrhosis; Misc. = miscellaneous diseases; SC = sclerosing cholangitis; PBC = primary biliary cirrhosis; Ca = carcinoma.
Source: Adapted from FA Bontempo, JH Lewis, MV Ragni, TE Starzl. The Perioperative Coagulation Pattern in Liver Transplant Patients. In PM Winter, YG Kang (eds), Hepatic Transplantation: Anesthetic and Perioperative Management. New York: Praeger, 1986;135–141.

Table 16-2. Mean Values (U/ml) of Coagulation Factors (Normal, 0.5–1.5 U/ml) of Patients Undergoing Liver Transplantation

Group	No.	II	V	VII	IX	X	XI	XII
PNC	20	0.33	0.35	0.27	0.43	0.56	0.44	0.65
Misc.	10	0.46	0.45	0.52	0.45	0.64	0.46	0.67
SC	8	1.13	0.64	1.42	1.02	1.43	0.63	1.00
PBC	16	0.95	1.00	1.00	0.90	0.95	0.76	1.07
Ca	10	0.81	1.10	0.92	1.05	0.80	1.00	1.11
All	64	0.68	0.68	0.74	0.73	0.81	0.63	0.87

PNC = postnecrotic cirrhosis; Misc. = miscellaneous diseases; SC = sclerosing cholangitis; PBC = primary biliary cirrhosis; Ca = carcinoma.
Source: Adapted from FA Bontempo, JH Lewis, MV Ragni, TE Starzl. The Perioperative Coagulation Pattern in Liver Transplant Patients. In PM Winter, YG Kang (eds), Hepatic Transplantation: Anesthetic and Perioperative Management. New York: Praeger, 1986;135–141.

survivors formed thrombi at or near femoral venotomy sites which had been used for the insertion of external bypass catheters; in all three, the eventual result was multiple pulmonary embolization.[71]

This clinical observation and animal studies led to the conclusion that liver transplantation "can cause hyperfibrinolysis, thrombocytopenia, and depression of various clotting factors . . . the extent of these changes are prognostic inasmuch as they are proportional to the magnitude of liver injury . . . the depression of clotting is not necessarily succeeded by hypercoagulability if thrombogenic agents are not administered." These findings have been confirmed by other investigators.[45, 72, 73]

During the preanhepatic stage, pre-existing coagulopathy is complicated by surgical bleeding that is caused by difficulties in the removal of the diseased liver. Bleeding is more severe in patients with portal hypertension, adhesions from previous abdominal surgery, and steroid-induced fragile tissues. Levels of all coagulation factors and the platelet count decrease gradually during this period, even in the presence of continuous infusion of coagulation factor–rich blood products (Figure 16-1). Patients with severe hepatocellular disease or who require a large amount of blood transfusion may develop fibrinolysis during this period. Gradual inadvertent hypothermia and massive blood transfusion–induced ionized hypocalcemia may impair coagulation as well. The coagulation system undergoes more significant changes during the anhepatic stage. The heparin effect may be observed when venovenous bypass is used because heparin solution (2,000–5,000 units of heparin) is

Table 16-3. Coagulopathy during Orthotopic Liver Transplantation

Stage	Coagulopathy
Preanhepatic	Pre-existing coagulopathy
	Dilution
	Fibrinolysis (mild)
	Ionized hypocalcemia
Anhepatic	Dilution
	Heparin effect (with venovenous bypass)
	Fibrinolysis (moderate)
	Intravascular coagulation
	Hypothermia
	Ionized hypocalcemia
Early neohepatic	Fibrinolysis (severe)
	Heparin effect
	Intravascular coagulation
	Dilution
	Hypothermia
	Ionized hypocalcemia
Late neohepatic	Gradual recovery

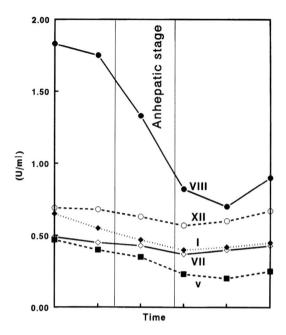

Figure 16-1. Intraoperative changes in coagulation factors. The levels of coagulation factors decrease during the anhepatic stage and reach nadir immediately on reperfusion, even with the administration of coagulation factor–rich blood (mixture of red blood cells to fresh frozen plasma to crystalloids = 300 to 200 to 250 ml, respectively). Normal baseline factor VIII level decreases rapidly during the same period, most likely from activation of fibrinolytic system. (Adapted from JH Lewis, FA Bontempo, SA Awad, et al. Liver transplantation: intraoperative changes in coagulation factors in 100 first transplants. Hepatology 1989;9:710–714.)

used to flush the cannulas. The heparin effect is observed as prolonged aPTT and reaction time, as measured by TEG; it disappears gradually within 30–60 minutes without treatment. Surgical bleeding and the absence of hepatic synthesis of coagulation factors result in further decreases in platelet count and coagulation factors. The release of tissue thromboplastin and the absence of hepatic clearance of activated coagulation factors may accelerate thrombin formation, as evidenced by gradual increases in thrombin–AT-III complex (TAT) and FDP.[74] However, clinically significant intravascular coagulation may rarely occur during the anhepatic stage. Fibrinolysis, caused by the release of tPA and the absence of its hepatic clearance, is seen in approximately 20% of patients during this period (Figure 16-2).[75] Thus, the combination of dilution, activation of coagulation, and fibrinolysis may decrease the coagulation factors and platelet count to an extremely low level and result in bleeding and oozing.

A severe coagulopathy, which is a component of postreperfusion syndrome, may occur on reperfusion of the grafted liver. The changes are prolonged PT, aPTT, reptilase time, and thrombin time; a generalized decrease in coagulation factor levels, including factors I, V, VII, and VIII; a sudden increase in tPA; thrombocytopenia; a shortened

euglobulin lysis time (ELT); and a moderate increase in FDP and TAT.[68, 73–77] Postreperfusion coagulopathy is believed to be multifactorial in etiology. A moderate to severe heparin effect is seen in approximately one-third of patients. The main source of heparin is endogenous heparin from the donor liver, although exogenous heparin administered during the donor procurement process may play some role. This heparin effect is seen as prolonged PT, thrombin time, and reaction time, and it may last for 60–120 minutes. The heparin effect is easily diagnosed by a shorter reaction time of TEG of blood treated with protamine sulfate or Heparinase I (Haemoscope Corp., Skokie, IL) compared to that of TEG of untreated blood (Figure 16-3).[78] It has been suggested that other coagulation inhibitors or a heparin-like substance plays a role in the development of the postreperfusion syndrome.[68]

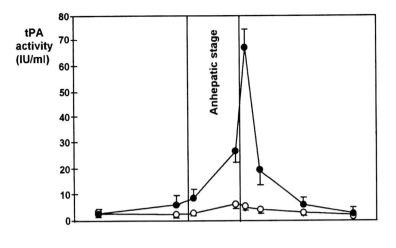

Figure 16-2. Intraoperative changes in tissue plasminogen activator (tPA) level of patients with and without fibrinolysis. Intraoperative levels of tPA activity (mean + standard error of mean) is much higher in patients with severe fibrinolysis (*solid circles*, n = 13) than in those with minimal fibrinolysis (*open circles*, n = 7). (Reprinted with permission from RJ Porte, FA Bontempo, EA Knot, et al. Systemic effects of tissue plasminogen activator-associated fibrinolysis and its relation to thrombin generation in orthotopic liver transplantation. Transplantation 1989;47:980.)

Fibrinolysis occurs in approximately 80% of patients, although severe fibrinolysis and generalized oozing are observed in approximately 40% of patients.[75] Fibrinolysis is believed to be caused by the massive release of tPA from the grafted liver, congested viscera, and lower extremities together with the reduction of plasminogen activator inhibitor (PAI) activity.[76, 77] Other potential causes of fibrinolysis include contact activation of fibrinolysis and activation of protein C or urokinase-type plasminogen activator.[79] Fibrinolysis observed during the anhepatic and neohepatic stages is primary in origin because of several factors, including an association between high tPA levels and primary fibrinolysis[76, 77]; a relatively steady level of AT-III[80]; only moderate levels of FDPs and D-dimers[45, 75]; an association between fibrinolysis and a selective decrease in factors I, V, and VIII[73]; the effectiveness of EACA without complications[75]; and no known microembolization. Fibrinolysis is confirmed by shortened ELT (as low as 0–15 minutes), an abrupt increase in tPA level, a very low level of PAI, a reduction in fibrinolysis time and maximum amplitude, and prolonged reaction time of TEG. Fibrinolysis is diagnosed by comparing the TEG of untreated blood with the TEG of blood treated with EACA (see Figure 16-3). Typically, the patient's untreated blood shows a hypocoagulable state, a prolonged reaction time, slow clot formation rate, small maximum amplitude, and measurable fibrinolysis time. Blood treated with EACA demonstrates an improvement in all variables of TEG. Fibrinolysis dissipates gradually during the next 2 hours as

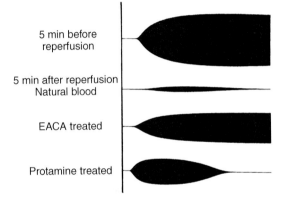

Figure 16-3. Fibrinolysis and the heparin effect on reperfusion. The first thromboelastograph (TEG) is taken 5 minutes before reperfusion. The next three TEGs are taken 5 minutes after reperfusion with untreated blood, blood treated with epsilon-aminocaproic acid (EACA) (0.3 mg), and blood treated with protamine sulfate (3 μg). Fibrinolysis and potential heparin effect are seen in the untreated blood, and their presence is confirmed by inhibition of fibrinolysis in the blood treated with EACA and shortened reaction time in the blood treated with protamine sulfate. (Reprinted with permission from YG Kang. Monitoring and Treatment of Coagulation. In PM Winter, YG Kang [eds], Hepatic Transplantation: Anesthetic and Perioperative Management. New York: Praeger, 1986;168.)

tPA level decreases and PAI level becomes detectable.[75, 77]

Excessive activation of coagulation and secondary fibrinolysis are known to occur, as evidenced by the increased levels of TAT complex, FDP, and fibrin monomers and the decreased levels of AT-III and PAI during the anhepatic stage and immediately after reperfusion.[74] These phenomena appear to be caused either by tPA-induced activation of platelet aggregation[81] or by extracellular release of lysosomal proteinases from macrophages (cathepsin B) and granulocytes (elastase).[82] Excessive activation of coagulation, which may result in consumption coagulopathy, peripheral venous thrombosis, and pulmonary thromboembolism, is receiving more attention from clinicians.[69, 83] DeWolf et al. reported that six patients developed clinical signs of pulmonary embolism immediately after reperfusion, with a clotted heparinized blood sample or sudden appearance of thrombus in the right side of the heart and pulmonary artery.[84] In another report, transesophageal echocardiography revealed a significant pulmonary thromboembolism within 60 seconds of reperfusion in 59% of patients without venovenous bypass and 11% of patients with venovenous bypass.[85] This excessive activation of coagulation may be caused by anoxic damage of endothelium, release of lysosomal proteinases from activated macrophages and platelets, or low AT-III level. Fatal pulmonary embolism occurs rarely, however, possibly because of ensuing severe fibrinolysis.

Quantitative and qualitative defects in platelets may cause reperfusion coagulopathy. Thrombocytopenia occurs in most patients on reperfusion,[86] and the transhepatic decrease in platelet count has been shown to be as much as 55%.[87, 89] Although the cause is unclear, reperfusion thrombocytopenia may be caused by extravasation of platelets into Disse's spaces in the perisinusoidal region of the liver or by phagocytosis by Kupffer's cells. Platelet function can be impaired by the loss of granulation[89] and decreased platelet aggregation.[90]

Reperfusion hypothermia (by 1–2°C), dilutional coagulopathy caused by an influx of preservation solution, and ionic hypocalcemia may also interfere with coagulation.[91] Additionally, it is possible that certain humoral substances released from the grafted liver may also inhibit coagulation.

Coagulopathy improves gradually as the grafted liver begins to function. Fibrinolysis and the heparin effect dissipate gradually within 2 hours, and the levels of coagulation factors and platelet count increase toward baseline levels by the end of surgery.[45] Bleeding or oozing may persist in some patients, however. Bleeding with persistent coagulopathy may be caused by insufficient replacement therapy or a poorly functioning graft liver with ischemic or immunologic injury-induced microvascular thrombosis. Coagulopathy associated with a nonfunctioning graft is caused by inadequate synthesis of coagulation factors and impaired clearance of activated clotting factors.[71, 83, 92] Bleeding with persistent low levels of factors I, V, and VIII may be a complication of fibrinolysis because plasminogen and plasmin selectively destroy these factors.[73] Oozing in the presence of an acceptable coagulation profile and TEG may indicate delayed bleeding. Improper polymerization of fibrin results in the formation of friable, soluble fibrin, which can be lysed or removed prematurely. More commonly, high plasmin content in the blood clot formed previously in the presence of fibrinolysis continues to dissolve the clot, even in the absence of active fibrinolysis. In the case of delayed bleeding, no specific treatment is helpful, and oozing stops when new clots form at the injured vessels.

The postoperative change of coagulation depends on graft function. In general, with adequate graft function, the coagulation factor level increases steadily toward normal values, and PT and aPTT return to normal values within 2 weeks.

Monitoring of Coagulation

The conventional coagulation profile includes the PT, aPTT, fibrinogen level, platelet count, ELT, and FDP level. Factor assays (I, V, VII, XII), reptilase time, thrombin time, and AT-III level can be determined for further information. A coagulation profile has limitations for clinical monitoring, namely, the lack of availability and difficulty in assessing blood coagulability in patients with dynamic and multiple coagulation defects.

TEG has been introduced to monitor wholeblood coagulation.[45, 93] TEG determines the sheer elasticity of fibrins formed continuously, assesses the interaction of all cellular and noncellular elements involved in coagulation, and is easily accessible. More important, TEG assists in making a differential diagnosis of coagulopathy and guides selective replacement and pharmacologic therapy.

Commonly determined TEG variables are shown in Figure 16-4. Reaction time (r) is the interval from the beginning of TEG trace to the point at which an

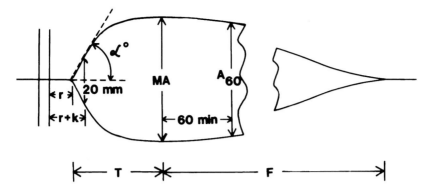

Figure 16-4. Variables and normal values measured by thromboelastography. (α = clot formation rate; r = reaction time; MA = maximum amplitude; T = time; F = fibrinolysis time; A_{60} = amplitude 60 minutes after maximum amplitude.) (Reprinted from YG Kang, DJ Martin, J Marquez, et al. Intraoperative changes in blood coagulation and thromboelastographic monitoring in liver transplantation. Anesth Analg 1985;64:891; by permission of the International Anesthesia Research Society.)

amplitude reaches 2 mm. It is the time taken to generate initial fibrin strands, primarily a function of the coagulation cascade. Maximum amplitude (MA), the largest amplitude reached, is a function of the platelets. Clot formation rate (α), the speed with which a solid clot forms, is a function of fibrinogen and platelets. The interval between the maximum amplitude and subsequent zero amplitude is the fibrinolysis time (F). The amplitude 60 minutes after maximum amplitude (A_{60}) is used to determine the fibrinolysis index (A_{60}/MA $\times$ 100). A fibrinolysis index less than 85% indicates fibrinolysis.

A normal TEG pattern is characterized by an initial latent period, followed by a gradual increase in fibrin shear elasticity or amplitude that reaches maximum amplitude in 30–60 minutes (Figure 16-5). The fibrinolysis index remains above 85%. In patients with hemophilia, the reaction time is prolonged and the clot formation rate is decreased because of the delayed formation of thrombin caused by insufficient activity of factor VIII. However, maximum amplitude (platelet function) is within the normal range because activation of more than the critical level of factor X results in normal clot formation. A similar TEG pattern is observed in patients with ionized hypocalcemia (less than 0.6 mmol/liter) or hypothermia (less than 34°C). In thrombocytopenia, the maximum amplitude is

Figure 16-5. Thromboelastographic patterns of normal and disease states. (Reprinted with permission from YG Kang. Monitoring and Treatment of Coagulation. In PM Winter, YG Kang [eds], Hepatic Transplantation: Anesthetic and Perioperative Management. New York: Praeger, 1986;155.)

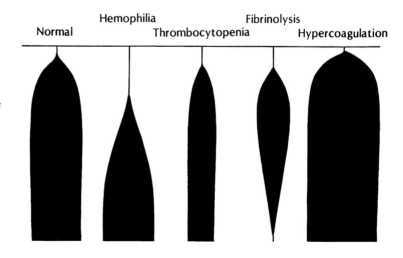

decreased. In addition, the reaction time is prolonged and the clot formation rate is decreased because coagulation cascade requires platelet phospholipids. In fibrinolysis, a rapid decrease in amplitude is accompanied by a prolonged reaction time and decreased maximum amplitude because fibrinolysis leads to the net decrease in fibrins as formed fibrins are destroyed. Hypercoagulation is characterized by a short reaction time, increased clot formation rate, and increased maximum amplitude.

For the differential diagnosis, TEGs of untreated and treated blood are compared. For the treated blood, 0.03 ml of FFP, cryoprecipitate, platelets, EACA (1% solution), protamine sulfate (0.01% solution), or Heparinase I (4 IU) is added to 0.33 ml of whole blood.

Perioperative Management of Coagulation

Preoperative Management

Preoperative optimization of coagulation by replacement therapy is not always successful because of continuous loss of coagulation factors. Preoperative management of coagulation should be tailored to the specific clinical circumstances, such as the degree and type of coagulation defects, the type of invasive procedure planned, the nature or location of bleeding, and the timing of surgery.

Vitamin K, a cofactor for posttranslational carboxylation, is required for hepatic synthesis of coagulation factors (II, VII, IX, and X). This lipid-soluble vitamin is either obtained directly from dietary intake requiring bile salts or produced by intestinal flora. Consequently, deficiency of vitamin K–dependent coagulation factors results from a poor dietary intake, inadequate production or excretion of bile salts, or suppression of normal intestinal flora by antibiotics. For a mild vitamin K deficiency, oral administration of vitamin K and bile salts is sufficient, and intramuscular or intravenous administration of vitamin K_1 (5 mg/day) is effective in correcting PT within 24–48 hours. Repeated administration of vitamin K_1 and coagulation factors may be necessary to treat bleeding tendency. Vitamin K may not be effective in patients with severe hepatocellular disease because of either an inadequate amount of coagulation factor precursors or incomplete carboxylation.[94]

FFP is administered to correct coagulation defects in patients with liver disease because it contains all coagulation elements and their inhibitors. It is generally accepted that FFP is given to patients with a prolonged PT (greater than 1.5 INR) before needle biopsy of the liver. FFP administration, however, improves coagulation only temporarily, and the large volume required to treat coagulopathy may cause fluid overloading.

Platelet transfusion is required for severe thrombocytopenia. The effectiveness of platelet transfusion is transient, however, because transfused platelets can be sequestered or destroyed by the spleen or liver. Clinical bleeding is not seen when the platelet count is greater than 75,000/μl, but satisfactory hemostasis can be obtained with lower platelet counts (greater than 40,000/μl).

Cryoprecipitate, containing fibrinogen and factors VIII and XIII, is indicated only when hypofibrinogenemia or fibrinolysis is present owing to a high level of factor VIII in patients with liver disease. One unit of cryoprecipitate contains 300 mg of fibrinogen, and the transfusion of 1 unit of cryoprecipitate increases the fibrinogen level approximately 10 mg/dl in a patient weighing 60 kg. The half-life of fibrinogen is approximately 3–4 days; repeated transfusion of cryoprecipitate is necessary to supplement the loss.

Anticoagulation therapy is rarely used in cirrhotic patients, although a subcutaneous injection of a small dose of heparin appears to be acceptable. Heparin can cause thrombocytopenia, and its effect may be exaggerated in the presence of thrombocytopenia. Oral anticoagulants are also not recommended because patient response is unpredictable.

Antifibrinolytic agents stabilize fragile hemostatic plugs in localized bleeding, such as a gastric mucosal ulcer or bleeding esophageal varices, and may decrease the bleeding tendency in patients without signs of fibrinolysis. However, EACA has been shown to be ineffective in improving coagulopathy in patients with liver disease.[95] Antifibrinolytic therapy should be used only for patients with demonstrable fibrinolysis to avoid thrombotic complications.

Plasmapheresis (30–40 ml/kg), in combination with replacement therapy, may improve coagulation by removing filterable humoral elements and coagulation inhibitors, particularly in patients with fulminant hepatic failure. Plasmapheresis of 36.8

ml/kg of blood has reportedly decreased PT from 28.3 to 17.7 seconds and aPTT from 64.8 to 43.3 seconds in patients awaiting liver transplantation.[96]

Intraoperative Management

Physiologic Therapy.   Hypothermia inhibits the activity of proteases involved in the coagulation cascade. It also prolongs the reaction time and decreases the clot formation rate of TEG.[91] A similar inhibition is seen in patients with ionized hypocalcemia because calcium ion is a cofactor of coagulation. Therefore, body temperature, tissue perfusion, gas exchange, acid-base state, and fluid-electrolyte balance should be optimized to maintain normal blood coagulability.

Replacement Therapy.   Replacement therapy is guided by the conventional coagulation profile or by TEG variables. Replacement guidelines based on conventional coagulation vary widely from institution to institution, ranging from specific guidelines (e.g., PT less than 1.5 INR; hematocrit, 30%; platelet count greater than 30,000/μl; and AT-III level greater than 70%)[97] to vaguer guidelines (e.g., hemoglobin greater than 9 gm/dl, FFP to correct coagulopathy, and platelet count greater than 100,000/μl).[98]

Most centers administer coagulation factor–rich blood (RBC to FFP = 1 to 1) to maintain sufficient coagulation factor level or to maintain PT less than 1.5–2.0 INR. The critical level of platelet count is considered to be approximately 40,000–50,000/μl.

At the University of Pittsburgh Medical Center, coagulation therapy is guided by TEG variables and by platelet count. In general, continuous replacement of coagulation factors is required to compensate for dilutional coagulopathy, excessive coagulation, and fibrinolysis. This is achieved by administering a mixture of blood products (RBC to FFP to crystalloids = 300 to 200 to 250 ml) containing 30–50% of normal levels of coagulation factors. Additional blood products may be administered according to TEG variables and platelet count. Platelets (10 units) are administered when maximum amplitude is less than 40 mm, thereby improving maximum amplitude as well as reaction time. Cryoprecipitate (6 units) is administered when clot formation rate is persistently less than 40 degrees even after platelet transfusion, particularly when fibrinolysis decreases the fibrinogen level.

Additional FFP (2 units) may be administered when reaction time is persistently longer than 15 minutes, even after the administration of platelets and cryoprecipitate.[99] However, the need for additional FFP is relatively rare.

During the anhepatic stage with venovenous bypass, aggressive administration of platelets and cryoprecipitate is avoided to prevent potential thromboembolism, unless bleeding is severe. However, platelet transfusion is commonly required after reperfusion because reperfusion is frequently associated with a remarkable decrease in platelet count. Furthermore, more aggressive replacement therapy may be needed during the neohepatic stage when surgical bleeding persists or when fibrinolysis or the heparin effect remains untreated. Untreated fibrinolysis may require replacement of a large quantity of factors I, V, and VIII by administration of cryoprecipitate and FFP. Additional platelet transfusion may be required in patients with poorly functioning grafted livers. In addition, alloimmunization to specific class I HLAs in highly sensitized patients may result in refractoriness to platelet transfusion.[100, 101] These patients may benefit from the transfusion of type-specific single-donor platelets.

Some centers recommended AT-III administration when the AT-III level was low because this may exacerbate activation of coagulation during the anhepatic and early neohepatic stages. However, its level remains relatively stable when FFP is adequately administered[80]; administration of AT-III neither improves the coagulation profile nor reduces blood loss and fibrinolytic activity.[102] Therefore, AT-III is reserved for patients with excessively low AT-III levels.

The TEG patterns and coagulation profile of a patient with fulminant hepatic failure are shown in Figure 16-6.[45] The baseline TEG pattern showed a prolonged reaction time, decreased maximum amplitude, and decreased clot formation rate, thereby indicating a generalized decrease in coagulation factors and platelets. Administration of 2 units of FFP improved reaction time. The administration of 10 units of platelets improved maximum amplitude, but mild fibrinolysis began to develop. Transfusion of 6 units of cryoprecipitate did not improve clot formation rate owing to the continuous deterioration of coagulation and fibrinolysis. The anhepatic stage II was characterized by pronounced fibrinolysis. On reperfusion (stage III), a

Case L.W.

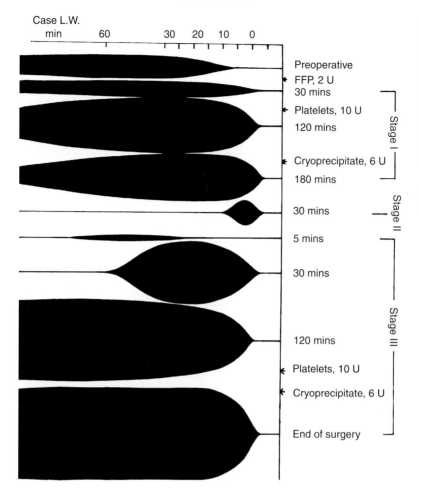

Figure 16-6. Thromboelasto-graphic patterns of a patient with fulminant hepatic failure during liver transplantation. (FFP = fresh frozen plasma.) (Reprinted from YG Kang, DJ Martin, J Marquez, et al. Intra-operative changes in blood coagulation and thromboelas-tographic monitoring in liver transplantation. Anesth Analg 1985;64:895; by permission of the International Anesthesia Research Society.)

severe coagulopathy was noted with a prolonged reaction time, decreased clot formation rate, decreased maximum amplitude, and signs of fibri-nolysis. Reperfusion coagulopathy gradually improved 2 hours after reperfusion. The adminis-tration of platelets and cryoprecipitate normalized the TEG by the end of surgery. Figure 16-7 shows the coagulation profile of the same patient.[103] The majority of coagulation tests were moderately or severely abnormal at the start of surgery. The coag-ulation profile gradually improved and was only moderately abnormal at the end of surgery, even in the presence of normal TEG.

Pharmacologic Therapy. Antifibrinolytic therapy has been tried since the early era of liver transplanta-tion to treat generalized oozing caused by fibrinoly-sis. EACA and tranexamic acid, which accelerate the conversion of plasminogen to plasmin and inhibit the formation of plasmin-fibrin(ogen) complex, are the most commonly used synthetic antifibrinolytic agents. EACA was used in the 1960s, but the clinical courses of three patients were complicated by fatal continuous bleeding or pulmonary embolism.[69] This experience led to the recommendation of no pharma-cologic coagulation therapy, although the antifibri-nolytic therapy was less than optimal. Indication for the treatment was unclear, the dosage was large (5-g loading dose followed by 1 g/hour), monitoring of coagulation was insufficient, and the treatment might not have caused the complications.

In one study of 79 patients, EACA (1 g) was administered to 20 patients who developed severe fibrinolysis (fibrinolysis time <120 minutes) (Figure 16-8).[75] All patients demonstrated complete inhibi-tion of fibrinolysis with improved maximum ampli-

Figure 16-7. Coagulation profile of a patient with fulminant hepatic failure during liver transplantation. (PT = prothrombin time; aPTT = activated partial thromboplastin time; FDP = fibrin degradation products; ELT = euglobulin lysis time.) (Reprinted with permission from Y Kang. Thromboelastography in liver transplantation. Semin Thromb Hemost 1995;21 [Suppl 4]:39.)

	Preanhepatic Stage		Anhepatic Stage		Neohepatic Stage		End
Platelet (K/μl)	28	109	92	85	107	110	125
PT (sec)	27.7	18.5	19.1	15.3	14.6	14	13.5
aPTT (sec)	47.1	43.4	72.9	41.3	40.9	39.3	33.3
Thrombin time (sec)	28.2	21.4	34.2	21.7	20.3	18.8	20.9
Reptilase time (sec)	33.5	24.1	24.6	24.4	23.4	21.6	23.1
Fibrinogen (mg/ml)	95	130	130	175	225	230	250
Factor II (U/ml)	0.17	0.24	0.24	0.31	0.33	0.35	0.43
Factor V (U/ml)	0.12	0.18	0.16	0.25	0.29	0.29	0.41
Factor VII (U/ml)	0.04	0.09	0.09	0.22	0.29	0.34	0.44
Factor VIII (U/ml)	2.75	1.95	1.75	1.9	0.15	1.25	1.4
Factor IX (U/ml)	0.31	0.36	0.33	0.52	0.62	0.58	1.15
Factor X (U/ml)	0.17	0.22	0.25	0.23	0.33	0.38	0.49
Factor XI (U/ml)	0.44	0.52	0.78	0.58	0.66	0.6	0.84
Factor XII (U/ml)	0.52	0.52	0.52	0.6	0.6	0.33	0.4
FDP (ug/ml)	0	0	0	0	0	0	20
ELT (h)	2	1	1	1	2.5	2.75	4

Figure 16-8. Thromboelastographic (TEG) patterns in a patient undergoing liver transplantation. Fibrinolysis developed during the anhepatic stage and became severe on reperfusion of the grafted liver. Administration of epsilon-aminocaproic acid (EACA) (1 g intravenously [IV]), after the inhibition of fibrinolysis was confirmed by TEG of blood treated with EACA, resulted in an improvement in fibrinolysis in subsequent TEGs. (Reprinted with permission from Y Kang, JH Lewis, A Navalgund, et al. Epsilon-aminocaproic acid for treatment of fibrinolysis during liver transplantation. Anesthesiology 1987;66:770.)

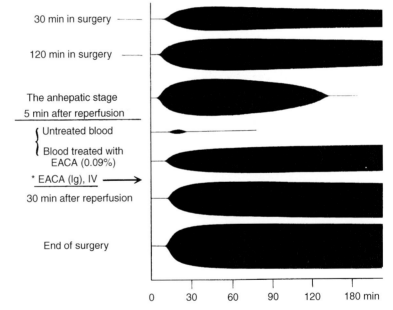

30 min in surgery

120 min in surgery

The anhepatic stage
5 min after reperfusion

{ Untreated blood

{ Blood treated with EACA (0.09%)

* EACA (Ig), IV →

30 min after reperfusion

End of surgery

0   30   60   90   120   180 min

tude and without thrombotic, hemorrhagic, or renal complications. An important finding of this study was that the small dose of EACA (1 g), compared to the conventional priming dose of 4–5 g followed by 1 g per hour to achieve a plasma level of 13 mg/dl, was effective in treating fibrinolysis.[104] It appears that a single, small dose of EACA is sufficient to treat severe but transient fibrinolysis, although its

short half-life may necessitate a second dose when an extremely high tPA level persists over a prolonged period or massive transfusion is required. An even smaller dose of EACA (250–500 mg) has been found to be effective in treating most types of fibrinolysis.[105] Early diagnosis and treatment of fibrinolysis appears to be beneficial. Reduction of bleeding minimizes RBC requirement; inhibition of plasmin

Table 16-4. Dosage of Aprotinin and Comparison of Red Blood Cell (RBC) Requirement

Study	Aprotinin Group			Control Group		
	No.	Aprotinin (10^6) KIU	RBC (U)	No.	Control	RBC (U)
Neuhaus et al.[110]	10	0.5×3	7.5	10	Historic	9.7
Grosse et al.[112]	40	2.0 + 0.5/hr	8.1	50	Historic	23.3
Mallet et al.[111]	20	2.0 + 0.5/hr	7.5	25	Historic	23.6
Groh et al.[115]	9	2.0 + 0.5/hr	18.0	9	Placebo	20.0
Himmelreich et al.[116]	10	0.2 – 0.4/hr	7.0	13	Placebo	8.0
Ickx et al.[118]	5	0.36/hr	7.0	5	Aprotinin (0.18×10^6 KIU/hr)	7.4
Suarez et al.[119]	13	2.0 + 0.5/hr	7.0	15	Placebo	11.6
Ickx et al.[109]	14	16 + 4/hr	7.2	16	Tranexamic acid (80 mg/kg + 40 mg/kg/hr)	7.5

KIU = kallikrein inhibition units.
Source: Adapted from H Riess. The Use of Aprotinin in Liver Transplantation. In R Plfarré (ed), Blood Conservation with Aprotinin. Philadelphia: Hanley & Belfus, 1995;349–358.

prevents destruction of factors I, V, and VIII to minimize the need for FFP and cryoprecipitate; and reduction of surgical hemostasis avoids unnecessary warm ischemia of the liver. Fibrinolysis can be diagnosed in its early stage by observing a significant improvement in TEG variables (reaction time and clot formation rate) in blood treated with EACA over untreated blood in the first 10–15 minutes of recording. The prophylactic use of EACA is not recommended, however, so as to avoid any potential thrombotic complications.[84, 106]

In a study of the routine use of tranexamic acid in children undergoing liver transplantation, Carlier et al. did not observe any complications associated with the antifibrinolytic therapy.[107] Similar results were reported in prospective, randomized clinical trials of tranexamic acid.[108, 109]

Aprotinin is a nonspecific inhibitor of serine protease. It inhibits coagulation, fibrinolysis, kallikrein, and complement cascade by inhibiting activation of the Hageman factor. It has been shown to decrease blood loss, operative time, and length of stay in the intensive care unit in patients undergoing liver transplantation,[110–114] although some studies fail to show the advantage of aprotinin (Table 16-4).[115–118] The beneficial effects of aprotinin appear to be related to reduced production of tPA and plasmin through inhibition of kallikrein and fibrinolysis.[112, 119] This antifibrinolytic effect is indirectly shown by the fact that patients receiving aprotinin and tranexamic acid have the same blood product require-

ments.[109] Furthermore, inhibition of the coagulation cascade by aprotinin is seen in the TEG of blood treated with aprotinin.[120] Therefore, the pharmacologic action of aprotinin in patients undergoing liver transplantation seems related to the inhibition of fibrinolysis and excessive activation of coagulation. The dosage of aprotinin varies by institution, ranging from a high dose (a bolus dose of 2 million kallikrein inhibition units [KIU] followed by 0.5 million KIU/hour) to a continuous infusion of a low dose (0.2–0.4 million KIU/hour).

Protamine sulfate (25–50 mg) is administered to approximately 30% of patients when a severe heparin effect is demonstrated by prolonged aPTT or by a significant improvement in the reaction time of blood treated with protamine sulfate or heparinase.[105]

Desmopressin acetate increases the levels of factor VIII, vWF, and plasminogen. It has been used in patients undergoing cardiac surgery[121] and in uremic patients[122] with platelet dysfunction to improve coagulation by increasing the vWF and promoting the endothelial release of factor VIII. Desmopressin appears to improve blood coagulability of patients undergoing liver transplantation in vitro, possibly by activating coagulation factors and platelets.[123]

Coagulation in Specific Conditions

Children undergoing liver transplantation have a relatively mild degree of coagulopathy compared to adults because cholestatic disease is more common, the duration of disease is shorter, and donor organs may have better function.[124] Some centers prefer minimal replacement and pharmacologic therapy because overtransfusion of clotting factors has been suggested as contributing to hepatic arterial thrombosis.[125] Coagulopathy is also less severe during heterotopic liver transplantation because the surgical technique avoids the anhepatic state. The hypercoagulable state of patients with Budd-Chiari syndrome may not require intraoperative anticoagulation therapy because of unavoidable dilutional and pathologic coagulopathy. The administration of a small dose of heparin (1,000–2,000 units) or warfarin, however, may be necessary postoperatively. Patients with hemophilia A or B require the specific coagulation factor to increase its level to more than 30% of normal during the preanhepatic and anhepatic stages. Additional treatment is unnecessary once the grafted liver begins to function.[126] Patients with protein C deficiency are prone to develop thromboembolism (heparin may be given until the grafted liver begins to produce protein C). Patients with familial AT-III deficiency may also develop thromboembolism; the administration of FFP or AT-III, or both, is required until the grafted liver begins to function.

Blood Transfusion

Hematopoiesis and Fluid Balance in Patients with End-Stage Liver Disease

Anemia (hematocrit, 25–35 vol%), which often occurs in patients with end-stage liver disease, is the result of iron and folic acid deficiency, impaired iron reuptake, sequestration and destruction of RBCs in patients with portal hypertension and hypersplenism, and blood loss from variceal and gastrointestinal bleeding. Additionally, normal hematopoietic response to anemia is reduced, and irreversible marrow failure may occur in some patients.

Ascites develops when an imbalance of Starling's forces in the hepatic sinusoids and splanchnic capillaries causes excessive lymph formation, thereby exceeding the capacity of the thoracic duct to return this lymph to general circulation. Normally, most newly formed albumin (11 mg/day/g of liver) is secreted through the hepatic sinusoidal wall into the plasma or directly into the ascitic fluid.[127] Hypoalbuminemia, together with ascites formation,

results in redistribution of plasma volume and contraction of circulating plasma volume. Subsequently, the diminished effective plasma volume and increased renal tubular absorption of sodium and water result in progressive ascites and peripheral edema. Plasma volume can be increased when water retention is excessive, but patients on diuretic therapy may develop hypovolemia.

Therefore, the goals of transfusion therapy consist of maintaining normal intravascular blood volume, oxygen-carrying capacity, colloid osmotic pressure, and blood coagulability and avoiding complications associated with massive blood transfusion.

Mode of Blood Transfusion

In general, RBCs are transfused to maintain an intraoperative hematocrit of 26–28 vol%. This relatively low hematocrit is preferred to reduce RBC requirements, improve microcirculation in potentially hypothermic patients, and avoid vascular thrombosis. A large volume of colloid and crystalloid is required to compensate for the continuous formation of ascites and third-space fluid loss and to maintain colloid osmotic pressure. This goal is met by administration of a fluid mixture of RBC, FFP, and crystalloids (300 ml, 200 ml, 250 ml, respectively)[45] containing consistent hematocrit (26–28%) and coagulation factors (30–50% of normal). Administration of this fluid mixture based on hemodynamic monitoring provides relatively constant hematocrit, colloid osmotic pressure, coagulation factor level, electrolyte balance, and hydration in patients with more than 5 liters of blood loss. When blood loss is less than 5 liters, additional colloids (FFP or 5% albumin) or crystalloids are necessary to avoid hemoconcentration.

Conventional pressurized transfusion devices with blood warmers have several major drawbacks when massive transfusion (more than 300 ml/minute) is required.[128] Transfusion speed is limited by the low flow rate (maximum flow rate less than 130 ml/minute) and the time required to spike blood bags. Hypothermia may result from limited blood-warming capacity (less than 25°C at a high flow rate); operation of several devices by multiple personnel may make fine adjustments of intravascular blood volume and composition difficult. Therefore, inadvertent hypovolemia or hypervolemia and variable levels of hemoglobin and coagulation factors are unavoidable with conventional transfusion devices.

To avoid these complications, a device that delivers a large volume of premixed, prewarmed blood on demand with minimal manpower is necessary. This goal is achieved by the homemade devices developed by various institutions or commercial massive transfusion devices, such as the Rapid Infusion System (Haemonetics, Inc., Braintree, MA)[129] or System 1025 (Level 1 Technologies, Inc., Rockland, MA).

The Rapid Infusion System includes a 2.5-liter cardiotomy reservoir lined with a 170-mm filter, a countercurrent heat exchanger, a roller pump, a 40-mm micropore filter, two air detectors, a temperature sensor, a pressure sensor, recirculation tubing, two large-bore transfusion tubes, and a control panel. The cardiotomy reservoir allows the rapid transfer of blood from the blood bags and removes large particles from the blood. A calcium-containing solution must not be used in the fluid mixture because adding calcium to the blood product results in clot formation in the reservoir. The heat exchanger column warms the blood effectively: In one pass, cold blood (less than 10°C) can be warmed to greater than 33°C, and warmer blood (20°C) can be warmed to greater than 36°C. The roller pump delivers fluids at a rate between 1 ml per hour and 1.5 liters per minute. The fluid-challenge mode delivers either 100 ml or 500 ml at a flow rate of 400 ml per minute. The recirculation tubing returns warmed blood to the reservoir (400 ml/minute) where it is mixed evenly and kept warm. The on-line micropore filter (40-mm) removes most of the aggregates. Two large-caliber (0.188-in., internal diameter) tubes are attached to two 8.5 French intravenous catheters for rapid delivery of the blood. Activation of the fluid-level sensor (fluid level less than 200 ml) and any one of the air sensors stops the roller pump. Low blood temperature (less than 36°C) and high pressure inside the system (more than 300 mm Hg) slows the infusion speed. The control panel includes variable control modes, warning displays, and infusion volume. A rechargeable battery is installed as a backup power source and for transfusion during transportation. The design and function of System 1025 is similar to but simpler than the Rapid Infusion System. Clinical outcome studies of any massive transfusion device are rare, although Dunham et al. reported that the use of the Rapid Infusion System was superior to conventional modes with respect to preser-vation of body temperature, improved cellular perfusion, and reduction of coagulopathy.[130] Massive transfusion devices have pitfalls: Addition of calcium-containing solution forms clots in the reservoir, filtration function can be lost when more than 50 units of RBCs are transfused, and operator error may cause fluid overloading.

Complications of Massive Blood Transfusion

Complications associated with blood transfusion are common during liver transplantation owing to the need for massive transfusion and negligible or absent hepatic function.

Ionic hypocalcemia (citrate intoxication), caused by inadequate hepatic clearance of citrate-calcium complex, invariably occurs during liver transplantation. The serum citrate level reaches the level in the banked blood and has an inverse relationship to the serum ionized calcium level. Ionic hypocalcemia (0.56 mmol/liter) is associated with decreased blood pressure, cardiac index, and stroke-work index. These negative hemodynamic changes are reversed by the administration of calcium preparation.[131] Because a prolonged Q-T interval is not a reliable indicator for ionized hypocalcemia, the ionic calcium level should be monitored frequently and normalized to prevent serious hemodynamic and coagulation complications. For the treatment of hypocalcemia, $CaCl_2$ and equimolar doses of calcium gluconate are equally effective.[132]

Ionic hypomagnesemia occurs during liver transplantation because citrate also binds with magnesium.[133] Ionic hypomagnesemia may lead to tachycardia, hypotension, seizures, a prolonged Q-T interval, myocardial depression, or sudden death.[134] Although the clinical significance of ionic hypomagnesemia during liver transplantation is unclear, $MgCl_2$ may be given if a magnesium deficiency is thought to be the cause of hemodynamic instability.

Progressive hyperkalemia (up to 7–8 mmol/liter) occurs when a large volume of the banked blood with a high potassium content is transfused rapidly, particularly in patients with renal dysfunction.[135] Hyperkalemia (more than 6 mmol/liter) reduces conduction velocity and myocardial contractility by decreasing the resting membrane potential and the number of open calcium channels during depolarization.[136] Hyperkalemia, seen as a tall, peaked T wave on the electrocardiogram, is effectively treated with the infusion of insulin (5–10 units) and glucose (12.5 g) within 15–30 minutes, even in the absence of hepatic function.[137] The transfusion of potassium-free blood should be considered when the serum potassium level increases progressively (more than 5.5 mmol/liter) even after the administration of insulin. Blood with low potassium content is available as washed RBCs at the blood bank. Alternately, it can be prepared by washing RBCs with saline solution using an autotransfusion system on site.[138, 139]

Progressive metabolic acidosis occurs when insufficient hepatic function cannot clear acid load from transfused blood. It should be treated aggressively (base deficit less than 5 mmol/liter) to preserve myocardial function, tissue perfusion, and cellular respiration. An incremental administration of $NaHCO_3$ is recommended to correct acidosis because the hyperosmolar solution $NaHCO_3$ may lead to myocardial depression and hypotension. In patients with hypernatremia and hyperosmolality, administration of tromethamine is preferred to prevent central pontine myelinolysis.[140]

Intraoperative Autotransfusion

Intraoperative autotransfusion has been used during liver transplantation,[141–143] although the effects of residual anticoagulants, contamination from tissue thromboplastin, dissemination of infection, electrolyte imbalance, and renal dysfunction can be a concern during liver transplantation.[144] One study demonstrated that the washing cycle of autotransfusion effectively removes most of the contaminants, including bilirubin, citrate, potassium, RBC fragments, coagulation factors (I, II, and VIII), platelets, FDP, and fibrin monomers.[145] Furthermore, plasma-free hemoglobin level and bacterial contamination are clinically insignificant. However, autotransfusion is not recommended for patients with potential systemic or intra-abdominal infection and malignancy.

Kidney and Pancreas Transplantation

Blood coagulation of patients undergoing pancreas transplantation is similar to that of patients with end-stage renal disease because most patients undergoing pancreas transplantation have diabetic nephropathy.

Coagulation in Patients with End-Stage Renal Disease

Patients with end-stage renal disease may have bleeding from mucous membranes, gastrointestinal bleeding, hemorrhagic pericardial effusions, or intracranial hemorrhage,[146, 147] but the levels of coagulation factors and platelet count are within the normal ranges. The most common bleeding tendency is caused by platelet dysfunction and is seen as prolonged bleeding time. Platelet dysfunction may be caused by reduced platelet factor 3[148]; inhibition of platelet-endothelium interaction by dialyzable plasma factors; inhibition of platelet aggregation by guanidinosuccinic acid,[149] phenol, and phenolic acid in the serum of uremic patients[150]; inhibition of the release of serotonin from platelets by middle molecules[151]; increased calcium ion level associated with the increased parathyroid hormonal activity[152]; and enhanced formation of antiaggregatory endoperoxides (prostacyclin, prostaglandin E_2, and prostaglandin I_2) of vessel walls.[153, 154] Other contributing factors are modified platelet membrane receptors for vWF binding and altered platelet production of beta-thromboglobulin, platelet factor 4 (antiheparin), and platelet growth factor.[155] Platelet dysfunction of patients with end-stage renal disease is commonly reversed by dialysis.[156]

The next most common coagulation abnormality is associated with hemodialysis. The residual heparin effect may increase bleeding tendency, although it is negligible when regional heparinization technique is used. Repeated hemodialysis may cause thrombosis and the activation of fibrinolysis.[157] The thrombotic tendency appears to be caused by recurrent platelet activation, imbalance between platelets and vascular prostaglandin, activation of fibrinolysis by the release of tPA from endothelial cells, and consumption of PAI.[158] Fibrinolytic activity is increased by the release of tPA as a result of complement activation,[159] platelet activation,[160] heparin administration,[161] or tissue hypoxia.[162]

Management of Coagulation

Bleeding time is considered the best screening test because it correlates with clinical bleeding.[154, 156] Dialysis is the treatment of choice for a prolonged bleeding time. Platelets may be administered to patients with a markedly prolonged bleeding time; cryoprecipitate may reduce bleeding time in certain patients.[163] The administration of desmopressin may also shorten bleeding time, possibly by improving the binding of vWF with platelet membranes.[164]

The residual heparin effect from hemodialysis can be detected by determination of the ACT, aPTT, or TEG and reversed by protamine sulfate (25–50 mg), although rebound heparinization can occur in some patients.[165] Antiplatelet agents (prostacyclin and sulfinpyrazone) may be used for patients on long-term dialysis to prevent activation of platelets and to maintain patency of the shunts,[166, 167] although the therapy may cause bleeding in patients with platelet dysfunction.[168]

Bleeding is not a clinical concern during kidney and pancreas transplantation because dialysis is usually performed preoperatively, and surgical bleeding is limited. Intra- or postoperative thrombocytopenia is commonly caused by hyperacute or acute rejection, and antiplatelet agents (e.g., prostacyclin) and immunosuppressants are reported to be effective in treating rejection-related thrombocytopenia.[169] In severe cases of thrombocytopenia with rejection, allograft nephrectomy improves thrombocytopenia. In addition, platelet dysfunction may result from depletion of serotonin from platelets,[170] activation of platelets by the circulating immune complex, and development of microvascular thrombosis.[171]

Blood Transfusion

Significant anemia (hematocrit less than 25 vol%) is caused by decreased erythropoietin production, bone marrow depression, shortened RBC survival from oxidizing drugs and microangiopathic lesions, iron deficiency with blood loss, decreased iron absorption due to phosphate-binding antacids, deficiency of folic acid and vitamins B_{12} and B_6, and secondary hyperparathyroidism.[172] Some degree of anemia (hematocrit 24–28 vol%) is considered satisfactory because patients with renal failure tolerate anemia easily by increasing the level of 2,3-diphosphoglycerate and cardiac output and by decreasing oxygen-hemoglobin affinity. On the other hand, RBC transfusion may increase alloantibodies to leukocyte antigens,[173] which may lead to febrile nonhemolytic reaction and hyperacute rejection or poor survival of the graft kidney.[174–176] Therefore, blood transfusion is minimized

during the perioperative period, and frozen deglycerolized RBCs containing a minimal volume of white blood cells is administered to patients with severe anemia. However, graft survival appears to improve when the patients receive 2–5 units of frozen deglycerolized RBCs 3 weeks to 6 months before transplantation.[177] The protective mechanism of RBC transfusion may be associated with the selection of better-matching grafts for patients with multiple cytotoxic antibodies after homologous blood transfusion.[178] In addition, RBC transfusion may modulate the immune response by nonspecific suppression of mixed lymphocyte culture reactivity and lymphocyte proliferative response to antigens,[179] proliferation of cells directed against antigens expressed by transfused cells,[180] overloading of the reticuloendothelial system,[181] and induction of anti-idiotypic antibodies against T lymphocytes.[182]

References

1. Hosenpud JD, Novick, RJ, Breen TJ, et al. The Registry of the International Society for Heart and Lung Transplantation: twelfth official report—1995. J Heart Lung Transplant 1995;14:805–815.
2. Dietrich W, Spannagl M, Schramm W, et al. The influence of preoperative anticoagulation on heparin response during cardiopulmonary bypass. J Thorac Cardiovasc Surg 1991;102:505–514.
3. Karck M, Haverich A. Heart transplantation under Coumadin therapy: friend or foe? Eur J Anaesthesiol 1994;11:475–479.
4. Edmunds LH. HIT, HITT, and desulfatohirudin: look before you leap. J Thorac Cardiovasc Surg 1995;110:1–3.
5. Khuri SF, Valeri R, Loscalzo J, et al. Heparin causes platelet dysfunction and induces fibrinolysis before cardiopulmonary bypass. Ann Thorac Surg 1995;60:1008–1014.
6. Dawkins KD, Jamieson SW, Hunt SA, et al. Long-term results, haemodynamics and complications after combined heart-lung transplantation. Circulation 1985;71:919–926.
7. McCarthy PM, Starnes VA, Theodore J, et al. Improved survival after heart-lung transplantation. J Thorac Cardiovasc Surg 1990;99:54–60.
8. Griffith BP, Hardesty RL, Trento A, et al. Heart-lung transplantation: lessons learned and future hopes. Ann Thorac Surg 1987;43:6–16.
9. Novick RJ, Menkis AH, McKenzie FN, et al. Reduction in bleeding after heart-lung transplantation: the importance of posterior mediastinal hemostasis. Chest 1990;98:1383–1387.
10. Sarris GE, Smith JA, Shumway NE, et al. Long-term results of combined heart-lung transplantation: the

Stanford experience. J Heart Lung Transplant 1994;3: 940–949.

11. Sharples LD, Scott JP, Dennis C, et al. Risk factors for survival following combined heart-lung transplantation. Transplantation 1994;57:218–223.

12. Vouhe PR, Dartevelle PG. Heart-lung transplantation: technical modifications that may improve the early outcome. J Thorac Cardiovasc Surg 1989;97:906–910.

13. Pasque MK, Cooper JD, Kaiser LR, et al. Improved technique for bilateral lung transplantation: rationale and initial clinical experience. Ann Thorac Surg 1990;49:785–791.

14. Hunt BJ, Sack D, Amin S, Yacoub MH. The perioperative use of blood components during heart and heart-lung transplantation. Transfusion 1992;32:57–62.

15. Peterson KL, deCampli WM, Feeley TW, Starnes VA. Blood loss and transfusion requirements in cystic fibrosis patients undergoing heart-lung or lung transplantation. J Cardiothorac Vasc Anesth 1995;9:59–62.

16. Zenati M, Keenan RJ, Landreneau RJ, et al. Lung reduction as bridge to lung transplantation in pulmonary emphysema. Ann Thorac Surg 1995;59: 1581–1583.

17. Detterbeck FC, Egan TM, Mill MR. Lung transplantation after previous thoracic surgical procedures. Ann Thorac Surg 1995;60:139–143.

18. Taylor KM. Perioperative approaches to coagulation defects. Ann Thorac Surg 1993;56:S78–S82.

19. Gravlee GP, Arora S, Lavender SW, et al. Predictive value of blood clotting tests in cardiac surgical patients. Ann Thorac Surg 1994;58:216–221.

20. Taborski U, Hofmann MR, Schupphaus S, et al. Autologous hemotherapy in heart transplantation: a case report [German]. Beitr Infusionsther Transfusionsmed 1991;28:335–336.

21. Goldfinger D, Capon S, Czer L, et al. Safety and efficacy of preoperative donation of blood for autologous use by patients with end-stage heart or lung disease who are awaiting organ transplantation. Transfusion 1993;33:336–340.

22. Etchason J, Petz L, Keeler E, et al. The cost effectiveness of preoperative autologous blood donations. N Engl J Med 1995;332:719–724.

23. Spiess BD, Sassetti R, McCarthy RJ, et al. Autologous blood donation: hemodynamics in a high-risk patient population. Transfusion 1992;32:17–22.

24. Sandler SG, Scaher RA. Preoperative autologous blood donations by high-risk patients. Transfusion 1992;32:1–2.

25. Tobe CE, Vocelka C, Sepulvada R, et al. Infusion of autologous platelet rich plasma does not reduce blood loss and product use after coronary artery bypass. J Thorac Cardiovasc Surg 1993;105:1007–1014.

26. Stover EP, Siegel LC. Platelet-rich plasma in cardiac surgery; efficacy may yet be demonstrated [letter]. J Thorac Cardiovasc Surg 1994;108:1148–1149.

27. Rosengart TK, Helm RE, Klemperer J, et al. Combined aprotinin and erythropoietin use for blood conservation:

results with Jehovah's Witnesses. Ann Thorac Surg 1994;58:1397–1403.

28. Shaddy RE, Bullock EA, Tani LY, et al. Erythropoietin alfa therapy in infants awaiting heart transplantation. Arch Pediatr Adolesc Med 1995;149:322–325.

29. Cheng DC, Demajo W, Sandler AN. Lung Transplantation. In AW Gelb, MD Sharpe (eds), Anesthesiology Clinics of North America. Philadelphia: Saunders, 1994;12:749–767.

30. Lemmer JH. Reporting the results of blood conservation studies: the need for uniform and comprehensive methods. Ann Thorac Surg 1994;58:1305–1306.

31. Blauhut B, Harringer W, Bettelheim P, et al. Comparison of the effects of aprotinin and tranexamic acid on blood loss and related variables after cardiopulmonary bypass. J Thorac Cardiovasc Surg 1994;108:1083–1091.

32. Horrow JC, Van Riper DF, Strong MD, et al. The dose-response relationship of tranexamic acid. Anesthesiology 1995;82:383–392.

33. Lemmer JH, Stanford W, Bonney SL, et al. Aprotinin for coronary bypass operations: efficacy, safety, and the influence on early saphenous vein graft patency. J Thorac Cardiovasc Surg 1994;107:543–553.

34. Royston D. High-dose aprotinin therapy: a review of the first five years' experience. J Cardiothoracic Vascular Surgery 1992;6:76–100.

35. Fremes SE, Wong BI, Lee E, et al. Metaanalysis of prophylactic drug treatment in the prevention of postoperative bleeding. Ann Thorac Surg 1994;58:1580–1588.

36. Royston D. Aprotinin therapy in heart and heart-lung transplantation. J Heart Lung Transplant 1993;12: S19–S25.

37. Kesten S, de Hoyas A, Chaparro C, et al. Aprotinin reduces blood loss in lung transplant recipients. Ann Thorac Surg 1995;59:877–879.

38. Bick RL. Hemostasis defects associated with cardiac surgery, prosthetic devices, and other extracorporeal circuits. Semin Thromb Hemost 1985;11:249–280.

39. Mammen EF, Koets MH, Washington BC, et al. Hemostasis changes during cardiopulmonary bypass surgery. Semin Thromb Hemost 1985;11:281–292.

40. Khuri SF, Wolfe JA, Josa M, et al. Hematologic changes during and after cardiopulmonary bypass and their relationship to the bleeding time and nonsurgical blood loss. J Thorac Cardiovasc Surg 1992;104:94–107.

41. Kirklin JK. The Postperfusion Syndrome: Inflammation and the Damaging Effects of Cardiopulmonary Bypass. In J Tinker (ed), Cardiopulmonary Bypass: Current Concepts and Controversies. Philadelphia: Saunders, 1989;131–146.

42. Hunter DN, Morgan CJ, Yacoub M, Evans TW. Pulmonary endothelial permeability following lung transplantation. Chest 1992;102:417–421.

43. Aeba R, Griffith BP, Kormos RL, et al. Effect of cardiopulmonary bypass on early graft dysfunction in clinical lung transplantation. Ann Thorac Surg 1994;57:15–22.

44. Francalancia NA, Aeba R, Yousem SA, et al. Deleteri-

ous effects of cardiopulmonary bypass on early graft function after single lung allotransplantation: evaluation of a heparin-coated bypass circuit. J Heart Lung Transplant 1994;13:498–507.

45. Kang YG, Martin DJ, Marquez J, et al. Intraoperative changes in blood coagulation and thromboelastographic monitoring in liver transplantation. Anesth Analg 1985;64:888–896.

46. Speiss BD, Ivankovich AD. Thromboelastography: A Coagulation-Monitoring Technique Applied to Cardiopulmonary Bypass. In N Ellison, DR Jobes (eds), Effective Hemostasis in Cardiac Surgery. Philadelphia: Saunders, 1988;163–181.

47. Wang JS, Lin CY, Hung WT, et al. Thromboelastogram fails to predict postoperative hemorrhage in cardiac patients. Ann Thorac Surg 1992;53:435–439.

48. Spiess BD, Tuman KJ, McCarthy RJ, et al. Thromboelastogram and postoperative hemorrhage [letters, and reply to editor]. Ann Thorac Surg 1992;54:810–813.

49. Ballard HS, Marcus AJ. Platelet aggregation in portal cirrhosis. Arch Intern Med 1976;136:316–19.

50. Canoso RT, Hutton RA, Deykin D. The hemostatic defect of chronic liver disease. Gastroenterology 1979; 76:540–547.

51. Aster RH. Pooling of platelets in the spleen: role in the pathogenesis of "hypersplenic" thrombocytopenia. J Clin Invest 1966;45:645–657.

52. Lindenbaum J. Folate and vitamin B_{12} deficiencies in alcoholism. Semin Hematol 1980;17:119–129.

53. Cowan DH. Effect of alcoholism on hemostasis. Semin Hematol 1980;17:137–147.

54. Thomas DP, Ream VJ, Stuart RK. Platelet aggregation in patients with Laennec's cirrhosis of the liver. N Engl J Med 1967;276:1344–1348.

55. Owen JS, Hutton RA, Day RC, et al. Platelet lipid composition and platelet aggregation in human liver disease. J Lipid Res 1981;22:423–430.

56. Karpatkin KS, Freedman ML. Hypersplenic thrombocytopenia differentiated from increased peripheral destruction by platelet volume. Ann Intern Med 1978; 89:200–203.

57. Martinez J, Palascak JE, Kwasniak D. Abnormal sialic acid content of the dysfibrinogenemia associated with liver disease. J Clin Invest 1978;61:535–538.

58. Green G, Thomson JM, Dymock IW, Poller L. Abnormal fibrin polymerisation in liver disease. Br J Haematol 1976;34:425–439.

59. Green AJ, Ratnoff OD. Elevated antihemophilic factor (AHF, factor VIII) procoagulant activity and AHF-like antigen in alcoholic cirrhosis of the liver. J Lab Clin Med 1974;83:189–197.

60. Colman RW, Rubin RN. Blood Coagulation. In IM Arias, WB Jakoby, H Popper, et al. (eds), The Liver: Biology and Pathobiology. New York: Raven Press, 1988;1033–1042.

61. Knot EAR, Drijfhout HR, ten Cate JW, et al. α_2-Antiplasmin inhibitor metabolism in patients with liver cirrhosis. J Lab Clin Med 1985;105:353–358.

62. Saito H, Goodnough LT, Boyle JM, Heimburger N. Reduced histidine-rich glycoprotein levels in plasmas of patients with advanced liver cirrhosis: possible implications for enhanced fibrinolysis. Am J Med 1982;73: 179–182.

63. Fletcher AP, Biederman O, Moore D, et al. Abnormal plasminogen-plasmin system activity (fibrinolysis) in patients with hepatic cirrhosis: its cause and consequences. J Clin Invest 1964;43:681–695.

64. Tyagt G, Collen D, DeBreker RR, Verstraete M. Investigators on the fibrinolytic system in liver cirrhosis. Acta Haematol (Basel) 1968;40:265–274.

65. Bontempo FA, Lewis JH, Ragni MV, Starzl TE. The Perioperative Coagulation Pattern in Liver Transplant Patients. In PM Winter, YG Kang (eds), Hepatic Transplantation: Anesthetic and Perioperative Management. New York: Praeger, 1986;135–141.

66. Seligsohn U, Shani M, Ramot B, et al. Dubin-Johnson syndrome in Israel. II. Association with factor-VII deficiency. QJM 1970;39:569–584.

67. Seligsohn U, Shani M, Ramot B. Gilbert syndrome and factor VII deficiency [letter]. Lancet 1970;1:1398.

68. Groth CG, Pechet L, Starzl TE. Coagulation during and after orthotopic transplantation of the human liver. Arch Surg 1969;98:31–34.

69. Von Kaulla KN, Kaye H, Von Kaulla E, et al. Changes in blood coagulation, before and after hepatectomy or transplantation in dogs and man. Arch Surg 1966;92:71–79.

70. Flute PT, Rake MO, Williams R, et al. Liver transplantation in man. IV. Haemorrhage and thrombosis. BMJ 1969;3:20–23.

71. Groth CG. Changes in Coagulation. In TE Starzl (ed), Experience in Hepatic Transplantation. Philadelphia: Saunders, 1969;159–175.

72. Owen CA Jr., Rettke SR, Bowie EJW, et al. Hemostatic evaluation of patients undergoing liver transplantation. Mayo Clin Proc 1987;62:761–772.

73. Lewis JH, Bontempo FA, Awad SA, et al. Liver transplantation: intraoperative changes in coagulation factors in 100 first transplants. Hepatology 1989;9:710–714.

74. Kratzer MAA, Dieterich J, Denecke H, Knedel M. Hemostatic variables and blood loss during orthotopic human liver transplantation. Transplant Proc 1991;23: 1906–1911.

75. Kang Y, Lewis JH, Navalgund A, et al. Epsilon-aminocaproic acid for treatment of fibrinolysis during liver transplantation. Anesthesiology 1987;66:766–773.

76. Porte RJ, Bontempo FA, Knot EA, et al. Systemic effects of tissue plasminogen activator-associated fibrinolysis and its relation to thrombin generation in orthotopic liver transplantation. Transplantation 1989;47: 978–984.

77. Virji MA, Aggarwal S, Kang Y. Alterations in plasminogen activator and plasminogen activator inhibitor levels during liver transplantation. Transplant Proc 1989;21(Suppl 3):3540–3541.

78. Kang YG. Monitoring and Treatment of Coagulation. In PM Winter, YG Kang (eds), Hepatic Transplantation:

Anesthetic and Perioperative Management. New York: Praeger, 1986;151–173.

79. Himmelreich G, Dooijewaard G, Breinl P, et al. Changes in urokinase-type plasminogen activator in orthotopic liver transplantation. Semin Thromb Hemost 1993;19:311–314.

80. Lewis JH, Bontempo FA, Ragni MV, Starzl TE. Antithrombin III during liver transplantation. Transplant Proc 1989;21:3543–3544.

81. Böhmgig HJ. The coagulation disorder of orthotopic hepatic transplantation. Semin Thromb Hemost 1977;4:57–82.

82. Riess H, Jochum M, Machliedt W, et al. Possible role of extracellularly released phagocyte proteinase in the coagulation disorder during liver transplantation. Transplantation 1991;52:482–490.

83. Starzl TE, Marchioro TL, von Kaulla KN, et al. Homotransplantation of the liver in humans. Surg Gynecol Obstet 1963;117:659.

84. DeWolf A, Gologorsky E, Scott V, et al. Intravascular and intracardiac thrombus formation and pulmonary thromboembolism immediately after graft reperfusion in six patients undergoing liver transplantation [abstract]. Liver Transplant Surg 1995;1:416.

85. Suriani RJ, Cutrone A, Cohen E, et al. Pulmonary thromboembolism during liver transplantation: is venovenous bypass protective [abstract]? Liver Transplant Surg 1995;1:416.

86. Hutchinson DE, Genton E, Porter KA, et al. Platelet changes following clinical and experimental hepatic homotransplantation. Arch Surg 1968;97:27–33.

87. Homatas J, Wasantapruek S, von Kaulla E, et al. Clotting abnormalities following orthotopic and heterotopic transplantation of marginally preserved pig livers. Acta Hepato-Spleno 1969;l2:14–27.

88. Porte RJ. Coagulation and fibrinolysis in orthotopic liver transplantation: current views and insights. Semin Thromb Hemost 1993;19:191–196.

89. Schlam SW, Terpstra JL, Achterberg JR, et al. Orthotopic liver transplantation. An experimental study on mechanisms of hemorrhagic diathesis and thrombosis. Surgery 1975;78:400–507.

90. Himmelreich GK, Hundt K, Neuhaus P, et al. Decreased platelet aggregation after reperfusion in orthotopic liver transplantation. Transplantation 1992;53:582–586.

91. Ferrara A, MacArthur JD, Wright HK, et al. Hypothermia and acidosis worsen coagulopathy in the patient requiring massive transfusion. Am J Surg 1990;160:515–518.

92. Machioro TL, Huntley RT, Waddell WR, Starzl TE. Extracorporeal perfusion of obtaining postmortem homografts. Surgery 1963;54:900–911.

93. Zuckerman L, Cohen L, Vagher JP, et al. Comparison of thrombelastography with common coagulation tests. Thromb Haemost 1981;46:752–756.

94. Blanchard RA, Furie BC, Jorgensen M, et al. Acquired vitamin K–dependent carboxylation deficiency in liver disease. N Engl J Med 1981;305:242–248.

95. Lewis JH, Doyle AP. Effect of epsilon aminocaproic acid on coagulation and fibrinolytic mechanism. JAMA 1964;188:56–63.

96. Munoz SJ, Ballas BE, Moritz MM, et al. Perioperative management of fulminant and subfulminant hepatic failure with therapeutic plasmapheresis. Transplant Proc 1989;21:3535–3536.

97. Azad SC, Kratzer MAA, Groh J, et al. Intraoperative monitoring and postoperative reevaluation of hemostasis in orthotopic liver transplantation. Semin Thromb Hemost 1993;19:233–237.

98. Ickx B, Pradier O, Degroote F, et al. Effect of two different dosages of aprotinin on perioperative blood loss during liver transplantation. Semin Thromb Hemost 1993;19:300–301.

99. Kang Y, Gelman S. Liver Transplantation. In S Gelman (ed), Anesthesia and Organ Transplantation. Philadelphia: Saunders, 1986;139–186.

100. Weber T, Marino IR, Kang YG, et al. Intraoperative blood transfusions in highly immunized patients undergoing orthotopic liver transplantation. Transplantation 1989;47:797–801.

101. Dutcher JP, Schiffer CA, Aisner J, Wiernik PH. Alloimmunization following platelet transfusion: the absence of dose-response relationship. Blood 1981;57:395–398.

102. Palareti G, Legagni C, Maccaferri M, et al. Coagulation and fibrinolysis in liver transplantation. The role of the recipient's disease and the use of antithrombin-III concentrates. Haemostasis 1991;21:68–76.

103. Kang Y. Thromboelastography in liver transplantation. Semin Thromb Hemost 1995;21(Suppl 4):34–44.

104. McNicol GP, Fletcher AP, Alkjaersig N, Sherry S. The absorption, distribution, and excretion of ε-aminocaproic acid following oral or intravenous administration to man. J Lab Clin Med 1962;59:15–24.

105. Kang Y. Coagulation and liver transplantation. Transplant Proc 1993;25:2001–2005.

106. Rake MO, Flute PT, Parnell G, Williams R. Intravascular coagulation in acute hepatic necrosis. Lancet 1970;1:533–537.

107. Carlier M, Veyckemans F, Scholtes JL, et al. Anesthesia for pediatric hepatic transplantation: experience of 33 cases. Transplant Proc 1987;19:3333–3337.

108. Klinck JR, Boylan JF, Sandler AN, et al. Tranexamic acid prophylaxis during liver transplantation: a randomized controlled trial [abstract]. Hepatology 1993;18:728.

109. Ickx B, Pierre S, Pradier M, et al. Comparison of two different antifibrinolytic treatments in the prevention of bleeding during orthotopic liver transplantation [abstract]. Liver Transplant Surg 1995;1:410.

110. Neuhaus P, Bechstein WO, Lefebre B, et al. Effect of aprotinin on intraoperative bleeding and fibrinolysis in liver transplantation. Lancet 1989;2:924–925.

111. Mallett SV, Cox D, Burroughs AK, Rolles K. Aprotinin and reduction of blood loss and transfusion requirements in orthotopic liver transplantation [letter]. Lancet 1990;336:886–887.

112. Grosse H, Lobbes W, Frambach M, et al. The use of

high dose of aprotinin in liver transplantation: the influence of fibrinolysis and blood loss. Thromb Res 1991; 63:287–297.

113. Himmelreich G, Kierzek B, Neuhaus P, et al. Fibrinolytic changes and the influence of the early perfusate in orthotopic liver transplantation with intraoperative aprotinin treatment. Transplant Proc 1991;23:1936–1937.

114. Riess H. The Use of Aprotinin in Liver Transplantation. In R Plfarré (ed), Blood Conservation with Aprotinin. Philadelphia: Hanley & Belfus, 1995;349–358.

115. Groh J, Welte M, Azad SC, et al. Does aprotinin really reduce blood loss in orthotopic liver transplantation? Semin Thromb Hemost 1993;19:306–308.

116. Himmelreich G, Muser M, Neuhaus P, et al. Different aprotinin applications influencing hemostatic changes in orthotopic liver transplantation. Transplantation 1992;53:132–136.

117. Ickx B, Pradier O, Degroote F, et al. Effect of two different dosages of aprotinin on perioperative blood loss during liver transplantation. Semin Thromb Hemost 1993;19:300–301.

118. Suarez M, Sangro B, Herrero J, et al. Effectiveness of aprotinin in orthotopic liver transplantation. Semin Thromb Hemost 1993;19:292–296.

119. Hunt BJ, Cottam S, Segal H, et al. Inhibition by aprotinin by tPA-mediated fibrinolysis during orthotopic liver transplantation. Lancet 1990;336:381.

120. Kang Y, DeWolf AM, Aggarwal S. In vitro study of the effects of aprotinin on coagulation during orthotopic liver transplantation. Transplant Proc 1991;23: 1934–1935.

121. Anderson TLG, Solem JO, Tengborn L, Vinge E. Effects of desmopressin acetate on platelet aggregation, von Willebrand factor, and blood loss after cardiac surgery with extracorporeal circulation. Circulation 1990;81:872–878.

122. Mannuccio PM, Vicente V, Vianello L, et al. Controlled trial of desmopressin in liver cirrhosis and other conditions associated with a prolonged bleeding time. Blood 1986;67:1148–1153.

123. Kang Y, Scott V, DeWolf A, et al. In vitro effects of DDAVP during liver transplantation. Transplant Proc 1993;25:1821–1822.

124. Kang Y, Borland LM, Picone J, Martin LK. Intraoperative coagulation changes in children undergoing liver transplantation. Anesthesiology 1989;71:44–47.

125. Massaferro V, Esquivel CO, Makowka L, et al. Hepatic artery thrombosis after pediatric liver transplantation: medical or surgical event? Transplantation 1989;47:971–977.

126. Bontempo FA, Lewis JH, Gorenc TJ, et al. Liver transplantation in hemophilia A. Blood 1987;69:1721–1724.

127. Zimmon DS, Oratz M, Kessler R, et al. Albumin to ascites: demonstration of a direct pathway bypassing the systemic circulation. J Clin Invest 1967;48:2074.

128. Dula DJ, Muller HA, Donovan JW. Flow rate variance of commonly used IV infusion techniques. J Trauma 1981;21:480–482.

129. Sassano JJ. The Rapid Infusion System. In PM Winter, YG Kang (eds), Hepatic Transplantation: Anesthetic and Perioperative Management. New York: Praeger, 1986;120–134.

130. Dunham CM, Belzberg H, Lyles R, et al. The rapid infusion system: a superior method for the resuscitation of hypovolemic trauma patients. Resuscitation 1991;21: 207–227.

131. Marquez J, Martin D, Kang YG, et al. Cardiovascular depression secondary to citrate intoxication during hepatic transplantation in man. Anesthesiology 1986; 65:457–461.

132. Martin TJ, Kang Y, Robertson KM, et al. Ionization and hemodynamic effects of calcium chloride and calcium gluconate in the absence of hepatic function. Anesthesiology 1990;73:62–65.

133. Scott V, Kang Y, DeWolf A, et al. Altered ionized magnesium level in plasma during orthotopic liver transplantation [abstract]. Hepatology 1993;18:725.

134. Altura BM, Altura BT. Mg, Na, and K interactions and coronary heart disease. Magnesium 1982;1:241–265.

135. Young LE. Complications of blood transfusion. Ann Intern Med 1964;61:136–146.

136. Schipperheyn JJ. The pathophysiology of potassium and magnesium disturbances. A cardiac perspective. Drugs 1984;28(Suppl 1):112–119.

137. DeWolf A, Frenette L, Kang Y, Tang C. Insulin decreases the serum potassium concentration during the anhepatic stage of liver transplantation. Anesthesiology 1993;78:677–682.

138. Belani KG, Estrin JA. Biochemical and hematologic effects of intraoperative processing of CPDA-1 and AS-1 packed red cells [abstract]. Anesthesiology 1987;67: A156.

139. Brown MR, Ramsay MA, Swygert TH. Exchange autotransfusion using the cell saver during liver transplantation. Anesthesiology 1989;70:168–169.

140. Videira R, Kang YG, Martinez J, et al. A rapid increase in sodium is associated with CPM after liver transplantation [abstract]. Anesthesiology 1991;75(3A):A222.

141. Lindop MJ, Farman JV, Smith MF. Anaesthesia: Assessment and Intraoperative Management. In RY Calne (ed), Liver Transplantation. London: Grune & Stratton, 1983;128–129.

142. Dzik WH, Jenkins R. Use of intraoperative blood salvage during orthotopic liver transplantation. Arch Surg 1985;120:946–948.

143. Van Voorst SJ, Peters TG, Williams JW, et al. Autotransfusion in hepatic transplantation. Am Surg 1985;51:623–626.

144. Hauer JM, Thurer RL. Controversies in autotransfusion. Vox Sang 1984;46:8–12.

145. Kang Y, Aggarwal S, Virji M, et al. Clinical evaluation of autotransfusion during transplantation. Anesth Analg 1991;72:94–100.

146. Kazatchkine M, Sultan YU, Caen JP, Bariety J. Bleeding in renal failure: a possible cause. BMJ 1976;2:612–615.

147. Carvalho, A. Bleeding in uremia—a clinical challenge [editorial]. N Engl J Med 1983;308:38–39.

148. Rabiner SF, Hrodek O. Platelet factor 3 in normal subjects and patients with renal failure. J Clin Invest 1968;47:901–912.

149. Horowitz HI, Stein IM, Cohen BD, White JG. Further studies on the platelet inhibitory effect of guanidinosuccinic acid: its role in uremic bleeding. Am J Med 1970;49:336–345.

150. Rabiner SF, Molinas F. The role of phenol and phenolic acids on the thrombocytopathy and defective platelet aggregation of patients with renal failure. Am J Med 1970;49:346–351.

151. Castaldi PA, Rosenberg MC, Stewart JH. Bleeding disorder of uraemia. Lancet 1966;2:66–69.

152. Gura V, Creter D, Levi J. Elevated thrombocyte calcium content in uremia and its correction by a 1 alpha (OH) vitamin D treatment. Nephron 1982;30:237–239.

153. Rao AK, Walsh PN. Acquired qualitative platelet disorders. Clin Haematol 1983;12:201–238.

154. DiMinno G, Martinez J, McKeann M, et al. Platelet dysfunction in uremia: multifaceted defect partially corrected by dialysis. Am J Med 1985;79:552–559.

155. Green D, Santhanam S, Krumlovsky FA, del Greco F. Elevated beta-thromboglobulin in patients with chronic renal failure; effect of hemodialysis. J Lab Clin Med 1980;95:679–685.

156. Stewardt JH, Castaldi PA. Uraemic bleeding: a reversible platelet defect corrected by dialysis. QJM 1967;36:409–423.

157. Jorgensen KA, Ingeberg S. Platelets and platelet function in patients with chronic uremia on maintenance hemodialysis. Nephron 1979;23:233–236.

158. Nakamura Y, Tomura S, Tachibana K, et al. Enhanced fibrinolytic activity during the course of hemodialysis. Clin Nephrol 1992;38:90–96.

159. Hakim RM, Breillatt J, Lazarus JM, Port FK. Complement activation and hypersensitivity reactions to dialysis membranes. N Engl J Med 1984;311:878–882.

160. Hakim RM, Schafer AI. Hemodialysis-associated platelet activation and thrombocytopenia. Am J Med 1985;78:57–80.

161. Speiser W, Wojta J, Korninger C, et al. Enhanced fibrinolysis caused by tissue plasminogen activator release in hemodialysis. Kidney Int 1987;32:280–283.

162. Tappy L, Hauert J, Bachmann F. Effects of hypoxia and acidosis on vascular plasminogen activator release in the pig ear perfusion system. Thromb Res 1984;33:117–124.

163. Janson PA, Jubelirer SJ, Weinstein MS, Beykin D. Treatment of bleeding tendency in uremia with cryoprecipitate. N Engl J Med 1980;303:1318–1322.

164. Mannucci PM, Remuzzi G, Pusineri F, et al. Deamino-8-D-arginine vasopressin shortens the bleeding time in uremia. N Engl J Med 1983;308:8–12.

165. Hampers CL, Blanfox MD, Merrill JP. Anticoagulant rebound after hemodialysis. N Engl J Med 1988;275:776–778.

166. Turney JH, Williams LC, Fewell MR, et al. Platelet protection and heparin sparing with prostacyclin during regular dialysis therapy. Lancet 1980;2:224–226.

167. Woods HF, Ash G, Weston MJ. Sulfinpyrazone reduced deposition of fibrin on dialyzer membranes [abstract]. Thromb Haemost 1979;42:401.

168. Lindsay RM, Prentice CRM, Davidson JF, et al. Hemostatic changes during dialysis, associated with thrombus formation on dialysis membrane. BMJ 1972;4:454–458.

169. Mundy AR, Bewick M, Moncada S, Vane JR. Short term suppression of hyperacute renal allograft rejection in presensitized dogs with prostacyclin. Prostaglandins 1980;19:595–603.

170. Capitanio A, Mannucci PM, Ponticelli C, Pareti F. Detection of circulating released platelets after renal transplantation. Transplantation 1982;33:298–301.

171. Moncada S, Vane, JR. Arachidonic acid metabolites and the interactions between platelets and blood vessel walls. N Engl J Med 1979;300:1142–1147.

172. Perkins HA. Transfusion of Patients with End-Stage Renal Disease. In LD Petz, SN Swisher (eds), Clinical Practice of Blood Transfusion. New York: Churchill Livingstone, 1981;485.

173. Dausset J. Leuko-agglutinins. IV. Leuko-agglutinins and blood transfusion. Vox Sang 1957;4:190.

174. Kissmeyer-Nielsen F, Olsen S, Petersen VP, Fjeldborg O. Hyperacute rejection of kidney allografts associated with pre-existing humoral antibodies against donor cells. Lancet 1966;1:662.

175. Patel R, Terasaki PI. Significance of the positive crossmatch test in kidney transplantation. N Engl J Med 1969;280:735.

176. Terasaki PI, Kreisler M, Michey RM. Presensitization and kidney transplant failures. Postgrad Med J 1971;47:89.

177. Feduska NJ, Amend WJ, Vincenti F, et al. Blood transfusions before and on the day of transplantation: effects on cadaver graft survival. Transplant Proc 1982;13:175.

178. Joysey VC. Some Effects of Blood Transfusion. In RY Calne (ed), Transplantation Immunology. London: Oxford University Press, 1984;278.

179. Maki T, Monaco AP. Impaired T-cell function after allogeneic blood transfusion in mice. Transplant Proc 1983;15:997.

180. Terasaki PI. The beneficial transfusion effect on kidney graft survival attributed to clonal deletion. Transplantation 1984;37:119–125.

181. Keown PA, Descamps B. Hypothesis: improved renal allograft survival after blood transfusion: a nonspecific, erythrocyte-mediated immunoregulatory process? Lancet 1979;1:20–22.

182. Singal DP, Joseph S. Role of blood transfusions on the induction of antibodies against recognition sites on T lymphocytes in renal transplant patients. Hum Immunol 1982;4:93–108.

Chapter 17
Biology of Immunosuppression and Immunosuppressive Agents

Debra A. Hullett, Dilly M. Little, and Hans W. Sollinger

Chapter Plan

Allograft rejection remains one of the most significant problems in transplantation despite the introduction of several new immunosuppressive agents. The ultimate goal of current strategies for developing new immunosuppressive agents and most of the basic research in transplant immunobiology is to develop graft-specific immunosuppression and peripheral tolerance. This chapter discusses the fundamentals of transplant immunobiology in the context of current organ transplantation and develops the idea of specific transplant tolerance.

Historic Aspects of Transplant Immunobiology

The phenomena of graft rejection was pioneered in the early 1900s by the studies of Tyzzer,[1] Little,[2] and Loeb,[3] who described the rejection of transplantable tumors in inbred strains of mice. Their work led to the concept of a biochemical difference between donor and recipient. The biochemical difference was later attributed to the independent segregation of multiple genes, which became known as histocompatibility genes.[4] Gorer's work provided the first evidence for an immune reaction to foreign tissue.[5] The presence of anti–donor-specific antibodies in the serum of mice who had rejected a tumor graft suggested the interaction of foreign tissue with the recipient's immune system. In the 1940s, however, Medawar and colleagues established that rejection is an active acquired immune response that is specific to the donor, is systemic, and involves the development of memory.[6, 7] Their conclusion was based on the accelerated or second-set rejection of a secondary skin allograft transplanted to recipients carrying a primary allograft from the same donor.

The concept of transplant tolerance was developed by the pioneering studies of Owen et al.[8] and

Medawar and colleagues.[9] Owen described tolerance of freemartin twin calves who shared hematopoietic circulation during fetal development. Medawar explored this further, describing neonatal tolerance.[9] Understanding of the immune system and its response to an organ allograft is greatly facilitated by the use of molecular biology techniques, which have been used to create transgenic and knockout recipients who lack or express specific components of the immune system. Thus, the understanding of the role of major histocompatibility complex (MHC) as antigens and the activation of T-helper lymphocytes as a result of presentation of antigens has greatly increased.

Transplant Immunobiology

The rejection of an organ allograft is a complex process involving the presentation and recognition of foreign antigen (transplanted organ), the involvement of costimulatory molecules, and the generation of effector cells or cytokines.

Cells Involved in Mediating an Immune Response

Allograft rejection is mediated by immunocompetent lymphocytes. These include T cells, B cells, macrophages, and NK cells. T cells can be defined both functionally and by the expression of cell surface glycoproteins. The majority of T-helper cells interact with class II–expressing, antigen-presenting cells (APCs) and express CD4 on their surface. The CD8 subpopulation of T cells interacts with MHC class I and is primarily responsible for cytotoxic effector function. The T-helper subpopulation can be further defined on the basis of the cytokine secretion pattern after activation. Th-1 helper cells secrete primarily interleukin-2 (IL-2) and interferon-gamma (IFN-γ) and provide the help necessary for the differentiation of cytotoxic T lymphocytes (CTLs) to cytolytic function. Th-1 helper cells are sensitive to inhibition by cyclosporine and tacrolimus (FK506). Th-2 helper cells secrete IL-4 and IL-10. This helper subset is primarily responsible for helping B cells differentiate into immunoglobulin-secreting plasma cells.

A second cell type involved in allograft rejection is the B lymphocyte. B lymphocytes interact with antigens via their surface immunoglobulin receptor, and with appropriate T-cell help, undergo class switch from immunoglobulin M (IgM) to IgG synthesis and secretion. Immunoglobulins play an important role in hyperacute rejection and may be involved in chronic rejection.

Macrophages and interstitial dendritic cells also play an important role in graft rejection. These cells function primarily in antigen presentation. In this capacity, antigen is processed or degraded by the APC and then displayed on the surface of the APC in association with MHC molecules. In addition, macrophages may play a role in cytotoxicity by being directly cytotoxic or by secreting cytotoxic lymphokines.

The Major Histocompatibility Complex and the Proteins Involved in Allograft Responses

The recognition of foreign protein occurs in the context of histocompatibility molecules. These molecules are cell-surface glycoproteins that vary between individuals of a species and result in incompatibility between donor and recipient. The primary locus involved in graft rejection is the major histocompatibility locus, although graft rejection can be stimulated by differences at minor histocompatibility loci. The MHC consists of three families of molecules: the class I, class II, and class III molecules. The class III molecules consist of members of the complement cascade and are not discussed further. Class I molecules are expressed on nearly all nucleated cells and consist of heterodimeric molecules. The class I heavy chain (45 kd) is highly polymorphic and is associated with a smaller, nonpolymorphic light chain called *beta$_2$-microglobulin*. Bjorkman and colleagues described the crystal structure for class I and introduced the concept of foreign antigen binding within a groove created by the alpha$_1$ and alpha$_2$ domains of class I.[10] The N-terminal portion of the class I heavy chain forms a platform, with a large groove consisting of eight antiparallel beta strands and two alpha helices. The groove is thought to provide the binding site for processed foreign antigen. The recognition of foreign antigen by T cells involves residues from the alpha helices and the peptide bound within the groove. In general, class I molecules bind peptides that are nine amino acids long. Initial characterization of peptides bound within

Figure 17-1. T-cell activation. After interaction of the T-cell receptor with major histocompatibility complex (MHC)/antigen (Ag) and costimulation by interaction of B7 with CD28, phosphorylation of the CD3 chain occurs. Phosphorylation is probably mediated by the src-family kinase Lck. This results in the activation of the syk-family kinase ZAP-70. Phosphorylation of phospholipase C (PLC) leads to the generation of second messengers that elevate intracellular calcium and protein kinase C. This results in the activation of several nuclear-binding factors (NF-AT, AP-1, NF-κB) and transcription factors required for cytokine gene expression. (APC = antigen-presenting cell.)

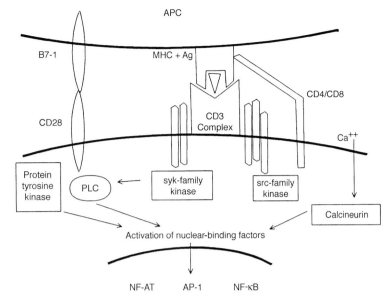

the groove has suggested the importance of certain sequence motifs.

Class II molecules are highly polymorphic, cell-surface glycoproteins expressed on a limited number of cell types. Class II is expressed on macrophages, dendritic cells, B cells, and, in some species, endothelial cells. Class II molecules are also expressed on T cells after activation. The class II surface structure is composed of a heterodimer containing a 35-kd and a 28-kd chain. The N-terminus of each chain is thought to form a helix. The peptide-binding groove consists of the alpha$_1$ domain of each chain. Compared to class I molecules, the peptide bound within the groove is longer (23 amino acids) and extends over the ends of the groove.

An important difference between class I and II molecules is the source of the peptides bound in the groove. Class I peptides derive primarily from cytoplasmic proteins, which are cleaved within the endoplasmic reticulum. Binding of peptide within the groove of class I peptide stabilizes the conformational structure, allowing interaction with beta$_2$-microglobulin and expression on the cell surface. In contrast, class II peptides derive primarily from extracellular proteins that undergo endocytosis by APC and are processed or degraded in endocytic vesicles. Because of the pH within the vesicle, invariant chain, which normally protects the peptide-binding site of class II, is released, and peptides are then bound. Bound peptide is then expressed on the APC surface in the context of class II.

T-Cell Receptor

The receptor on the surface of the T cells for class I- or class II-containing bound peptide consists of a heterodimer, called the *alpha* and *beta chains*, which are cell surface glycoproteins of approximately 40–50 kd. Like the MHC molecules, the T-cell receptor (TcR) is extremely polymorphic. MHC polymorphism, along with the genomic structure of the TcR, is responsible for the specificity of T cell recognition and for the variation in foreign antigen (alloantigen) responsiveness. The TcR exists on the cell surface as a complex with several other proteins, which together make up the CD3 complex. These proteins are primarily responsible for signal transduction leading to T cell activation after recognition of MHC and foreign antigen on the surface of an APC. The structure of the TcR and subsequent signaling events are shown in Figure 17-1.

Costimulatory Molecules

Lafferty and Cunningham[11] and Bretscher and Cohn[12] have demonstrated that two signals are required for lymphocyte activation. The first signal is the recognition of antigen in the context of MHC by the TcR. The second signal is a costimulatory signal provided by metabolically active APC. One of the important second signals is provided by the interaction of CD28 with B7-1. Other molecules implicated in providing costimulatory signals include CTLA4,

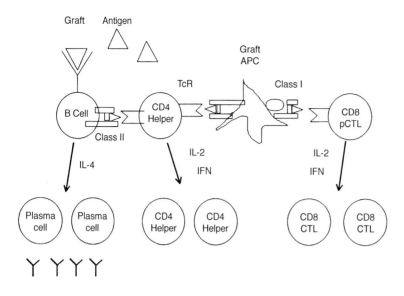

Figure 17-2. Model of allograft rejection. Graft alloantigen presented by either donor antigen-presenting cells (interstitial dendritic cells) or recipient antigen-presenting cells (macrophages, dendritic cells, or B cells) may result in the direct activation of cytotoxic T lymphocytes (CTL) or T helper cells, or both. Activated T and B cells undergo differentiation and clonal expansion in response to increased cytokine synthesis to become effector cells. Cytokines act both in an autocrine and paracrine fashion. (APC = antigen-presenting cell; IFN = interferon; IL = interleukin; TcR = T-cell receptor; pCTL = precursor cytotoxic T lymphocyte.)

heat-stable antigen, and B7-2. The interaction of the TcR with MHC and antigen in the absence of a costimulatory signal results in the functional inactivation of the responding T cell, a process termed *anergy.*

The interaction of responding T cell with donor APC or recipient APC presenting processed foreign antigen is strengthened by the interaction of several accessory molecules. Included in these accessory interactions are the interaction of CD4 and MHC class II, CD8 with MHC class I, and leukocyte function–associated antigen-1 (LFA-1) with the intracellular adhesion molecules 1 and 2 (ICAM-1, ICAM-2). These molecules contribute to cell adhesion, activation, and specific effector functions.

Route of Antigen Presentation

The recognition of alloantigen can occur through two pathways. One pathway is the recognition of MHC directly by either CD4+ or CD8+ T cells on professional donor APC that are able to provide signal 2 (costimulation) and are present in the graft. This has been termed the *direct pathway*, or *pathway 2*. The recognition of allopeptide in the context of self (recipient) class I or II molecules has been termed the *indirect pathway*. Some results from numerous laboratories have suggested that both pathways are involved in graft rejection.

Mechanisms of Graft Rejection

The process of graft rejection is complex and involves several cell types. There is considerable controversy regarding the role of antibody, cytotoxic T cells, NK cells, and delayed type hypersensitivity (DTH) in the destruction of the graft. The schematic shown in Figure 17-2 gives an overview of the possible mechanisms of graft rejection. The first step in graft rejection is the recognition of alloantigen on either donor or recipient APC. This interaction results in the activation of the responding T cells, which then undergo differentiation and induction of cytokine synthesis. Cytokines play an important role in the upregulation of MHC class I and II expression (IFN-γ), cell activation and clonal expansion of cytotoxic T cells and NK cells (IL-2 and IFN-γ), the activation and differentiation of B cells to antibody-secreting plasma cells (IL-4 and IL-6), and the activation of cytocidal macrophages (tissue necrosis factor). In the second step of graft rejection, the responding cells undergo clonal proliferation and expansion under the influence of IL-2, IFN-γ, and IL-4. In the final step, differentiation to effector populations occurs. This involves the production of serine esterases in cytotoxic T cells, DTH response in the CD4+ population, and antibody synthesis and secretion from plasma cells.

Tolerance in Transplant Immunobiology

Tolerance can be defined as the long-term stable acceptance of an allograft in the absence of immunosuppressive therapy. The objective of the transplant immunobiologist is to achieve long-term graft-specific peripheral tolerance. Peripheral tolerance may result from one of three pathways: clonal deletion, anergy, or the development of regulatory cells. Although clonal deletion readily occurs in the thymus during the education of emerging T cells (the clones with overreactivity to self are deleted), peripheral clonal deletion is controversial.[13] Kroemer and Martinez have suggested that clonal deletion in the periphery results from the irregular activation of T cells.[14] Cross-linking of the CD3/TcR complex without APC, simultaneous cross-linking of CD3/TcR and class I, or independent cross-linking of CD3/TcR and CD4 are examples of irregular activation.

The interaction of TcR with MHC and peptide in the absence of costimulatory signal results in the functional inactivation of the responding T cell, a process termed *anergy*. The anergic T cell resists subsequent challenge with antigen and metabolically functional APC. However, anergy can be overcome by IL-2 addition.[15, 16] Guerder and Matzinger have suggested that peripheral T cell tolerance results from the recognition of signal 1 in the absence of signal 2 when presented by naive B cells.[17] In contrast, Th-2 CD4+ cells may be activated by B cells.

Some experiments have suggested that anergy varies in different T-cell subsets.[17, 18] Anergic Th-1 CD4+ T cells do not proliferate or produce IL-2 in response to antigenic challenge. Anergic Th-2 CD4+ T cells proliferate in response to antigenic challenge but fail to secrete lymphokines. Studies have suggested that CD8+ cytolytic T cells may also become anergic.[18] Anergy in this case probably results from the absence of CD4+ T-cell help (IL-2).

The third route for achieving peripheral tolerance is through the generation of regulatory cells (suppression). The generation of regulatory cells may be achieved through three pathways:

1. A CD8+, class I+, class II−, or low, bone-marrow-derived veto-like cell of donor origin has been described by Thomas and colleagues in a nonhuman primate model of renal allograft tolerance.[19]
2. An autoreactive CD4+ or CD8+ T cell has been described in a syngeneic graft-versus-host disease

model[20] and in the downregulation of autoimmunity in an experimental allergic encephalomyelitis model.[21]
3. A CD4+ T suppressor cell.[22, 23] Veto cell activity has been suggested as the mediator of prolonged graft survival after blood transfusion.[24]

Wood and colleagues have used anti-CD4 antibody treatment in combination with donor-specific transfusion before transplantation to induce tolerance to heart grafts.[22] In this study, the mechanism of tolerance was suggested to be a disruptive interaction of TcR/CD4 with donor APC as a result of the presence of anti-CD4 antibody (steric hindrance). These studies suggest a pivotal role for CD4+ T cells in the development of peripheral tolerance. Alternatively, Waldmann and colleagues have described a process termed *infectious tolerance*.[23] Tolerance in this model also depended on the presence of CD4+ T cells. Moreover, these T cells were capable of transferring tolerance to a naive population.

Graft Rejection

Broadly defined, rejection is an immunologic response elicited by a genetic disparity between donor and recipient, resulting in injury to the engrafted organ. In transplantation biology, the most important genetic differences are antigens of the MHC and major blood groups, and possibly tissue-specific antigens, such as those expressed on endothelial and reticuloendothelial cells. Like other immune responses, rejection demonstrates both specificity and memory, whereby re-exposure to previously encountered antigens results in a more rapid and vigorous response. Therefore, the clinical and pathophysiologic manifestations of rejection depend on the context in which the process develops.

Traditionally, allograft rejection has been classified into the distinct phases of hyperacute, acute, and chronic rejection. This may be a somewhat artificial classification of a process that frequently manifests considerable overlap, at least clinically.

Hyperacute Rejection

Hyperacute rejection results from preformed cytotoxic antibodies directed against graft antigen. With the institution of pretransplantation cross-match, its incidence has been dramatically reduced. Clinically, hyperacute rejection is characterized by rapid and widespread intravascular thrombosis occurring after vascular reperfusion of the organ. The engrafted organ suddenly appears cyanotic or mottled in color and fails to function. Immunofluorescence of graft biopsy may reveal IgG, IgM, or complement deposition in the vascular walls and in the thrombi. Characteristically, the thrombi incorporate polymorphonuclear cells.

Hyperacute rejection must be differentiated from other causes of extensive intravascular graft thrombosis, such as physical perfusion-related injury to vascular endothelium and injury related to cold agglutinins. Both these conditions may result in acute intragraft thrombosis in the immediate postoperative period. Hemolytic-uremic syndrome, either recurring in the graft or associated with a cyclosporine-induced thrombotic microangiopathy, generally manifests later in the posttransplant period.[25]

Acute Rejection

Approximately 50% of allograft recipients have at least one episode of acute allograft rejection during the lifetime of the transplanted organ.[26] Acute rejection can occur at any time after transplantation and is characterized clinically by rapid deterioration in graft function. Obviously, this presents a diagnostic dilemma because a number of other factors, such as drug toxicity, allograft infarction, systemic infection, or even dehydration, may adversely affect graft function.

Because early diagnosis and appropriate treatment of an acute rejection episode is mandatory to preserve long-term graft function, accurate and reliable diagnosis must be made. Depending on the organ involved, a number of clinical and biochemical parameters are used to monitor for rejection (Table 17-1). However, histologic examination of a graft biopsy specimen remains the diagnostic gold standard. The pathologic appearance of acute allograft rejection is generally characterized by an acute inflammatory response within the transplanted organ associated with a dense cellular infiltrate, predominantly composed of lymphocytes (Figure 17-3).

Table 17-1. Frequently Used Diagnostic Tests to Clinically Monitor and Diagnose Acute Allograft Rejection in Transplanted Organs

Organ	Diagnostic Test
Heart	Ejection fraction per electrocardiogram
	Coronary angiography
	Endomyocardial biopsy
Kidney	Serum creatinine
	Glomerular filtration rate
	Biopsy
Liver	Serum bilirubin
	Liver function tests
	Biopsy
Lung	Pulmonary function tests
	Bronchoscopy
	Bronchoalveolar lavage
	Transbronchial biopsy
Pancreas	Blood glucose, HbA_{1C}
	Glucose tolerance test
	Insulin release assay
Intestine	Urinary amylase (if exocrine secretions drain into urinary bladder)
	Random endoscopic biopsy

HbA_{1C} = glycosylated hemoglobin.

Chronic Rejection

The clinical entity of chronic vascular rejection was first described by Hume et al. in a 6-month human renal allograft.[27] With improved diagnosis and treatment of acute rejection, chronic rejection is emerging as a significant cause of allograft dysfunction and loss.[28, 29] Current definitions of chronic rejection have been hampered by the lack of universally applied diagnostic criteria. A working definition has to take into consideration both clinical and pathologic parameters because neither set of criteria in isolation is sufficient. Clinically, chronic allograft rejection is defined as a gradual but progressive functional deterioration of the allograft, typically occurring months or years after transplantation and ultimately leading to graft failure. Morphologically, chronic rejection is characterized by the progressive narrowing of hollow structures within the graft, regardless of whether they are vessels, bile ducts, or bronchioles. Whether the process is vanishing bile duct syndrome (Figure 17-4) in liver allografts, progressive glomerulosclerosis in kidney allografts, bronchi-

Figure 17-3. Hematoxylin-eosin stain of biopsy specimen of a transplanted kidney showing obliteration of arterial lumen (L) with inflammatory cells (*large arrows*) and endothelial proliferation (*small closed arrows*) consistent with severe acute cellular rejection. Note the propensity of inflammatory cells (plasma cells and lymphocytes) in the interstitium (*small open arrows*). (Courtesy of Dr. C. Guiraudon, London Health Sciences Centre, London, Ontario, Canada.)

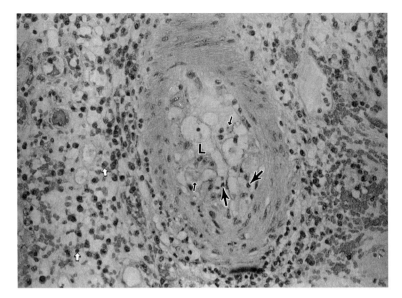

olitis obliterans in lung allografts, or accelerated atherosclerosis (Figure 17-5) in heart allografts, the common pathologic feature observed in all chronically rejecting grafts is progressive arterial intimal thickening with eventual vascular occlusion.

Tissue and Blood Group Typing

Blood Group Typing

Similar to blood transfusion incompatibility, the ABO blood group antigens behave as strong transplantation antigens. Transplantation across ABO barriers usually leads to rapid hyperacute rejection of the allograft and systemic hemolysis. It is assumed that rejection is caused by antibody reacting with blood group A or B antigens (or both) on the vascular endothelium.[30] There have been a number of reports of successful ABO-incompatible renal transplants, however. Successful cadaveric renal transplantation from blood group A_2 donors to blood group O recipients have been reported.[31] This may reflect a reduced recipient IgM anti-A_2 titer as well as low donor antigen expression seen in the "low-secretor" phenotype. Antibodies to blood group antigens other than ABO can be relevant to transplantation. For example, antibodies directed against the Ii system can cause hyperacute rejection of cooled donor organs.[32]

Major Histocompatibility Complex

The human MHC, otherwise termed the *HLA complex*, is encoded by a series of genes located on the short arm of chromosome 6. The concentration of HLA genes in one defined area of the chromosome allows these genes to be inherited as a packet or haplotype. Each individual inherits a haplotype of HLA genes from each parent, which together constitute the individual's HLA profile.

As previously outlined, the HLAs can be divided into two classes based on their structure and cellular distribution. Class I molecules are named HLA-A, -B, and -C and are expressed on all nucleated cells. Class II molecules are named HLA-DP, -DQ, and -DR and are expressed on most B and activated T lymphocytes, monocytes, dendritic cells, renal glomerular and tubular cells, and capillaries. In clinical transplantation, the A, B, and DR antigens are considered the most important. The remarkable degree of polymorphism exhibited by these antigens accounts for the difficulty in accurate tissue matching. Since the 1970s, the recognized HLA specificities have been classified according to nomenclature designated by the World Health Organization.[33] Through international cooperation, a large number of HLA specificities have been identified by standard serologic microcytotoxicity assay and typed. Matching of antigens against this known database of recog-

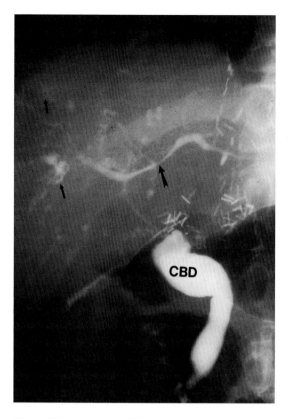

Figure 17-4. Radiograph of liver transplant after percutaneous transhepatic cholangiogram showing diffuse narrowing (*large arrow*) and absence of intrahepatic ducts and ectasia of smaller bile ducts (*small arrows*) consistent with chronic rejection (vanishing bile duct syndrome). The native common bile duct (CBD) appears normal. (Courtesy of Dr. W. Wall, London Health Sciences Centre, London, Ontario, Canada.)

nized tissue antigens provides the basis of the current practice of tissue typing.

In most instances, T lymphocytes are capable of recognizing processed foreign antigen only in the context of MHC molecules expressed on the surface of the target cell. Therefore, accurate matching of these antigens between donor and recipient should theoretically prevent or at least reduce the incidence of allograft rejection. In practice, however, because of the high degree of polymorphism exhibited by the HLA and the presence of "minor" histocompatibility antigens, absolute matching can be achieved only in homozygous twins. In fact, tissue typing has been demonstrated to significantly improve long-term graft outcome in the case of renal transplantation, in which successful matching of HLA-DR in particular appears to confer a benefit.[34, 35] The positive benefits of HLA tissue typing in other solid-organ transplantations remain inconclusive.[36]

Tissue-Typing Techniques

Lymphocytes are generally used for tissue typing because of the high level of surface expression of HLA antigens. The basic test used is the "cytotoxicity reaction," which types a cell depending on the binding of a specific antibody to the cell surface in the presence of complement, to cause cell lysis. Testing for class I specificities is performed on peripheral blood lymphocytes. Class II typing requires B lymphocytes.

The Microlymphocytotoxicity Test

This serologic test is the most common method of determining class I antigens. Lymphocytes from the person to be typed are tested against a panel of antisera defining each of the HLA types under standard conditions. Maternal antibodies produced against fetal antigens present in the serum of pregnant women are the primary source of antibodies used. After addition of rabbit complement and incubation, cell lysis is determined using eosin exclusion staining.

Mixed Lymphocyte Culture

When lymphocytes from one individual are mixed in culture with those of an unrelated individual, both groups of cells proliferate. This phenomenon is the basis of the mixed lymphocyte reaction and is determined by mismatching at the class II locus. This test is therefore used for typing of class II loci: Test lymphocytes are mixed in tissue culture with homozygous typing cells that have been irradiated to prevent their proliferation in response to the test cells. The test cells that lack the specificities of the typing cells recognize them as foreign and are stimulated to undergo proliferation (recognized by the uptake of [³H] thymidine into DNA) and transformation (recognized visually).

The application of molecular biology techniques to the HLA complex has made possible new and more precise methods of HLA typing. Restriction endonuclease digestion of HLA genes produces patterns that depend on the restriction endonuclease,

Figure 17-5. Mowat's stain of epicardial artery showing obliteration of lumen (L) with marked intimal proliferation (*arrow*) consistent with chronic rejection. (M = media.) (Courtesy of Dr. C. Guiraudon, London Health Sciences Centre, London, Ontario, Canada.)

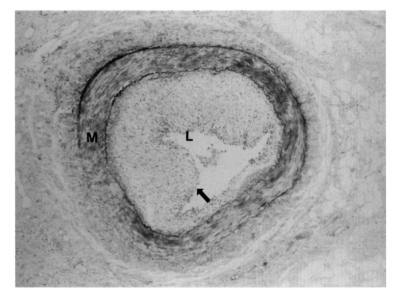

HLA gene, and probe used. These restriction patterns may correlate with particular HLA types; therefore, HLA typing can be performed by this method.

Oligonucleotide typing has emerged as a prime candidate for HLA typing. Because each HLA allele has a unique nucleotide sequence that differentiates it from every other allele, it is possible to synthesize an oligonucleotide that will hybridize only to this unique sequence. A set of tagged oligonucleotides corresponding to various alleles at a given locus can then be tested for hybridization to an individual's DNA, identifying the allele he or she possesses.

Cross-Matching

The pretransplant lymphocyte cross-match detects preformed HLA antibodies in the serum of the transplant recipient directed against the lymphocytes of the proposed donor. This test has assumed paramount importance because transplant of an organ in the presence of a positive cross-match invariably results in hyperacute rejection. In a modification of the cytotoxicity assay, recipient serum and donor lymphocytes are co-incubated at either 5°C (cold cross-match) or 37°C (warm cross-match). After addition of complement, cell lysis indicates a positive cross-match. False-positive cross-match results may be produced by antibodies that are typically reactive at low temperatures. In general, these antibodies are IgM "autoantibodies" or "non-HLA antibodies." They are more common in patients with autoimmune disease (e.g., systemic lupus erythematosus). Performing the cross-match test at 37°C or using a reducing agent, such as dithiothreitol, can reduce the incidence of these false positives.

The flow cytometric cross-match, which was introduced in 1983, is reported to have a 30- to 250-fold greater sensitivity than the standard cytotoxicity assay.[37] Because it also detects low-level, non–complement-binding antibodies, however, the clinical relevance of such "positive" results have been questioned. Multiple studies have helped to define the clinical significance of the flow cytometry to the point that it is now considered a useful component of the pretransplant evaluation of the sensitized patient.[38]

Panel-Reactive Antibodies

To determine whether a potential organ recipient is likely to have a positive cross-match against a donor at the time of transplantation, the microlymphocytotoxicity test can be used to screen for preformed anti-HLA cytotoxicity antibodies. The patient's serum is incubated at different temperatures with B and T cells from a panel of donors selected to represent the HLA specificities. Complement is added and cell lysis detected as previously described. The results are usually expressed as the percentage of panel cells that show positive antibody activity, or "panel-reactive antibodies" (PRA). Previous blood transfusion or transplantation and pregnancy are the most common source of these antibodies.[38] The

Table 17-2. Immunosuppressive Agents

Cyclosporine
Tacrolimus (FK506)
Mycophenolate (RS-61443)
Prednisone
Azathioprine
Antilymphocyte globulin
OKT3
Investigational immunosuppressive agents
    Rapamycin
    Leflunomide
    Deoxyspergualin
    Monoclonal antibodies specific for CD4, LFA-1,
       ICAM-1, and CTLA4

Table 17-3. Commonly Used Drugs That Affect Cytochrome P-450 Activity

Drugs that induce cytochrome P-450 activity
    Anticonvulsants
        Carbamazepine
        Phenobarbitone
        Phenytoin
        Primidone
    Isoniazid
    Nafcillin
    Norfloxacin
    Rifampin
Drugs that inhibit cytochrome P-450 activity
    Azole antifungals
        Fluconazole
        Itraconazole
        Ketoconazole
    Calcium channel blockers
        Diltiazem
        Nicardipine
        Verapamil
    Fluoroquinolones (e.g., ciprofloxacin)
    Macrolide antibiotics (e.g., erythromycin)
    Metoclopramide
    Oral contraceptives

higher the patient's percentage PRA, the more difficult it is to find a cross-match negative.

Immunosuppressive Agents

Currently Used Immunosuppressive Agents

Currently used immunosuppressive agents include cyclosporine, tacrolimus, mycophenolate mofetil (RS-61443), prednisone, azathioprine, antilymphocyte globulin (ALG), and OKT3 (Table 17-2).

Cyclosporine

Cyclosporine (as well as tacrolimus) is an early T-cell activation inhibitor. Its primary mechanism of interaction is to interfere with calcium-mediated signaling events after delivery of signal 1 and signal 2 to the T cell. Thus, they are especially effective in preventing T cell–mediated graft rejection, such as development of CTL or DTH effector functions associated with acute rejection. In addition, because they interfere with IL-2 and IL-2 receptor expression, they are effective in preventing the clonal expansion of alloreactive T cells.

In blood, 30% of absorbed cyclosporine is found in plasma, bound primarily to lipoproteins. Most of the remaining drug is bound to erythrocytes. The parent drug has a half-life of approximately 8 hours and is metabolized to at least 15 metabolites by the cytochrome P-450 hepatic microsomal enzyme system. Therefore, numerous drug interactions may

occur between many commonly used drugs that either induce or depress this metabolic system (Table 17-3). Tacrolimus is also metabolized by the P-450 system. Therapeutic blood levels are therefore used to assess and modify the drug dosage of these immunosuppressive agents and to monitor for toxicity. Apart from the obvious side effects of any immunosuppressive drug (i.e., an increased risk of infection), nephrotoxicity is the most important and frequent side effect of cyclosporine (Table 17-4). Hepatotoxicity is a dose-dependent phenomenon manifested by a reversible increase in bilirubin, liver enzymes, and alkaline phosphatase; a reduction in the cyclosporine dose usually resolves these changes. Neurotoxicity may manifest as headache, tremor, peripheral neuropathy, and seizures (which may be triggered by hypomagnesemia due to renal loss). Electrolyte disturbances may include hyperkalemia, hypomagnesemia, and hyperuricemia.

Tacrolimus

Tacrolimus is a macrolide antibiotic and has a mechanism of action similar to cyclosporine. It is almost entirely metabolized by the cytochrome P-

Table 17-4. Side Effects of Immunosuppressive Agents

Agent	Side Effects
Cyclosporine	Nephrotoxicity
	Hypertension
	Hepatic dysfunction
	Neurotoxicity: headaches, tremor, seizures, peripheral neuropathy
	Gingival hypertrophy
	Hyperkalemia
	Hypomagnesemia
	Hyperuricemia
	Lymphoproliferative disease
Tacrolimus (FK506)	Nephrotoxicity
	Hyperkalemia
	Neurotoxicity: headache, tremor
	Nausea and vomiting
	Flushing
	Hyperglycemia
	Psychological disturbances: nightmares, mood changes
Mycophenolate (RS-61443)	Bone marrow depression: leukopenia
	Nausea, vomiting, diarrhea
Azathioprine	Bone marrow suppression: leukopenia, thrombocytopenia, macrocytic anemia
	Bleeding
	Hepatic dysfunction
	Pancreatitis
	Nausea, vomiting, diarrhea
OKT3	Fever, chills
	Nausea, vomiting
	Pulmonary edema
	Hypotension, hypertension
	Neurotoxicity: headache, seizures, aseptic meningitis
	Nephrotoxicity
Polyclonal antiserum (ALG/ATG)	Fever, chills
	Serum sickness
	Thrombocytopenia
	Phlebitis, erythema
	Anaphylaxis
	Nephrotoxicity
	Lymphoproliferative disease
Steroids	Salt and water retention
	Hyperglycemia
	Hypertension
	Electrolyte disorders: hypokalemia, hypocalcemia
	Peptic ulceration
	Infection
	Osteoporosis
	Myopathy
	Psychological disturbances: insomnia, euphoria, depression, mood swings, steroid psychosis
	Cataracts
	Cushingoid features

450 system; therefore, concomitant administration of drugs known to affect cytochrome P-450 activity (see Table 17-2) affects plasma levels of tacrolimus. Side effects include nausea or vomiting and flushing, which may occur shortly after intravenous administration and last approximately 1 hour. Like cyclosporine, tacrolimus is nephrotoxic and occasionally may cause hyperkalemia. Hyperglycemia may occur due to the ability of tacrolimus (and cyclosporine) to inhibit insulin release.

Mycophenolate

Mycophenolate mofetil (and azathioprine) are antimetabolites that interfere with cell proliferation by depleting nucleotides required for DNA synthesis. These agents are selective for lymphocytes because lymphocytes are not efficient users of nucleotide salvage pathways and primarily depend on de novo nucleotide synthesis. RS-61443, a morpholino ester of mycophenolic acid, noncompetitively inhibits the enzyme inosine monophosphate dehydrogenase, a key enzyme involved in de novo purine nucleotide biosynthesis, leading to a depletion of guanine nucleotides. Both drugs may give rise to profound leukopenia due to bone marrow suppression. Drug action is monitored by daily white blood cell (WBC) count in the immediate posttransplant period and regular outpatient monitoring of WBC levels while the patient remains on the drug.

Azathioprine

Azathioprine has a similar mechanism of action to mycophenolate: It interferes with the proliferative response of WBC to antigenic stimulation. Specifically, it inhibits phosphoribosyl pyrophosphate aminotransferase, an enzyme involved in purine metabolism. Profound bone marrow suppression resulting in leukopenia and thrombocytopenia increases the risk of infection and bleeding, respectively. Occasionally, azathioprine is associated with significant hepatotoxicity and pancreatitis, necessitating withdrawal of the drug. As for mycophenolate, WBC counts are monitored regularly while the patient remains on the drug.

OKT3

OKT3 and ALG are immunoglobulin reagents that specifically interact with T cells. OKT3 is a mono-clonal antibody specific for an epitope in the TcR/CD3 complex targeting the CD3-ε chain. Its mechanism of action is not fully understood. Studies suggest that OKT3 may block the TcR interaction with MHC or antigen, however, resulting in modulation of CD3 complex expression. Alternatively, it may induce the complement-dependent clearance of T cells.

Significant, potentially life-threatening adverse reactions may occur during the first days of treatment with OKT3. These adverse reactions occur as the percentage of potent T cells plummets and a series of T cell-derived cytokines, including tumor necrosis factor, IL-2, and IFN-γ, are released into the circulation. This cytokine release syndrome is normally clinically manifest as fever, pulmonary edema, deteriorating renal function, and neurologic sequelae, ranging from mild headache to seizures. Because this cytokine release may occur after the first dose of OKT3, obvious caution must be exercised if the initial induction dose is administered during the course of the transplant procedure itself because many of the clinical signs may then be masked by anesthesia.

A further drawback to the use of OKT3 is the generation of an antimouse immunoglobulin humoral response because OKT3 is a murine monoclonal antibody. Studies are currently under way to determine the efficacy of a humanized OKT3 monoclonal antibody. In these studies, a fusion protein was genetically engineered to contain the constant region of human immunoglobulin fused with the variable region from OKT3. Several other monoclonal antibodies directed against the TcR/CD3 complex, including BMA 031, T10B9.1A-31, and BC3, are currently in clinical trials.

Polyclonal Antisera

ALG and ATG are polyclonal antisera specific for T cells, usually derived from rabbit or horse serum. Their mechanism of action is thought to be complement-dependent depletion of T cells. Most of the side effects of polyclonal antibodies relate to the release of foreign protein. Chills, fever, and arthralgia are common, although the severe first-dose reactions seen with OKT3 tend not to occur. There have been occasional reports of anaphylaxis and a serum sickness–like illness occurring during prolonged treatment.

Because of the potent immunosuppressive effects of these agents, patients treated with either

OKT3 or ALG preparations are at considerable risk of developing infection and neoplasia. In particular, the risk of posttransplant lymphoproliferative disease increases significantly.

Steroids

Prednisone is widely used as an immunosuppressive and anti-inflammatory agent and is often used in high doses to reverse acute rejection. Its mechanism of action was thought to be interference with antigen presentation by disruption of IL-1 metabolism. Some studies have suggested that prednisone and other glucocorticoid drugs mediate suppression of the immune response by preventing a nuclear binding protein (NF-kB) required for expression of numerous cytokines from reaching the nucleus. Active NF-kB is bound by a cytoplasmic inhibitor IkBα. Prednisone upregulates the synthesis of IkBα. Clinically, all the well-documented side effects of steroid administration (see Table 17-4) are associated with prolonged administration. The usual precautions with regard to anesthesia must be applied to these patients.

New Immunosuppressive Agents

Currently, more than 25 immunosuppressive agents are under investigation for the prevention of acute allograft rejection (see Table 17-2). These include rapamycin; leflunomide; deoxyspergualin; monoclonal antibodies specific for CD4, LFA-1, and ICAM-1; and CTLA4-Ig (a fusion protein that binds B7-1). In addition, several studies are investigating the potential of class I–derived peptides and soluble class I for the prevention of graft rejection and the induction of recipient tolerance. At the time of this writing, a clinical trial is under way to determine the efficacy of class I peptide therapy.

Rapamycin

Rapamycin is a macrocyclic antibiotic that is structurally similar to FK506. Although rapamycin also binds to the FK506-binding proteins, its mechanism of action does not appear to involve inhibition of calcineurin activity. The exact mechanism remains to be identified. Rapamycin blocks cell proliferation by inhibiting growth factor–dependent signaling, such as interfering with IL-2

receptor signaling events. It appears to block cells at the G1/S interface of the cell cycle. This activity may be mediated by rapamycin-mediated inhibition of the ribosomal protein S6 kinase, which is involved in G1 cell cycle progression. One of the most important aspects of rapamycin-mediated immunosuppression may be its ability to inhibit chronic rejection.

Leflunomide

Leflunomide is an isoxazole derivative that is rapidly converted to a water-soluble derivative with a half-life of 10–30 hours. Evidence has suggested that leflunomide is a tyrosine kinase inhibitor. This would account for its ability to inhibit both cell proliferation and the response to cytokines.

Deoxyspergualin

The agent 15-deoxyspergualin (a peptide-like molecule) is a derivative of spergualin isolated from the bacterium *Bacillus laterosporus*. Its mechanism of action appears to be different from that of other T-cell immunosuppressive agents. Evidence suggests that it does not act directly on lymphocyte proliferation but prevents the differentiation to effector function. In addition, deoxyspergualin inhibits both T-cell–dependent and T-cell–independent humoral responses. Finally, in vitro studies suggest that deoxyspergualin may interact directly with APCs, inhibiting their ability to process and present peptides. The primary protein interaction of deoxyspergualin in the cytoplasm is with Hsc70, a member of the heat shock protein 70 family. Because heat shock proteins may be involved in transport of peptides within the cell, interferences with this pathway may prevent antigen presentation. The ability to inhibit humoral responses along with limited toxicity makes deoxyspergualin a promising new immunosuppressive therapy.

Monoclonal Antibodies

Prolongation of allograft survival with monoclonal antibody to CD4 (OKT4) treatment was first observed in cynomolgus monkeys in 1980. As with the OKT3 antibody, OKT4 has been humanized by combining the binding site of OKT4 with a variable-region framework and constant region of either human IgG1 or IgG4 (OKT4a). Significant graft prolongation has been achieved in cynomolgus monkeys with these infusion proteins. An advantage to anti-CD4 immunosuppressive therapy is the potential for induction of donor-specific tolerance. Studies in rodents suggest this possibility. Studies by Wood and colleagues and Waldmann and colleagues using anti-CD4 treatment before allografting demonstrate not only graft prolongation but also specific tolerance.[22, 23] Tolerance in both models is thought to depend on the continued presence of CD4[+] T cells. It has been suggested that the mechanism of tolerance is a disruption of the interaction of the TcR/CD4 molecule with donor APC as a result of the presence of the anti-CD4 antibody.

Adhesion molecules facilitate the interaction of lymphocytes with the extracellular environment, endothelium, cytotoxic T cell targets, and APCs. The role of adhesion molecules in multiple steps of the immune response makes them excellent candidates for targeted immunosuppressive therapy. LFA-1, a member of the beta$_2$ integrin family along with its receptor, ICAM-1, has been the subject of extensive study. In animal models, treatment with antibodies to LFA-1 or ICAM-1 has shown graft prolongation. Induction of specific donor tolerance has been variable. Although the exact mechanism is unknown, one possible route for tolerance induction with anti-LFA-1/ICAM-1 therapy is disruption of adhesion molecule interaction during antigen presentation and delivery of signal 2 costimulation, resulting in the development of anergy. Although anti-LFA-1 or anti-ICAM-1 therapy alone have been shown to prolong graft survival, combined therapy with both antibodies is most effective. Limited clinical trials with anti-LFA-1/ICAM-1 therapy have shown reduced incidence of rejection, but large doses of antibody were required to achieve therapeutic levels.

Stimulation of an immune response requires not only recognition of foreign antigen in the context of MHC (signal 1) but also the delivery of signal 2 costimulation mediated by the interaction of CD28 with B7-1/B7-2. Delivery of signal 1 in the absence of signal 2 results in T-cell anergy. Other molecules implicated in the delivery of signal 2 include CTLA4. Linsley and colleagues created a fusion protein consisting of the extracellular domains of CD28 and the constant region of human immunoglobulin, termed *CTLA4Ig*.[39] This molecule binds effectively to B7-1. In vitro blocking studies

have demonstrated inhibition of alloreactivity. In vivo studies have demonstrated prolonged human islet allograft in mice and heart allograft survival in rats. Other studies have suggested that combination therapy with donor-specific transfusion may result in long-term graft survival and the induction of donor-specific tolerance.

Conclusions

Although many new immunosuppressive agents have been developed and are currently being investigated for their therapeutic effect, the objective remains to develop agents that specifically suppress the allograft response in a donor-specific manner. To this end, new approaches involving the use of class I peptides, soluble class I molecules, or gene therapy to express donor class I in thymus provide hope that donor-specific tolerance can be achieved.

References

1. Tyzzer EE. A study of inheritance in mice with reference to their susceptibility to transplantable tumors. Am J Pathol 1909;21:519–573.
2. Little CC. The genetics of tissue transplantation in mammals. J Cancer Res 1924;8:75–95.
3. Loeb L. Transplantation and individuality. Physiol Rev 1930;10:547–616.
4. Snell GD. Methods for the study of histocompatibility genes. J Genetics 1948;49:87–103.
5. Gorer PA. The genetic and antigenic basis of tumour transplantation. J Pathol Bacteriol 1937;44:691–697.
6. Medawar PB. The behaviour and fate of skin autografts and skin homografts in rabbits. J Anat 1944;78:176–199.
7. Medawar PB. Immunity to homologous grafted skin. II. The relationship between the antigens of blood and skin. Brit J Exp Pathol 1946;27:15–24.
8. Owen RD. Immunogenetic consequences of vascular anastomoses between bovine twins. Science 1945;102:400.
9. Billingham RE, Brent L, Medawar PB. "Actively acquired tolerance" of foreign cells. Nature 1953;172:603–606.
10. Bjorkman PJ, Saper MA, Samaraoni B, et al. Structure of the human class I histocompatibility antigen, HLA-A2. Nature 1987;329:506.
11. Lafferty KJ, Cunningham AJ. A new analysis of allogeneic interactions. Aus J Exp Biol Med Sci 1975;53:27.

12. Bretscher P, Cohn M. A theory of self-non-self discrimination. Science 1970;169:1042.

13. Bloom BR, Modlin RL, Salgame P. Stigma variations: observations on suppressor T cells and leprosy. Ann Rev Immunol 1992;10:453.

14. Kroemer G, Martinez AC. Mechanisms of self-tolerance. Immunol Today 1992;13:401.

15. Jenkins MK. Relevance of the two signal model of T cell activation to transplantation biology. Transplant Sci 1993;3:33.

16. Krummel MF, Allison JP. CD28 and CTLA-4 have opposing effects on the response of T cells to stimulation. J Exp Med 1995;182:459.

17. Guerder S, Matzinger P. A fail-safe mechanism for maintaining self-tolerance. J Exp Med 1992;176:553.

18. Otten GR, Germain RN. Split anergy in a CD8+ T cell: receptor-dependent cytolysis in the absence of interleukin-2 production. Science 1991;251:1228.

19. Thomas JM, Carver FM, Kasten-Jolly J, et al. Transplantation tolerance in nonhuman primates: a case for veto cells. Transplant Sci 1993;3:69.

20. Herber-Katz H. The autoimmune T cell receptor epitopes, idiotopes, and malatopes. Clin Immunol Immunopathol 1990;55:1.

21. Kumar V, Secarz EE. The involvement of T cell receptor peptide-specific regulatory CD4+ T cells in recovery from antigen-induced autoimmune disease. J Exp Med 1993;178:909.

22. Bushell A, Pearson TC, Morris PJ, Wood KJ. Donor-recipient microchimerisn is not required for tolerance induction following recipient pretreatment with donor-specific transfusion and anti-CD4 antibody. Transplantation 1995;59:1367.

23. Qin S, Cobbold SP, Pope H, et al. "Infectious" transplantation tolerance. Science 1993;259:974.

24. Burlingham WJ. The blood transfusion effect. In D Thirus, A Waldman (eds), Pathology and Immunology of Renal Transplantation. Oxford, UK: Blackwell (in press).

25. Van Buren D, Van Buren CT, Flechner SM, et al. De novo haemolytic uremic syndrome in renal transplant recipients immunosuppressed with cyclosporine. Surgery. 1985;98:54–62.

26. Gulanikar AC, MacDonald AS, Sungurtekin U. Belitsky P. The incidence and impact of early rejection episodes on graft outcome in recipients of first cadaver kidney transplants. Transplantation. 1992;53:323–328.

27. Hume DM, Merrill JP, Miller BF, Thorn GW. Experiences with renal homotransplantation in the human: report of nine cases. J Clin Invest 1955;34:327.

28. Cook D. Clinical Transplantation. Los Angeles: UCLA Tissue Typing Laboratory, 1987;277.

29. Land W. Kidney transplantation—state of the art. Transplant Proc 1989;21:1425.

30. Paul LC, van Es LA, Brutel de la Riviere G, et al. Blood group B antigen on renal endothelium as a target for rejection in an ABO-incompatible recipient. Transplantation 1978;26:268–271.

31. Alexander GPJ, Latinne D, Carlier M, et al. ABO-incompatibility and organ transplantation. Transplant Rev 1991;5:230–240.

32. Belzer FO, Kountz SL, Perkins HA. Red cell cold agglutinins as a cause of failure of renal allotransplantation. Transplantation 1971;11:422–424.

33. Bodmer JG, Marsh SGE, Albert ED, et al. Nomenclature for factors of the HLA system 1990. Tissue Antigens 1991;37:97–104.

34. Held PJ, Kahan BD, Hunsicker LG, et al. The impact of HLA mismatches on the survival of first cadaveric kidney transplants. N Engl J Med 1994;331:765–770.

35. Takemoto S, Carnahan E, Terasaki PI. A report of 504 six antigen-matched transplants. Transplant Proc 1991;23:1318–1320.

36. Pollack MS, Ballantyne CM, Payton-Rous C, et al. HLA match and other immunological parameters in relation to survival, rejection severity, and accelerated coronary artery disease after heart transplant. Clin Transplant 1990;269:269–275.

37. Garovoy MR, Rheinschmidt M, Bigos M, et al. Flow cytometry analysis: a high technology cross-match facilitating transplantation. Transplant Proc 1983;15:1939–1941.

38. Scornik JC, Brunson ME, Howard RJ, Pfaff WW. Alloimmunization, memory, and the interpretation of crossmatch results for renal transplantation. Transplantation 1992;54:389–394.

39. Larson CP, Elwood ET, Alexander DZ, et al. Long-term acceptance of skin and cardiac allografts after blocking CD40 and CD28 pathways. Nature 1996;381:434–438.

Chapter 18

Infections in the Transplant Patient

Sally H. Houston, Julie A. Larkin, and John T. Sinnott

Chapter Plan

Maintaining a chronic state of immunosuppression is vital to the success of transplantation but carries with it risks of infection, drug toxicity, and malignancy. Although advances in diagnosis and management of infection have been achieved, infectious complications continue to be the major cause of morbidity and mortality in the allograft recipient.[1] More than 80% of renal transplant patients experience an infectious complication,[2] and infection remains the leading cause of death after heart transplantation.[3, 4] Miller et al. reviewed acute infection in 814 consecutive heart transplant patients and found that the rate of infection during the 6 months after transplantation was 34%.[5] By 18 months, 31% of heart transplant recipients had one or more episodes of infection, with an overall mortality of 13% per episode. Aggressive immunosuppression with the aim of preventing rejection escalates the incidence and severity of infection in this population.[6] Other factors that increase the risk of infection in the heart transplant population include age, compliance, and the etiology of the underlying heart disease. Patients transplanted for ischemic heart disease tend to have a higher frequency of infection than do those transplanted for other reasons. An older mean age may explain this trend.[7] Heart-lung transplants average 2.74 infections per patient, 61% of which involve the lungs.[8] Liver transplantation centers report infection rates of 47–80%, a mean of 0.8–2.5 infectious episodes per patient, and an infection related mortality of 20–30%.[9–12] Risk factors for infection in liver recipients include postoperative dialysis, age older than 20 years, gastrointestinal or vascular complications, intensive care unit (ICU) stay longer than 15 days, and a low preoperative serum albumin.[10] The duration of the operation and the number of previous procedures also affect the infection risk in these patients.[13] Infection is the most frequent complication and the major cause of death in pancreatic transplant patients; a mean of 2.1 serious infections in 79% of patients has been reported. This high infection rate may occur because pancreatic transplantation is associated with a high incidence of allograft rejection, necessitating prolonged high doses of immunosuppressive drugs.[14]

Table 18-1. Pretransplantation Screening Tests

Organ donor
    HIV-1 and HIV-2 Ab
    HTLV-1 and HTLV-2 Ab
    HBsAg and anti-HBc
    HCV Ab
    RPR or VDRL
    CMV titers
    Toxoplasmosis titers
    EBV titers
    HSV and VZV titers
Organ recipient
    HIV-1 and HIV-2 Ab
    HBsAg and anti-HBc
    HCV Ab
    RPR or VDRL
    CMV titers
    Toxoplasmosis titers
    EBV titers
    HSV and VZV titers
    Purified protein derivative

Ab = antibody; HIV = human immunodeficiency virus; HTLV = human T-cell lymphotropic virus; HBsAg = hepatitis B surface antigen; HCV = hepatitis C virus; anti-HBc = hepatitis B core antibody; RPR = rapid plasma reagent; CMV = cytomegalovirus; EBV = Epstein-Barr virus; HSV = herpes simplex virus; VZV = varicella-zoster virus.

The chronic risk of infection after transplantation with its diagnostic challenges and potentially fatal outcome demands that transplant practitioners have an appreciation for the complexity of transplant-associated infections. Early infectious disease consultation is advisable. This chapter gives an overview of frequently encountered infections, before and after transplant, and an approach to the prevention, diagnosis, and management of these infections.

Preoperative Management

Donor Selection and Screening

Careful screening of potential organ donors for evidence of infection is of paramount importance (Table 18-1). Human immunodeficiency virus (HIV), viral hepatitis, and other organisms can be transmitted through transplantation; therefore, detailed protocols for donor evaluation are mandatory. Although serologic testing constitutes the major screening tool, the value of a thorough history, physical examination, and autopsy findings of active infections or tumor in the donor should not be overlooked. Evidence of tuberculosis, bacteremia, or organ-specific infection should be carefully sought. All donors should have premortal blood cultures done to exclude occult bacteremia. The following serologic tests should be obtained: HIV-1 and -2, hepatitis B (HBV) and C (HCV), syphilis (VDRL), human T-cell lymphotropic virus-I (HTLV-1), cytomegalovirus (CMV), Epstein-Barr virus (EBV), herpes simplex virus (HSV), varicella-zoster virus (VZV), and toxoplasmosis.[15] These results aid in preventing, recognizing, and managing infections after transplantation and also in selecting appropriate blood products for transfusion. For example, a patient who is seronegative for CMV should receive CMV-negative blood products to minimize the risk of primary CMV, which carries a higher risk of mortality than do reactivation or secondary CMV infections.[16]

Serologic testing has limitations. Uremia, hemodilution from massive transfusions or fluid resuscitation, and autoimmune diseases can affect results. Improper collection and storage of samples and exposure to heat, air, or ethylenediaminetetraacetic acid may further confound results.

Recipient Selection and Management

Transplantation centers should have a standardized recipient screening protocol in place to ensure that potential infectious complications are avoided. A detailed history is the first part of this evaluation. Patients should be screened for any evidence of active infection (e.g., cough, dysuria). Active infection is generally a contraindication to transplantation because it is associated with poor outcome, although Anguita et al. have reported successful cardiac transplantation in a small number of infected recipients.[17] A medical and travel history to document tuberculosis exposure, parasitic infection, underlying immunodeficiency (frequent sinopulmonary infections), foreign bodies (artificial valve, shunts, or orthopedic hardware), and exposure to endemic fungi is vital.

Recipient laboratory screening includes serologic tests for the following (see Table 18-1): VDRL or rapid plasma reagent, VZV, HIV-1 and -2,

HTLV-I, *Toxoplasma gondii*, CMV, HBV, HCV, HSV, and EBV titers. A purified protein derivative skin test with control should be done. Stool samples for ova and parasites are collected if indicated by the history.[18] Patients infected with *Strongyloides* (parasites) should be treated with thiabendazole before transplantation. Vaccinations must be current, including tetanus, pneumococcal vaccine,[19] and influenza (autumn and winter months). If the patient has had a splenectomy, vaccinations for pneumococcus and probably *Haemophilus influenzae* type b and *Neisseria meningitidis* should be given. The VZV vaccine should be strongly considered in candidates with negative VZV titers.[20] A study conducted in a group of pediatric renal transplant recipients found the varicella vaccine safe and effective in this population.[21] A live attenuated CMV vaccine shows promise for CMV-negative recipients of CMV-positive grafts.[22] A dental evaluation with any required intervention should also be included in the pretransplant workup.[23]

For tuberculin reactors, isoniazid (INH) should be considered in patients at risk of reactivation of tuberculosis. This applies to patients with a history of exposure to an active tuberculosis case, patients inadequately treated for tuberculosis in the past, patients with evidence of past infection who did not receive prophylaxis, recent skin test converters, people born in a foreign country with a high prevalence of tuberculosis, and those with underlying medical conditions associated with an increased risk of tuberculosis (e.g., malnutrition, achlorhydria, diabetes mellitus).[24, 25] The benefit of INH prophylaxis must outweigh the potential toxicity because the risk of hepatotoxicity is higher compared to nontransplant patients.[25] Therapy should be continued for 6–12 months. For patients with a high probability of infection with multi–drug-resistant strains of tuberculosis, preventive regimens of ethambutol and pyrazinamide or pyrazinamide plus a quinolone for 6 months are reasonable alternatives.[24]

Patients who are hospitalized awaiting transplantation require careful attention to prevention of nosocomial infections. Indwelling lines and catheters must be monitored meticulously to detect infection. Early interventions, such as elective intubation of the encephalopathic liver transplant candidate to reduce aspiration risk, may prevent complications.

Perioperative Management

Perioperative management of the transplant patient entails a multifaceted approach. Ensuring the delivery of prophylactic antibiotics is of paramount importance. Regimens vary, but most centers use a first-generation cephalosporin, such as cefazolin, for renal cases and cefoxitin in liver cases. A 24- to 48-hour course of cefuroxime is frequently used in cardiac patients at our center. In potential heart recipients who have had a prolonged pretransplant hospitalization awaiting a donor, we consider the use of vancomycin and ceftazidime. Vancomycin may be administered to patients with penicillin allergy or if methicillin-resistant *Staphylococcus aureus* (MRSA) is a problem. Selective bowel decontamination to reduce gram-negative and fungal colonization may precede liver transplantation.[26] Prophylaxis with an antipseudomonal antibiotic is given before surgery and continued for approximately 5 days after. Clotrimazole or nystatin is used for concurrent fungal prophylaxis.[23, 27] Trials using fluconazole and itraconazole prophylaxis in liver transplant recipients are under way.

Recovery in a designated transplant unit with experienced health care personnel is optimal to minimize postoperative complications and hasten patient recovery. In general, salads and fresh fruits are avoided to decrease gram-negative colonization, particularly in bone marrow cases. Intravenous lines and Foley catheters must be monitored meticulously and removed as soon as possible. Environmental exposures are reduced by enforcing strict hand washing on the transplant unit and isolating the recipient from patients and visitors with potentially contagious disease, such as upper respiratory tract illnesses, infections, or colonization with resistant organisms (i.e., MRSA, vancomycin-resistant *Enterococcus* spp.) or chickenpox.[27] Health care workers with respiratory infections should not care for transplant patients. In unavoidable situations, the worker must wear a mask. Fresh floral arrangements are prohibited in the hospital room. Outbreaks of legionellosis and aspergillosis require prompt epidemiologic investigation. Decontamination of hot water supplies and filtering of air may be required in certain instances to control such outbreaks.

On a long-term basis, we advise our patients to avoid contact with potential zoonotic vectors, such as birds (*Chlamydia psittacosis*) or cats and litter

Table 18-2. Syndromes That May Mimic Infection

| | Rejection | | | | | Antilymphocyte |
	Lung	Liver	Heart	Kidney	Infection	Antibody
Fever	+	+	+	+	+	+
Arthralgias and myalgias	+	+	+	+	+	+
Headache	—	—	—	—	+	+
Leukocytosis	+	+	+	+	+	+
Hypotension	—	—	+	—	+	+
Cough or dyspnea	+	—	+	—	+	+
Gastrointestinal symptoms	—	+	+	—	+	+
Dysuria	—	—	—	—	+	—

boxes (toxoplasmosis). For the first 6 months post transplant, we advise patients to wear a mask during exposure to crowds. Any travel should be preceded by a travel medicine consultation because infection with pathogens, such as *Salmonella* spp., has significant implications for the transplant patient. Patients meeting the American Heart Association guidelines should receive endocarditis prophylaxis when indicated. Although data are limited, we recommend continuing this practice for life.

General Principles of Infection

Diagnostic Challenges

The presentation of infection in transplant patients can be quite vague. The immunosuppressive regimens impair the host's inflammatory response resulting in a paucity of physical signs and atypical manifestations of infectious processes. As a result, serious infections may present insidiously yet progress rapidly, so that a prompt, thorough evaluation should be undertaken early in the course of any febrile illness. A comprehensive physical examination with emphasis on the patient's mucous membranes and skin is important. A complete blood count, urinalysis, chest radiograph, and appropriate cultures of blood, urine, and sputum are indicated. The empiric initiation of broad-spectrum antibiotics is reasonable in patients with suspected bacterial infection or sepsis. Several syndromes can mimic infection in the transplant patient, thereby obscuring the diagnosis (Table 18-2). For example, allograft rejection may present with fever, myalgia,

arthralgia, hypotension, and leukocytosis, thus simulating infection.

In the liver transplant recipient, in whom infection is the most important determinant of morbidity and mortality, securing a diagnosis of infection is often difficult because of the similarities between the presentation of infection and rejection.[28] Abdominal pain, malaise, anorexia, fever, increased prothrombin time, and elevated liver enzymes with organ dysfunction are seen with acute rejection,[28] but these symptoms may suggest intra-abdominal sepsis. Findings on liver biopsy (the gold standard for diagnosing rejection) can be altered in the face of infection, making a histologic diagnosis of rejection uncertain.[10]

Rejection in cardiac transplant patients may present with fever and hypotension secondary to graft dysfunction, suggesting septic shock. The possibility of rejection should be considered during all febrile episodes in transplant patients, but it should not interfere with the initiation of empiric antibiotic therapy after appropriate cultures have been obtained.

Medication side effects may also resemble infection. OKT3 can cause fever, chills, and a capillary leak syndrome that resembles sepsis. Aseptic meningitis may occur in patients receiving OKT3.[29] Cyclosporine, azathioprine, halothane, and enflurane may cause drug-induced hepatitis, and these must be differentiated from infectious causes.

Continued Immunosuppression

The key to minimizing infections in the transplant patient is achieving an immunosuppressive regimen that prevents rejection yet allows successful treatment of potential infections. In most cases, immunosuppression must be continued even in the face of severe infection because loss of the graft could culminate in death of the patient. An exception to this is the renal transplant recipient. Because dialysis and retransplantation are viable alternatives, immunosuppression can be withdrawn in the face of overwhelming infection. This approach has been applied to other solid-organ transplant groups. In a small group of 31 liver transplant patients who developed severe infection, temporary withdrawal of immunosuppression allowed successful recovery in 18 patients. Four of these 18 developed rejection, which was readily controlled with reinstitution of baseline immunosuppression. Of the 13 patients who died of infectious complications, eight autopsy examinations were available, none of which revealed rejection.[30]

Time Frame for Infections

Although infections may vary according to the type of transplant, some general guidelines allow the practitioner to predict potential infectious syndromes based on the interval since transplantation. During the first 30 days post transplantation, nosocomial infections predominate. The early transplant period (1–6 months) is marked by infection with opportunistic pathogens, and the late transplant period (after 6 months) is characterized by the usual community-acquired infections of immunocompetent hosts.[31] Infections in liver transplant recipients are less predictable because the graft is an "immunologic" organ. Although these are helpful guidelines, it is important to realize that they are not all-inclusive. Most of the infections discussed in the following sections could occur at any time after transplantation.

Infectious Complications in the Transplant Patient

Days 0–30

Infections in the early period fall into three categories. Nosocomial pathogens are the most common cause of infections during this period, and they are frequently the etiology of fever in the patient with a prolonged postoperative hospitalization or ICU stay.[31] Infection can be transmitted by the allo-graft, or occult infection present before the operation may be revealed by the stress of surgery and immunosuppression.

Nosocomial Infections

Indwelling Lines.   Intravenous lines, both peripheral and central, are a common cause of postoperative fever. As with all patients, indwelling vascular devices should be meticulously inserted, changed regularly, and removed as soon as feasible. Although the practice is controversial, we recommend changing central catheters every 72 hours or sooner if the patient is febrile without an identifiable source. Isolation of more than 15 colonies from a semiquantitative culture of the central line tip indicates line infection.[32] *S. aureus* and *S. epidermidis* are the most frequent pathogens, but gram-negative organisms and *Candida* spp. may be encountered, particularly during prolonged ICU stays. Pacing wires should be pulled as soon as practicable.

Wound Infections.   Although reduction of wound infection rates has had a major impact on transplantation success, wound infections remain a significant source of morbidity. The classic signs of warmth, pain, erythema, and fever may be absent or minimal in the transplant patient; a high index of suspicion must be maintained to recognize wound infections promptly. In suspected cases, a biopsy or Gram's stain of the wound and culture as well as blood cultures should be obtained. The deepest and most "active" part of the wound should be sampled, after surface decontamination.

In the renal transplant recipient, most wound infections can be linked to technical complications that result in hematoma, lymphocele formation, or urine leakage from the ureteral anastomoses.[33, 34] Most of these infections are caused by *Staphylococcus* spp. or gram-negative enteric organisms. With the use of intraoperative antibiotics and improved surgical techniques, the incidence of wound infection can be reduced to approximately 1%.[33] When evaluating a suspected wound infection, a plain film to exclude soft tissue or perirenal gas and a sonogram or computed tomographic (CT) scan looking for perinephric fluid should be considered. Some perirenal fluid is expected around a newly transplanted kidney. If no other source of fever is apparent, however, an attempt to aspirate a sample of fluid for Gram's stain and culture is indicated because extension of infection into the perinephric space necessitates a transplant nephrectomy in up to 75% of cases.[2]

Surgical wound infections are uncommon in the heart transplant recipient, but the morbidity associated with mediastinitis makes this a grave complication. Superficial wound infections tend to occur early postoperatively, whereas mediastinitis usually presents near the end of the first postoperative month. The causative organisms are usually *Staphylococcus* spp., but gram-negative organisms, such as *Serratia* spp., *Pseudomonas* spp., and *Enterobacter* spp., are also important. Rare causes of mediastinitis include atypical mycobacteria (*Mycobacterium chelonae* and *M. fortuitum*), *Aspergillus* spp., and *Mycoplasma hominis*. Diagnostically, a CT scan of the chest with aspiration of any fluid collections is indicated when mediastinitis is suspected. Sternal debridement and intravenous antibiotics are required for sternotomy infections.[35] Cultures from an intraoperative bone biopsy are mandatory and should guide antimicrobial therapy. Mycobacterial and fungal cultures should be submitted in addition to routine bacterial cultures and histopathology. Patients who have required a left ventricular assist device or total artificial heart as a bridge to transplantation may be at a higher risk of mediastinitis.[20]

Pancreatic transplantation is associated with a high rate of wound infection (33% in one study).[36] Damage and necrosis of adjacent tissues as a result of the liberated digestive enzymes is thought to play a role in the higher infection rate. Coagulase-negative staphylococci and *Candida* spp. were the most common pathogens in one series, but enteric gram-negative organisms are often present as well. Drainage of the pancreatic secretions into the bladder rather than the small intestine decreases wound infections, especially those caused by *Candida* spp. Deep wound infections commonly lead to graft loss despite aggressive therapy.[36]

Urinary Tract Infection. Nosocomial urinary tract infections (UTIs) are particularly common in kidney recipients in whom the urinary tract is the prime site of infection for the first 90 days post transplant.[33] The incidence of UTI in the renal patient varies from 35% to 79%, and more than 50% of bacteremia cases have a urinary source.[2] Gram-negative rods infecting an indwelling catheter are the major pathogens.

Asymptomatic bacteriuria in the renal transplant recipient requires antimicrobial therapy. A minimum 10-day course of oral antibiotics followed by repeat culture is optimal. Mild, asymptomatic UTIs should be treated with a 4- to 6-week course of therapy.[37] In severe cases, intravenous antibiotics may be used initially, completing the course with oral trimethoprim-sulfamethoxazole (TMP-SMX) or a quinolone. The prophylactic use of TMP-SMX for 6 months after renal transplantation has been shown to reduce the incidence of UTI in patients without anatomic abnormalities and is widely used.[6, 38] This regimen also protects against infections with *Pneumocystis carinii*, *Listeria monocytogenes*, and *Nocardia* spp. For *Candida* spp. UTIs, fluconazole is effective in most cases, and significant interactions with cyclosporine are rare. A search for a drainable focus should be undertaken. Rarely, amphotericin B may be required for UTIs with *Candida* spp. resistant to fluconazole. A short course of intravenous amphotericin B may suffice (250–500 mg). Bladder irrigation may be effective for treatment of cystitis; however, it is difficult to exclude graft involvement.

Intra-Abdominal Infection. Intra-abdominal infections are most commonly seen after liver and pancreas transplantation. Due to the technical complexity of liver transplantation, there is a high rate of surgical complications. Sites of vascular and enterobiliary anastomoses are especially vulnerable. Vascular anastomoses can become thrombosed and infected during the first postoperative week, particularly in children. Hepatic gangrene with secondary abscess formation may ensue. Hepatic or portal vein thrombosis may occur, leading to bacteremia. Fever may be the only clinical manifestation, although these patients may present with ascites and elevated liver enzymes.[28]

Biliary anastomoses may become infected with normal gastrointestinal flora if leaks or obstruction occur. The complications are diverse and include bacteremia, abscess formation, and cholangitis.[28] Postoperative ileus may put increased pressure on the biliary anastomoses, increasing the risk of rupture and subsequent infection. All patients with a fever of unclear etiology should undergo abdominal ultrasound and, if negative, a CT scan to look for abscess or ductal dilation. Abscesses require drainage and intravenous antibiotics. Significantly, because the biliary system becomes colonized soon after surgery, antibiotic prophylaxis before biopsy or cholangiogram is essential and should be continued for at least 48 hours after the procedure.

Liberation of enzymatic secretions increases the risk of intra-abdominal infections in pancreatic transplant patients. *Candida* spp., anaerobic organisms, and gram-negative enteric organisms are the usual pathogens, although use of selective gastrointestinal decontamination protocols has led to a predominance of gram-positive infections in some centers.[14] Drainage and antibiotics may be successful, but extensive infections often result in graft loss.

Pneumonia.   Nosocomial pneumonia is a frequent postoperative complication in the transplant patient. Prolonged intubation and altered mental status increase the risk of aspiration and pneumonia. Clinical entities such as postoperative atelectasis, adult respiratory distress syndrome, pulmonary hemorrhage, congestive heart failure, and pulmonary emboli or infarction may resemble pneumonia and must be considered in the diagnosis. A stepwise approach to the transplant patient with presumed pulmonary infection is listed in Table 18-3. Evaluation includes careful examination of a chest radiograph, sputum Gram's stain and culture, blood culture, and bronchoscopic specimens when indicated. Although postoperative pleural effusions are common, especially in the heart and lung recipient, diagnostic thoracentesis is indicated if the etiology of fever remains unclear. Antibiotic selection for nosocomial pneumonia is based on the clinical setting, Gram's stain results, culture and local susceptibility patterns. In the absence of a specific pathogen, piperacillin-tazobactam, imipenem, or an antipseudomonal cephalosporin are reasonable initial choices.

Other Nosocomial Infections.   Sinusitis and prostatitis are other less common but important causes of nosocomial infection. Sinusitis is often related to nasogastric or nasotracheal intubation. Fever is often the only manifestation. A CT scan of the sinuses or Water's view radiograph confirms the diagnosis. Removal of the tube and local sinus sprays, such as oxymetazoline 0.5% or phenylephrine, may be sufficient, but most cases require systemic antibiotics; pathogens may be gram-negative, gram-positive organisms, or anaerobes. Antral puncture for drainage and culture is indicated in persistent cases.

Table 18-3. Stepwise Approach to Pulmonary Infections in the Transplant Patient

History: Clinical onset and characteristics
Other: Travel, occupational, or animal exposure
    Vaccination (pneumococcal, influenza)
    Ill contacts
    ? PCP prophylaxis
    Immunosuppressive regimen
    ? Recipient and donor status
      CMV, HSV, VZV, EBV
    Toxoplasmosis
Laboratory
  CBC, SMAC, LFTs, ABG, blood cultures
  Sputum studies
    Gram's stain and culture
    AFB smear and culture
    Legionella smear and culture
  Other laboratory tests
    Cryptococcal antigen
    Legionella urinary antigen
    CXR: current and follow-up examinations
Empiric antimicrobial therapy for the following:
  Bacterial pathogens: ticarcillin-clavulanate, piperacillin-tazobactam, third-generation cephalosporin ± vancomycin
  If clinically indicated, consider the following:
    Trimethoprim-sulfamethoxazole for PCP
    Macrolide or fluoroquinolone for *Legionella*
If severely ill, immediate bronchoscopy
If clinically stable, watch for 24–48 hours, then bronchoscopy if no improvement
Immunosuppressed protocol for bronchoscopy (preferable to have BAL *and* biopsy):
  Gram's stain and bacterial culture
  KOH prep and fungal culture
  AFB smear and culture
  Nocardia smear and culture
  Legionella smear and culture
  CMV and HSV smear and culture
  Respiratory viral panel: smear and culture
    Influenza virus
    Respiratory syncytial virus
    Adenovirus
    Parainfluenza virus
  Silver stain for PCP and toxoplasmosis
  Cytology (may also detect *Strongyloides*)
If no diagnosis and no improvement, consider the following:
  Repeat bronchoscopy
  Transthoracic aspiration or biopsy
  Open lung biopsy or thorascopic biopsy

PCP = *Pneumocystis carinii* pneumonia; CMV = cytomegalovirus; EBV = Epstein-Barr virus; HSV = herpes simplex virus; VZV = varicella-zoster virus; CBC = complete blood count; SMAC = Sequential Multiple Analyzer Computer; LFTs = liver function tests; ABG = arterial blood gas; AFB = acid-fast bacillus; CXR = chest x-ray; BAL = bronchoalveolar lavage.

Prostatitis, when present, usually follows prolonged bladder catheterization. Pus may drain around the catheter, and a rectal examination reveals a tender, boggy prostate. In some cases, the pathogen may be determined by culture of the expressed prostatic fluid. TMP-SMX or a quinolone are good therapeutic choices, and a minimum of 4 weeks of therapy is required. Cyclosporine levels should be followed if TMP-SMX is used, and renal function should be monitored during treatment with quinolones.[39]

Infections Transmitted by the Graft

Infections can be transmitted by the allograft. Pyelonephritis developing soon after kidney transplantation is a prime example of this. The graft may be seeded hematogenously or by retrograde spread before harvesting.[40] Organs from donors who have been in the ICU for more than a week pose the greatest risk. Contamination of the graft during preservation and handling probably occurs more frequently than donor-transmitted infection. Culture of the graft and kidney perfusate can identify recipients at risk of infection. Recipients of a culture-positive kidney or perfusate should receive 7–14 days of antibiotics depending on the pathogenic potential of the cultured organism and its sensitivity.[31, 41]

Other infections that may be transmitted by the graft include HIV-1 and -2, HTLV-I, HBV, HCV, EBV, CMV, toxoplasmosis, syphilis, and tuberculosis (see Table 18-1). Transplantation of a heart seropositive for toxoplasmosis into a seronegative recipient requires a 6-week prophylactic course of pyrimethamine (25 mg/day) and folinic acid. Seronegative recipients who seroconvert after transplant should receive 4–6 weeks of pyrimethamine, sulfadiazine, and folinic acid.[20]

Reactivation of Prior Infection

CMV may reactivate after transplantation, and it generally causes symptoms after 30 days. Preexisting tuberculosis can disseminate after the start of immunosuppressive therapy and lead to miliary disease, meningitis, or other manifestations. Undetected *Strongyloides stercoralis* infestation can evolve into a hyperinfection syndrome, with pulmonary infiltrates and polymicrobial bacteremia. The manifestations are often protean, and mortality

approaches 70%.[18] Thiabendazole is the treatment of choice.[42] Screening of the stool (more than four samples), sputum, and duodenal aspirate allows identification of larvae in more than 90% of cases.[43]

Early Posttransplantation Period (1–6 Months)

Various infections characterize the early posttransplantation period (Table 18-4).

Viral Infections

Cytomegalovirus. CMV is a member of the herpesvirus family. It is ubiquitous and causes asymptomatic or very mild illness in the general population. In the solid-organ transplant patient, however, CMV is the single most important pathogen. CMV is a cell-associated virus that is able to establish latency at an unknown site in the host. In the transplant patient, three potential CMV syndromes may be encountered. Primary CMV infection occurs in the previously uninfected recipient who receives CMV-infected cellular blood products or an organ from a CMV-seropositive donor. Reactivation CMV occurs when a latently infected patient loses the ability to contain viral replication in the face of immunosuppression. Superinfection occurs when the latently infected recipient is infected with a different strain of CMV via blood products or the donor organ.[44] Primary disease generally follows a more severe course than reactivation disease or superinfection.

In discussing CMV, it is important to distinguish between CMV infection and CMV disease. A positive culture for CMV (from blood, urine, sputum, or stool) or positive titers for CMV in an asymptomatic patient is consistent with CMV infection. CMV disease is defined as symptomatic or invasive illness. Histopathologic evidence of CMV with viral inclusions on biopsy specimens indicates CMV disease (Figure 18-1).

CMV becomes a major consideration approximately 30 days after transplantation. The major risk factor for the development of CMV is the serostatus of the donor and recipient. CMV-seronegative recipients of seropositive organs (CMV mismatch) are at the highest risk of disease.[45] In one analysis of heart transplant patients, CMV mismatch resulted in a 64–92% chance of CMV disease, whereas seroneg-

Table 18-4. Major Pathogens of Infections in Transplant Patients

Organ System	Major Pathogens	Uncommon Pathogens
Central nervous system	*Cryptococcus*	PML
	Listeria	
	Toxoplasma	
	Nocardia	
	Aspergillus	
Skin or soft tissue	*Staphylococcus aureus*	Histoplasmosis
	Streptococcus spp.	Coccidiomycosis
	Atypical *Mycobacteria*	Blastomycosis
	Cryptococcus	
	HSV, VZV	
	Human papillomavirus	
	Nocardia	
Wound	*S. aureus*	*Aspergillus*
	Streptococcus sp.	Atypical *Mycobacteria*
	Gram-negative bacteria	
Lung	Bacterial	RSV
	PCP	HSV
	Legionella	Adenovirus
	CMV	Parainfluenza
	Aspergillus	Histoplasmosis
	Toxoplasmosis	Coccidiomycosis
	Cryptococcus	Blastomycosis
	Influenza	*Strongyloides*
	Tuberculosis	
	Nocardia	
Heart	Toxoplasmosis	Trypanosomiasis
Gastrointestinal	CMV	
	HSV	
	Candida	
	EBV	
	Aspergillus	
Genitourinary	Bacterial	CMV
	Tuberculosis	Adenovirus
	Cryptococcus	BK virus
Disseminated	Bacterial sepsis	Tuberculosis
	CMV	
	Toxoplasmosis	
	Candida	

PML = progressive multifocal leukoencephalopathy; HSV = herpes simplex virus; VZV = varicella-zoster virus; PCP = *Pneumocystis carinii* pneumonia; CMV = cytomegalovirus; EBV = Epstein-Barr virus; RSV = respiratory syncytial virus.
PML is associated with JC virus, a polyomavirus that causes a rare demyelinating disease. BK virus is another polyomavirus that has been associated with ureteral ulcers and strictures in renal transplant recipients and hemorrhagic cystitis in bone marrow transplant patients.

ative recipients of seronegative organs had a 15% risk of disease.[46] CMV-seronegative recipients of seronegative grafts are at the lowest risk of developing CMV disease. The degree of immunosuppression also plays a role in the development of CMV disease. Specifically, the use of antilymphocyte preparations (especially OKT3) is associated with a

higher risk of CMV disease.[45, 47] It is hypothesized that systemic cytokine release resulting from antilymphocyte preparations may allow reactivation of latent CMV infection in the transplant patient.[48]

The clinical presentation of CMV disease in the transplant patient can be protean. Fever is commonly the only manifestation of the disease. In some

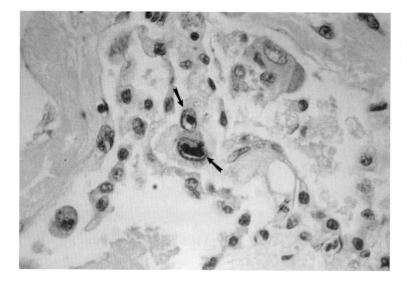

Figure 18-1. Peroxidase stain of transbronchial biopsy showing cytomegalovirus inclusions (*arrows*).

patients, a nonspecific illness occurs, characterized by fever and mononucleosis-like symptoms of malaise, arthralgia, and anorexia. Alternatively, CMV can be very aggressive, involving one or more organ systems. CMV pneumonitis and gastrointestinal involvement are probably most commonly encountered, but pancreatic involvement, myocarditis, and encephalitis may also occur. CMV pneumonia presents with respiratory symptoms and bilateral diffuse infiltrates on the chest radiograph. Gastrointestinal disease usually manifests as gastroduodenal ulceration or colitis, but any site along the gastrointestinal tract can be affected. Hepatitis may ensue, and liver enzyme abnormalities are common.[48]

In addition to clinical syndromes attributable to CMV, the virus also exhibits immunomodulatory properties. Although elevated levels of tumor necrosis factor are thought to lead to CMV reactivation,[49] studies have demonstrated that CMV infection may in turn result in production of immunosuppressive cytokines, which depress lymphocyte and macrophage function.[50] Other alterations in immune response include inversion of CD4 to CD8 ratios and suppression of cytotoxic T-cell activity.[51-53] Patients with CMV disease seem predisposed to superinfection with other opportunistic pathogens, especially disseminated fungal infections with *Candida* and *Aspergillus* spp.[54, 55]

CMV is implicated in the development of allograft dysfunction and rejection[56, 57] and seems to play a role in the development of coronary artery disease after heart transplantation.[55, 58, 59] Essentially, there are two postulated mechanisms by which CMV induces immune injury of the graft. CMV infection enhances production of interferon-gamma, which upregulates expression of class I and II major histocompatibility complex (MHC) antigens, resulting in rejection.[60-62] Another mechanism of injury has been described in which host cellular and humoral responses mistake HLA-DR for CMV. Sequence homology has been demonstrated between HLA-DR and CMV and between MHC class I and a glycoprotein produced by CMV-infected cells.[63, 64] This is one proposed mechanism for cardiac allograft vasculopathy. Supporting this are several reports suggesting that closer matching between graft and recipient at the HLA-DR locus increases the risk of CMV infection and rejection.[65-68]

Diagnosis of CMV disease may be problematic. Most patients develop leukopenia, some with an atypical lymphocytosis. Hemolytic anemia and thrombocytopenia may develop but are nonspecific. Definitive diagnosis requires histopathologic evidence of CMV cytopathic effects on a biopsy specimen. A biopsy is not always feasible, however, and alternative methods of diagnosing CMV must be used. Serologic testing for the virus is available. A positive immunoglobulin M (IgM) suggests recent exposure to CMV, whereas a positive IgG signifies past exposure. Detection and quantification of viral antigen in blood, urine (urine more sensitive than blood), and other body fluids are very useful, particularly in assessing patients for prophylactic or preemptive therapies; however, these techniques are not universally available.[69, 70] Antigen assays may be less sensitive than polymerase chain reaction (PCR),[71] but detection of CMV antigen in bronchoalveolar lavage (BAL) fluid has shown promise in rapid, early diagnosis of CMV pneumonia.[72] The presence of viremia correlates fairly well with invasive disease.[73] Viremia was the only identifiable virologic risk factor for the development of CMV pneumonia in one study; this group found that positive cultures for CMV from BAL, urine, or throat washings correlated poorly with the subsequent development of CMV pneumonia.[74] A quantitative culture method has also been developed that may be valuable in distinguishing infection from disease.[73] PCR for CMV is available in many laboratories. Although PCR is very sensitive, there is concern over the specificity of the technique, with a specificity and positive predictive value of only 42.9% and 58.6%, respectively, in one study of liver transplant patients.[75] However, PCR for CMV is helpful in excluding this diagnosis because the negative predictive value approaches 100%.[76] In general, the diagnosis of CMV is based on a compatible clinical picture with a combination of the aforementioned studies.

The clinical management of CMV disease requires a multifaceted approach encompassing early recognition and diagnosis, reduction in immunosuppression when possible, optimization of nutritional status, surveillance for rejection and other opportunistic infections, and use of antiviral medication. There are currently two medications for the treatment of CMV: ganciclovir and foscarnet. Ganciclovir is a virustatic nucleoside analogue that acts by inhibiting DNA chain elongation and DNA polymerase activity. The usual dose is 5 mg/kg every 12 hours for 3 weeks. Dose reduction is required for renal insufficiency. The major toxicity of ganciclovir is leukopenia, which can usually be controlled with use of a granulocyte colony-stimulating factor. Thrombocytopenia and anemia occur infrequently. Studies reveal that ganciclovir reduces sperm counts in animals; fertility in humans may be diminished. Foscarnet is a pyrophosphate analogue that also acts to inhibit CMV DNA polymerase. It is used less frequently than ganciclovir because of increased toxicities, such as renal insufficiency; electrolyte abnormalities, including hypocalcemia, hypophosphatemia, and hypokalemia; and occasionally, liver function enzyme abnormalities.

CMV hyperimmune globulin (CMVIG; CytoGam) is a selective antibody preparation pooled from blood donors with high antibody titers to CMV. The role of CMVIG in the treatment of CMV disease in the solid-organ transplant remains ill defined. In the bone marrow transplant population, CMV pneumonia responds poorly to therapy and requires a combination of ganciclovir or foscarnet plus CMVIG. In the solid-organ transplant, CMV pneumonia is more responsive to single therapy, but many authorities use CMVIG plus antiviral therapy in severe cases of pneumonia or gastrointestinal disease. Some research suggests that CMVIG should be added to antiviral therapy in refractory or recurrent disease.[77]

Prophylactic therapy for patients at high risk of CMV disease is evolving. Primary CMV infection leads to more frequent and more severe manifestations of CMV disease, making effective prevention strategies for high-risk patients (seropositive donor and seronegative recipient) essential.[71] Prophylactic regimens may involve single or combination therapy. It is likely that each organ transplant population will require unique strategies for CMV prophylaxis.[78]

SINGLE-AGENT PROPHYLAXIS.   High-dose oral acyclovir has shown benefit in a small group of renal recipients but has been unsuccessful in the prevention of primary CMV and CMV disease in liver transplant recipients.[79-82] Prophylaxis using ganciclovir has met with variable success, with some studies demonstrating efficacy[82, 83] and others failing to show benefit.[84] It seems that administration of prophylactic ganciclovir delays the onset of CMV disease and attenuates the disease course.[83, 85] Regimens using intravenous ganciclovir for 2 weeks followed by high-dose oral acyclovir have met with similar results but appear to be more effective than high-dose acyclovir alone.[81] Administration of CMVIG has resulted in a decreased incidence and severity of CMV disease and a concomitant decline in the incidence of opportunistic infections and rejection in transplants recipients.[82-85] Moreover, patients who receive CMVIG have improved graft and overall survival rates compared to patients who do not receive CMVIG.[86] Metselaar's group found that CMVIG was beneficial in the high-risk group of CMV-mismatched heart transplant recipients.[46]

PREEMPTIVE THERAPY.   Disappointed by ineffective prophylaxis regimens against CMV disease, several researchers have examined the role of preemptive therapy in aborting CMV disease. Several studies have demonstrated the efficacy of initiating ganciclovir in patients receiving antilymphocyte globulin therapy. These high-risk patients have a lower incidence of CMV disease and tend to have milder manifestations of disease than patients on antilymphocyte therapy alone.[87–90] Interest is intense in using early markers of infection, such as quantitative antigenemia or PCR to determine when to initiate preemptive therapy.

COMBINATION THERAPY. Combination regimens using CMVIG with ganciclovir or acyclovir appear to offer added benefit over single-agent regimens in preventing severe CMV disease in the high-risk patient.[81, 91–98] Ganciclovir in combination with CMVIG has been shown to reduce CMV disease in lung, liver, and kidney recipients. Owing to the significance of CMV disease and the attendant risk of rejection, prophylaxis with CMVIG and ganciclovir should be considered in CMV-mismatched[99] and all CMV-seropositive solid-organ transplant recipients, regardless of donor serostatus.

Epstein-Barr Virus. EBV, a herpesvirus, causes infectious mononucleosis in the immunocompetent host and is associated with nasopharyngeal carcinoma and Burkitt's lymphoma in genetically susceptible populations. Approximately 90% of the adult population have serologic evidence of previous exposure to EBV. In the transplant patient, EBV disease can range from a mild febrile illness to a life-threatening posttransplant lymphoproliferative disorder (PTLD). As with CMV, EBV infection occurs when EBV-positive blood or tissue is transplanted into a naive host or when the recipient's latent virus reactivates.[100] Seronegative individuals may also be exposed through family members and other close associates. Mild infections can mimic CMV and present with fever, malaise, leukopenia, and sometimes adenopathy and splenomegaly. Chronic graft dysfunction has also been described.[101]

PTLD is a complex process initiated by EBV that results in abnormal proliferation of B cells.[102, 103] Although the pathogenetic mechanism is unclear, it is hypothesized that EBV-driven B-cell proliferation, which is normally controlled in part by cytotoxic T cells, is allowed to go unregulated in the face of transplant immunosuppressive regimens. PTLD occurs in 1–3% of renal, 5–13% of cardiac, 9% of

heart-lung, 12% of pancreatic, and 2% of liver transplant patients.[14, 104] The process is best thought of as a spectrum of disease. The process begins as a polyclonal expansion of B cells that responds to a reduction in immunosuppression 90% of the time, but 10% of cases evolve into an aggressive malignant monoclonal B-cell proliferation, with a mortality of 70%. Risk factors for the development of PTLD include EBV seronegativity or mismatch at transplantation, the use of antilymphocyte globulin therapy (especially OKT3), cyclosporine use, CMV mismatch at the time of transplantation, and coexistent infections, such as CMV.[105–107] EBV seronegativity and CMV mismatch are the two most important risk factors for PTLD culminating in a greater than 100-fold chance of PTLD compared to recipients without these risk factors.[107]

Clinically, the lymphoma most commonly involves lymph nodes and other lymphoid tissue, the gastrointestinal tract, lung, kidney, central nervous system (CNS), and the graft itself. The syndrome can range from isolated organ involvement to widely disseminated multiorgan disease. Fever is the cardinal manifestation with other symptoms of PTLD related to dysfunction of the involved organ systems.[104] Smooth muscle tumors are another EBV-associated disorder that has been described in three children after liver transplantation.[108]

The diagnosis of PTLD is made by tissue biopsy. The histopathologic classification of PTLD is complex, and hyperplasia, lymphoma, or immunoblastic changes in a polyclonal or monoclonal pattern may suggest PTLD.[109] Detection of EBV DNA in tissue by PCR provides further evidence of PTLD. Serologic studies generally are not helpful, although a trend of rising titers may be a clue to the diagnosis. In suspected cases, radiologic studies, such as a CT scan, may suggest abnormalities and identify appropriate areas for tissue biopsy.

Treatment of PTLD has met with limited success. A high index of suspicion and prompt diagnosis are essential as the syndrome may be reversible in the early polyclonal stages or when limited to a single organ. Initial therapy for PTLD includes a reduction in the immunosuppressive regimen, which may lead to regression of approximately 40% of lesions, usually within 2 weeks.[107, 110] Antiviral therapy with acyclovir or ganciclovir may provide additional benefit by inhibiting viral replication. Localized symptomatic lesions can be surgically excised. Patients with severe systemic involvement unresponsive to initial treatment may be candidates for chemotherapy or radiation therapy. Additional reported approaches include the use of specific B-cell monoclonal antibodies, infusion of nonirradiated donor leukocytes (in bone marrow transplants), infusion of EBV-specific cytotoxic T-cells, and interferon-alpha in combination with intravenous immunoglobulin.[110-113] Despite intervention, the survival rate for PTLD remains only 31%.[104] The benefit of prophylactic acyclovir in preventing PTLD is being investigated.

Herpes Simplex Virus. HSV infections are common after transplantation. Most HSV infections represent reactivation of previous disease and generally occur in the first 2 months. Approximately 50% of kidney recipients reactivate cutaneous herpetic lesions within 30–60 days of the operation.[31] A major determinant of the incidence and severity of HSV infection is the type and intensity of immunosuppressive therapy. Lympholytic preparations (OKT3, antilymphocyte globulin) prompt earlier reactivation of the virus.

Herpes labialis is characterized by oral mucosal ulceration or lesions along the vermilion border. In the transplant patient, oral ulceration can be extensive, prohibiting nutritional intake. Endotracheal and nasogastric tubes may allow spread of the virus, precipitating nasal or esophageal ulcers and pneumonitis. Esophageal herpes can mimic *Candida* esophagitis radiographically. Lesions often become superinfected with *Candida* spp.[37]

Anogenital lesions due to HSV-2 are less common but can lead to painful, extensive ulceration with an atypical appearance. Direct immunofluorescence or viral culture is helpful. Severe cases can become superinfected with gastrointestinal flora and serve as a portal of entry for bacteremia.

Visceral dissemination of HSV can involve the hepatic, pulmonary, or gastrointestinal systems. This form of HSV is typically rapidly progressive and difficult to diagnose. In one review of 12 cases of HSV hepatitis after solid-organ transplant, five patients developed disseminated intravascular coagulation (DIC) and eight patients died.[114]

Treatment of HSV infection requires oral or parenteral acyclovir, depending on the severity of illness.[23] The use of prophylactic acyclovir after solid-organ transplant may decrease the incidence of severe HSV outbreaks and invasive disease and is routinely used in many centers.[114] Foscarnet may be useful for resistant viruses.

Varicella-Zoster Virus. Primary varicella infection (chickenpox) is rare in the transplant patient because most adults have had the illness during childhood. In the immunosuppressed patient, primary varicella can be catastrophic. In addition to cutaneous manifestations, pneumonitis, hepatitis, CNS involvement, and DIC may ensue. Transplant recipients who are seronegative for VZV should receive prophylaxis with varicella-zoster immune globulin (VZIG) if exposed to the virus. VZIG decreases the severity of infection but also increases the incubation period from 21 to 28 days. If infection occurs, high-dose intravenous acyclovir (15 mg/kg every 8 hours if normal renal function) should be initiated promptly.[31]

Zoster, or shingles, represents reactivation of latent VZV, and is quite common in the transplant population. Typically, the rash is contained within 1–2 dermatomes. Dissemination is rare. Treatment with acyclovir or famciclovir enhances healing and decreases the incidence of postherpetic neuralgia. Early diagnosis is imperative for ocular or otic disease. With normal renal function, a dose of 15 mg/kg every 8 hours is recommended. Immunosuppressive regimens do not need to be adjusted in most cases. All patients with varicella require isolation until the lesions crust over.[23]

Hepatitis B Virus. HBV infection in transplantation continues to be a complex issue. Categorization of transplant-associated HBV disease according to organ transplanted (hepatic vs. nonhepatic) is appropriate.

NONHEPATIC TRANSPLANTS. Transmission of HBV via solid-organ allografts has been documented. Recipients of HBV surface antigen (HBsAg)–positive kidneys who are already immune to HBV, either through previous exposure or vaccination, seem to have a low risk of developing hepatitis. In one study, 0 of 10 previously immune recipients of HBsAg-positive kidneys developed evidence of acute HBV infection, and it was concluded that transplantation of HBsAg-positive kidneys into immune donors is an acceptable practice.[115] Data also suggest that transplantation of kidneys from an HBsAg-positive donor to a susceptible recipient does not result in severe hepatitis and does not affect graft or patient survival, despite a higher risk of hepatitis.[116, 117] Passive immunization with hepatitis B immune globulin (HBIG) or HBIG plus vaccination have successfully prevented seroconversion in seronegative recipients of HBV-positive kidney and heart transplantations and should be used in these instances.[116, 118, 119] The presence of hepatitis B early antigen in the donor confers a higher risk of recipient seroconversion and morbidity related to hepatitis. It is also known that HBV rarely can be transmitted from organs that are solely HBV core antibody–positive (negative surface antigen and antibody). The transmission rate and severity of infection in this circumstance appear to be greatest in liver recipients.[120] Most centers transplant nonhepatic grafts into HBV-positive recipients as long as there is no evidence of active liver disease.[121]

HEPATIC TRANSPLANTS.   The greatest controversy surrounds liver transplantation in patients with chronic HBV infection. Recurrence of HBV is high in this population, and retransplantation is associated with high mortality.[122–124] Candidates who have detectable early antigen or viral DNA may have a higher risk of recurrence—as high as 81% in one study.[125] Patients with both HBV and hepatocellular carcinoma have particularly poor outcomes after transplantation, but coexistence of the delta agent has a protective effect and results in a more favorable prognosis.[122, 123, 125] Patients with fulminant hepatitis pretransplantation are less likely to have recurrence post transplantation than those who are transplanted for chronic hepatitis.[126] Long-term use of HBIG after transplantation may prevent recurrence.[123, 125] The benefit of interferon-alpha and ganciclovir to treat posttransplant hepatitis has not been demonstrated, but one case report using prostaglandin E and famciclovir significantly reduced viral replication and resulted in histologic improvement.[127, 128]

Hepatitis C.   HCV is another complex issue in transplantation. Understanding of this virus in the immunocompetent host is in its infancy; therefore, the implications of HCV for the transplant patient are sketchy at best. Currently, it is clear that HCV can be transmitted via grafts from seropositive donors to seronegative recipients.[129–132] Findings have varied, however, regarding patient and graft outcomes in this patient population. The Centers for Disease Control and Prevention recommend that blood or tissue from HCV-positive donors not be transfused or transplanted. This view is supported by several studies[129, 130, 133, 134]; however, many researchers have concluded that discarding all HCV-positive grafts unnecessarily wastes precious resources. Some think that HCV-positive organs should be transplanted in limited circumstances, such as when the donor is HCV antibody–positive but has no other risk factors for HCV and has normal liver histopathology.[135] Use of HCV-positive grafts has also been advocated for recipients who are HCV positive or United Network of Organ Sharing status 1 transplant candidates.[136–138] A few studies support transplantation of HCV-positive organs into HCV-negative recipients because the potential long-term complications seem not to outweigh the shorter-range benefits.[121, 131, 139] Transplantation of the HCV-positive graft into an HCV-positive donor carries the risk of reinfection because there are several strains of HCV.[137] Milfred et al. surveyed 48 programs that perform heart, lung, or heart-lung transplants to determine their policies on HCV-positive donors and recipients.[140] Sixty-four percent of the 45 responding centers accept HCV-positive transplant candidates. Organs seropositive for HCV are transplanted into HCV-positive recipients or status 1 candidates at 45% of centers.[140]

Recurrence of HCV post transplantation is another concern and can be seen with hepatic or nonhepatic grafts as a result of immunosuppression. Review of the literature suggests that although the incidence of HCV recurrence is high, the short-term risk of hepatitis, cirrhosis, and hepatic failure is low.[141–145] In hepatic transplant patients, HLA matching between graft and recipient increases the risk of recurrent HBV and HCV after transplant.[146] Although many investigators have found that posttransplant HCV runs a fairly benign course, others have observed lower graft survival in HCV-positive renal transplant recipients.[147] Long-term follow-up is not available for these patients. Membranoproliferative glomerulonephritis has been described in seropositive renal transplant patients in whom circulating immune complexes of HCV antigen and antibody have been demonstrated.[148] Monitoring of the disease course during HCV infection is hindered by the poor correlation between liver enzyme levels and liver histopathology.[149]

As in the immunocompetent host, treatment of HCV infection has been disappointing, although studies are contradictory on this point. A few groups have demonstrated the efficacy of interferon

Figure 18-2. Gram's stain of blood culture showing preponderance of *Listeria monocytogenes* (*arrows*).

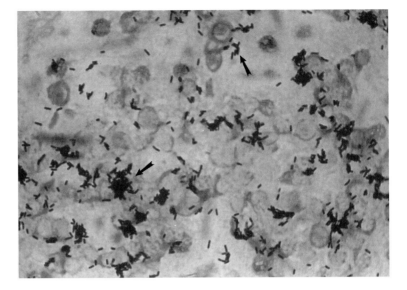

therapy,[126, 150] whereas others report a high relapse rate and risk of interferon-induced renal failure in HCV-positive renal transplant recipients.[141, 151, 152] Many investigators express concerns about induction of rejection with interferon, but a few studies found no increase in the incidence of rejection and a good response to routinely used antirejection therapies.[126, 141, 150]

Human Papillomavirus.   Human papillomaviruses (HPVs) are the etiologic agents of human warts. Warts can be classified as nongenital (common, flat, plantar) or anogenital. Nongenital warts occur frequently in transplant patients; up to 40% of renal transplant recipients are affected. These warts can evolve into large, disfiguring lesions, and malignant transformation can occur, especially in sun-exposed areas.[31] Control of the lesions may require reduction of immunosuppression and cryosurgery. Dermatologic consultation is advised.

HPV also causes anogenital warts or condyloma acuminata and is associated with malignant transformation. In one study of 133 renal allograft recipients, HPV 16 was detected in 27% of anal biopsy specimens, and histologic evidence of HPV or anal intraepithelial neoplasia was present in 24%. Of note, 81% of these patients were asymptomatic.[153] Fairley et al. evaluated 69 female kidney recipients and found evidence of HPV DNA in 21.7% of cervical specimens.[154] Immunosuppression puts these patients at a higher risk of HPV infection as well as vulvar, cervical, perineal, and anal carcinoma.

Bacterial Infections

Bacterial infections during the early posttransplant period are similar to those experienced in the immunocompetent patient. Skin infections, especially cellulitis caused by *Staphylococcus* spp., streptococci, or, less commonly, gram-negatives, are more frequent because of steroid-induced skin fragility. Intra-abdominal processes, such as cholecystitis and diverticulitis, must be sought because steroid use often masks the severity of symptoms, thus delaying diagnosis.

Bacterial meningitis in the transplant patient is most commonly caused by *L. monocytogenes* (Figure 18-2 and Color Plate 18-2). Presentation is similar to other types of bacterial meningitis, with fever, headache, and nuchal rigidity. A CT scan should be performed initially in subacute presentation to rule out other causes of CNS infection, such as brain abscess, cryptococcosis, and toxoplasmosis as well as noninfectious causes. Acute meningitis mandates immediate lumbar puncture. Various regimens of initial antimicrobial coverage exist, including ampicillin and gentamicin or, for the penicillin-allergic patient, intravenous TMP-SMX, and ampicillin or vancomycin plus a third-generation cephalosporin. The low doses of TMP-SMX used for *P. carinii* pneumonia (PCP) prophylaxis provide some protection against listeriosis.

Legionella.   Legionellosis is encountered with significant geographic and environmental variability in

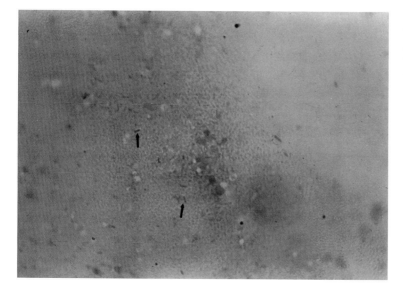

Figure 18-3. Gram's stain of sputum showing *Legionella pneumophila* (*arrows*). It is exceptional to capture this organism on Gram's stain.

transplant patients and is most common in heart recipients. Victims present with fever, dry cough, dyspnea, and often confusion or diarrhea. The most typical chest radiograph appearance is a progressive, patchy, interstitial process, but cavitation may develop.[35]

The diagnosis of legionellosis can be made by culture or direct fluorescent antibody studies of pulmonary secretions (Figure 18-3 and Color Plate 18-3); bronchoscopy specimens are optimal for these tests.[2] Serologic studies can be useful. A single titer of greater than 1:256 is presumptive evidence of legionellosis, and a fourfold rise in paired sera is diagnostic.[155] Detection of urinary antigen is the preferred diagnostic technique because it is both sensitive and specific and can be done early in the course of disease.[155]

High-dose erythromycin (4–6 g/day) is the treatment of choice for *Legionella*. Intravenous therapy should be given for 1–2 weeks, followed by oral erythromycin (2 g/day) to complete a 21-day course. Reversible hearing loss may occur with high-dose intravenous erythromycin. Cyclosporine levels must be followed closely because erythromycin elevates cyclosporine levels. Addition of rifampin may provide synergistic benefit in severe or refractory cases, but it complicates cyclosporine maintenance.[156] Ofloxacin, ciprofloxacin, doxycycline, and the newer macrolides, azithromycin and clarithromycin, also appear to have good activity against *Legionella* spp. Studies of the interaction of azithromycin or clarithromycin and cyclosporine

are anticipated. Currently, we use ofloxacin or doxycycline to avoid the pitfalls associated with the combined use of erythromycin and cyclosporine.

Nocardia. *Nocardia* infections in transplant patients are usually caused by either *N. asteroides* or *N. brasiliensis*. The patient's lung and skin are the most common sites of involvement. Pulmonary nocardiosis is characterized by fever, cough, and pneumonia, with variable radiographic findings. Lymphocutaneous nocardiosis is typified by subcutaneous nodules, lymphangitis, and cellulitis. In the immunosuppressed patient, nocardiosis may be rapidly progressive and has a propensity to disseminate. Disseminated *Nocardia* principally involves the CNS, but any organ may be involved. The appearance of ulcerative skin lesions and pulmonary infiltrates should heighten suspicion for nocardiosis. With the routine use of TMP-SMX for PCP prophylaxis, the incidence of *Nocardia* infections has declined.

Expectorated sputum cultures for the diagnosis of *Nocardia* spp. have a yield of only 30%.[157] Tissue or bronchoscopic specimens for culture and histopathologic examination are optimal. The finding of branching, beaded, gram-positive or acid-fast organisms is presumptive evidence for nocardiosis (Figure 18-4 and Color Plate 18-4). The diagnosis is confirmed by culture.

Sulfa drugs represent the mainstay of treatment for *Nocardia* spp. Other potentially useful agents include

Figure 18-4. Gram's stain of sputum showing beaded morphology of *Nocardia* species (*arrow*).

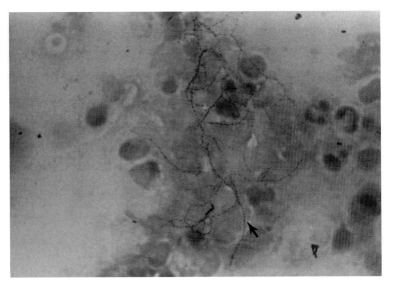

Figure 18-5. Gram's stain of throat swab showing fungal elements (mycelia [*arrows*]) typical of *Candida albicans* (thrush).

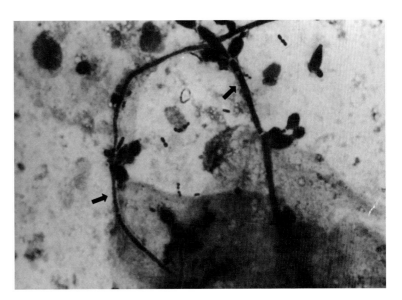

amikacin, imipenem, third-generation cephalosporins, minocycline, and the quinolones.[158, 159] Antimicrobial sensitivity testing is available at many laboratories. The duration of therapy in this population is not well defined. Short courses have resulted in relapse; therefore, a minimum of 4–6 months is advised.

Fungal Infections

Candida. *Candida* infections are very common in the transplant population. The most benign presentation of *Candida* infection is oral thrush, which is usually easily controlled with topical clotrimazole or nystatin (Figure 18-5 and Color Plate 18-5). Other syndromes include esophagitis, colitis, wound infection, tracheobronchitis, folliculitis, and UTI. Wound infections are most often seen in liver or pancreatic recipients and are often polymicrobial. Pulmonary involvement, although it is unusual, typically occurs in heart-lung recipients.

Systemic infection is the most serious manifestation of *Candida* infection. Nearly any organ can be involved in disseminated disease. Commonly affected organs include the lungs, spleen, liver, and

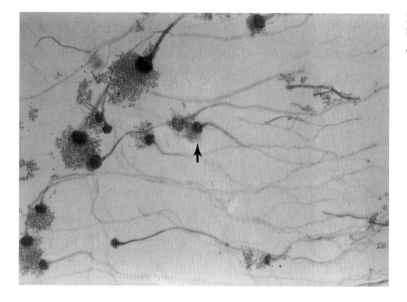

Figure 18-6. Lactophenol cotton blue staining of *Aspergillus fumigatus* (*arrow*) culture.

kidneys (native or graft). Liver recipients are particularly prone to systemic *Candida* infection. In one study, 24% of liver recipients developed significant fungal infections, 84% of which were due to *Candida* spp.[160] In an effort to avoid the risk of nephrotoxicity, fluconazole is the drug of choice, particularly if the species is routinely sensitive to this drug, such as *C. albicans*. Severe or refractory *Candida* infections may require intravenous amphotericin B. Nephrotoxicity occurs with increased frequency in patients receiving cyclosporine. Lipid complex amphotericin B (ABLC) has been an effective alternative in our experience, although increases in serum creatinine may arise. ABLC was made available January 2, 1996, in the United States.

Aspergillus.   *Aspergillus* spp. are ubiquitous fungi found in soil, decaying vegetation, and stored grains. Although exposure to *Aspergillus* occurs frequently, it is a very uncommon pathogen in immunocompetent hosts. In immunocompromised patients, *Aspergillus* spp. can cause a wide array of clinical syndromes. Prolonged neutropenia in cancer patients poses the greatest risk, but transplant recipients are also at risk. The usual portal of entry is inhalation of aerosolized spores. Outbreaks of aspergillosis have occurred in cancer and transplant patients during hospital construction and renovation.[161, 162]

The most common and serious manifestation of aspergillosis in this population is invasive disease.

Invasive pulmonary aspergillosis presents with fever, cough, and dyspnea. Pleuritic chest pain and hemoptysis may follow, resembling pulmonary embolism. The radiographic findings are nonspecific, and focal or diffuse infiltrates can be seen in any lobe. Invasive aspergillosis may involve the sinuses, CNS, gastrointestinal tract, and other areas. Dissemination to the skin occurs in approximately 10–15% of cases.[37]

Invasive aspergillosis is a rapidly progressive, often fatal process. Early diagnosis must be aggressively sought. Sputum cultures are helpful in less than 10% of cases. Definitive diagnosis requires histopathologic review and cultures of tissue samples (Figure 18-6). Stains (KOH preparation) and culture of material obtained by needle aspiration (e.g., sinuses, CNS lesions) are helpful.[163] Invasive disease is characterized histopathologically by fungal invasion of vessels, leading to thrombosis, infarction, and necrosis.

Primary cutaneous aspergillosis is a form of localized invasive disease. Direct inoculation is the usual mode of acquisition, and cases have been associated with intravenous catheter sites, intravenous arm boards, and gauze dressings. The lesions begin as small violaceous papules, which ulcerate and form a black, necrotic eschar. Other potential manifestations of aspergillosis in the transplant patient include ulcerative tracheobronchitis in lung transplant recipients and fatal surgical wound infections mimicking necrotizing fasciitis in liver recipients.[164, 165]

Figure 18-7. Gomori's methenamine silver stain of sputum showing *Pneumocystis carinii* (*arrow*).

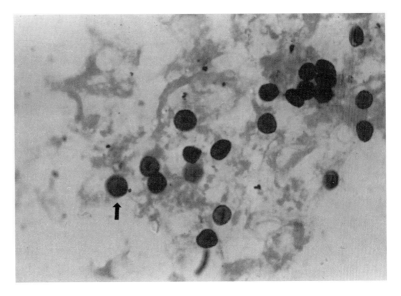

The treatment of aspergillosis requires a multipronged approach. Surgical debulking when feasible is of paramount importance and should endeavor to remove all affected tissue. Medical therapy of invasive disease uses high-dose amphotericin B (1.0 mg/kg/day). The addition of rifampin or itraconazole to amphotericin therapy has shown benefit in anecdotal reports, but combining azoles and amphotericin has been questioned.[166] As mentioned previously, ABLC is a less nephrotoxic alternative to currently available amphotericin B preparations. Itraconazole is not recommended as initial therapy for severe disease, but it may be useful for selected cases of localized disease or as subsequent therapy in cases that have responded to an initial course of amphotericin.

Pneumocystis carinii.   The incidence of PCP in transplant recipients has decreased significantly with the routine use of TMP-SMX prophylaxis. Patients who are unable to tolerate sulfa prophylaxis due to gastrointestinal effects, severe rash, or cytopenia should receive alternative prophylaxis with inhaled pentamidine, but the inferiority of this substitute regimen should be recognized. The usual clinical presentation of PCP is a dry cough with progressive shortness of breath. Diffuse infiltrates are characteristic on chest radiograph, but focal abnormalities may be seen. Diagnosis can be made by silver staining of sputum or bronchoscopic specimens, but biopsy specimens are more sensitive (Figure 18-7 and Color Plate 18-7). BAL is more than 90% sensitive for the diagnosis of PCP.[167] TMP-SMX is the drug of choice. Alternative therapies include intravenous pentamidine, dapsone and pyrimethamine, trimethoprim, or clindamycin and primaquine. Mortality due to PCP in the transplant population is low due to aggressive management with early bronchoscopy for pulmonary infiltrates.

Zygomycetes.   *Rhizopus* spp. are the most common cause of zygomycosis in the transplant patient. Other pathogenic species include *Mucor, Cunninghamella*, and *Absidia* spp. These fungi may cause a broad range of disease. Rhinocerebral disease, characterized by thrombosis and necrosis, may involve the turbinates, palate, and in extreme cases extend to involve the orbits and cerebrum. Other manifestations of zygomycosis include pulmonary nodules or infiltrates, skin and soft tissue infection, gastrointestinal involvement, and a highly fatal disseminated form. The use of steroids for prevention and treatment of rejection and diabetes are predisposing factors in this population. The overall mortality for these infections is 56%.[168] Limited infections may respond to surgical debridement and antifungal therapy with amphotericin B; early diagnosis is critical.

Protozoal Infections

Toxoplasmosis.   *Toxoplasma gondii* is an intracellular protozoal parasite. In the organ transplant recipient, acute toxoplasmosis usually occurs as a result of reactivation of latent disease or newly acquired infection transmitted by the donor organ. The latter occurs in patients who are seronegative for *T. gondii* before transplantation and receive an organ from a seropositive donor. Heart transplant patients are at highest risk of organ-transmitted toxoplasmosis because of the propensity of the protozoan to maintain latency in myocardial tissue. Although rare, toxoplasmosis has been transmitted by renal and hepatic grafts.[169, 170] A nonspecific febrile illness with CNS disease is the most frequent clinical presentation of acute toxoplasmosis in the transplant patient. CNS involvement in this population is usually more diffuse than in HIV patients. Meningoencephalitis with seizure or mental status changes and lack of focal findings on brain CT scan are typical. Myocarditis, cytopenia, and pneumonitis may also occur with disseminated disease. Toxoplasmosis may mimic rejection, especially in the cardiac recipient.

The diagnosis of toxoplasmosis is often difficult and may only be made at postmortem examination. Serologic tests may be of some use if seroconversion after transplantation is documented and IgM levels are elevated. *Toxoplasma* trophozoites or cysts may be demonstrated in BAL specimens, bone marrow aspirates, myocardial biopsy specimens, and other tissues.[169] In disseminated disease, trophozoites may be observed in urine by dark field examination or by Giemsa stain.

Treatment of toxoplasmosis is most successful if initiated early. Pyrimethamine and sulfadiazine along with a reduction in the immunosuppressive regimen is optimal therapy. For sulfa-allergic patients, pyrimethamine plus clindamycin is an alternative. Pretransplant determination of donor and recipient serologic status may help to identify those at highest risk for toxoplasmosis. Prophylactic treatment with pyrimethamine in high-risk heart patients has been shown to decrease donor-transmitted disease.[171]

Late Posttransplantation Period (Beyond 6 Months)

General

Generally, the late posttransplant period is a time of low-level maintenance immunosuppression. Infections in this period are of three types: community acquired, chronic viral, and an occasional opportunistic infection. Community-acquired diseases predominate, such as skin and soft tissue infections, pneumonia, bronchitis, UTIs, influenza, and other viral illnesses. Chronic hepatitis B and C are examples of viral infections acquired early after transplantation that may cause disease in the late posttransplant period. Opportunistic infections are discussed in the following sections.

Mycobacterial Infections

Mycobacterium tuberculosis.   The incidence of tuberculosis in the transplant population is greater than in immunocompetent hosts. In one study, the annual incidence of tuberculosis in renal transplant patients was 50 times higher than that of the general population.[172] Although often recognized later post transplant, tuberculosis can actually develop any time after transplantation,[173] with a mean of 76 days reported in one analysis of cardiac transplant recipients.[174] The most common forms of tuberculosis are disseminated and pulmonary. One review found that 43% of transplant patients with tuberculosis develop disseminated disease.[175]

M. tuberculosis (MTB) in the transplant recipient poses a diagnostic challenge because of its protean manifestations and insidious onset. Radiographically, apical fibronodular infiltrates, with cavitation or a miliary pattern, are the most common findings in pulmonary tuberculosis. However, any pattern may be seen. In miliary tuberculosis, liver, spleen, and bone marrow involvement are common. Extrapulmonary tuberculosis in transplant recipients include genitourinary, skeletal, or pancreatic involvement; brain abscess; and pyomyositis.[176–179]

The diagnosis of MTB must be aggressively sought in any transplant patient with pulmonary infiltrates or fever of unknown etiology. The skin test is rarely useful because most recipients become anergic within 2–4 weeks of initiating daily steroids. Sputum studies should be obtained. Bronchoscopy should be performed in any transplant patient with a pulmonary process if clinical improvement has not occurred within 24–48 hours after initiation of antimicrobial therapy. Lung transplant recipients require early biopsy to exclude the possibility of rejection. Collection of expectorated sputum for acid-fast bacilli smear and culture

Figure 18-8. Ziehl-Neelsen stain of sputum showing acid-fast bacilli, subsequently cultured and identified as *Mycobacterium tuberculosis* (*arrows*).

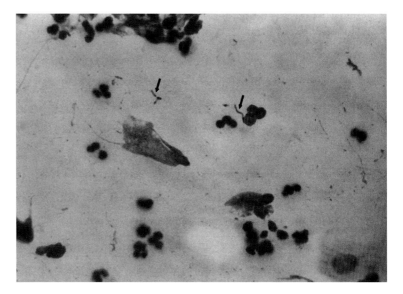

should be continued after bronchoscopy because there may be an increased yield of mycobacteria after the procedure (Figure 18-8).[180] In disseminated disease, a biopsy of the bone marrow or other involved tissues is useful.

As in the immunocompetent host, treatment of tuberculosis in the transplant patient requires multidrug regimens and should be based on sensitivity data. Isoniazid, pyrazinamide, ethambutol, and streptomycin generally can be used safely with immunosuppressive drugs. Rifampin is a potent inducer of the hepatic P-450 system and therefore decreases cyclosporine levels significantly. Rifampin may also increase the clearance of prednisone and has been associated with organ rejection.[181] It may be prudent to avoid the use of rifampin when possible. The optimal duration of treatment for tuberculosis in the transplant patient is unknown. Although a 9-month course may be sufficient, longer courses may be prudent in this population.[23, 174]

Nontuberculous Mycobacterial Infections. Nontuberculous mycobacterial (NTM) infections in the transplant recipient are well described and tend to occur a mean of 48 months post transplant.[182] Most cases have been described in renal or heart recipients. Unlike tuberculosis, NTM in the transplant population is rarely disseminated. The most common manifestations are cutaneous lesions of the extremities, tenosynovitis, and arthritis. Skin lesions usually begin as erythematous subcutaneous nodules, which progress to purulent ulcers. Systemic manifestations are uncommon. The pathogen most frequently associated with skin and soft tissue disease is *M. fortuitum/M. chelonae* complex. Sternotomy wound infections with NTM have been described.

Pulmonary involvement occurs in 28% of cases and may be accompanied by skin or soft tissue lesions.[182] Single or multiple pulmonary nodules or infiltrates are the usual findings. *M. kansasii* is the most common pulmonary pathogen, but others, such as *M. scrofulaceum*, have also been reported.[183]

The treatment of NTM infections in the transplant patient is not well delineated. For skin and soft tissue infections, debridement in conjunction with antimycobacterial therapy is usually required. For a single pulmonary nodule, resection may be adequate therapy. Rifampin, isoniazid, ethambutol, and streptomycin are the primary therapeutic choices. Clarithromycin has excellent in vitro activity against most NTM and will probably play an important role in treatment. Therapeutic agents should be chosen on the basis of sensitivity testing.

Fungal Infections

Cryptococcosis. Cryptococcosis occurs worldwide and is a frequent cause of opportunistic infection in the immunocompromised host. Fever, headache, and altered mental status usually develop in a subacute or chronic fashion. Hydrocephalus can complicate severe disease. Skin lesions are fairly common in cryptococcal disease and may provide a clue to the diagnosis. The lesions are usually nodular, but cellulitis may be seen. Diagnosis of cryptococcal disease uses cryptococcal antigen testing and culture of cerebrospinal fluid, both of which are very sensitive and specific. Other sites (blood, urine, sputum) may also demonstrate positive cultures. Biopsy of skin lesions may appear early, yielding a diagnosis before meningitis develops. In critically ill patients, an initial course of amphotericin B followed by fluconazole is justified despite the risk of nephrotoxicity with amphotericin B. Once the patient stabilizes, oral fluconazole should be given for at least 3 months. Indolent disease, which is a very common presentation, usually responds to fluconazole. In severe cases, the addition of flucytosine may be necessary, but routine use of this agent is discouraged because of renal and bone marrow toxicity in patients receiving cyclosporine and azathioprine. Repeat cultures and cryptococcal antigen studies should be negative before cessation of antifungal agents.[31]

Endemic Fungi. Endemic fungi (e.g., those causing coccidioidomycosis, histoplasmosis, and blastomycosis) uncommonly cause disease in the transplant patient. Pulmonary, CNS, and disseminated disease, often with skin involvement, are the usual manifestations. A thorough history regarding areas of previous residence, travel, and occupation helps to identify patients at risk for these diseases. Treatment of severe infections may require amphotericin B. Fluconazole has demonstrated efficacy against coccidioidomycosis, whereas itraconazole seems to be effective treatment for blastomycosis and histoplasmosis.[184, 185] In transplant recipients who have a pretransplant history of coccidioidomycosis, antifungal therapy should be strongly considered post transplantation to prevent reactivation.[186]

Conclusions

Managing transplant patients is demanding yet rewarding. Transplant medicine remains a frontier, posing unfamiliar challenges involving new surgical techniques, drugs, infections, and ethical dilemmas. The physician facing these perplexities must be mindful of a few simple concepts to ensure success. When infection is suspected, always rule out rejection or drug reaction. Determine the immunosuppressive regimen, history of rejection, and period since transplantation. This information is invaluable in narrowing the differential diagnosis. If there is any doubt as to the diagnosis, seek early consultative assistance, and be aggressive in obtaining tissue specimens for microbiological and histologic examination. There is a great deal of satisfaction to be gained when working with patients who have received a new lease on life.

References

1. United Network for Organ Sharing. UNOS Update. UNOS Scientific Registry 1995;11(11):34.
2. Rubin RH, Wolfson JS, Cosimi AB, et al. Infection in the renal transplant recipient. Am J Med 1981;70: 405–411.
3. Bourge RC, Naftel DC, Cosanzo-Nordin MR, et al. Pretransplantation risk factors for death after heart transplantation: a multi-institutional study. J Heart Lung Transplant 1993;12:549–562.
4. Behrendt DM, Billingham ME, Boucek MM, et al. Session IV. Rejection/infection: the limits of heart transplantation success. J Heart Lung Transplant 1991;10:841–847.
5. Miller LW, Naftel DC, Bourge RC, et al. Infection after heart transplantation: a multi-institutional study. J Heart Lung Transplant 1994;13:381–393.
6. O'Connell JB, Bourge RC, Costanzo-Nordin MR, et al. Cardiac transplantation: recipient selection, donor procurement, and medical follow-up. A statement for health professionals from the Committee on Cardiac Transplantation of the Council on Clinical Cardiology, American Heart Association. Circulation 1992;86: 1061–1079.
7. Cooper DK, Lanza RP, Oliver S, et al. Infectious complications after heart transplantation. Thorax 1983;38: 822–828.
8. Kramer MR, Marshall SE, Starnes VA, et al. Infectious complications in heart-lung transplantation. Arch Intern Med 1993;153:2010–2016.
9. Paya CV, Herman PE, Washington JA, et al. Incidence, distribution, and outcome of episodes of infection in 100 orthotopic liver transplantations. Mayo Clin Proc 1989;64:555–564.
10. Colonna JO II, Winston DJ, Brill JE, et al. Infectious complications in liver transplantation. Arch Surg 1988;123:360–364.
11. Mora NP, Gonwa TA, Goldstein RM, et al. Risk of postoperative infection after liver transplantation: a univariate and stepwise logistic regression analysis of risk factors in 150 consecutive patients. Clin Transplant 1992;46:443.
12. Saint-Vil D, Luks FI, Lebel P, et al. Infectious compli-

cations of pediatric liver transplantation. J Pediatr Surg 1991;26:908–913.

13. Kusne S, Dummer JS, Singh N, et al. Infections after liver transplantation. An analysis of 101 consecutive cases. Medicine 1988;67:132–143.

14. Lumbreras C, Fernandez J, Velosa S, et al. Infectious complications following pancreatic transplantation: incidence, microbiological, and clinical characteristics, and outcome. Clin Infect Dis 1995;20:514–520.

15. Perlroth MG. The role of organ transplantation in medical therapy. In E Rubenstein, DD Federman (eds), Scientific American Medicine. New York: Scientific American Books, 1989;1–16.

16. Keating MR, Wilhelm MP, Walker RC. Strategies for prevention of infection after cardiac transplantation. Mayo Clin Proc 1992;67:676–684.

17. Anguita M, Arizon JM, Valles F, et al. Results of heart transplantation in recipients with active infection. J Heart Lung Transplant 1993;12:808–809.

18. DeVault GA Jr, King JW, Rohr MS, et al. Opportunistic infections with *Strongyloides stercoralis* in renal transplantation. Rev Infect Dis 1990;12:653–671.

19. Amber JI, Gilbert EM, Schiffman G, et al. Increased risk of pneumococcal infections in cardiac transplant recipients. Transplantation 1990;49:122–125.

20. Petri WA. Infections in heart transplant recipients. Clin Infect Dis 1994;18:141–148.

21. Zamora I, Simon JM, Da Silva ME, Piqueras AI. Attenuated varicella virus vaccine in children with renal transplants. Pediatr Nephrol 1994;8:190–192.

22. Brayman KL, Dafoe DC, Smythe WR, et al. Prophylaxis of serious cytomegalovirus infection in renal transplant candidates using live human cytomegalovirus vaccine. Arch Surg 1988;123:1502–1508.

23. Peterson PK, Anderson RC. Infection in renal transplant recipients. Am J Med 1986;81(Suppl 1A):2–10.

24. American Thoracic Society. Treatment of tuberculosis and tuberculosis infection in adults and children. Am J Respir Crit Care Med 1994;149:1359–1374.

25. Naqvi SA, Hussain M, Askari H, et al. Is there a place for prophylaxis against tuberculosis following renal transplantation? Transplant Proc 1992;24:1912.

26. Wiesner RH, Hermans P, Rakela J, et al. Selective bowel decontamination to prevent gram-negative bacterial and fungal infection following orthotopic liver transplantation. Transplant Proc 1987;19:2420–2423.

27. Rubin RH. The indirect effects of cytomegalovirus infection on the outcome of organ transplantation. JAMA 1989;261:3607–3609.

28. Busuttil RW, Goldstein LI, Danovitch GM, et al. Liver transplantation today [clinical conference]. Ann Intern Med 1986;104:377-389.

29. Adair JC, Woodley SL, O'Connell JB, et al. Aseptic meningitis following cardiac transplantation: clinical characteristics and relationship to immunosuppressive regimen. Neurology 1991;41:249–252.

30. Manez R, Kusne S, Linden P, et al. Temporary withdrawal of immunosuppression for life-threatening infections after liver transplantation. Transplantation 1994;57:149–164.

31. Rubin RH. Infection in the organ transplant recipient. In RH Rubin, LS Young (eds), Clinical Approach to Infection in the Compromised Host (3rd ed). New York: Plenum, 1994;629–705.

32. Maki DG, Weise CE, Sarafin HW. A semi-quantitative culture method for identifying intravenous catheter-related infection. N Engl J Med 1977;296:1305–1309.

33. Cuvelier R, Pirson Y, Alexandre G. Late urinary tract infection after transplantation: prevalence, predisposition and morbidity. Nephron 1985;40:76–78.

34. Tilney NL, Strom TB, Vineyard GC, Merrill JP. Factors contributing to the declining mortality rate in renal transplantation. N Engl J Med 1978;299:1321–1325.

35. Gentry LO, Zeluff B. Infection in the cardiac transplant patient. In RH Rubin, LS Young (eds), Clinical Approach to Infection in the Compromised Host (2nd ed). New York: Plenum, 1988;623–644.

36. Everett JE, Wahoff DC, Statz C, et al. Characterization and impact of wound infection after pancreas transplantation. Arch Surg 1994;129:1310–1317.

37. Auchincloss H Jr, Rubin RH. Clinical management of the critically ill renal transplant patient. In JE Parillo, H Masur (eds), The Critically Ill Immunosuppressed Patient. Rockville, IL: Aspen, 1987;347–376.

38. Simmons RL, Migliori RJ. Infection prophylaxis after successful organ transplantation. Transplant Proc 1988; 20:7–11.

39. Peters C, Peterson P, Marabella P, et al. Continuous sulfa prophylaxis for urinary tract infection in renal transplant recipients. Am J Surg 1983;146:589–593.

40. Bijnen AB, Weimmar W, Bijlstra AM, Jeekel J. Infections after transplant of a contaminated kidney. Scand J Urol Nephrol 1985;92(Suppl):49–51.

41. Gottesdiener KM. Transplanted infections: donor-to-host transmission with allograft. Ann Intern Med 1989; 110:1001–1016.

42. Morgan JS, Schaffner W, Stone WJ. Opportunistic strongyloidiasis in renal transplant recipients. Transplantation 1986;42:518–524.

43. Smith JW, Bartlett MS. Diagnostic parasitology: introduction and methods. In EH Lennette, A Balows, WJ Hausler Jr, HJ Shadomy (eds), Manual of Clinical Microbiology (4th ed). Washington, DC: American Society for Microbiology, 1985;596.

44. Smyth RL, Sinclair J, Scott JP, et al. Infection and reactivation with cytomegalovirus strains in lung transplant recipients. Transplantation 1991;52:480–481.

45. Stratta RJ. Clinical patterns and treatment of cytomegalovirus infection after solid-organ transplantation. Transplant Proc 1993;25(Suppl 4):15–21.

46. Metselaar HJ, Balk AHMM, Mochtar B, et al. Cytomegalovirus seronegative heart transplant recipients: prophylactic use of anti-CMV immunoglobulin. Chest 1990;97:396–399.

47. Kirklin JK, Naftel DC, Levine TB, et al. Cytomegalovirus

after heart transplantation. Risk factors for infection and death: a multi-institutional study. J Heart Lung Transplant 1994;13:394–404.

48. Fietze E, Prosch S, Reinke P, et al. Cytomegalovirus infection in transplant recipients. Transplantation 1994; 58:675–680.

49. Docke WD, Prosch S, Fietz E, et al. Cytomegalovirus reactivation and tumour necrosis factor. Lancet 1994; 343:268–269.

50. Paya CV. Opportunistic infections: risk factor or virus-associated complication? Transplant Proc 1994;26 (Suppl 1):12–15.

51. Carney WP, Rubin RH, Hoffman RA, et al. Analysis of T-lymphocyte subsets in cytomegalovirus mononucleosis. J Immunol 1981;126:2114–2116.

52. Schooley RT, Hirsch MS, Colvin RB, et al. Association of herpesvirus infections with T-lymphocyte subset alterations, glomerulopathy, and opportunistic infections after renal transplantation. N Engl J Med 1983;308:307–313.

53. Dummer JS, Ho M, Rabin BP, et al. The effect of cytomegalovirus and Epstein-Barr virus infection on T-lymphocyte subsets in cardiac transplant patients on cyclosporine. Transplantation 1984;38:433–435.

54. Chatterjee SN, Fiala M, Weiner J, et al. Primary cytomegalovirus and opportunistic infections: incidence in renal transplant recipients. JAMA 1978;240:2446–2471.

55. Abramson JS, Mills EL. Depression of neutrophil function induced by viruses and its role in secondary microbial infections. Rev Infect Dis 1988;10:326–341.

56. Tolkhoff-Rubin NE, Rubin RH. The interaction of immunosuppression with infection in the organ transplant recipient. Transplant Proc 1994;26(Suppl 1):16–19.

57. Basadonna G, Feria A, Perez R, et al. Incidence of infection and acute rejection after cytomegalovirus immune globulin prophylaxis in renal transplantation. Transplant Proc 1994;26(Suppl 1):52–53.

58. Kendall TJ, Wilson JE, Radio SJ, et al. Cytomegalovirus and other herpes viruses: do they have a role in the development of accelerated coronary arterial disease in human heart allografts? J Heart Lung Transplant 1992;11:514–520.

59. Pouteil-Noble C, Chossegros P, Caillette A, et al. Influence of chronic cytomegalovirus and hepatitis B virus infections on the outcome of renal transplantation. Transplant Proc 1990;22:1820–1821.

60. Reinke P, Fietze E, Ode-Hakim S, et al. Late-acute renal allograft rejection and symptomless cytomegalovirus infection. Lancet 1994;344:1737–1738.

61. von Willebrand E, Pettersson E, Ahonen J, et al. CMV infection, class II antigen expression, and human kidney allograft rejection. Transplantation 1986;42:364–367.

62. van Dorp W, Jonges E, Burggeman CA, et al. Direct induction of MHC class I, but not class II, expression on endothelial cells by cytomegalovirus infection. Transplantation 1989;48:469–472.

63. Fujinami RS, Nelson JA, Walker L, et al. Sequence homology and immunologic cross-reactivity of human cytomegalovirus with HLA-DR beta chain: a means for graft rejection and immunosuppression. J Virol 1988;62:100–105.

64. Beck S, Barrell BG. Human cytomegalovirus encodes a glycoprotein homologous to MHC class I antigens. Nature 1988;331:269–272.

65. Martin S, Morris D, Dyer PA, et al. The association between cytomegalovirus-specific antibodies, lymphocytotoxic antibodies, HLA-DR phenotype, and graft outcome in renal transplant recipients. Transplantation 1991;51(6):1303–1305.

66. Salmela K, Hockerstedt K, Koskimies S, et al. Is the susceptibility to recurrent CMV infection linked to certain HLA antigens in renal transplant patients? Clin Transplant 1990;4:216–219.

67. Harfmann P, Dittmer R, Tenschert W, et al. Association of HLA-A1, A-3, and B-15 with CMV disease in cytomegalovirus IgG-positive recipients of renal allografts. Transplant Proc 1991;23:2660–2661.

68. O'Grady JG, Alexander GJ, Sutherland S, et al. Cytomegalovirus infection and donor/recipient HLA antigens: interdependent co-factors in pathogenesis of vanishing bile-duct syndrome after liver transplantation. Lancet 1988;2(8606):302–305.

69. Iberer F, Halwachs-Baumann G, Rodl S, et al. Monitoring of cytomegalovirus disease after heart transplantation: persistence of anti-cytomegalovirus IgM antibodies. J Heart Lung Transplant 1994;13:405–411.

70. Grossi P, Minoli L, Percivalle E, et al. Clinical and virological monitoring of human cytomegalovirus infection in 294 heart transplant recipients. Transplantation 1995; 59:847–851.

71. Wunderli W, Auracher JD, Zbinden R. Cytomegalovirus detection in transplant patients: comparison of different methods in a prospective survey. J Clin Microbiol 1991; 29:2648–2650.

72. Heurlin N, Markling L, Barkholt L, et al. Rapid detection of cytomegalovirus antigen on alveolar cells in bronchoalveolar fluid from transplant patients with cytomegalovirus pneumonia. Clin Transplant 1994;8: 466–473.

73. Bailey TC, Buller RS, Ettinger NA, et al. Quantitative analysis of cytomegalovirus viremia in lung transplant recipients. J Infect Dis 1995;171:1006–1010.

74. Slavin MA, Gooley TA, Bowden RA. Prediction of cytomegalovirus pneumonia after marrow transplantation from cellular characteristics and cytomegalovirus culture of bronchoalveolar lavage fluid. Transplantation 1994;58:915–919.

75. Brainard JA, Greenson JK, Vesy CJ, et al. Detection of cytomegalovirus in liver transplant biopsies. Transplantation 1994;57:1753–1757.

76. Schmidt CA, Oettle H, Peng R, et al. Comparison of polymerase chain reaction from plasma and buffy coat with antigen detection and occurrence of immunoglobulin M for the demonstration of cytomegalovirus infec-

tion after liver transplantation. Transplantation 1995; 59:1133–1138.

77. Waid TH, McKeown JW. Cytomegalovirus hyperimmune globulin for CMV disease refractory to ganciclovir in renal transplantation. Transplant Proc 1995;27(Suppl 1):46.

78. Winston DJ. Prevention of cytomegalovirus disease in transplant recipients [commentary]. Lancet 1995;346: 1380–1381.

79. Balfour HH Jr, Chace BA, Stapleton JT, et al. A randomized, placebo-controlled trial of oral acyclovir for the prevention of cytomegalovirus disease in recipients of renal allografts. N Engl J Med 1989;320:1381–1387.

80. Wong T, Lavaud S, Toupance O, et al. Failure of acyclovir to prevent cytomegalovirus infection in renal allograft recipients. Transplant Int 1993;6(Suppl 5):285–290.

81. Martin M, Manez R, Linden P, et al. A prospective randomized trial comparing sequential ganciclovir-high dose acyclovir to high dose acyclovir for prevention of cytomegalovirus disease in adult liver transplant recipients. Transplantation 1994;7:779–785.

82. Winston DJ, Wirin D, Shaked A, et al. Randomised comparison of ganciclovir and high-dose acyclovir for long-term cytomegalovirus prophylaxis in liver-transplant recipients. Lancet 1995;346:69–74.

83. Merigan TC, Renlund DG, Keay S, et al. A controlled trial of ganciclovir to prevent cytomegalovirus disease after heart transplantation. N Engl J Med 1992;326: 1182–1186.

84. Kelly JL, Albert RK, Wood DE, et al. Efficacy of a 6-week prophylactic ganciclovir regimen and the role of serial cytomegalovirus antibody testing in lung transplant recipients. Transplantation 1995;59:1144–1147.

85. Rondeau E, Bourgeon B, Peraldi MN, et al. Effect of prophylactic ganciclovir on cytomegalovirus infection in renal transplant recipients. Nephrol Dial Transplant 1993;8:858–862.

86. Snydman DR. Review of the efficacy of cytomegalovirus immune globulin in the prophylaxis of CMV disease in renal transplant recipients. Transplant Proc 1993;5 (Suppl 4):25–26.

87. Prokurat S, Drabik E, Grenda R, et al. Ganciclovir in cytomegalovirus prophylaxis in high-risk pediatric renal transplant recipients. Transplant Proc 1993;25:2577.

88. Singh N, Yu VL, Mieles L, et al. High-dose acyclovir compared with short-course preemptive ganciclovir therapy to prevent cytomegalovirus disease in liver transplant recipients. Ann Intern Med 1994;120:375–381.

89. Hibberd PL, Tolkhoff-Rubin NE, Conti D, et al. Preemptive ganciclovir therapy to prevent cytomegalovirus disease in cytomegalovirus antibody-positive transplant recipients. Ann Intern Med 1995;123:18–26.

90. van Son WJ, van den Berg AP, The TH, et al. Preemptive therapy with ganciclovir for early high-risk CMV infection allows effective treatment with antithymocyte globulin of steroid-resistant rejection after renal transplantation. Transplant Proc 1993;25:1436–1438.

91. Carrieri G, Jordan ML, Shapiro R, et al. Acyclovir/cytomegalovirus immune globulin combination therapy for CMV prophylaxis in high-risk renal allograft recipients. Transplant Proc 1995;27:961–963.

92. Prian GW, Koep LJ. Elimination of cytomegalovirus disease in liver transplant patients treated prophylactically with combination cytomegalovirus hyperimmune globulin and ganciclovir. Transplant Proc 1994;26(Suppl 1): 54–55.

93. Uber L, Cofer J, Baliga P, et al. Effectiveness of combination prophylaxis with cytomegalovirus hyperimmune globulin and acyclovir in the high-risk kidney transplant recipient. Transplant Proc 1995;26(Suppl 1): 42–43.

94. Maurer JR, Snell G, de Hoyas A, et al. Outcomes of lung transplantation using three different cytomegalovirus prophylactic regimens. Transplant Proc 1993;25(Pt 2): 1434–1435.

95. Nicol DL, MacDonald AS, Belitsky P, et al. Reduction by combination prophylactic therapy with CMV hyperimmune globulin and acyclovir of the risk of primary CMV disease in renal transplant recipients. Transplantation 1993;55:841–846.

96. Stratta RJ, Shaeffer MS, Cushing KA, et al. Successful prophylaxis of cytomegalovirus disease after primary CMV exposure in liver transplant recipients. Transplantation 1991;51:90–97.

97. Ham JM, Shelden SL, Godkin RR, et al. Cytomegalovirus prophylaxis with ganciclovir, acyclovir, and CMV hyperimmune globulin in liver transplant patients receiving OKT3 induction. Transplant Proc 1995;27(Suppl 1):31–33.

98. Valenza M, Czer LS, Pan SH, et al. Combined antiviral and immunoglobulin therapy as prophylaxis against cytomegalovirus infection after heart transplantation. J Heart Lung Transplant 1995;14:659–665.

99. Valentine HA. Prevention and treatment of cytomegalovirus disease in thoracic organ transplant patients: Evidence for a beneficial effect of hyperimmune globulin. Transplant Proc 1995;27(Suppl 1):49–57.

100. Straus SE, Cohen JI, Tosato G, et al. NIH conference. Epstein-Barr virus infections: biology, pathogenesis, and management. Ann Intern Med 1993;118:45–58.

101. Telent A, Smith TF, Ludwig J, et al. Epstein-Barr virus and persistent graft dysfunction after liver transplantation. Hepatology 1991;14:282–286.

102. Patton DF, Wilkowski CW, Hanson CA, et al. Epstein-Barr virus determined clonality in posttransplant lymphoproliferative disease. Transplantation 1990;49: 1080–1084.

103. Cen H, Williams PA, McWilliams HP, et al. Evidence for restricted Epstein-Barr virus latent gene expression and anti-EBNA antibody response in solid organ transplant recipients with posttransplant lymphoproliferative disorders. Blood 1993;81:1393–1403.

104. Cohen JI. Epstein-Barr virus lymphoproliferative disease associated with acquired immunodeficiency. Medicine 1991;70:137–160.

105. Chen JM, Barr ML, Chadburn A, et al. Management of lymphoproliferative disorders after cardiac transplantation. Ann Thorac Surg 1993;56:527–538.

106. Penn I (moderator). Immunosuppression and Lymphoproliferative Disorders Roundtable. Cincinnati. Raritan, NJ: Ortho Biotech, 1992.

107. Walker RC, Marshall WF, Strickler JG, et al. Pretransplantation assessment of the risk of lymphoproliferative disorder. Clin Infect Dis 1995;20:1346–1353.

108. Lee ES, Locker J, Nalesnik M, et al. The association of Epstein-Barr virus with smooth-muscle tumors occurring after organ transplantation. N Engl J Med 1995;332:19–25.

109. Craig FE, Gulley ML, Banks PM. Posttransplantation lymphoproliferative disorders. Am J Clin Pathol 1993;99:265–276.

110. Benkerrou M, Durandy A, Fischer A. Therapy for transplant-related lymphoproliferative diseases. Hematol Oncol Clin North Am 1993;7:467–495.

111. Papadopoulos EB, Ladanyi M, Emanuel D, et al. Infusions of donor leukocytes to treat Epstein-Barr virus-associated lymphoproliferative disorders after allogeneic bone marrow transplantation. N Engl J Med 1994;330:1185–1191.

112. Rooney CM, Smith CA, Ng CY, et al. Use of gene-modified virus-specific T lymphocytes to control Epstein-Barr virus-associated lymphoproliferation. Lancet 1995;345:9–13.

113. Taguchi Y, Purtilo DT, Okano M. The effect of intravenous immunoglobulin and interferon-alpha on Epstein-Barr virus-induced lymphoproliferative disorder in a liver transplant recipient. Transplantation 1994;57:1813–1815.

114. Kusne S, Schwartz M, Breinig MK, et al. Herpes simplex virus hepatitis after solid organ transplantation in adults. J Infect Dis 1991;163:1001–1007.

115. Bedrossian J, Akposso K, Metivier F, et al. Kidney transplantations with HBsAg+ donors. Transplant Proc 1993;25:1481–1482.

116. Chan PCK, Lok ASF, Cheng IKP, et al. The impact of donor and recipient hepatitis B surface antigen status on liver disease and survival in renal transplant recipients. Transplantation 1992;53:128–131.

117. Roy DM, Thomas PP, Dakshinamurthy KV, et al. Long-term survival in living related donor renal allograft recipients with hepatitis B infection. Transplantation 1994;58:118–119.

118. Turik MA, Markowitz SM. A successful regimen for the prevention of seroconversion after transplantation of a heart positive for hepatitis B surface antigen. J Heart Lung Transplant 1992;11:781–783.

119. Kiyasu PK, Ishitani MB, McGory RW, et al. Prevention of hepatitis B "rerecurrence" after a second liver transplant—the role of maintenance polyclonal HBIG therapy. Transplantation 1994;58:954–955.

120. Wachs ME, Amend WJ, Ascher NL, et al. The risk of transmission of hepatitis B from HBsAg(–), HBcAb(+), HBIgM(–) organ donors. Transplantation 1995;59:230–234.

121. Schweitzer EJ, Bartlett ST, Keay S, et al. Impact of hepatitis B or C infection on the practice of kidney transplantation in the United States. Transplant Proc 1993;25:1456–1457.

122. Eason JD, Freeman RB, Rohrer RJ, et al. Should liver transplantation be performed for patients with hepatitis B. Transplantation 1994;57:1588–1593.

123. Konig V, Hopf U, Neuhaus P, et al. Long-term follow-up of hepatitis B virus-infected recipients after orthotopic liver transplantation. Transplantation 1994;58:553–559.

124. Crippin J, Foster B, Carlen S, et al. Retransplantation in hepatitis B—a multicenter experience. Transplantation 1994;57:823–826.

125. Lake JR, Wright T, Ferrell L, et al. Hepatitis C and B in Liver Transplantation. Transplant Proc 1993;25:1006–1009.

126. Van Thiel DH, Fagiuoli S, Caraceni P, et al. Recurrence of hepatitis C following liver transplantation: treatment with interferon. Transplant Sci 1994;4(Suppl 1):S26–S28.

127. Yoshida EM, Wolber RA, Mahood WA, et al. Attempted resolution of acute recurrent hepatitis B in a transplanted liver allograft by the administration of ganciclovir. Transplantation 1994;58:956–958.

128. Boker KH, Ringe B, Kruger M, et al. Prostaglandin E plus famciclovir—a new concept for the treatment of severe hepatitis B after liver transplantation. Transplantation 1994;57:1706–1708.

129. Pereira BJG, Milford EL, Kirkman RL, et al. Transmission of hepatitis C virus by organ transplantation. N Engl J Med 1991;325:454–460.

130. Pereira BJG, Wright TL, Schmid CH, et al. A controlled study of hepatitis C transmission by organ transplantation. Lancet 1995;345:484–487.

131. Tesi RJ, Waller K, Morgan CJ, et al. Transmission of hepatitis C by kidney transplantation—the risks. Transplantation 1994;57:826–831.

132. Zucker K, Cirocco R, Roth D, et al. Prospective longitudinal assessment of hepatitis C virus infection after renal transplantation. Transplant Proc 1995;27:943–944.

133. Huang CC, Lai MK, Lin MW, et al. Transmission of hepatitis C virus by renal transplantation. Transplant Proc 1993;25:1474–1475.

134. Manfro RC, Karohl C, Gonclaves LF, et al. Liver function tests in hepatitis C virus infected kidney transplant recipients. Transplant Proc 1995;27:1821–1822.

135. Aswad S, Obispo E, Mendez RG, et al. HCV+ donors: should they be used for organ transplantation? Transplant Proc 1993;25:3072–3074.

136. Kiberd BA. Should hepatitis C-infected kidneys be transplanted in the United States? Transplantation 1994;57:1068–1072.

137. Sanchez-Tapias JM, Rodes J. Dilemmas of organ transplantation from anti-HCV-positive donors. Lancet 1995;345:469–470.

138. Sheiner PA, Mor E, Schwartz ME, et al. Use of hepatitis C-positive donors in liver transplantation. Transplant Proc 1994;25:3071.

139. Neu L, Brown MG, Korb S, et al. Clinical implications

of transplanting hepatitis C-positive donor organs. Transplant Proc 1993;25:2472–2473.

140. Milfred SK, Lake KD, Anderson DJ, et al. Practices of cardiothoracic transplant centers regarding hepatitis C-seropositive candidates and donors. Transplantation 1994;57:568–572.

141. Rostaing L, Izopet J, Baron E, et al. Treatment of chronic hepatitis C with recombinant interferon alpha in kidney transplant recipients. Transplantation 1995;59:1426–1431.

142. Wright TL, Donegan E, Hsu H, et al. Recurrent and acquired hepatitis C viral infection in liver transplant recipients. Gastroenterology 1992;103:317–322.

143. Ponz E, Campistol JM, Bruguera M, et al. Hepatitis C infection among kidney transplant recipients. Kidney Int 1991;40:748–751.

144. Shiffman ML, Contos MJ, Luketic VA, et al. Biochemical and histologic evaluation of recurrent hepatitis C following liver transplantation. Transplantation 1994;57:526–532.

145. Belli LS, Alberti A, Rondinara GF, et al. Recurrent hepatitis C after liver transplantation. Transplant Proc 1993;25:2635–2637.

146. Manez R, Mateo R, Tabasco J, et al. The influence of HLA donor-recipient compatibility on the recurrence of HBV and HCV hepatitis after liver transplantation. Transplantation 1995;59:640–642.

147. Ihara H, Ikoma F. Influence of anti-hepatitis C virus antibody on kidney transplant survival in a single Japanese center [letter; comment]. Transplantation 1994;57:781.

148. Roth D, Cirocco R, Zucker K, et al. De novo membranoproliferative glomerulonephritis in hepatitis C virus-infected renal allograft recipients. Transplant Proc 1995;59:1676–1682.

149. Boletis J, Delladetsima J, Psimenou E, et al. Liver biopsy is essential in anti-HCV(+) renal transplant patients irrespective of liver function tests and serology for HCV. Transplant Proc 1995;27:945–947.

150. Durlik M, Gaciong Z, Rancewicz Z, et al. Renal allograft function in patients with chronic hepatitis B and C treated with alpha interferon. Transplant Proc 1995;27:958–959.

151. Thervet E, Pol S, Legendre C, et al. Low-dose recombinant leukocyte interferon-alpha treatment of hepatitis C viral infection in renal transplant recipients. Transplantation 1994;58:625–628.

152. Hanafusa T, Ichikawa Y, Kyo M, et al. Long-term impact of hepatitis virus infection on kidney transplant recipients and a pilot study of the effects of interferon alpha on chronic hepatitis C. Transplant Proc 1995;27:956–957.

153. Ogunbiyi OA, Scholfield JH, Raferty AT, et al. Prevalence of anal human papillomavirus infection and intraepithelial neoplasia in renal allograft recipients. Br J Surg 1994;81:365–367.

154. Fairley CK, Chen S, Tabrizi SN, et al. Prevalence of HPV DNA in cervical specimens in women with renal transplants: a comparison with dialysis dependent patients and patients with renal impairment. Nephrol Dial Transplant 1994;9:416–420.

155. Peters JB. Use and Interpretation of Tests in Medical Microbiology (2nd ed). Santa Monica, CA: Specialty Laboratories, Inc., 1990;84.

156. Saravolatz LD, Burch KH, Fisher E, et al. The compromised host and Legionnaires' disease. Ann Intern Med 1979;90:533–537.

157. Palmer DL, Harvey RL, Wheeler JK. Diagnostic and therapeutic considerations in *Nocardia asteroides* infections. Medicine (Baltimore) 1974;53:391–401.

158. Kim J, Minamoto GY, Hoy CD, et al. Presumptive cerebral *Nocardia asteroides* infection in AIDS: treatment with ceftriaxone and minocycline. Am J Med 1991;90:656.

159. Garlando F, Bodmer T, Lee C, et al. Successful treatment of disseminated nocardiosis complicated by cerebral abscess with ceftriaxone and amikacin: case report. Clin Infect Dis 1992;15:1039–1040.

160. Castaldo P, Stratta RJ, Wood RP, et al. Fungal infections in liver allograft recipients. Transplant Proc 1991;23:1967.

161. Arnow PM, Andersen RL, Mainoues PD, et al. Pulmonary aspergillosis during hospital renovation. Am Rev Respir Dis 1978;118:49–53.

162. Sarubbi FA, Kopf HB, Wilson MB, et al. Increased recovery of *Aspergillus flavus* from respiratory specimens during hospital construction. Am Rev Respir Dis 1982;125:33–38.

163. Britt RH, Enzmann DR, Remington JS. Intracranial infection in cardiac transplant recipients. Ann Neurol 1981;9:107.

164. Kramer MR, Denning DW, Marshall SE, et al. Ulcerative tracheobronchitis after lung transplantation: a new form of invasive aspergillosis. Am Rev Respir Dis 1991;144:552–556.

165. Pla MP, Berenguer J, Arzuaga JA, et al. Surgical wound infection by *Aspergillus fumigatus* in liver transplant recipients. Diagn Microbiol Infect Dis 1992;15:703–706.

166. Denning DW, Stevens DA. New drugs for systemic fungal infections. BMJ 1989;299(6696):407–408.

167. Levine SJ, Stover DE. Bronchoscopy and Related Techniques. In J Shelhamer, PA Pizzo, JE Parillo, H Masur (eds), Respiratory Disease in the Immunosuppressed Host. Philadelphia: Lippincott, 1991;73–93.

168. Singh N, Gayowski T, Singh J, et al. Invasive gastrointestinal zygomycosis in a liver transplant recipient: case report and review of zygomycosis in solid-organ transplant recipients. Clin Infect Dis 1995;20:617–620.

169. Jacobs F, Depierreux M, Goldman M, et al. Role of bronchoalveolar lavage in diagnosis of disseminated toxoplasmosis. Rev Infect Dis 1991;13:637–641.

170. Mayes JT, O'Connor BJ, Avery R, et al. Transmission of *Toxoplasma gondii* infection by liver transplantation. Clin Infect Dis 1995;21:511–515.

171. Wreghitt TG, Gray JJ, Pavel P, et al. Efficacy of pyrimethamine for the prevention of donor-acquired *Toxoplasma gondii* infection in heart and heart-lung transplant patients. Transplant Int 1992;5:197–200.

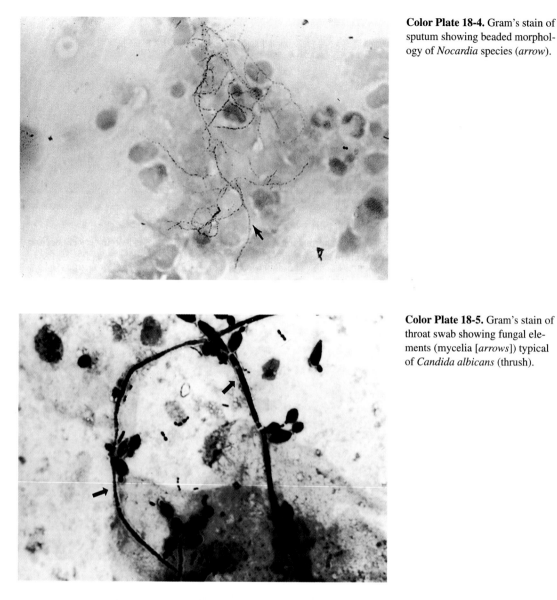

Color Plate 18-4. Gram's stain of sputum showing beaded morphology of *Nocardia* species (*arrow*).

Color Plate 18-5. Gram's stain of throat swab showing fungal elements (mycelia [*arrows*]) typical of *Candida albicans* (thrush).

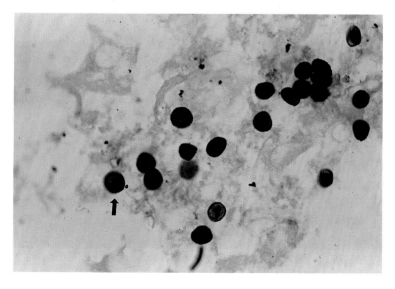

Color Plate 18-7. Gomori's methenamine silver stain of sputum showing *Pneumocystis carinii* (*arrow*).

Chapter 19
Principles of Pharmacokinetics

David J. Freeman

Chapter Plan

This chapter presents an overview of pharmacokinetic concepts and measurements that are commonly used to describe the time course of drug disposition in the body. For many drugs, pharmacologic effects are interpreted from concentrations measured in blood, plasma, or serum and in some cases, saliva and urine. These biological fluids are chosen for their ease of access, and it is assumed that the observed temporal changes in drug concentration more or less parallel those that occur at the receptor sites in target tissues. It is also generally accepted that only free drug can diffuse out of the bloodstream into extravascular tissues to cause a pharmacologic effect. This concept is based on the work of Brodie et al., who demonstrated the importance of lipid solubility and protein binding on the diffusion of various drugs from blood into the cerebrospinal fluid.[1] Protein binding of a drug and factors that may affect binding are therefore important considerations in interpreting pharmacokinetic data.

Measurements, such as clearance (CL), terminal half-life (t½), and volume of distribution (Vd) are commonly used for developing dosing schedules and for therapeutic monitoring of agents with narrow therapeutic ranges. Changes in the values of these parameters aid the objective assessment of pharmacokinetic drug interactions and study of the effect of diseases and physiologic changes on the body's ability to absorb, metabolize, and eliminate drugs. Although this chapter deals with the description, use, and derivation of pharmacokinetic parameters, the reader should be aware that appropriate experimental design for the acquisition of drug concentration data is essential for their calculation. Meaningful interpretation of data can be achieved only when drug assays are accurate, precise, and sensitive. For example, to calculate t½ from blood concentrations measured after a single dose, it is essential that the drug assay be sensitive enough to accurately measure the low concentration normally encountered during the later stages of terminal disposition. Along similar lines, blood sampling must be sufficiently frequent during the early part of an intravenous bolus dis-position curve to enable observation of the rapid distribution phase of a drug with two-compartment characteristics or to measure the absorption com-ponent of an orally administered drug.

Another cautionary note in pharmacokinetic cal-culations is that, historically, drug concentrations have been measured in plasma or serum on the assumption that the ratio of blood-to-plasma con-centration is 1. In many cases, this assumption is correct. With cyclosporine and tacrolimus (FK506), however, the ratios are greater than 1, with the result that values for some kinetic parameters, such as CL and Vd, are smaller when derived from blood data than when derived from plasma or serum data.

Physiologic Basis of Pharmacokinetics

Absorption and Bioavailability

The most common routes of drug administration are intravenous and oral. When a drug is given as a bolus or by infusion directly into the peripheral blood-stream, the whole dose reaches the systemic circula-tion. Thus, the bioavailability, defined as the fraction of the dose that reaches the systemic circulation in the unchanged form, is 100%. This is not always true for drugs given orally or by other extravascular routes. When given by mouth, drug bioavailability may range from 100% to 0, depending on its physio-chemical properties and the potential for presystemic drug elimination by the gut and liver.

Physiochemical Properties of Drugs

As a general rule, the ability of a drug to permeate biological membranes is a function of its polarity, molecular size, and charge. Small molecules (100–600 molecular weight [MW]) diffuse more readily than larger ones (greater than 600 MW). Nonpolar lipophilic drugs diffuse across lipoidal bio-logical membranes more readily than across polar hydrophilic ones. Drug molecules can be chemically divided into three categories: basic, acidic, and neu-tral. Weak acids (e.g., salicylate) and bases (e.g., pro-pranolol) have functional groups whose degree of ionization and thus polarity are altered by changes in pH. The polarity of neutral drugs, such as pred-nisone, cyclosporine, and tacrolimus, are unaffected

by pH, and therefore their pharmacokinetics are not influenced by changes in pH. The degree of ioniza-tion of a weak acid or base depends on the pH of the immediate environment and the ionization con-stant (pK_a) of the molecule being considered. The pK_a is a characteristic of each drug and is the pH at which an aqueous solution of drug is 50% ionized. Table 19-1 lists a selection of acidic and basic drugs with their pK_a values.

The gastric contents are normally acidic (pH 1–3). In such an environment, weak acids, such as salicy-late (pK_a 3.0), exist as a protonated, nonionized species with relatively lipophilic characteristics, thereby enhancing absorption in the stomach. On the other hand, propranolol, a weak base (pK_a 9.4), exists as a positive ion with relatively polar, hydrophilic properties. The environmental pH rises to between 6 and 8 when the gastric contents enter the small intes-tine. Under these conditions, weak bases tend to become nonionized (lipophilic) and thus more readily absorbed, whereas weak acids ionize and become less easily absorbed. Again, the degree to which this hap-pens for a particular drug depends on its pK_a value. The fraction of ionized molecules in aqueous solu-tions can be calculated with the well-known Hender-son-Hasselbalch equation:

For acidic drugs
$$\frac{\log[\text{ionized}]}{[\text{nonionized}]} = pH - pK_a$$

For basic drugs
$$\frac{\log[\text{nonionized}]}{[\text{ionized}]} = pH - pK_a$$

Although one can theorize about the effect of pH on the ability of drug molecules to diffuse across lipid membranes, in reality, most drugs are absorbed from the small intestine no matter what their degree of ionization. This is because of the large surface area of the lumen and its extensive blood supply, which maintains a consistently high concentration gradient across the intestinal wall. The more ionized a drug is, however, the slower its rate of absorption.

Physical Barriers to Drug Absorption

Although the duodenum and jejunum are the major sites of drug absorption, the epithelial cells lining the luminal surface form tight junctions, which block channeling of drug molecules through the extracellular spaces between cells. In this sense, the epithelial cells behave in a similar fashion to the endothelial cells of the blood-brain barrier. Pores that exist in the membrane are usually too small for most drug molecules to pass through. Therefore, drugs diffuse across the cell membrane according to their lipid solubility.

Bile plays an important role in the absorption of highly lipophilic drugs, such as cyclosporine and the fat-soluble vitamins. Bile salts act as a detergent that forms micelles from aqueous fluids and drug molecules in the duodenum. Drugs packaged in this manner are readily absorbed when they contact the gut wall. In the absence of bile, bioavailability can be drastically reduced, with much of the drug being excreted unchanged in the feces. This has been demonstrated for cyclosporine in liver transplant patients by comparing absorption with biliary tract T-tubes, open and closed.[2–4] These studies showed a large increment in blood cyclosporine levels when oral doses were administered with closed T-tubes.

First-Pass Effect

Drugs administered orally are subject not only to the solubility and permeation barriers presented by the gut wall but also to the first-pass effect or presystemic elimination (reviewed by Pond et al.[5] and Tam[6]). The first-pass effect is a process in which a relatively large proportion of absorbed drug is metabolized in the intestinal wall or liver during its passage to the systemic circulation. As a consequence, the fraction of dose actually available for therapeutic action may be sufficiently reduced to require intravenous or other routes of administration to improve bioavailability. It is difficult to predict the extent of this effect from the chemical structure of a particular drug. However, a first-pass effect is suspected if there is a reduction in the bioavailability of a drug given orally compared to the intravenous route when administered in equal doses. As noted earlier, a drug given by the intravenous route is completely available, whereas drugs given by mouth may have bioavailability values ranging from 100% to 0. Table 19-2 lists a number of drugs with significant first-pass elimination by the liver, intestine, or both.

The therapeutic consequence of first-pass effect is decreased oral bioavailability and should be

Table 19-1. Negative Logarithm of Acid Ionization Constant (pK_a) Values of Some Acidic and Basic Drugs

Drugs	pK_a
Acids	
Penicillins	2.7
Acetylsalicylic acid	3.5
Ibuprofen	4.4, 5.2
Glutethimide	4.5
Chlorpropamide	4.8
Warfarin	5.0
Naproxen	5.0
Glibenclamide	5.3
Tolbutamide	5.3
Phenobarbital	7.4
Thiopental	7.6
Phenytoin	8.3
Theophylline	8.8
Propofol	11.0
Bases	
Caffeine	0.8
Diazepam	3.3
Etomidate	4.2
Quinidine	4.3, 8.5
Chlordiazepoxide	4.6
Midazolam	6.2
Propoxyphene	6.3
Trimethoprim	6.4
Alfentanil	6.5
Ketamine	7.5
Lidocaine	7.9
Morphine	7.9
Sufentanil	8.0
Isoproterenol	8.6
Fentanyl	8.4
Meperidine	8.6
Erythromycin	8.8
Diphenhydramine	9.0
Procainamide	9.2
Propranolol	9.4
Imipramine	9.5
Nitrazepam	10.8
Oxazepam	11.5

Source: Adapted from LZ Benet, N Massoud, JG Gambertoglio (eds). Pharmacokinetic Basis for Drug Treatment. New York: Raven Press, 1984;1–28; M Rowland, TN Tozer. Principles of Applied Pharmacokinetics (3rd ed). Baltimore: Williams & Wilkins, 1995; and CJ Hull. Pharmacokinetics for Anaesthesia. Boston: Butterworth–Heinemann, 1991.

Table 19-2. Drugs with Low Bioavailability due to High First-Pass Elimination

Alprenolol
Coumarin
Desipramine
Dextromethorphan[a]
Diltiazem
Doxepin
Felodipine
Hydralazine
Ketamine
Lidocaine
Meperidine
Mercaptopurine
Methylphenidate
Metoclopramide
Morphine
Nifedipine
Pentazocine
Propafenone
Propoxyphene
Propranolol
Terfenadine[b]
Verapamil

[a]SJ Veticaden, BE Cabana, VK Prasad, et al. Phenotypic differences in dextromethorphan metabolism. Pharm Res 1989;6: 13–19.
[b]KT Kivisto, PJ Neuvonen, U Klotz. Inhibition of terfenadine metabolism. Clin Pharmacokinet 1994;27:1–5.
Source: Adapted from YK Tam. Individual variation in first-pass metabolism. Clin Pharmacokinet 1993;25:300–328.

viewed in the context of whether the administered drug is itself active or is an inactive prodrug. In the former case, metabolic conversion of active drug to inactive metabolites by enzymes in the gut wall or liver is an obvious disadvantage (e.g., diltiazem, felodipine). In the latter case, an inactive prodrug would be metabolized during the first pass to an active product (e.g., azathioprine, dextromethorphan, terfenadine).

Distribution

Distribution and elimination occur simultaneously as drug reaches the systemic circulation. Distribution into peripheral tissues is a complex function of blood perfusion, drug lipophilia (a function of pK_a), and the extent of binding to blood proteins and extravascular tissues. Uptake of drug continues until equilibrium is achieved between the transfer of free (unbound) drug to the tissues and the back-diffusion of free drug from tissues to blood. Protein binding is an important factor in the distribution process and in the pharmacokinetics of drugs in general. Drug molecules bind reversibly and to varying degrees with proteins in the bloodstream, a process that has been extensively discussed by other authors.[7, 8] Acidic drugs bind mainly to albumin, whereas basic drugs, although able to bind to albumin, bind mostly to alpha-acid glycoprotein. Highly lipophilic drugs, such as cyclosporine, rapamycin, and tacrolimus, can also accumulate in the lipid core of lipoproteins and bind to erythrocytes (Table 19-3). Indeed, tacrolimus and rapamycin are taken up into red cells so extensively that the blood-to-plasma concentration ratios are greater than 10.[9, 10] The effect of protein binding and partitioning into blood components is to maintain the drug in a nondiffusible state in the vascular compartment. Consequently, drug molecules are unable to distribute to extravascular tissues. Protein binding can be altered in renal and hepatic diseases so that changes in drug kinetics significantly affect drug action. This aspect of kinetics is considered in Factors That Affect Drug Pharmacokinetics.

Drug distribution may be altered by enterohepatic cycling, whereby parent drug is eliminated in the bile but is subsequently transported to the duodenum, from which it is reabsorbed. This movement of drug falls under the heading of distribution rather than elimination because drug molecules are not actually removed from the body; rather, they are moved from the blood to another site within the Vd. Reabsorption of this recycled drug back into the blood at a later time can give a characteristic biphasic pattern to the early part of the concentration-time profile.

The rate at which equilibrium is achieved depends on the blood flow to individual organs and tissues (Table 19-4). The highly perfused tissues, such as the lungs, liver, and kidney, tend to reach equilibrium earlier than the more slowly perfused organs (e.g., bone, brain, fat, and inactive muscle).

Volume of Distribution

The pharmacokinetic parameter linking blood concentrations to administered dose is the apparent Vd. As the term *apparent* implies, Vd does not repre-

Table 19-3. Protein Binding of Various Drugs

Drug	% Bound	Drug	% Bound
Warfarin	99.0	Propranolol	89.0
Naproxen	99.0	Tacrolimus[b]	88.0
Diazepam	99.0	Prednisone	85.0
Ketoconazole	99.0	Thiopental	85.0
Mycophenolic acid	98.5	Fentanyl	84.0
Chlorpromazine	98.0	Carbamazepine	82.0
Clorazepate	98.0	Triamterene	82.0
Rapamycin[a]	98.0	Methylprednisolone	78.0
Propofol	98.0	Propoxyphene	76.0
Clofibrate	97.0	Trimethoprim	67.0
Dicloxacillin	97.0	Pentobarbital	66.0
Cyclosporine[a]	96.0	Benzylpenicillin	66.0
Furosemide	95.0	Sulfamethoxazole	66.0
Phenylbutazone	95.0	Meperidine	58.0
Cloxacillin	95.0	Chloramphenicol	51.0
Bupivacaine	95.0	Methotrexate	46.0
Flucloxacillin	94.0	Vecuronium	39.0
Sufentanil	93.0	Morphine	35.0
Alfentanil	92.0	Vancomycin	30.0
Valproate	92.0	Digoxin	25.0
Salicylate	92.0	Mercaptopurine[c]	19.0
Desipramine	90.0	Ranitidine	15.0
Quinidine	90.0	Cyclophosphamide	13.0
Phenytoin	90.0	Ketamine	12.0
Verapamil	89.0	Pancuronium	7.0

Note: Values are approximate.
[a]Binding to blood.
[b]Binding to plasma.
[c]Initial metabolic product of azathioprine.
Source: Data adapted from JG Gambertoglio. Effects of Renal Disease: Altered Pharmacokinetics. In LZ Benet, N Massoud, JG Gambertoglio (eds), Pharmacokinetic Basis for Drug Treatment. New York: Raven Press, 1984;149–171; A Fahr. Cyclosporin clinical pharmacokinetics. Clin Pharmacokinet 1993;24:472–495; DH Peters, A Fitton, GL Plusker, D Faulds. Tacrolimus: a review of its pharmacology and therapeutic potential in hepatic and renal transplantation. Drugs 1993;46: 746–794; CJ Hull. Pharmacokinetics for Anaesthesia. Boston: Butterworth–Heinemann, 1991; LS Goodman, A Gilmans. Goodman and Gilman's CD-ROM (9th ed). New York: McGraw-Hill, 1996; F Bochner, G Carruthers, J Kampmann, J Steiner. Handbook of Clinical Pharmacology. Boston: Little, Brown, 1983; R Yatscoff, P Wang, K Chan, et al. Rapamycin: distribution, pharmacokinetics and therapeutic range investigations. Ther Drug Monit 1995;17:666–670; and I Nowak, LM Shaw. Mycophenolic acid binding to human serum albumin: characterization and relationship to pharmacodynamics. Clin Chem 1995;41: 1011–1017.

sent an identifiable physiologic volume but rather a fluid volume into which the dose would have to diffuse and equilibrate to give a concentration the same as that measured in blood. For comparison, the blood volume of a 70-kg man is approximately 5 liters, the extracellular volume is approximately 12 liters, and total body water is approximately 42 liters. Some drugs have Vd values that fall within this range (5–42 liters); many others have volumes much larger (Table 19-5).

For drugs with large Vds, therefore, it is evident that when distribution is complete, much of the drug is not in the blood but rather is accumulated in peripheral tissues, presumably at concentrations considerably higher than those in blood. Although it seems reasonable in some cases to associate Vd with a physiologically identifiable volume (i.e., 42 liters is equal to total body water), it cannot be assumed that a drug is actually located in this physiologic space. The volume, in fact, is the net result

Table 19-4. Relative Organ Weights and Blood Flow in a 70-kg Person

Organ	% of Body Volume	Blood Flow (ml/min)
Adrenal gland	0.03	25
Bone	16.0	250
Brain	2.0	700
Fat	10.0	200
Heart	0.5	200
Kidneys	0.4	1,100
Liver	2.3	1,350
Portal vein		1,100
Hepatic artery		300
Lungs	0.7	5,000
Muscle	42.0	750
Skin	18.0	300
Total body	100.0	5,000

Source: Adapted from M Rowland, TN Tozer. Principles of Applied Pharmacokinetics (3rd ed). Baltimore: Williams & Wilkins, 1995.

of distribution into a heterogeneous group of organs and tissues, which, by coincidence, measure 42 liters. Vd may also change with age, body composition, and disease, but, in all these cases, the underlying cause is alteration in drug binding to tissue and blood proteins and changes in partitioning of drug between fatty and lean tissues. For example, water occupies a greater proportion of the body weight of neonates (88%) than of adults (60%), and a greater proportion is extracellular. This has clinical relevance for drugs such as the penicillins and cephalosporins because weight-normalized doses may have to be increased to maintain therapeutic tissue concentrations. The practical application of this parameter is that once Vd is known for a particular drug, it is a relatively simple task to calculate the dose required to achieve a therapeutic concentration. Calculation of Vd based on blood concentration data is considered under Pharmacokinetic Models.

Drug Metabolism and Elimination

Drug-metabolizing enzymes are present in many tissues, including liver, gut, lung, and kidney, but the major metabolic activity occurs in the liver.[11] Metabolism takes two forms: the oxidative transformation of the drug molecule (phase I) and conjugative transformations (phase II), such as acetylation, glucuronidation, and sulfation. The great majority of phase I metabolism is catalyzed by a heterogeneous family of enzymes known as *cytochrome P-450*.[12] The individual variability in the activity of these enzymes is under genetic and environmental control, which gives rise to wide biological variability. Disturbances in drug metabolism can occur with drugs that are coadministered and metabolized by the same isozymes.[13–15] For instance, the metabolism of several drugs, including cyclosporine, tacrolimus, and rapamycin, may be inhibited to a clinically relevant degree when they are coadministered with erythromycin or ketoconazole; all these drugs are metabolized by P-450-3A (Table 19-6).

This list is by no means complete and continues to expand as more isozymes and their corresponding drug substrates are identified and characterized. The extent of interaction, however, is not always predictable and depends, in part, on the affinities of interacting drugs for the metabolizing enzyme as well as the concentration of each drug at the metabolic site. For example, cyclosporine metabolism is strongly inhibited by nifedipine in vitro but not in vivo. This appears to be due to the relatively low concentrations of circulating nifedipine that occur during therapy, which therefore do not effectively compete with cyclosporine for hepatic metabolism.

The process of enzyme induction by environmental factors (cigarette smoking) or other drugs is another factor responsible for increasing drug metabolism. Phenytoin, rifampin, and phenobarbital are commonly associated with enzyme induction and have been shown to reduce serum concentrations of many drugs, including cyclosporine[16] and tacrolimus.[17] Elimination of nonvolatile drugs from the blood is due mainly to hepatic metabolism and renal excretion. Other mechanisms include enzyme hydrolysis in the bloodstream by plasma cholinesterases (e.g., suxamethonium[18]) and nonenzymatic chemical decomposition (e.g., atracurium undergoes Hoffmann degradation to laudanosine[19]). Volatile agents, such as gaseous anesthetics, are eliminated to a large extent by the lungs, but the more lipid-soluble agents (e.g., halothane) may also distribute into tissues and may be eliminated by the same metabolic mechanisms as nonvolatile drugs. Elimination is commonly measured in terms of CL and t½.

Table 19-5. Volumes of Distribution of Selected Drugs for a 70-kg Person*

Drug	Vd (liters/kg)	Vd (liters)	Drug	Vd (liters/kg)	Vd (liters)
Heparin	0.06	4.2	Indomethacin	1.0	70
Dicloxacillin	0.08	5.6	Prednisone	1.0	70
Furosemide	0.10	7.0	Sufentanil	1.7	119
Warfarin	0.10	7.0	Ondansetron	1.9	133
Aspirin	0.14	9.8	Cimetidine	2.0	140
Probenecid	0.14	9.8	Procainamide	2.0	140
Aminosalicylate	0.23	16	Vecuronium	2.1	147
Gentamicin	0.23	16	Naloxone	2.1	147
Kanamycin	0.25	17	Nitrazepam	2.3	161
Pancuronium	0.26	18	Thiopental	2.5	172
Chlordiazepoxide	0.30	21	Quinidine	2.8	196
Omeprazole	0.34	24	Amphotericin B	3.0	210
Cloxacillin	0.35	24	Morphine	3.0	210
Sulfadiazine	0.35	24	Ketamine	3.1	214
Tubocurarine	0.39	27	Propranolol	4.0	280
Methotrexate	0.40	28	Verapamil	4.0	280
Vancomycin	0.45	31	Cyclosporine	4.0	280
Prednisolone	0.50	35	Fentanyl	4.3	300
Theophylline	0.50	35	Meperidine	4.4	305
Mercaptopurine	0.60	42	Etomidate	5.4	380
Oxazepam	0.65	45	Tubocurarine	5.7	400
Phenytoin	0.65	45	Amitriptyline	8.0	560
Atenolol	0.70	49	Digoxin	10.0	700
Erythromycin	0.70	49	Propofol	11.0	771
Lithium	0.80	56	Tacrolimus	19.0	1,330
Phenobarbital	0.80	56	Chlorpromazine	20.0	1,400
Midazolam	0.90	63	Haloperidol	25.0	1,750
Acetaminophen	1.00	70	Fluoxetine	28.0	1,960
Bupivacaine	1.00	70	Amiodarone	60.0	4,200
Chloroquine	200.0	14,000			

Vd = volume of distribution.

*Volumes vary between individuals; values are approximate.

Source: Adapted from LZ Benet, N Massoud, JG Gambertoglio (eds). Pharmacokinetic Basis for Drug Treatment. New York: Raven Press, 1984;1–28; M Rowland, TN Tozer. Principles of Applied Pharmacokinetics (3rd ed). Baltimore: Williams & Wilkins, 1995; and CJ Hull. Pharmacokinetics for Anaesthesia. Boston: Butterworth–Heinemann, 1991.

Clearance

CL is a constant describing the rate of drug elimination from the body (hepatic, renal, and other) to observed blood concentrations at steady state. Whole-body CL is therefore the sum of hepatic CL (CL_H), renal CL (CL_r), and clearances from other sites. It is defined as the volume of blood from which all drug is removed in unit time and thus has units of ml per minute or liters per hour. Note that CL is based on removal of drug from blood, not from plasma or serum. Nevertheless, values calculated from plasma (serum) and blood are the same provided the blood-to-plasma (serum) concentration ratio is 1 (i.e., the measured drug concentration is the same in whole blood and in plasma or serum). With knowledge of CL and a measurement of drug concentration in the blood, the actual rate of drug elimination can be calculated.

$$\text{Rate of elimination} \left(\frac{\text{wt}}{\text{unit time}}\right) =$$

$$\text{CL} \left(\frac{\text{vol}}{\text{unit time}}\right) \times \text{Concentration} \left(\frac{\text{wt}}{\text{vol}}\right)$$

Table 19-6. Selected Drug Substrates for Cytochrome P-450 Enzymes

P-450-3A	P-450-1A2	P-450-2D6	P-450-2C9	P-450-2C19	P-450-2E1
Lidocaine	Theophylline	Amitriptyline	Phenytoin	Diazepam	Acetaminophen*
Diltiazem	Caffeine	Haloperidol	Tolbutamide	Hexobarbital	Ethanol
Verapamil	Phenacetin	Clozapine (?)	Diclofenac	Imipramine*	Enflurane
Erythromycin	Acetaminophen*	Propranolol*	Ibuprofen	Mephenytoin	Chlorzoxazone
Cyclosporine	Antipyrine	Metoprolol	Naproxen	Omeprazole*	
Tacrolimus		Propafenone	Warfarin	Propranolol*	
Rapamycin		Flecainide			
Ketoconazole		Codeine			
Quinidine		Dextromethorphan			
Glyburide		Phenformin			
Nicardipine		Debrisoquine			
Nifedipine		Imipramine*			
Nisoldipine		Fluoxetine			
Felodipine					
Cortisone					
Midazolam					
Triazolam					
Terfenadine					
Taxol					
Alfentanil					
Lovastatin					
Omeprazole*					

*These drugs are metabolized by more than one P-450 isozyme.
Source: Adapted from J Brockmoller, I Roots. Assessment of liver metabolic function. Clin Pharmacokinet 1994;27:216–248; and PF Guengerich. Human Cytochrome P450 Enzymes. In PR Ortiz de Montellano (ed). Cytochrome P450 (2nd ed). New York: Plenum, 1995;473–535.

Under stable physiologic conditions, CL for a particular drug does not change and therapeutic blood concentrations can be manipulated by matching rate drug input to the rate of elimination. However, factors such as disease and drug interactions may alter CL of a particular drug to an extent that dosages may require adjustment to maintain therapeutic concentrations.

The CL of a drug is a function of the blood flow to the eliminating organ and the ability of the organ to extract unbound drug from the blood perfusing it. If we consider the liver as an example, CL_H is related to blood flow and the metabolic activity by this formula:

$$CL_H = Q \times ER_H$$

where Q is the blood flow and ER_H is the extraction ratio. ER_H is simply the proportion of drug irreversibly removed from the blood during transit through the liver and has a value between 0 and 1.

For instance, if all incoming drug is metabolized (i.e., no parent drug exits the liver in the venous blood), then 100% of the drug is extracted and value for ER_H is 1. The maximum CL_H is then the rate at which the drug is presented to the site of metabolism (i.e., the hepatic blood flow) or approximately 1,300 ml per minute. On the other hand, if no drug were extracted on its passage through the liver, ER_H would be 0 and thus CL_H would be 0.

The CL_H of drugs with high hepatic extraction ratios (>0.7) is relatively unaffected by protein binding because drug molecules are avidly extracted from the blood by the hepatocyte regardless of protein binding, and ER_H remains constant. The CL_H of such drugs is therefore influenced more by hepatic blood flow than by protein binding and is said to be perfusion rate limited. On the other hand, the CL_H of low-extraction drugs (<0.3) is metabolically rate limited such that the equilibrium between free and bound drug is not greatly disturbed, and only unbound drug is extracted. The net result is that CL_H of these drugs is influenced by changes in protein binding but relatively unaffected by changes in blood flow.

CL_r can be viewed in much the same way as CL_H, but in this case, drug is excreted into the urine.

$$CL_r = \frac{\text{Amount of drug excreted in urine per time interval}}{\text{Conc}_{ave}\text{ in blood over time interval}}$$

where $conc_{ave}$ is the average concentration. As with any CL term, the unit is volume per unit time.

The removal of drug from the blood by the kidney is the net result of four processes: glomerular filtration, active tubular secretion, active tubular reuptake, and passive tubular resorption. The renal handling of some common substances gives a reasonable idea of the normal interplay between these processes. For instance, creatinine, inulin, and mannitol are non–protein-bound substances that are filtered almost exclusively by the glomerulus. CL_r is therefore equal to glomerular filtration rate (GFR), which is normally approximately 125 ml per minute. Urea and uric acid are filtered at the glomerulus but are also passively resorbed by the tubules; thus, CL_r is less than GFR. Glucose, Na, and K are filtered at the glomerulus but are actively resorbed; therefore, CL_r is essentially 0. Hippurate and para-aminohippurate are completely removed from renal blood in one pass through the kidney ($CL_r \approx 1,200$ ml/minute). Such high clearances can only be achieved with combined filtration and secretion. Probenecid is actively secreted by the renal tubule and is capable of competing with other drugs, particularly acids, that are also actively secreted into the tubule (e.g., some penicillins). CL_r of these drugs is therefore reduced and elimination from the body slowed. Passive resorption of drugs by the renal tubule is influenced by their lipid solubility; therefore, by appropriate pharmacologic alteration of urine pH to maintain the drug molecules in an ionized (polar) form, the reabsorption of weak acids or bases can be reduced. For example, administration of sodium bicarbonate alkalinizes the urine and increases the excretion of salicylate, a weak acid.

Terminal Half-Life

The rate at which drug is eliminated from the blood is reflected by its $t\frac{1}{2}$. This parameter is defined as the time required to reduce the amount of drug in the body (or the concentration in blood or plasma) by a factor of 1/2. The rate of decline is a function of two independent factors already considered: CL and Vd.

$$t\frac{1}{2} = \frac{Vd \times 0.693}{CL}$$

This relationship must be kept in mind when interpreting changes in blood concentrations based only on measurement of $t\frac{1}{2}$. A change in $t\frac{1}{2}$ may reflect an alteration in metabolic rate, in Vd, or in both.

Linear and Nonlinear Kinetics

For most therapeutic agents, the rate of metabolic conversion in the body depends on drug concentration in the blood. This relationship is generally described by the Michaelis-Menton equation:

$$\text{Rate of metabolism (V)} = \frac{Vm \times Cu}{Km + Cu}$$

where Vm is the maximum metabolic rate, Km is the drug concentration at which the metabolic rate is 1/2 Vm, and Cu is the concentration of unbound drug in blood.

For most drugs, the therapeutic free drug concentrations are usually well below Km (Km » Cu) and V in this case reduces to (Vm/Km) × Cu. Under these circumstances, drug metabolism is not rate limited, CL (reflected by Vm/Km) and $t\frac{1}{2}$ remain constant, and drug concentrations rise (or fall) linearly with increasing (or decreasing) doses. Drugs with these characteristics are said to display linear or dose-independent kinetics. On the other hand, if therapeutic concentrations of a drug are significant relative to Km (Cu ≥ Km), the ability of the enzymes to metabolize the drug becomes increasingly rate limited and finally plateaus at Vm. At this point, an increase in dose is accompanied by a disproportional increase in concentration, as is seen with phenytoin and theophylline in the therapeutic range. When metabolism becomes rate limiting in this way, CL and $t\frac{1}{2}$ are no longer constant; essentially, they become meaningless.

Pharmacokinetic Models: First-Order Processes

Almost all movement of drug between blood and body tissues is governed by processes that are driven by concentration gradients. The steeper the

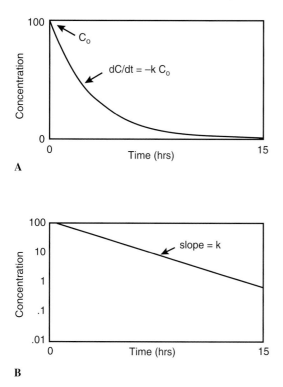

A

B

Figure 19-1. Concentration-time profile for drug displaying first-order elimination from a single compartment. **A.** The relationship between the rate of decline of drug concentration (dC/dt) and the initial concentration (C_o) after an intravenous bolus injection. k is the elimination rate constant. **B.** Same data but plotted as the natural logarithm concentration versus time. The straight line is characteristic of a drug with single-compartment pharmacokinetics. The slope is k.

gradient, the greater the amount of drug transferred per unit time. Such processes are quite common in nature. They are called *first order* because the rates of transfer (e.g., drug molecules crossing a semipermeable membrane) can be shown mathematically to depend on concentration raised to the first power. The general equation is as follows:

$$\frac{dC}{dt} = -kC^n$$

where dC/dt is the change in concentration as a function of time, C is the concentration at the site of highest concentration, k is the diffusion or transfer rate constant, and n is an exponent. In this equation, if n = 0, then C = 1, and the equation reduces to

$$\frac{dC}{dt} = -k$$

In this case, the rate of change is independent of C and is called *zero order*. For a first-order process, n = 1, and thus the equation becomes:

$$\frac{dC}{dt} = -kC$$

Integration of this equation gives this one:

$$C_t = C_0\, e^{-kt}$$

which is an exponential relationship (e) relating the concentration (C_t) to the elapsed time (t) when the initial concentration is C_o. This relationship is fundamental to pharmacokinetic modeling of drugs in blood or plasma as a function of time and, as it stands, is the equation commonly used to describe the concentration-time curve for a one-compartment drug (Figure 19-1A). When concentrations are converted to their natural logarithms (ln), the equation becomes:

$$\ln C_t = \ln C_o - kt$$

Thus, a plot of lnC versus time (the semi-ln plot) is a straight line with a slope of –k (i.e., concentrations are decreasing), as shown in Figure 19-1B.

Compartmental Models

Pharmacokinetic modeling is useful for generating dosing schedules and for assessing the mechanism of drug interactions that involve changes in pharmacokinetic profiles. The kinetics of most therapeutic agents can be described by a two-compartment model. However, a spectrum of "compartmentality" exists, such that, for practical purposes, a single-compartment model may be adequate for some drugs, whereas others may require a more complex model. The appropriate model is usually chosen after graphical assessment of drug concentration-time data that are obtained from preclinical animal studies or from clinical phase I and II studies. These studies also determine whether a drug displays linear kinetics with increasing doses (i.e., dose-independent kinetics).

One-Compartment Model

The one-compartment model is the simplest pharmacokinetic model, in which the decline in drug concentration after an intravenous bolus dose behaves as though the body were a single homogeneous volume from which drug is eliminated. In this case, the slope of the line reflects elimination of drug.

A single-compartment model is described by the following first-order relationship:

$$C_t = C_o \, e^{-kt}$$

C_t is the concentration at time t, C_o is the drug concentration at time 0, and k is the elimination rate constant. The negative sign indicates loss of drug over time.

Two-Compartment Model

The two-compartment model can be envisioned as a rapidly exchanging central compartment (including the blood), into which drug is administered, and a more slowly exchanging deep or peripheral compartment in which drug accumulates during the distribution process (Figure 19-2), where k12 and k21 are transfer constants describing the back-and-forth movement of drug between the central and peripheral compartments, and k is the elimination rate constant from the central compartment.

For simplicity, it is normally assumed that all drug is irreversibly eliminated from the central compartment. Therefore, any drug in the peripheral compartment must first diffuse back into the central compartment before elimination can occur. In this model, the concentration profile after an intravenous bolus is characterized by an initial rapid decline in concentration, usually associated with drug distribution, followed by a slower terminal decline reflecting irreversible elimination of drug from the blood (Figure 19-3).

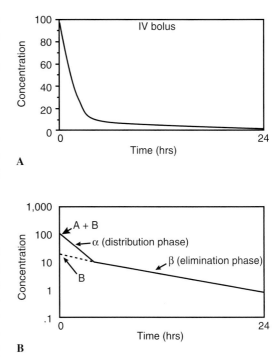

A

B

Figure 19-3. Concentration-time profile for a drug displaying two-compartment kinetics. **A.** Declining concentrations after an intravenous (IV) bolus. **B.** The natural logarithm concentration showing the two compartments: an initial fast distribution phase (α) and slower terminal elimination phase (β). As plotted, the rapid decline contains both distribution and elimination components until the inflection point is reached. A and B are concentrations at time 0 for each compartment. The extrapolated concentration, B, can be used to calculate volume of distribution.

The decline in concentration over time in the central compartment can be described by the sum of two first-order processes:

$$C_t = Ae^{-\alpha t} + Be^{-\beta t}$$

where C_t is the concentration in blood or plasma after an elapsed time t, A and B are initial concentrations derived by back-extrapolation to t = 0, and α and β are hybrid constants (derived from the rate constants k12, k21, and k in Figure 19-2) representing the slopes of the distribution and terminal phase, respectively.

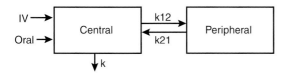

Figure 19-2. A two-compartment pharmacokinetic model composed of a central and peripheral compartment. Drug is administered into the central compartment and distributes from there into the peripheral compartment. The drug movement between these compartments is governed by the first-order rate constants k12 and k21. Elimination occurs from the central compartment with a rate constant, k. Volume of distribution will be the sum of the volumes for each compartment.

Noncompartmental Methods

The number of compartments required to best describe the decline of drug concentrations after an intravenous

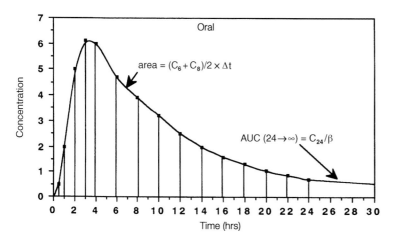

Figure 19-4. Calculation of total area under the curve (AUC) by the trapezoidal method. The area for each trapezoid is calculated as shown from the concentration-time plot and then summed over time (t). The residual area from the time point (24 hours) to infinity is determined by dividing the concentration by β, the slope of the terminal component. This procedure can be applied to all concentration-time plots regardless of the route of drug administration.

bolus dose can sometimes be difficult to determine. This can arise from the experimental design of the pharmacokinetic study, particularly with regard to the timing and frequency of blood samples. Conflicting results using compartmental analysis has led to the increasing use of statistical moments. This analytic approach is applicable to all drugs and is based on the amount of time drug molecules appear to reside in the body. Moment analysis looks at the body as a whole and does not attempt to create structural models, as in compartmental analysis. When considering the arithmetic plot of concentration versus time for an intravenous bolus drug (see Figure 19-1A), the *zero moment* of the plot is the conventional area under the curve (AUC), whereas the *first moment* is the area under the product of concentration and elapsed time versus time plot (AUMC). These two parameters are then used to calculate the mean residence time (MRT), CL, and Vd at steady state (Vd_{ss}). If a drug is given orally, the mean absorption time can also be calculated from the difference of MRT_{IV} and MRT_{oral}. A more detailed description of moment analysis is presented by Gibaldi[20] and Rowland and Tozer.[21]

Derivation of Common Pharmacokinetic Parameters from Blood and Plasma Data

Bioavailability

Oral bioavailability (F) of drug is calculated from the ratio of AUCs for equal doses of intravenous and orally administered drug. Thus:

$$F = \frac{AUC_{oral}}{AUC_{IV}}$$

Table 19-2 lists examples of drugs with low F due to first-pass effect (i.e., metabolized in liver, gut, and so forth). Other causes of low F may be malabsorption from the gut (e.g., cyclosporine and tacrolimus), poor dissolution of solid oral formulations, and chemical or enzymatic degradation of drug within the stomach or small intestine (e.g., penicillin G, erythromycin).

The AUC is usually derived from the sum of trapezoids (Figure 19-4), with the residual area from the last time point to infinity being estimated from the following relationship:

$$Area(residual) = \frac{C_t}{\beta}$$

where Ct is the last measured concentration and β is the terminal rate constant.

Volume of Distribution

In theory, Vd should be determined after drug accumulation has reached a plateau (i.e., blood or plasma concentrations are at steady state), but this is impractical in many instances.

In practice, Vd can be calculated from a single intravenous dose by several methods, three of which are shown below.

$$1.\ Vd_{extrap} = \frac{Dose_{IV}}{C_o}$$

$$2.\ Vd_{area} = \frac{Dose}{AUC \times \beta}$$

$$3.\ Vd_{ss} = \frac{IV\ dose \times AUMC}{(AUC)^2}$$

For a one-compartment drug, the values for Vd are identical by each method. For a two-compartment drug, however, methods 1 and 2 overestimate Vd. The most robust means of calculating Vd is method 3. This technique gives an estimate of Vd_{ss} even though it is calculated from a single intravenous bolus dose. In addition, there is no need to specify a particular model, as is necessary for compartmental analysis.

Vd can also be derived from oral doses in the same manner, but the amount of drug that reaches the systemic circulation (i.e., the bioavailability, or F) must be known before a relevant volume can be calculated.

Elimination Half-Life

The t½ of a drug is derived from the slope of the ln concentration versus time plot (i.e., k for one compartment and β from the terminal component of a two-compartment model):

$$\text{Slope }(\beta) = \frac{(\ln c - \ln c_{0.5})}{\Delta t} = \frac{\ln \dfrac{c}{c_{0.5}}}{\Delta t}$$

where C is drug concentration, $C_{0.5}$ is one-half of initial drug concentration, and Δt is time taken for concentration of drug to decrease by half.

By definition, however,

$$\frac{c}{c_{0.5}} = 2$$

Therefore,

$$\Delta t = \frac{(\ln 2)}{\beta} = t^{1/2}$$

Because ln 2 = 0.693,

$$t^{1/2} = \frac{0.693}{\beta}$$

Total Clearance

CL can be calculated in two ways, depending on the model used:

$$1.\ CL = Vd \times k \ (\text{one compartment})$$

$$CL = Vd \times \beta \ (\text{two compartment})$$

or

$$2.\ CL = \frac{Dose}{AUC}$$

Derivation of these formulas can be found elsewhere.[21]

Equation 2 is the most convenient means of calculating CL because it does not depend on specifying a model. As noted earlier for Vd_{ss}, CL cannot be calculated from an oral dose unless the bioavailability (F) is known. However, it is not unusual to see oral CL reported as CL/F. This is a way of compensating for an unknown F, but it assumes, rightly or wrongly, that F remains constant and only CL changes.

Pharmacokinetic Parameters Related to Oral Dosing

At this point, it is worth mentioning some descriptive parameters commonly used to describe the kinetics of a drug given orally and by other extravascular routes. Figure 19-5A shows typical concentration versus time and ln concentration versus time plots. Maximum concentration (C_{max}) and the time required to achieve C_{max} (t_{max}) reflect the amount of drug absorbed and the rate of absorption, respectively. Also characteristic of orally administered drugs is a delay (lag time) in the appearance of the drug in peripheral blood. The lag time, which may vary between a few minutes to several hours, is usually associated with gastric retention or, in the case of enteric formulations, with both gastric retention and dissolution of the enteric coating in the small intestine.[22]

Multiple Dosing and Drug Accumulation

The kinetics of single intravenous or oral doses of drugs have thus far been considered and parameters were derived. The most important of these are CL, t½, and Vd. From such information, dosing schedules can be derived to maintain blood levels within a therapeutic range.

The steady-state concentrations (C_{ss}) of any drug having first-order kinetics is reached after four to five half-lives of repeated oral doses or continuous intravenous infusion. This is demonstrated in Table 19-7 for a drug that is given as an intravenous bolus every t½.

Unlike the smooth concentration curve obtained with intravenous infusions, oral dosing is characterized by a sawtooth appearance of peak (C_{max}) and trough (C_{min}) levels, with an average concentration (C_{ave}) falling somewhere between these two extremes. For therapeutic monitoring, the dose

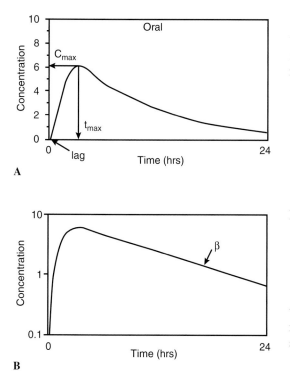

A

B

Figure 19-5. Typical concentration true plot for oral dose. **A.** Parameters associated with oral dose–maximum concentration (C_{max}), the time required to achieve C_{max} (t_{max}), and the delay (lag). **B.** The natural logarithm concentration-time profile and the slope, β, of the terminal phase (assuming two-compartment model).

adjustments are normally based on trough concentrations that define the lower limit of the therapeutic range. C_{max}, on the other hand, is maintained at a level that minimizes adverse events.

At steady state, as the term implies, the rate at which drug enters the bloodstream, either from intravenous infusion or oral dosing, is equal to the rate at which it is removed.

For intravenous infusion,

$$\text{Infusion rate} = \text{Elimination rate}$$
$$\text{Since elimination rate} = CL \times C_{ss}$$
$$\text{then infusion rate} = CL \times C_{ss}$$
$$\text{and } C_{ss} = \frac{\text{infusion rate}}{CL}$$

For oral dosing,

$$\text{Rate of drug input} = \frac{\text{dose}(F)}{\tau}$$
$$\text{Rate of drug output} = C_{ave} \times CL$$

where F is the oral bioavailability, τ is the dosing interval, and C_{ave} is the average concentration at steady state.

Therefore,

$$C_{ave} = \frac{\text{dose}(F)}{CL \times \tau}$$

From these relationships, it can be seen that if CL (and F for an oral dose) remain unchanged, serum concentration during intravenous infusion is directly proportional to infusion rate or the amount and frequency of oral dosing. It must be remembered that the time to achieve a new steady state, no matter in which direction the dose is changed, is four to five half-lives. For this reason, many pharmacokinetic studies comparing two or more drugs by a crossover design allow

Table 19-7. Accumulation of a Drug When 100-mg Dose Is Repeated Every Terminal Half-Life (t½)

Time (t½)	Doses					Trough Total[a]	Peak Total[b]
	First	Second	Third	Fourth	Fifth		
0	100	—	—	—	—	0	100
1	50	100	—	—	—	50	150
2	25	50	100	—	—	75	175
3	12.5	25	50	100	—	87	187
4	6.2	12.5	25	50	100	94	194
5	3.12	6.25	12.5	25	50	97	197
6	1.56	3.12	6.25	12.5	25	99	199

[a]Amount in body before next dose (trough).
[b]Current dose plus drug remaining in the body from previous doses.

lengthy washout periods between each phase. Furthermore, a loading dose may be required for drugs with long half-lives to cover the period between initiation of dosing and attainment of therapeutic concentrations.

Factors That Affect Drug Pharmacokinetics

Hepatic Dysfunction

The effect of liver disease on pharmacokinetics is apparent only for drugs that are predominantly eliminated by the liver. Nevertheless, there is mounting evidence to suggest that the hepatorenal syndrome (renal impairment linked only to severe hepatic failure) is present even in modest liver dysfunction and that reduced renal excretion of drugs can occur.[23]

The effect of liver dysfunction on CL is not always predictable due to the various types of hepatic disease and the effect they may have on metabolic enzyme activity, blood flow, and protein binding. For drugs such as fentanyl ($ER_H = 0.8$) and sufentanil ($ER_H = 1$), the CL_H is sensitive to alterations in blood flow, whereas CL_H of alfentanil ($ER_H = 0.4$) is influenced more by changes in protein binding and metabolic enzyme activity.[24] With few exceptions, CL of a drug is decreased in chronic diseases, such as cirrhosis, chronic hepatitis, and obstructive jaundice. In acute viral hepatitis, there is a range of effects in which the CL of some drugs does not change while for others it increases (see reviews by Wilkinson and Schenker,[25] Bass et al. 1988,[26] McLean and Morgan,[27] and Morgan and McLean[23]). Any reduction in hepatic metabolism is restricted to oxidative processes (phase I); conjugation (phase II) reactions appear to be little affected.[27]

To assess changes in hepatic metabolic capability, it is not uncommon to measure the t½ of drugs. However, t½ measurements alone may lead to inappropriate dose changes. If an increase in t½ is due to reduced CL, a dose reduction may be necessary. However, t½ is also increased by expansion of Vd, but in this case, dose reduction is not required because the main determinant of steady-state drug concentration is CL.

A reduction in protein binding is commonly seen in liver disease as a result of reduced hepatic synthesis of albumin and alpha$_1$-acid glycoprotein.[28, 29] This has varied effects on the half-lives of drugs, depending on their hepatic extraction ratios. In general, a reduction in protein binding increases CL of drugs that have low hepatic extraction ratios (<0.3) (metabolizing enzymes are rate limited by available free drug). However, Vd may also increase because unbound drug tends to redistribute to extravascular tissues. An increase in Vd is more noticeable if it is relatively small to start with (<15 liters); if Vd is initially large, the impact of reduced protein binding will be small.[30]

Drugs with high hepatic extraction ratios normally show a high first-pass effect, which can be affected by two mechanisms in liver disease. The first is reduced hepatic extraction due to declining enzyme activity (in other words, the extraction ratio declines). The second is intra- or extrahepatic portocaval shunting, which decreases first-pass metabolism by allowing drug to bypass the liver during the absorption process. These mechanisms result in increased oral bioavailability and steady-state concentrations; therefore, doses may have to be reduced. Propranolol is often used as a model for high-extraction drugs. A study of intravenous and oral doses of this drug in patients with cirrhosis revealed a threefold increase in steady-state free drug concentrations compared to normal subjects due to a decrease in first-pass effect, reduced intrinsic CL or portasystemic shunting, and decreased systemic CL. Protein binding was decreased, consequently expanding Vd. The combined changes in CL and Vd resulted in the t½ of propranolol increasing by a factor of approximately 3.[31] Other drugs that behave in a similar way are pentazocine, meperidine, and salicylamide. These are high–first-pass analgesic agents that show increased bioavailability and reduced CL in patients with cirrhosis.[32]

Tacrolimus kinetics must be interpreted with care due to a high but variable blood to plasma ratio (13.4–114.0). Although the drug has low bioavailability (approximately 25%) and is extensively metabolized by the liver,[33] its CL based on plasma analysis is high (1,974 ml/minute); based on blood, however, CL is low (63 ml/minute).[34] The Vd is likewise affected by the high blood to plasma ratio (see Table 19-5). It is likely that rapamycin kinetics must be interpreted with similar caution because it, too, has a high blood to plasma ratio (approximately 11).[10] The impact of these observations on therapeutic monitoring is not clear, but the situation is highly reminiscent of that confronting cyclosporine monitoring when the problems of temperature-dependent plasma concentrations and variable blood to plasma ratios were first recognized.[35]

Patients with defective graft function were found to have unexpectedly high plasma tacrolimus concentrations relative to those with normally functioning grafts or to patients with kidney and heart transplants. The degree of increase correlated with serum bilirubin concentrations and was sufficient to require dose reductions.[36] Because these observations were made with intravenous dosing, it is reasonable to attribute the changes to reduced CL_H.

Although the posttransplant CL_H of cyclosporine may be reduced with increasing severity of liver dysfunction, the reduction would be relatively small because of its low hepatic extraction ratio (0.3). Of greater impact on the dose-concentration relationship and therapeutic monitoring is the characteristic erratic absorption of cyclosporine, however, which can severely reduce bioavailability during this period. In a controlled study in patients with biliary cirrhosis, the systemic CL of cyclosporine was not altered compared to that in patients with psoriasis,[37] but others have noted a large variability in pharmacokinetic results from such patients.[38]

Hepatic diseases in which bile flow is compromised can have a large impact on highly lipophilic oral drugs that require emulsification with bile before absorption from the small intestine. In such cases, oral bioavailability is decreased due to poor absorption, and much of the drug is excreted in the feces. In the field of transplantation, this is a particularly perplexing problem with oral formulations of cyclosporine. Shortly after transplantation, when liver and intestinal function are temporarily compromised due to surgical procedures, cyclosporine bioavailability can be extremely low with current oil-based formulations. For this reason, intravenous infusions are given until oral absorption improves. The important role of bile has been directly demonstrated in patients with biliary diversion via open T-tubes[2–4] and in pharmacokinetic studies with a microemulsion formulation of cyclosporine (Neoral) in liver transplant patients.[39] Significantly, although tacrolimus is highly lipophilic and has similar bioavailability to cyclosporine, its absorption does not appear to depend on biliary excretion.[40]

Transplantation procedures result in gastric and intestinal dysfunction that is reflected in a reduction in the rate and extent of absorption of orally administered drugs. The absorption process is hindered by slowed gastric emptying or reduced intestinal motility. Studies with the prokinetic agent metoclopramide in kidney transplant patients revealed that cyclosporine bioavailability was improved by 29%, presumably by increasing the rate of drug delivery to the small intestine and improving mixing in the gut lumen.[16] Improved bioavailability was also reported with concomitant use of cisapride, another prokinetic agent.[41] In the case of tacrolimus, in vitro studies suggest that the drug is unstable in solutions of magnesium oxide and is readily adsorbed to aluminum hydroxide.[17] It is likely, therefore, that coadministration of these antacids with tacrolimus to transplant patients could reduce its bioavailability. Other antacids (sodium bicarbonate) also appear to reduce tacrolimus bioavailability to varying degrees.[17] The mechanism of interaction with magnesium oxide and sodium bicarbonate has been attributed to the instability of tacrolimus at alkaline pH.

Renal Dysfunction

The major impact of renal failure affects the urinary excretion of drugs and their metabolites that are primarily eliminated by the kidney. Meperidine and morphine, for example, are metabolized by the liver to active compounds (normeperidine and morphine-6-glucuronide) that are excreted by the kidney. Both metabolites can accumulate in the blood and cause significant side effects (seizures and respiratory depression, respectively) during renal insufficiency.[42] Drugs that are eliminated by other routes are generally little affected by renal impairment unless CL by those routes is influenced by renal-induced changes in protein binding (e.g., CL_H of phenytoin). Cyclosporine, tacrolimus, and rapamycin are eliminated by hepatic metabolism and therefore are essentially unaffected by kidney dysfunction. Renal failure affects GFR as well as tubular secretion and resorption.[43] Therefore, the CL_r of all drugs eliminated by this route is reduced regardless of extraction efficiency. The CL of creatinine (CL_{cr}), a commonly used marker of renal function, shows an inverse linear relationship with increasing severity of renal dysfunction. This has been demonstrated for several drugs, including cefepime,[44] gabapentin,[45] and the antibiotics (reviewed by St. Peter et al.[46]). The antiepileptic agent, gabapentin, is essentially unbound and is eliminated entirely by renal excretion. Changes in total CL and $t\frac{1}{2}$ as a function of declining renal function (CL_{cr}) are shown in Table 19-8.

Renal failure was the first pathologic condition to be associated with abnormalities in drug binding to plasma proteins.[47] Most acidic drugs bind to albumin, whereas basic drugs bind mostly to alpha₁-acid glycoprotein, an acute-phase reactant that increases in the blood during several circumstances, including stress (burn injury), myocardial infarction, trauma, surgery, carcinoma, inflammatory disease, and infection (reviewed by Piafsky 1980[7]). Neutral drugs bind to a variety of blood components, including plasma proteins, red cells, and lipoproteins.

Binding of acidic drugs to albumin in uremic patients is decreased due to accumulation of endogenous substances that compete with drug molecules for protein binding sites. In addition, there is evidence to suggest that the molecular structure of albumin is altered such that binding affinity is reduced.[47] With increased free fraction of drug in the circulation, the CL_H of low-extraction acidic drugs and their Vd may increase with a consequent reduction in t½. For example, the binding of phenytoin to plasma proteins declines from 90% in individuals with normal renal function to 80% when creatinine levels rise to 10–12 mg/dl. The resulting increase in CL_H and Vd lowers total blood concentration by as much as 50%. Nevertheless, seizure control in uremic patients is adequate without dose changes because the unbound concentration remains within the therapeutic range (1–2 μg/ml). The unbound fraction of several other acid drugs (warfarin, furosemide, salicylate, diazoxide, clofibrate, and some sulfonamides) may also increase in uremia due to endogenous competitors, even though albumin levels are normal.

In contrast to acidic drugs, the protein binding of basic drugs in uremic patients is either unchanged or only slightly decreased.[7]

CL_r of a drug depends on the interplay between filtration, tubular secretion, and tubular resorption. In uremic patients, it appears that all these functions decline in parallel due to an absolute loss (≈ 90%) of functioning nephrons. In nephrotic patients, however, plasma albumin is lost in the urine, but CL_{cr} remains relatively normal. In this situation, the effect of decreased plasma protein binding on CL_r is reasonably predictable based on renal extraction ratios. Only unbound drug is filtered at the glomerulus; thus, decreased protein binding increases the elimination rate of drugs by filtration. Acidic drugs, such as penicillins, are rapidly secreted into the renal tubule even though they are highly protein bound and would be relatively unaffected by changes in protein binding.

Table 19-8. Gabapentin Elimination after Oral Administration to Patients with Renal Failure

CL_{cr} (ml/min)	CL_r*	CL/F*	Terminal Half-Life (hrs)*
>60	79	160	9.2
30–59	36	63	14.0
<30	11	24	40.0

CL_{cr} = creatinine clearance; CL_r = renal clearance; CL/F = apparent oral clearance.
*Values are medians.
Source: Adapted from RA Blum, TJ Comstock, DA Sica, et al. Pharmacokinetics of gabapentin in subjects with various degrees of renal function. Clin Pharmacol Ther 1994;56:154–159.

protein binding. Similarly, glucuronide and sulfate conjugates of many drugs are highly extracted by the renal tubule and are likely to be unaffected by reduced concentrations of plasma albumin. Between these extremes are drugs that are poorly secreted and are more affected by protein binding.

Cardiovascular Dysfunction

Reduction in hepatic blood flow may also result from conditions that compromise cardiac output, such as shock and congestive heart failure. Reduced tissue perfusion can potentially affect hepatic CL of highly extracted drugs. This was shown for lidocaine in patients with mild and severe congestive heart failure.[48]

Reduced perfusion of the splanchnic bed may also reduce absorption from the small intestine or other routes of administration. Studies in humans have suggested that general anesthesia slows the absorption of cyclosporine in liver transplant patients if an oral dose is given within a 4-hour period before surgery.[49] This was confirmed in fasted anesthetized rats (albeit with normal liver function), in which the rate, and probably the extent, of oral cyclosporine absorption was decreased by isoflurane.[50]

Drug Interactions

Pharmacokinetic drug interactions are an important consideration in therapies requiring the administration of more than one drug. In the field of transplantation, drug interactions are an ever-present

Table 19-9. Drug Interactions with Cyclosporine or Tacrolimus

Drug	Proposed Mechanism	Cyclosporine	Tacrolimus
Pharmacokinetic interactions that decrease concentrations			
Carbamazepine	Increased metabolism	√	—
Nafcillin	Increased metabolism	√	—
Phenobarbitone	Increased metabolism	√	—
Phenytoin[a]	Increased metabolism		—
	Decreased absorption	√	—
Rifampin	Increased metabolism	√	√[b]
Somatostatin analogue	Increased absorption	√	—
Sulfonamide/trimethoprim	Increased metabolism (?)	√	—
Pharmacokinetic interactions that increase concentrations			
Danazol	Inhibited metabolism	√	√[c]
Diltiazem	Inhibited metabolism	√	—
Erythromycin[a]	Inhibited metabolism	√	—
	Increased absorption	√	—
Ketoconazole	Inhibited metabolism	√	√
Methyltestosterone	Inhibited metabolism	√	—
Methylprednisolone	Inhibited metabolism	√	√[b]
Metoclopramide	Increased absorption	√	—
Nicardipine	Inhibited metabolism	√	—
Norfloxacin	Inhibited metabolism	√[d]	—
Oral contraceptives	Inhibited metabolism	√	—
Verapamil	Inhibited metabolism	√	—
Grapefruit juice	Inhibited metabolism	√[e]	—
Pharmacodynamic interactions that increase nephrotoxicity			
Aminoglycosides	—	√	—
Amphotericin B	—	√	—
Cimetidine/ranitidine	—	√	—
Co-trimoxazole	—	√	—

[a]Both mechanisms have been reported.

[b]V Furlan, L Perello, E Jacquemin, et al. Interaction between FK506 and rifampicin or erythromycin in pediatric liver recipients. Transplantation 1995;59:1217–1218.

[c]R Shapiro, R Venkataramanan, US Warty, et al. FK506 interaction with Danazol. Lancet 1993;341:1344–1345.

[d]RA McLellan, RK Drobitch, DH McLellan, et al. Norfloxacin interferes with cyclosporine disposition in pediatric patients undergoing renal transplantation. Clin Pharmacol Ther 1995;58:322–327.

[e]MP Ducharme, LH Warbasse, DJ Edwards. Disposition of intravenous and oral cyclosporine after administration with grapefruit juice. Clin Pharmacol Ther 1995;57:485–491.

Source: Adapted from GC Yee, TR McGuire. Pharmacokinetic drug interaction with cyclosporine (part 1). Clin Pharmacokinet 1990;19:319–332; and GC Yee, TR McGuire. Pharmacokinetic drug interactions with cyclosporine (part 2). Clin Pharmacokinet 1990;19:400–415.

danger to recipients of organ transplants. The key immunosuppressants, cyclosporine and tacrolimus, are both metabolized by CYP 3A4, an isoenzyme of the cytochrome P-450 family, which is found in abundance in the gut wall and liver. The steady-state blood concentrations these drugs are subject to clinically important changes when coadministered with agents that induce or inhibit metabolism. Interactions that inhibit metabolism may cause increases in concentrations sufficient to cause nephro- or hepatotoxicity, whereas drug-induced metabolism

may reduce concentrations to the extent that rejection occurs. In both cases, dose adjustments based on careful evaluation of trough levels must be made to compensate for changes in elimination rates of the immunosuppressants.

In vitro screening studies with both cyclosporine and tacrolimus confirm the potential for interaction with drugs that are metabolized by CYP 3A4.[13–15, 51] It should be kept in mind, however, that some of these interactions may not be clinically important in vivo (e.g., nifedipine). Table 19-9 is a compilation of reported interactions with cyclosporine and tacrolimus in transplant patients.

Conclusions

The movement of drug within the various tissues of the human body is difficult or impossible to study directly. Pharmacokinetic models have therefore been developed based on drug and metabolite movements in readily accessible biological fluids and expired air. These models are now used routinely to examine and quantify the effects of disease, genetics, and polypharmacy on drug kinetics and to guide the clinician in therapeutic drug monitoring.

It is clear that some drugs are more difficult to get a pharmacokinetic "handle" on than are others. The current immunosuppressive drugs, particularly cyclosporine, tacrolimus, and rapamycin, are cases in point. It is evident that predicting dosing changes and maintaining effective steady-state drug concentrations based on trough concentrations has been anything but easy, particularly in the immediate posttransplant period and several weeks thereafter.

Nevertheless, the effective use of current immunosuppressive drugs in transplantation depends, in part, on recognizing the various factors that can alter the pharmacokinetics of these agents in the patient. Monitoring drug concentrations based on knowledge of potential problems (e.g., drug interactions, disease states) continues to be a key component of clinical management of transplant patients.

References

1. Brodie BB, Kurz H, Schanker LJ. The importance of dissociation constants and lipid solubility on influencing the passage of drugs into the CSF. J Pharmacol Exp Ther 1960;130:20–25.
2. Mehta M, Venkataramanan R, Burkart GJ, et al. Antipyrine kinetics in liver disease and liver transplantation. Clin Pharmacol Ther 1986;39:372–377.
3. Levy G, Asfar S, Rochon J, et al. Cyclosporine Neoral in liver transplant recipients. Transplant Proc 1994;26:2949–2952.
4. Trull AK, Tan KKC, Tan L, et al. Absorption of cyclosporin from conventional and new microemulsion oral formulations in liver transplant recipients with external billiary diversion. Br J Clin Pharmacol 1995;39:627–631.
5. Pond SM, Tozer TN. First pass elimination: basic concepts and clinical consequences. Clin Pharmacokinet 1984;9:1–25.
6. Tam YK. Individual variation in first-pass metabolism. Clin Pharmacokinet 1993;25:300–328.
7. Piafsky KM. Disease-induced changes in the plasma binding of basic drugs. Clin Pharmacokinet 1980;5:246–262.
8. Herve F, Urien S, Albengres EE, et al. Drug binding in plasma: a summary of recent trends in the study of drug and hormone binding. Clin Pharmacokinet 1994;26:44–58.
9. Peters DH, Fitton A, Plosker GL, Faulds D. Tacrolimus: a review of its pharmacology and therapeutic potential in hepatic and renal transplantation. Drugs 1993;46:746–794.
10. Yatscoff R, Wang P, Chan K, et al. Rapamycin: distribution, pharmacokinetics and therapeutic range investigations. Ther Drug Monit 1995;17:666–670.
11. Watkins P. Drug metabolism by cytochromes P450 in the liver and bowel. Gastroenterol Clin North Am 1992;21:511–526.
12. Guengerich PF. Human Cytochrome P450 Enzymes. In PR Ortiz de Montellano (ed), Cytochrome P450 (2nd ed). New York: Plenum Press, 1995;473–535.
13. Pichard L, Fabre I, Domergue J, et al. Screening for inducers and inhibitors of cytochrome P450 (cyclosporin A oxidase) in primary cultures of human hepatocytes and in liver microsomes. Drug Metabol Dispos 1990;18:595–606.
14. Iwasaki K, Matsuda H, Nagase K, et al. Effects of twenty-three drugs on the metabolism of FK506 by human liver microsomes. Res Commun Chem Pathol Pharmacol 1993;82:209–216.
15. Prasad TNV, Stiff DD, Subbotina N, et al. FK506 (tacrolimus) metabolism by rat liver microsomes and its inhibition by other drugs. Res Commun Chem Pathol Pharmacol 1994;84:35–46.
16. Wadhwa NK, Schroeder TJ, Pesce AJ, et al. Cyclosporine drug interactions: a review. Ther Drug Monit 1987;9:399–406.
17. Venkataramanan R, Swaminathan A, Prasad T, et al. Clinical Pharmacokinetics of Tacrolimus. Clin Pharmacokinet 1995;29:404–430.
18. Hobbinger F, Peck AW. Hydrolysis of suxamethonium by different types of plasma. Br J Pharmacol 1969;37:258–271.
19. Nigrovic V, Pandya JB, Klaunig JE, Fry K. Reactivity and toxicity of atracurium and its metabolites in vitro. Can J Anaesth 1989;36:262–268.
20. Gibaldi M. Biopharmaceutics and Clinical Pharmacokinetics (4th ed). Philadelphia: Lea & Febiger, 1991;17.
21. Rowland M, Tozer TN. Principles of Applied Pharmacokinetics (3rd ed). Baltimore: Williams & Wilkins, 1995.
22. Mojaverian P, Rocci ML, Conner DP, et al. Effect of food on the absorption of enteric-coated aspirin: correlation with gastric residence time. Clin Pharmacol Ther 1987;41:11–17.
23. Morgan DJ, McLean AJ. Clinical pharmacokinetic and pharmacodynamic considerations in patients with liver disease. Clin Pharmacokinet 1995;29:370–391.

24. Scholz J, Steinfath M, Schulz M. Clinical pharmacokinetics alfentanil, fentanyl and sufentanil. Clin Pharmacokinet 1996;31:275–292.

25. Wilkinson GR, Schenker S. Drug disposition in liver disease. Drug Metabol Rev 1975;4:139–175.

26. Bass NM, Williams RL. Guide to drug dosage in hepatic disease. Clin Pharmacokinet 1988;15:396–420.

27. McLean AJ, Morgan DJ. Clinical pharmacokinetics in patients with liver disease. Clin Pharmacokinet 1991; 21:42–69.

28. Blaschke TF. Protein binding and kinetics of drugs in liver disease. Clin Pharmacokinet 1977;2:32–44.

29. Tillement JP, Lhoste F, Guidicelli JF. Diseases and drug protein binding. Clin Pharmacokinet 1978;3:144–154.

30. Rowland M. Protein binding and drug clearance. Clin Pharmacokinet 1984;9(Suppl 1):10–17.

31. Wood AJ, Carr K, Vestal RE, et al. Direct measurement of propanolol bioavailability during accumulation to steady-state. Br J Clin Pharmacol 1978;6:345–350.

32. Neal A, Meffin PJ, Gregory PB, Blaschke TF. Enhanced bioavailability and decreased clearance of analgesics in patients with cirrhosis. Gastroenterology 1979;77:96–102.

33. Venkataramanan R, Jain A, Cadoff E, et al. Pharmacokinetics of FK506: preclinical and clinical studies. Transplant Proc 1991;22(Suppl 1):52–56.

34. Jusko WJ, Piekoszewski W, Klintmalm GB, et al. Pharmacokinetics of tacrolimus in liver transplant patients. Clin Pharmacol Ther 1995;57:291–290.

35. Shaw LM, Yatscoff RW, Bowers LD, et al. Canadian consensus meeting on cyclosporine monitoring: report of the consensus panel. Clin Chem 1990;36: 1841–1846.

36. Abu-Elmagd K, Fung JJ, Alessiana M, et al. The effect of graft function on FK506 plasma levels, dosages and renal function, with particular reference to the liver. Transplantation 1991;52:71–77.

37. Beukers R, De Rave S, Van Den Berg JWO, Schalm SW. Oral pharmacokinetics of cyclosporine in patients with primary biliary cirrhosis and patients with skin diseases. Aliment Pharmacol Ther 1992;6:459–468.

38. de Groen PC, McCallum DK, Moyer TP Wieser RH.

39. Freeman D, Grant D, Levy G, et al. Pharmacokinetics of a new oral formulation of cyclosporine in liver transplant patients. Ther Drug Monit 1995;17:213–216.

40. Furokawa H, Imventarza O, Venkataramanan R, et al. The effect of bile duct ligation and bile diversion on FK506 pharmacokinetics in dogs. Transplantation 1992;53:722–725.

41. Finet L, Westeel PF, Hary L, et al. Effects of cisapride on the intestinal absorption of cyclosporine in renal transplant patients. Gastroenterology 1991;100:A209.

42. Davies G, Kingswood C, Street M. Pharmacokinetics of opioids in renal dysfunction. Clin Pharmacokinet 1996;13:410–422.

43. Dettli L, Spring P, Ryter S. Multiple dose kinetics and drug dosage in patients with kidney disease. Acta Pharmacol Toxicol (Copenh) 1971;29(Suppl 3):211–224.

44. Barbhaiya RH, Knupp CA, Forgue ST, et al. Pharmacokinetics of cefepime in subjects with renal insufficiency. Clin Pharmacol Ther 1990;48:268–276.

45. Blum RA, Comstock TJ, Sica DA, et al. Pharmacokinetics of gabapentin in subjects with various degrees of renal function. Clin Pharmacol Ther 1994;56:154–159.

46. St. Peter WL, Redic-Kill KA, Halstenson CE. Clinical pharmacokinetics of antibiotics in patients with impaired renal function. Clin Pharmacokinet 1992;22:169–210.

47. Reidenberg MM, Drayer DE. Alteration of drug protein binding in renal disease. Clin Pharmacokinet 1984;9 (Suppl 1):18–26.

48. Zito RA, Reid PR. Lidocaine kinetics predicted by indocyanine green clearance. N Engl J Med 1978; 298:1160–1163.

49. Brown MR, Brajtbord D, Johnson D, et al. Efficacy of oral cyclosporine given prior to liver transplantation. Anesth Analg 1989;69:773–775.

50. Gelb AW, Freeman DJ, Robertson KM, Zhang C. Isofluorane alters the kinetics of oral cyclosporine. Anesth Analg 1991;72:801–804.

51. Burke MD, Omar G, Thomson AW, Whiting PH. Inhibition of the metabolism of cyclosporine by human liver microsomes by FK506. Transplantation 1990;50:901–902.

Chapter 20
Ethical Issues in Transplantation*

Calvin R. Stiller and Cate Abbott

Chapter Plan

Ethical dilemmas have occurred throughout the history of transplantation, since the first successful transplant in 1954, when a man donated one of his kidneys to his identical twin. At that time, the likelihood of operative mortality and the long-term risks of living with one kidney were unknown. Transplant surgery proceeded based on the recipient's and donor's consent and the belief that greater psychological risk might result from not donating than from the medical risk of donation.[1]

Since then, most ethical issues have resulted from the unmet need for organs. Many of these issues would be resolved if enough organs were donated or if organs could be mechanically constructed to reduce the disparity between the great demand and the limited supply. Ethical debates will continue as attempts are made to allocate the limited number of organs fairly and to increase the organ supply through scientific advances and new technology.[1]

To increase the number of organs, transplant specialists are considering compensation to the donor's next of kin, increased living donation, xenotransplantation, artificial support devices, and non–heart-beating donors. Ethical theory and principles—such as autonomy, justice, utility, beneficence, and nonmaleficence—must be applied to these scientific advances and policy changes, thereby demonstrating not only technical skill but also ethical accountability.

Ethical Theories and Principles

Ethics—the study of standards for conduct and moral judgment[1]—help as options are considered and moral actions chosen, and bioethics is the application of ethics to medicine and medical research. Few ethicists believe that absolute moral standards of right and wrong exist because ethical judgment can vary among cultures. In multicultural

*Portions of this chapter have previously appeared in Anesthesiology Clinics of North America 1994;12:845-855. © W. B. Saunders Co. Reprinted by permission.

societies, which consist of many different perspectives, ethics do not provide only one answer. Some problems require ethical analysis at the bedside; others require involvement at a broader level, such as policy.[2] A course of action is chosen when it is thought to satisfy certain rules or principles.[3]

Two traditional approaches to ethics are deontology and teleology. Deontologic theory focuses on people's motives or the goodness of their intention. Because humans are seen as rational beings, moral rules are based on reason and logic, so the rules are applicable to everyone as laws of nature. For example, all people have inherent dignity and deserve to be treated with respect. This rule translates as follows: People should be treated as ends in themselves rather than as a means to help someone else. Because we have a duty to treat each other and ourselves in this way, certain actions may be wrong. Actions should be limited when they are incompatible with respect for people, even if the outcome is beneficial. Given this approach, there are limits to high-tech medicine. Just because we are capable of doing something does not necessarily mean that we should do it.

Teleology is based on the principle of utility with the focus on the ultimate end or outcome. Often called *utilitarianism*, this theory determines the goodness of an action by the overall good or value that results for the greatest number of people. With this approach, the value of an action may be based on patient or graft survival rates, quality of life, or cost-benefit analysis.[4–8]

Other, less well-known ethical theories include virtue ethics (people are predisposed to act in the right way), situation ethics (moral action depends on each situation), and a biologically based ethics of suffering (sentient creatures can suffer).[5] Accepted principles for bioethical decision-making include autonomy (patient self-determination and involvement in health care decisions), beneficence (obligation to help and care for patients), nonmaleficence (obligation to avoid harming patients), justice (obligation to provide medical care in an equitable way), and utility (obligation to provide medical care with the greatest good for the greatest number).[4, 9]

Ethical Decision-Making in Transplantation: Organ Allocation

In the early years of transplantation, the sickest patients were often selected as recipients according to a "lifeboat ethics formula"[10]: If death was inevitable and imminent, an attempt to save those patients' lives using a new, unproved treatment was seen as a legitimate alternative. As transplantation became successful and available organs failed to meet the demand, allocation criteria became necessary. Although physicians would like to transplant all patients who need a new organ, there are not enough donated organs. Therefore, organs need to be allocated in a fair way that also maximizes the benefit, as shown by good survival rates and improved quality of life. This dilemma illustrates the basic difference between deontology (the duty to meet each patient's needs) and teleology (the duty to use the resource for the best outcome) and underscores the ethical conflict inherent in organ allocation. The conflict for physicians is how they can fulfill their duty to do all that is possible for a patient when they are constrained by a shortage of organs. Their duty to act as an advocate for each patient does not override their duty to provide the best for groups of patients.

Because there are not enough organs to transplant all potential recipients, and to help deal with this conflict, the principle of justice guides organ allocation so that patients are given equal concern and respect and organs are distributed in a more or less equitable way. Distribution can be based on financial factors (i.e., ability to pay), the efficacy principle (i.e., best medical outcome), the rescue principle (i.e., transplanting the sickest, most urgent patients), the egalitarian principle (i.e., first-come, first-served), the lottery principle (i.e., random chance or luck), or the "squeaky-wheel" principle (i.e., lobbying determines recipient selection).[7, 11]

The allocation system must be equitable to maintain public willingness to fund transplantation among competing demands. The quality of life after transplantation should be relatively high compared to other medical care to offset the expense of transplantation.[12] Comparative data, including quality-of-life and cost figures, must be available as governments and hospitals evaluate and assign funding priority to various health care treatments. Although some recipients may experience difficulties with work, finances, and side effects of long-term drug treatment, many studies confirm that transplant patients experience an improved lifestyle, rating their quality of life at a level comparable to that of the general public. Most patients with successful transplants are physically active and able to return to work. Reports on the percentage of patients who return to work vary, but recipients' employment rates appear to be similar to those of other patients who have experienced life-threatening illness and surgery. Patients older than 60 years also report excellent quality of life after transplant, similar to the age-matched population. Most children return to school and an active lifestyle, which includes catch-up growth and normal development. Before the transplant, parents of pediatric patients need accurate information about the current state of transplantation because they give consent for their child's transplant. Some parents may choose compassionate care rather than transplantation for a child who is born with a lethal defect (such as hypoplastic left heart syndrome) if they think the success rate or quality of life is insufficient.[13] Patient refusal of transplantation may be upsetting for the transplant team, but they must acknowledge patient autonomy and accept the patient's decision.

For an equitable distribution system, patients must have impartial access to organs. Donated organs belong to the community, and transplant staff are the trustees who use selection criteria that reflect justice and utility. Social aspects should not be considered. The tremendous value of agreed-on medical criteria for organ distribution, rather than social factors, is that they help lessen the bias against certain individual patients. Organs cannot be rationed as they were in the early years of transplantation or as dialyzers were rationed in treating renal disease. Hospital selection committees once chose patients who they thought had the greatest need for dialysis. With a large patient population and a limited number of dialysis machines, biases resulted when selection criteria included social factors, such as the patient's sex, marital status, number of dependents, occupation, education, income, and age.[14] Typically, men were offered dialysis because it was assumed that they had families to support. Older patients were not offered dialysis because younger patients would receive greater benefit in terms of years. Similarly, with transplantation, patients older than age 50 years were not accepted on waiting lists at one time. This age restriction has since been removed, and the success rate among older patients is approximately the same as that of younger patients.[15–17]

On the other hand, if medical utility is assessed in terms of years of life added, then age may be a relevant criterion. A successful transplant provides more years of life to a younger patient than to an older patient; therefore, if the goal is to increase the number of years of life per transplant, medical utility may consider the potential recipient's age. Age may also be considered using the principle of justice. Although two patients are equally in need at a particular time, the younger patient has had less opportunity for well-being than an older patient simply because of age. The younger patient may then have a greater claim to the organ.[18]

With the inadequate number of available organs and ever-increasing waiting lists, the criteria for allocation have become even more important. Medical selection criteria should be the same for all patients, aiming for an acceptable outcome in survival and quality of life while considering medical urgency and waiting time. Transplant programs in North America use computer algorithms to select the most suitable recipients. A point system, which recognizes factors such as the patient's current medical condition, the length of waiting time, and suitable matching by blood type, size, and weight, provides equitable access to organs based on a combination of the efficacy, egalitarian, and rescue principles. A system based on only one of these factors would result in injustice. If, for example, success rates were the only criterion, then such a system would be unfair because it ignores the needs of other patients, such as the critically ill and the highly sensitized, who tend to have lower success rates.[19]

As equitable as this system tries to be, medical criteria can also produce inequities. An emphasis on tissue matching for kidney transplants means that minority groups are disadvantaged because they are underrepresented in the donor pool. Data from research studies indicate that tissue matching may not be as important for improved success rates as was once believed. Such a policy, therefore, unfairly penalizes those with rare tissue types.[20] At the same time, an explicit policy directing more organs to minority groups is unacceptable because the United Network for Organ Sharing (UNOS) forbids gender, race, and other ethnic considerations when determining allocation policy.

The role of UNOS is to determine how available organs should be allocated among patients in the United States. With a board of directors composed of scientists, doctors, patients and their families, recipients, donor families, and the public, UNOS aims to enhance organ availability, to allocate organs based on medical criteria while considering utility and justice issues, to minimize waiting-time disparities, and to respect patient autonomy.[19]

Other Issues in Organ Allocation

Alcohol-Induced Liver Disease

Should an organ transplant be given to people who could have prevented their disease, such as patients with cirrhosis due to alcoholism? Most transplant programs do not categorically exclude these patients in need of a liver transplant: They are accepted if they demonstrate abstinence for a specified period. Patients who continue with destructive behavior forfeit their claim to a transplant if the behavior will likely lead to organ loss. This approach recognizes the need to provide health care for the patient and the need to maximize a valuable, limited resource. Transplantation for alcoholic liver disease and for older patients is becoming less controversial because these patients have excellent survival and good quality of life after transplant. Transplantation for other diseases, such as hepatitis B or primary liver cancer, remains controversial because recurrent disease is common.[21]

Multiple Listing

When a potential recipient's name is placed on more than one center's waiting list, it is referred to as *multiple listing*. Although allowed, it may be unethical because this opportunity does not extend to all transplant patients. When patients have their name on more than one list, they have financial resources to travel to more than one center for assessment. As long as some patients die waiting for an organ, other patients should not be able to increase their likelihood of a transplant by multiple listing. Although patient choice is important, equity must be given priority. This also holds true for designated organ donation. Although donor families may want the choice of designating the recipient, this practice contravenes the agreed-on ranking of patients. It seems unfair to allow designated donation in a public system of allocation. The physician's obligation is to transplant the organ according to the prescribed order, which supports the principles of equality and justice.

No Health Insurance

In the United States, when a transplant is not covered by public or private insurance, the ability to pay enters into the decision about candidacy. Equitable access remains an issue as long as admissibility to the waiting list is determined by ability to pay. Wealthy patients and those with medical insurance have a better chance of being referred and accepted for transplant.[20] Because of the social aspect of donation, however, it is unfair to ask all people to donate if access to those donated organs is restricted according to ability to pay rather than medical need, waiting time, and likelihood of success. There has been strong condemnation of commercialization in organ procurement (i.e., buying an organ for transplant), and a similar perspective may oppose commercialization in organ distribution so that ability to pay is not a factor in allocation.[22]

International Transfer of Organs

Should organs be given to foreign patients who come to a country specifically for medical treatment? Should organs be sent to other countries for transplant? Debate has focused on whether patients from other nations should be denied access to waiting lists, whether they should be transplanted only if suitable Americans are unavailable, or whether quotas should be established.[23] In an attempt to balance the principles of beneficence, justice, and utility, nonresident aliens are not excluded. For most types of transplant, eligibility depends on no American citizen or resident being suitable. For kidney transplants, eligibility depends on the patient being part of the quota allowed on the waiting list and receiving equal treatment regardless of nationality.[22] The international export of organs happens only after all attempts to place the organs nationally have failed. This practice protects the rights of Americans to their own resources in preference to an open international exchange.[23]

Repeat Transplants

Patients with failed transplants may be placed on the waiting list again, and existing allocation policies distribute between 10% and 20% of hearts and livers to patients who need a second or third transplant.[24] But is this fair, considering that other waiting patients may die without receiving their first transplant? The dilemma consists of choosing one patient when an obligation to both is felt. There is an understandable reluctance to bypass patients who need another transplant. According to the principle of justice, whether a patient needs a first or repeat transplant, they have equal claims to the organ. Utilitarianism favors the patient most likely to benefit in terms of living longer or enjoying a better quality of life. This principle expresses a duty to the donor and to society to try to achieve the best results in quantity and quality of life. Accordingly, repeat transplantation has been challenged on the basis that primary transplant patients have better survival with lower costs.[24, 25]

Commercialization

Organ trafficking in some countries has led to organs being distributed in an inequitable way based on financial gain. The media have documented that people have sold their kidneys, usually in countries without any or only newly developed cadaveric transplant programs. Without cadaver organs available and with widespread poverty, the rich were able to buy kidneys from living donors, who seized the opportunity to improve their own impoverished conditions. Under these circumstances, the donor's health was often poor from malnutrition, and the quality of the kidney was not assessed before transplant. Without adequate follow-up care, the donor's health was further jeopardized. Recipients also had unacceptably high levels of mortality or morbidity, including infection with human immunodeficiency virus.[26] The person who benefited the most was the "broker," who charged a fee to arrange for the "donation." The International Transplantation Society responded with guidelines[27] forbidding commercialization, based on nonmaleficence and noncommercialization of the body. Many legislative organizations passed laws to prevent the buying and selling of body parts.

In North America, there is no ethical justification for living donors to sell kidneys because there are well-established transplant programs and, even without adequate cadaveric donors, other medical services are available, such as dialysis. Can the ethical decisions of developed countries, such as the United States and Canada, apply equally well to developing nations with limited or no access to cadaveric transplant programs? As long as there are regions (e.g., in India) where the poor can make much more by selling a kidney ($7,000 U.S. currency) than their annual salary ($900)[28] and that have limited cadaveric transplant programs, commercialization will likely continue, as demonstrated by a transplant surgeon who said, "Either I buy, or they [the patients] die."[29]

North American culture may reject a commercial market for organs and tissues because it treats human bodies as commodities. The culture may also perceive payment for organs as a coercive factor in the decision to donate, with resulting unfairness because the rich are able to gain special access. Donors, however, may argue their right to sell a kidney as their own personal property[30] and that they are victimized, not by selling their kidney, but by another culture's ethical judgment. Paradoxically, whereas transplant personnel have generally condemned payment for organs from living donors, some have advocated payment or compensation to the cadaver donor's next of kin.

Compensation to the Donor Family

Compensation to the deceased patient's next of kin may encourage organ donation by providing an incentive, such as payment for burial expenses, a tax rebate, or a direct cash payment.[31] Should compensation to families be prohibited, or can a regulated system increase the organ retrieval rate while safeguarding ethical principles?

Family compensation may undermine the foundation of the altruistic system because families may not donate organs if they can be sold. If the body is treated as a commodity, altruism may be replaced by the "utilitarian business ethics of the marketplace,"[32] such as selling to the highest bidder. The result (presumably more organs) could justify family compensation from a utilitarian perspective. From the deontologic perspective, perhaps noncommercialization of the body is more important and, therefore, family compensation cannot be justified even if it increases the number of organs for transplant.

It is ironic that, as other countries are condemned for trying to increase the number of organs through payment to living donors, the same strategy through payment to the next of kin is being considered. Payment for cadaveric organs may be just as morally offensive because the family gains financially from treating the body as a commodity.

Living Donors

When compensation is not a potentially coercive factor and medical criteria have assessed the living donor as suitable, the donation process aims to ensure the donor's genuine motivation without coercion from family members or health care workers.[33] Informed consent from the donor requires mental competence to decide; voluntary choice; and disclosure of the risks, benefits, and alternatives.[23]

Although living-related kidney donation can potentially harm one person to save another, the increased advantage to the recipient has usually outweighed the minimal risk to the donor.[33] At one time, that increased advantage meant approximately a 30% better survival rate.[34] As a result of improved immunosuppression and better survival rates for cadaveric transplantation, some have questioned if living donation is still justified.[34] The wide range of incidence for living-related transplants may reflect professional perceptions of donor risk and the inadequacy of donor consent. Yet, if physicians make the decision for the potential donor about the acceptable level of risk and do not offer donation as an option, are they not restricting the patient's autonomy? Living-related kidney transplants are still approximately 15–20% more successful than cadaveric transplants.[35] Even if cadaveric transplants were as successful as living-related donations, related donations would remain an important avenue to reduce the organ shortage.

Without living donors, more patients would be denied transplantation, so some transplant programs accept unrelated kidney donors. If living-related donors can safely donate a kidney, genetically unrelated people can also donate, as long as the donation is motivated by altruism instead of profit. This scenario is possible, as shown by successful national and international registries of altruistic bone marrow donors for patients who do not have a relative with matching marrow. When unrelated kidney donors have been used (i.e., altruistic donation when the donor's health and organ quality are assessed), results have been excellent. Four-year graft survival (85%) is significantly better than graft survival from cadaveric donors (76%).[36] Although living-related kidney donation is well accepted, the impetus is to expand living kidney donation beyond spouses and friends, who are emotionally related to the recipient, to include altruistic strangers.[37]

Ethical concerns also arise about living donation of liver, lung, and intestinal segments. The benefits and risks for both recipient and donor must be considered because complication rates are higher than with kidney transplants.[38–40] The advantages for the recipient are obvious: His or her life is saved without an extended time waiting for a suitable cadaveric organ and its accompanying increased morbidity and mortality. The major disadvantage is that only a segment of the organ is grafted rather than the whole organ. At least for liver transplantation, however, patient and graft survival rates are better than survival rates using cadaveric organs.[38] For the donor, risks include operative death or postoperative complications. The major advantage for the donor is psychological. Donors (usually parents) think that they have done their best to save their child. Because parents are likely to try anything to save their child's life, however, can they give informed consent if they feel internal pressure to donate, which may be heightened, especially if the medical situation is urgent? Do the donors understand the risk to themselves? If they apparently understand the risks and still consent to the donation, can their donation be refused when the alternative for the recipient may be a long waiting period with possibly no available organ?

Living donation remains an ethical choice when it is not obligatory but rests on the principles of autonomy and altruism.[41] Although people have a duty to help others, they are not obligated to go beyond ordinary means of doing so. Using these principles as a basis for decision-making, people should be able to choose their own actions. Because potential donors can give informed consent, based on understanding the risks, alternatives, and realistic benefit, living donors will likely be used to a greater extent in the future.

Xenotransplantation

Living donation cannot solve the organ donor shortage. Another strategy to increase the number of organs is xenotransplantation (cross-species transplants). Is there a reasonable scientific basis for transplanting patients with animal organs? Have patients given their informed consent to the procedure, knowing what alternative treatment options exist? Research has shown that nonhuman organs can support human life. Rejection can be reversed and long-term survival may be possible because of improved antirejection drugs. Eventually, xenografts may provide an answer to the inadequate number of cadaveric donors while also sparing relatives the risk of living donation.[35]

Transgenic animals are being developed for these cross-species transplants. These donor animals, such as the pig, are genetically manipulated so that patients are less likely to reject the transplanted organ.[42] But is genetic manipulation to create a new breed that could supply organs for transplant without risk? Some of the potential consequences of introducing a new species, which goes far beyond traditional breeding technology, must be considered.[43, 44] Some see cross-species genetic transfers as the ultimate offense to human dignity, saying "prolonged and expanded use of these cross-species engineering feats could mean the end of the natural world as we know it."[44]

Does the scarcity of human organs make it morally right to use animals as a source of replacement parts? Utilitarian theory excludes the interests of animals to focus on the outcome that best serves the interests of patients or human society. Deontologic theory divides the universe into people and things. Because animals are not people, they have no value in their own right, so we are allowed to use them. Human needs are given precedence because of our special moral status. A modified deontologic perspective argues that, although animals are not "moral agents," they deserve our concern and respect because they have their own inherent value (J. B. Dossetor, M.D., personal communication, May 1993). Interspecies transplantation could still be justified: As long as animals receive humane care and are killed without pain, scientists are respecting animals as sentient beings. Although animals may have "moral standing," they are not morally equivalent to humans.[45, 46]

We have generally excluded animals from our moral community because animals are members of other species. Their interests are secondary to humans. This approach has now been rejected by some people, who emphasize animal rights instead of animal welfare.[47] Because animals have inherent rights and should be given respect, we cannot kill them for human purposes. Instead, we may have to accept the organ shortage or to resolve the shortage in other ways.

Two opposite views summarize this issue. "Eco-holistic world views of human beings as a part of the whole with no preeminence in it are ultimately a stumbling block for medical progress and the human good"[46] because our first obligation is to our own species. Those who endorse species egalitarianism counter that "we are animals ourselves, large omnivorous primates, very precocious to be sure, but just big monkeys, nevertheless. We are therefore a part of nature, not set apart from it."[43] These views illustrate the wide diversity of opinion underlying this complex ethical debate.

Artificial Support Devices

The first patient to survive an artificial heart as a bridge to a human heart transplant was an American, implanted with a Jarvik-7 in 1985. Although bridge-to-transplant heart patients have a lower 1-year survival rate than do other heart transplant recipients,[48] artificial hearts may become even more popular as a way to support patients until a human organ can be transplanted. For example, many patients with acute myocardial infarction could be candidates for an artificial device as a bridge to transplant. Artificial liver support systems have also been used as a bridge for liver transplant recipients. Although it is not a permanent option, temporary support is provided so that patients can be transplanted when a liver becomes available, or patients may be supported until their own liver function improves, if transplantation is not an option.[49, 50]

Artificial support systems as a bridge to transplant are ethically justified on two counts: (1) The physician is acting as the patient's advocate in trying to save his or her life or at least to improve his or her quality of life, and (2) the patient understands the risks and potential benefits and has given informed consent.[51, 52] Informed consent is essential because patients must not be misled or given false hope about the outcome. For procedures that involve continuing treatment, informed consent should be an ongoing agreement rather than a one-time event. The question remains whether terminally ill patients or parents of critically ill children are "coerced" into experimentation because it gives them some hope. Before patients are asked for their informed consent to experimental procedures, the procedure must be assessed as to whether it is reasonable to perform on humans. A patient's consent cannot change an unacceptable experiment into an acceptable treatment.[53]

Using mechanical devices may be unethical because they save no extra lives but only shuffle the waiting list of patients, thereby subverting the fairness of the waiting-list system.[51] Greater emphasis is placed on the rescue principle at the expense of efficacy (best medical outcome) and egalitarian (first-come, first-served) principles. The probable outcome is that a successful transplant is less likely and that other potential recipients will have to wait longer while their own health may worsen. If a totally implantable, permanent organ could be manufactured, the organ shortage could be alleviated, but long-term reliability and risk of infection are unknown.

Non–Heart-Beating Donors

If permanent artificial organs are not yet a realistic alternative, can more human organs become available by using non–heart-beating donors? Although the early history of transplantation was based on using non–heart-beating donors, the development of brain death criteria in the late 1960s meant that brain-dead donors were preferred. Organs from brain-dead donors provided better function and improved graft survival because a ventilator supported organ function artificially. Today, improved techniques for organ cooling reduce the time that organs are ischemic and the chance of organ damage, so non–heart-beating donors as one alternative are being reconsidered given the severe shortage of brain-dead donors.[54] Because organ recovery from these donors is unconventional, with perhaps a higher risk of complications, potential recipients should be told that their transplant program may use organs from non–heart-beating donors to ensure patients' informed consent.

Non–heart-beating donors are declared dead after cessation of heartbeat; for example, after life support systems have been withdrawn at the request of the next of kin. Other times, non–heart-beating donors are undergoing brain death determination when the heart suddenly stops functioning. Some hospitals have inserted catheters into the patient's femoral artery so that organs remain usable.[54, 55] This approach allows time to locate the next of kin and to inform them of the option to donate. Although this approach safeguards the family's right to make an informed decision about organ donation and the procedure is nondeforming, family consent for organ perfusion is not obtained before the procedure.[54]

Is it morally acceptable to perform an invasive procedure on dead patients to benefit others? Again, we are faced with the basic conflict between two ethical perspectives. Is it the intention to use the dead patient only as a means to benefit others, or is the outcome to ensure that the next of kin has the option to donate and possibly save a recipient's life? North American culture has generally resisted the routine removal of organs after death because this may violate the dignity of the deceased and his or her family's wishes. In this light, perhaps the routine insertion of perfusion catheters, which holds no benefit for the individual patient and may be treating him or her as a means to help others, should be resisted. On the other hand, once patients are dead, they no longer have "primary worth"—that is, they are not capable of suffering. Because they cannot be either harmed or benefited, the main ethical obligation then may be to help others.[56] This approach, however, fails to recognize that people can be wronged (by having their wishes thwarted after death) even when they are not harmed.[22]

The next of kin and the public must be assured that the patient's status as a potential donor has not influenced his or her care, including the clinical decision of when to stop resuscitation efforts. To minimize any possible conflict of interest, a separation must be maintained between health professionals responsible for the critically ill patient's care and those responsible for the transplantation process.[57] Just as there are policies and procedures to ensure that physicians who declare brain death are not involved in the transplant procedure, there must be similar guidelines to ensure that patient care is not compromised by the need for organs. Although non–heart-beating donors could increase the donor pool five- to 10-fold,[54] these ethical issues must be addressed. Public trust and support for transplantation may falter if the public perceives this practice as acting in physicians' own self-interest by gaining easier access to organs.

Anencephalic Infants

Similar ethical issues prevail when discussing the appropriateness of using organs retrieved from anencephalic infants.[58] Infants born with anencephaly (a congenital neural tube malformation in which the whole brain does not form) have brain stem function only. Some have suggested that these infants could become organ donors by being placed in a special category of death.[59, 60] By separating the cognitive and vegetative brain functions, the lack of consciousness or cognition would be redefined as death.

Although these infants never achieve cognitive brain function, their "brain absence" cannot be equated with brain death. The application of unique brain-death criteria is inappropriate. As long as these infants have some brain function, they do not meet the definition of death and they cannot be organ donors. If humans who are not brain dead are considered as organ donors (i.e., anencephalic babies), one begins to descend a slippery slope, on which one may find that people with limited or lost cognitive ability are also considered organ donors (i.e., severely mentally defective or vegetative patients).

According to the utilitarian perspective, the greatest good would result from using the organs so that recipients, who may otherwise die, will live and the anencephalic infant's parents may lessen their sense of loss. If the end result is beneficial, this argument goes, the means may be justified. The means may include meeting defined brain-death criteria, altering patient care to optimize the usefulness of the organs, classifying these infants as "nonpersons" (because they have no self-awareness or cognitive function), or declaring death so that organs can be retrieved even while the infant is still breathing.[61, 62] But if moral duty is to the individual rather than the outcome, the concern is that these infants are treated with routine, compassionate care. Patient care would not be altered to enhance organ viability. The moral rule that each person has inherent dignity means that these infants are important as ends in themselves and should not be treated differently to benefit others.

Fetal Tissue

The fetus, too, may be seen as a means to benefit others, especially if purposely conceived to provide tissue for treatment or research, thus becoming a "pharmaceutical commodity."[63] If abortion is a legal option, however, the presumption is that abortions will be done. Is it then acceptable to use this tissue to benefit others? From the deontologic perspective, the use of fetal tissue from abortion would be unacceptable because the fetus is attributed full human status and therefore has inherent dignity. The utilitarian would approve the use of tissue to treat diseases because whatever wrong is attached to using aborted fetal tissue is balanced by the benefit for patients. The use of fetal tissue may be ethically justified on the basis of the recipient's informed consent and the physician's role of helping the patient (beneficence).[64] Although the primary ethical issue has been the use of fetal tissue from abortions, another issue is the use of public resources to fund this research.[65]

Conclusions

Transplantation and clinical research must be evaluated by ethical principles. No clear-cut answers exist, however, because ethical theories themselves value certain principles above others (e.g., the individual patient versus the outcome). This conflict is illustrated by the dual responsibility in organ allocation of meeting each patient's needs yet maximizing the benefit from limited resources. In a pluralistic society, in which some favor pure utilitarianism and others favor egalitarianism, consideration of each principle is a fair, workable compromise.

It can only be anticipated that further scientific advances will occur and more technology will be developed as the transplant community tries to reduce the imbalance between organ supply and patient need. Physicians must remember, however, that their enthusiasm for the possibility of saving lives and providing new treatment cannot overshadow the basic responsibility to prevent suffering. At times, the preservation of life at all costs is not justified.[66] At other times, even if the outcome is beneficial, the means may not be ethical. With so many options, one must consider ethical theories and principles and apply them, thereby making ethical choices.

References

1. Diethelm AG. Ethical decisions in the history of organ transplantation. Ann Surg 1990;211:505–520.

2. Vevaina JR, Nora LM, Bone RC. Issues in biomedical ethics. Dis Mon 1993;39:869–925.

3. Loewy EH. Textbook of Medical Ethics. New York: Plenum, 1989;ix–xiii.

4. Biedermann CL, Layon AJ, D'Amico R. Ethics in the intensive care unit. Anesthesiol Clin North Am 1991;9: 423–435.

5. Loewy EH. Textbook of Medical Ethics. New York: Plenum, 1989;15–36.

6. Mappes TA, Zembaty JS. Biomedical Ethics (2nd ed). New York: McGraw-Hill, 1986;1–46.

7. O'Connell DA. Ethical implications of organ transplantation. Crit Care Nurs Q 1991;13:1–7.

8. Rakich JS, Longest BB, Darr J. Managing Health Services Organizations (2nd ed). Philadelphia: Saunders, 1985;80–107.

9. Gillon R. Transplantation: a framework for analysis of ethical issues. Transplant Proc 1990;22:902–903.

10. Surman OS, Purtilo R. Reevaluation of organ transplantation criteria. Allocation of scarce resources to borderline candidates. Psychosomatics 1992;33:202–212.

11. Dossetor JB, Kjellstrand CM. Ethics Issues in Selection for Dialysis and Transplantation: The Duty of Advocacy. In JB Dossetor, CM Kjellstrand (eds), Ethical Problems in Dialysis and Transplantation. Dordrecht: Kluwer Academic, 1992;37–52.

12. Busschbach JJ, Horikx PE, van den Bosch JM, et al. Measuring the quality of life before and after bilateral lung transplantation in patients with cystic fibrosis. Chest 1994;105:911–917.

13. Zahka KG, Spector M, Hanisch D. Hypoplastic left-heart syndrome: Norwood operation, transplantation, or compassionate care. Clin Perinatol 1993;20:145–154.

14. Fox RC, Swazey JP. The Courage to Fail: A Social View of Organ Transplants and Dialysis (2nd ed). Chicago: University of Chicago Press, 1978;226.

15. Andreu J, de la Torre M, Oppenheimer F, et al. Renal transplantation in elderly patients. Transplant Proc 1992;24:120–121.

16. Pirsch JD, Kalayoglu M, D'Alessandro AM, et al. Orthotopic liver transplantation in patients 60 years of age and older. Transplantation 1991;51:431–433.

17. Miller LW, Vitale-Noedel N, Pennington G, et al. Heart transplantation in patients over fifty-five years. J Heart Transplant 1988;7:254–257.

18. United Network for Organ Sharing, Ethics Committee. General principles for allocating human organs and tissues. Transplant Proc 1992;24:2227–2235.

19. Benenson E. The UNOS statement of principles and objectives of equitable organ allocation. UNOS Update 1994;10(8):20–38.

20. Caplan AL. Problems in the policies and criteria used to allocate organs for transplantation in the United States. Transplant Proc 1989;21:3381–3387.

21. Keefe EB, Esquivel CO. Controversies in patient selection for liver transplantation. West J Med 1993;159:586–593.

22. Childress JF. Ethical criteria for procuring and distributing organs for transplantation. J Health Polit Policy Law 1989;14:87–112.

23. Simmons RG, Abress L. Ethics in Organ Transplantation. In GJ Cerilli (ed), Organ Transplantation and Replacement. Philadelphia: Lippincott, 1988;691–701.

24. Ubel PA, Arnold RM, Caplan AL. Rationing failure. The ethical lessons of the retransplantation of scarce vital organs. JAMA 1993;270:2469–2474.

25. Kankaanpaa J. Cost-effectiveness of liver transplantation—how to apply the results in resource allocation. Prev Med 1990;19:700–704.

26. Daar AS. Organ donation—world experience; the Middle East. Transplant Proc 1991;23:2505–2507.

27. Morris PJ, Tilney NL, Bach JF, et al. Commercialisation in transplantation: the problems and some guidelines for practice [for the Council of The Transplantation Society]. Lancet 1985;2:715–716.

28. Schneider A, Flaherty MP. The Challenge of a Miracle: Selling the Gift. Pittsburgh: Pittsburgh Press, 1985;12–13.

29. Bailey R. Should I be allowed to buy your kidney? Breakthroughs 1991;2:36–41.

30. Fox RC, Swazey JP. Spare Parts: Organ Replacement in American Society. New York: Oxford University Press, 1992;43–72.

31. Kittur DS, Hogan MM, Thukral VK, et al. Incentives for organ donation? [for the United Network for Organ Sharing Ad Hoc Donations Committee]. Lancet 1991;338:1441–1443.

32. Dossetor JB, Manickavel V. Ethics in organ donation: contrasts in two cultures. Transplant Proc 1991;23: 2508–2511.

33. Neely S, Davis NS. Legal and Ethical Issues. In KM Sigardson-Poor, LM Haggerty (eds), Nursing Care of the Transplant Recipient. Philadelphia: Saunders, 1990; 395–421.

34. Starzl TE. Will live organ donations no longer be justified? Hastings Cent Rep 1985;15:5.

35. Benenson E. Living-related transplants: are we advancing or regressing? UNOS Update 1993;9(6):11–12.

36. Benenson E. Living unrelated kidney donation advocated. UNOS Update 1992;8(10):6.

37. Spital AL. Unrelated living donors: should they be used? Transplant Proc 1992;24:2215–2517.

38. Piper JB, Whitington PF, Woodle ES, et al. Pediatric Liver Transplantation at the University of Chicago Hospitals. In PI Terasaki, JM Cecka (eds), Clinical Transplants 1992. Los Angeles: Regents of the University of California, 1992;179–189.

39. Shaw LR, Miller JD, Slutsky AS, et al. Ethics of lung transplantation with live donors. Lancet 1991;338: 678–681.

40. Singer PA, Siegler M, Whitington PF, et al. Ethics of liver transplantation with living donors. N Engl J Med 1989;321:620–621.

41. Caplan A. Must I be my brother's keeper? Ethical issues in the use of living donors as sources of liver and other solid organs. Transplant Proc 1993;25:1997–2000.

42. Barker CF, Markmann JF. Xenografts: is there a future? Surgery 1992;112:3–5.

43. Callicott JB. La nature est morte, vive la nature! Hastings Cent Rep 1992;22:16–23.

44. Rifkin J, Kimbrell A. Let's not be playing God with the genetic code [for the Foundation for Economic Trends in the United States]. London Free Press 1993;July 24:E5.

45. Caplan A. Is xenografting morally wrong? Transplant Proc 1992;24:722–727.

46. Post SG. Baboon livers and the human good. Arch Surg 1993;128:131–133.

47. Francione GL. Xenografts and animal rights. Transplant Proc 1990;22:1044–1046.

48. Goodman ER, Hardy MA. Transplantation 1992: The Year in Review. In PI Terasaki, JM Cecka (eds), Clinical Transplants 1992. Los Angeles: The Regents of the University of California, 1992;285–297.

49. Dixit V. Development of a bioartificial liver using isolated hepatocytes. Artif Organs 1994;18:371–384.

50. Benenson E. Artificial liver machine successfully "bridges" patients to transplant. UNOS Update 1993;9(5):15–16.

51. Levine RJ. Mechanical circulatory support systems: ethical considerations. Transplant Proc 1990;22:969–970.

52. Simmons PD. Ethical considerations of artificial heart implantations. Ann Clin Lab Sci 1986;16:1–12.

53. Annas GJ. Death and the magic machine: informed consent to the artificial heart. West N Engl Law Rev 1987;9:89–112.

54. Anaise D, Rapaport FT. Use of non–heart-beating cadaveric donors in clinical organ transplantation—logistics, ethics, and legal considerations. Transplant Proc 1993;25:2153–2155.

55. Anaise D. The non-heartbeating cadaveric donor: a solution to the organ shortage crisis. UNOS Update 1992;8(10):32–34.

56. Loewy EH. Textbook of Medical Ethics. New York: Plenum, 1989;109–121.

57. Youngner SJ, Arnold RM. Ethical, psychosocial, and public policy implications of procuring organs from non–heart-beating cadaver donors. JAMA 1993;269:2769–2774.

58. Churchill LR, Pinkus RLB. The use of anencephalic organs: historical and ethical dimensions. Milbank Q 1990;68:147–169.

59. Harrison MR. The anencephalic newborn as organ donor. Hastings Cent Rep 1986;16(2):21–22.

60. Truog RD, Fletcher JC. Anencephalic newborns: can organs be transplanted before brain death? N Engl J Med 1989;321:388–391.

61. Fries ES. The ethical issues of transplanting organs from anencephalic newborns. MCN Am J Matern Child Nurs 1989;14:412–414.

62. Leggans T. Anencephalic infants as organ donors: legal and ethical perspectives. J Legal Med 1988;9:449–465.

63. Jones D. Halifax hospital first in Canada to proceed with controversial fetal-tissue transplant. CMAJ 1992;146:389–391.

64. Strong C. Fetal tissue transplantation: can it be morally insulated from abortion? J Med Ethics 1991;17:70–76.

65. Hoffer BJ, Olson L. Ethical issues in brain-cell transplantation. Trends Neurosci 1991;14:384–388.

66. Chantler C. Transplantation—a new dimension for paediatrics. Eur J Pediatr 1992;151(Suppl 1):581–584.

Chapter 21
Psychosocial Issues of Organ Transplantation

Robert M. House, Thomas P. Beresford,
Michael Talamantes, and Jeremy Katz

Chapter Plan

Technical advances in surgery, intensive care, and pharmacology have increased the success of solid-organ transplantation, which is now a viable treatment option for patients with end-stage organ disease. Similarly, psychiatry's understanding of and contribution to this process has grown dramatically. Psychiatric consultation is often requested at all stages of the transplant process: the initial evaluation, pre- and posttransplant care, and rehabilitation. In the past, psychiatry was often involved to exclude patients with existing psychiatric disorders or those considered at psychiatric risk. The focus now is identifying potential psychological problems, instituting appropriate treatment, and assessing the impact of such disorders on receiving a grafted organ. Although the ability to identify and treat psychiatric disorders has improved dramatically, the ability to predict compliance and other behaviors does not yet approach the level desired. Nowhere is this more evident than the evaluation of patients with an addictive disorder, especially those that have led to the patient's organ failure.[1, 2]

This chapter focuses on issues of evaluation and patient selection, common clinical psychiatric problems that arise during the transplant process, the function of support groups, and quality-of-life concerns, including religious and financial issues. Substance abuse is addressed at some length because of its increasing importance in the selection of patients. Although each organ system has its own unique psychological meaning, most clinical and psychosocial concerns are common to all types of solid-organ transplants.

Psychiatric Exclusion Criteria

One of the most difficult tasks in psychiatric evaluation of patients for transplantation is deciding on the selection criteria. There are no universally accepted criteria indicating how psychiatric history, psychological testing, or mental status examination data should be incorporated in the selection process. The decision to transplant must be made on an individual basis. Patients with psychiatric disorders that would have excluded them in the past, such as schizophrenia, bipolar disorder, and mental retarda-

Table 21-1. Preoperative Assessment

Basic patient profile, including relationships, support network, educational history, occupational history, and legal history

Style of coping with his or her illness to date

Expectations of surgery

Current psychiatric diagnosis and treatment

Drug, alcohol, and tobacco history

Mental status examination (may include formal neuropsychological testing)

Understanding of proposed surgery and treatment recommendations, along with the consequences of treatment versus no treatment

tion, have been successfully transplanted, although they have been carefully evaluated.[3–5]

Pertinent factors include the availability of a support network, evidence of medical compliance, a willingness to comply with the demands of the procedure, and a willingness to make necessary lifestyle changes or an absence of behaviors that would be incompatible with transplantation. Patients with an identified or pre-existing psychiatric disorder must be ready to follow through with recommended psychiatric care.

There are few absolute psychiatric contraindications for excluding a candidate from transplantation. Common exclusions include chronic psychosis that is refractory to treatment, severe mental retardation, drug and alcohol disorders in which there is a high risk for recidivism (see Addictions), and irreversible cognitive disorders, such as Alzheimer's disease. Patients requiring a more extensive evaluation are those with severe personality disorders, such as borderline personality disorder and antisocial personality disorder, in whom compliance and impulsivity may be a significant concern.[4]

Preoperative Evaluation

In addition to helping with the selection process, the preoperative evaluation can serve as a baseline for comparison should future problems arise (Table 21-1). Involving family members in this process provides an opportunity to assess the support available to the patient and to provide education. When an illness is of long standing, a sense of stability often develops that may be upset when the trans-

plant recipient regains a state of health. Denial is a common first response when a patient is told that there is a need for transplantation. It is often followed by a bargaining stage, often with the patient's physician, in hopes that the illness will reverse itself. In an attempt to change the outcome, patients may alter their eating patterns or lifestyle (e.g., the alcoholic who stops drinking). When the hoped-for improvement in health does not occur, there is often a sense of resignation and acquiescence to the evaluation process and treatment recommendations.

Support Groups

The group model for the emotional support of transplant patients and their families has developed as a standard at most transplant centers. In addition to providing support to transplant recipients and their families, the sharing of information, resources, and education and the enhancement of a common social network can all be benefits of the group process. Group members often reinforce information or share an emotional or physical symptom, which can be extremely reassuring. A group can increase patients' coping abilities by letting them share different ways to solve problems.

Support group meetings can be organized in various ways. Many use a psychoeducational model, in which didactic sessions are held and members of the transplant team (e.g., anesthesiologist, surgeon, nurse coordinator) make various educational presentations. The opportunity can be provided for patients to share experiences and support each other as they deal with common stressors. Open groups allow recipients, candidates, and families to receive support and information as needed. Social support cannot be overemphasized because it minimizes the loneliness and fear that most patients encounter.[6] This is particularly true for patients in outlying regions, who may be the only transplant recipient in the area. The World Wide Web and Internet are becoming more of a support and source of information for patients and families.

Assisting patients and their families in finding the support, information, and resources to get through the transplant experience is crucial for a successful outcome.[7, 8] Whether through hospital or professional staff, hospital- or community-based support groups, or community and national foundations, intervention for patients should be sought wherever their personal needs can best be met. Besides transplant-related issues, other fears common to any long-term illness may also arise with transplant patients, including loss of control and fears of dependency, pain, isolation, or death. These issues should be explored to ensure that patients are coping as well as possible.

Financial Impact

The financial implications and the resulting stress on families of transplant patients has been well documented.[9, 10] In addition to the transplant itself, costs include procurement, organ transplantation fees, professional fees, hospital charges, and medication. Other costs include lodging, travel, and meal expenses for the patient and family members so that they may be near the transplant center, especially at the time of discharge. Loss of income from employers could also hinder a patient's financial status during follow-up, before the patient is healthy enough to return to work.

As medical costs are more closely scrutinized, cost-effectiveness and accountability are issues that transplant centers must address. The effects of managed care and capitation of hospital and physician fees influences transplant centers through cost, resource use, and patient selection.[11] The patient's insurance status in resolving financial issues is a serious concern. This is less an issue in countries where there is a national or universal health insurance plan.

Religion

A central aspect of most theological systems has to do with the belief in an afterlife, the sanctity of the body, and the relationship between the body and the soul.[12] A common feature of most religions is the value placed on life and the value placed on benevolence. Dixon[13] described various religious traditions (e.g., Judaism, Islam, Christianity, Hinduism, Buddhism, Shinto, Taoism, and Confucianism) as having a "permissive approach" to organ donation and transplantation. Jehovah's Witnesses present a unique situation: Their religious beliefs allow the acceptance of an organ transplant, but receiving blood or blood products is prohibited. In this circumstance, the transplant committee must make a decision because most anesthesiologists and surgeons think that this prohibition severely limits their ability to provide optimal medical care at the time of surgery.

Most transplant patients are struggling with issues of life and death—their own and that of the potential donor. Many patients with a terminal illness who also face high-risk surgery may experience a crisis in their faith. Some may respond with an increase in their religious belief, but others may feel betrayed. Some patients feel a sense of guilt, that they are being punished for some sin or transgression by their organ failure. In either circumstance, a hospital chaplain or other religious leader may offer valued support and encouragement.

Postoperative Phase

Euphoria and a sense of well-being often follow a successful transplant. Postoperative complications may make this feeling short-lived. Acute mental status changes may occur in up to 50–70% of patients.[14–16]

Delirium

Delirium is the most common psychiatric problem before and after transplant, with an incidence as high as 50%.[17–19] Key diagnostic features include a disturbance of concentration, impairment in cognition, or the development of a perceptual disturbance that cannot be attributed to a pre-existing dementia. Drug toxicity (Table 21-2), infection, electrolyte imbalance, and organ rejection are the most common causes. Anesthetic agents must also be considered as causes in the immediate postoperative period. Treatment consists of correction of any underlying medical or surgical problems that contribute to this behavior. Patients at risk of harming themselves through their behavior may require restraints and pharmacotherapy (Table 21-3). High-potency neuroleptic agents should be considered. Haloperidol can be given orally, intramuscularly, or intravenously and has minimal extrapyramidal side effects.[20, 21] Benzodiazepines can be helpful in providing sedation. Preference should be given to agents with a shorter half-life (e.g., lorazepam or

Table 21-2. Neuropsychiatric Effects of Immunosuppressant Agents

Agent	Neuropsychiatric Effects
Cyclosporine	Anxiety, delirium, hallucinations, seizures, tremor, paresthesias, and hirsutism
FK506	Anxiety, delirium, insomnia, tremor, paresthesias
Mycophenolate	Anxiety, depression, somnolence
Muromonab-CD3 (OKT3)	Aseptic meningitis, seizures, tremor, myalgia, photophobia
Corticosteroids	Delirium, euphoria, depression, mania, insomnia, tremor, irritability
Azathioprine	Meningitis-type syndrome (rare)
Lymphocyte immuneglobulin (Atgam)	Confusion, disorientation
Ganciclovir	Nightmares, agitation, anxiety, depression, euphoria, mania, psychosis, decreased libido

oxazepam), beginning with lower doses to minimize making delirium worse.

Depression

The incidence of clinically significant depression is high both before transplant (up to 60%)[22] and afterward (up to 80%).[16] Pretransplant depression is generally a reactive depression that may be made worse by long waiting lists, continued physical deterioration, and fear that a transplant will not occur in time. Posttransplant depression is most often an organically based condition precipitated by complications, such as drug toxicity or side effects and metabolic disturbances. Prolonged stays in the intensive care unit (ICU) or the hospital in general can precipitate or worsen an existing depression. Patients enter into transplant surgery with the expectation that they will regain their health. Postoperative complications that necessitate a longer hospital stay, especially in the ICU, may cause patients to have second thoughts about the transplant because they have not achieved the desired state of improved health. Depressive symptoms resulting from such setbacks are often short-lived and respond to emotional support. However, the team must be alert for a worsening of depressive symptoms. Symptoms to be especially concerned about include a significant decrease in energy, lack of motivation, lack of cooperation with rehabilitation care, refusal or disinterest in eating, and self-destructive behaviors, such as refusal to take medications. Attention must first be given to readily correctable causes, including drug toxicity, infection, or metabolic disturbance. Pharmacologic interventions can then be considered (Table 21-4). Methylphenidate has the advantage of rapid response, safety, and easily measurable responses.[17] At a therapeutic dose, the patient begins to report an increased interest in their state of health and well-being, including an interest in eating, dressing changes, an increase in motivation, and increased

Table 21-3. Pharmacologic Management of Delirium

Agent	Oral Dosage Range (mg)	Dosage Form	Comments
Neuroleptics			
Haloperidol	0.5–5.0	PO, IM, IV	High potency, low incidence of extrapyramidal side effects. Effective for agitation and behavioral dyscontrol without significant orthostatic hypotension.
Loxapine	5.0–10.0	PO, IM	Low potency; may be substituted for patients
Thiothixene	2.0–10.0	PO, IM, IV	with extrapyramidal side effects rather than add an anticholinergic agent.
Anxiolytics			
Lorazepam	1.0–6.0	PO, IM	Most commonly used benzodiazepines for
Oxazepam	15.0–90.0	PO	delirium. Rapid response; half-life 10–12 hours; do not require hepatic metabolism.

Table 21-4. Pharmacologic Management of Depression

Drug	Dose Range (mg)	Sedation	Anticholinergic Effects	Comments
Atypical agent				
Methylphenidate	5–60	None	None	Especially safe for the medically ill patient; rapid response; use with caution with patients who have history of addiction
Selective serotonin reuptake inhibitors				
Fluoxetine	20–80	Minimal	Minimal	Insomnia and headache common
Paroxetine	20–50	Low	Minimal	Agitation common, as is sexual dysfunction
Sertraline	50–200	Minimal	Minimal	Very low overdose risk
Phenyl piperazine				
Trazodone	300–600	High	Minimal	A good sleep medication at 50- to 100-mg range
Tricyclic antidepressants				
Amitriptyline	150–300	High	High	Amitriptyline available IM; at low doses can help manage chronic pain; sedation and anticholinergic effects may lower compliance; must be titrated to a therapeutic dose; blood levels available
Desipramine	150–300	Low	Low	—
Nortriptyline	50–150	Low	Low	—
Monoamine oxidase inhibitor				
Phenelzine	45–90	Low	Low	Patients must be educated on dietary restrictions; monitor closely for hypertension

cooperation with rehabilitation efforts. For most patients, the starting dose is 5–10 mg given in a divided dose, morning and noon. If there is no response, the dose is increased to 10 mg: 5 mg in the morning and 5 mg at noon the second day. The dose should be increased by 5 mg each day up to a daily dose of 30 mg. Doses greater than 30 mg are seldom helpful. Methylphenidate should be discontinued by the time of discharge from the hospital. More traditional antidepressants can be considered for significant depressions or in conjunction with methylphenidate. The new selective serotonin reuptake inhibitors (SSRIs) offer a wide range of safety with a minimum of side effects. Some SSRIs, such as fluoxetine and paroxetine, offer the advantage of once-a-day dosing. Common side effects include disturbance of sleep, sexual dysfunction, and agitation. The more traditional tricyclic antidepressants are especially helpful for patients with a sleep disturbance or agitation. They can also promote weight gain. Tricyclic agents must be started at low doses and gradually titrated to a therapeutic level. Nortriptyline and desipramine are especially helpful because they have fewer anticholinergic side effects than most. The disadvantage of all antidepressants is the 10- to 14-day delay before an optimal response is achieved. Often, a patient is given both methylphenidate for its immediate effect and an antidepressant for longer-term management. An additional disadvantage is that, with the exception of amitriptyline, all are available only for oral administration. A parenteral form of amitriptyline is available, but a therapeutic level is difficult to achieve. Patients may present to surgery while being treated pharmacologically for depression. This may include a single antidepressant or an antidepressant and a mood stabilizer, such as carbamazepine, lithium carbonate, or valproic acid.

Depression continues to be a very treatable disorder, even for the seriously medically ill patient. For the anesthesiologist, it is important to be aware of these medications and their interaction with anesthetic agents (Table 21-5). As a result of advances in technology, the increased understanding of drug interactions by anesthesiologists, and the improved safety of the new antidepressants, there is rarely a need to discontinue psychiatric medications before surgery. These are not benign agents, however, and they can cause or worsen delirium.

Anxiety

Along with depression, generalized anxiety and panic disorders are common. Prevalence may range as high as 40%.[19, 23] Cyclosporine is particularly problematic, especially at the higher doses often seen immediately after transplantation. Physiologic concerns that must be addressed include cardiac arrhythmias, hypoglycemia, hypocalcemia, and hypoxia. Before beginning any form of anxiolytic treatment, these factors should be ruled out. Similarly, the newer immunosuppressant FK506 is known to precipitate anxiety.[24] Benzodiazepines are safe drugs with few drug interactions. Conjugated agents, such as lorazepam and oxazepam, allow for rapid regulation because of their short half-life. Lorazepam also has the advantage of intravenous, intramuscular, and sublingual forms. Midazolam has a very short half-life and rapid onset of action. It is not suitable for long-term administration, but for anxiety associated with procedures it can be very effective. In some patients, it also has an amnestic quality that can be beneficial.

Addictions

One of the most controversial areas in providing solid-organ transplants to patients with end-organ failure is organ failure brought on by the patient's own behavior, such as pulmonary failure and nicotine dependence or liver failure and alcohol abuse.[1, 25] Most of these conditions involve the anesthesiologist only from the aspect of assessing physiologic parameters that affect successful induction and recovery from anesthesia during the operative procedure (Table 21-6).

Behind the physical sequelae of such self-injurious behavior lies the dependency disorders themselves. These states have relevance to anesthetic practice in several ways. First, substance dependency disorders or addictive disorders include the development of tolerance to the particular substance in question. In some cases, tolerance may affect the induction phase of operative anesthesia, as in a patient who is tolerant to central nervous system depressants, such as alcohol, benzodiazepines, or other sedative compounds. This may result in longer induction time and use of more sedative drugs than one might normally need. Second, along with tolerance, most dependency disorders include withdrawal syndromes. The classic case is that of a patient undergoing delirium tremens (DTs) in the immediate postoperative period when an anesthetic agent has worn off, thereby unmasking the underlying physiologic process. Third, a further indication of cross-tolerance may appear postoperatively in the need for postoperative sedative or analgesic agents far beyond the normal period during which these agents are used.

In such cases, unless the addictive disorder is attended to, treatment teams may find themselves in the uncomfortable position of attempting to regulate habit-forming drugs in people already addicted to or dependent on them. Finally, the dependence disorder raises questions in the minds of most physicians as to the propriety of allocating scarce resources to those whose behavior has resulted in the destruction of the organ with which they were born (for further discussion, see Alcohol-Induced Liver Disease in Chapter 20). In the following sections, each of these issues is considered.

Tolerance

The addictive disorders all share four clinical phenomena: the development of tolerance, the presentation of withdrawal symptoms on abrupt cessation of the substance, an inability to control the quantity or length of use, and social or physical decline directly attributed to uncontrolled use of a psychoactive substance. In the first case, it is important clinically to establish the history of tolerance in a patient identified as having an addictive disorder. Tolerance is elicited in the history by demonstrating that an increase in frequency and quantity of substance use has developed over time from a naive

Table 21-5. Interactions between Psychiatric Agents and Anesthetic Agents

Psychiatric Drugs	Anesthetic Agents										
	Inhalational Agents	Propofol	Ketamine	Etomidate	Thiopental	Benzodiazepines	Opioids	Anticholinergic Agents	Local Anesthetics	Sympathomimetics	Muscle Relaxants
Cyclic Antidepressants	Avoid enflurane; increased anesthetic agent requirements	Increased propofol requirements	—	Increased etomidate requirement	Augments sedative aspects of barbiturates*		Augments analgesic and respiratory depressant effects of opioids*	May increase incidence of postoperative confusion	Avoid local anesthetics with added epinephrine	Avoid indirect-acting sympathomimetics	Pancuronium associated with dysrhythmias
SSRIs	—	—	—	—	—	Decreased clearance of diazepam	—	—	—	—	—
MAOIs	Use of inhalational agents considered safe	—	—	—	May potentiate sedative effect of barbiturates*	Considered safe with MAOIs	Avoid meperidine; reduce other narcotic doses	Anticholinergic agents considered safe	Local anesthetics well tolerated, except cocaine	Avoid indirect-acting sympathomimetics	Avoid pancuronium (theoretical contraindication)
Butyrophenone and Haloperidol	Potentiates CNS depression	Potentiates CNS depression	Potentiates CNS depression	Potentiates CNS depression	—	Potentiates CNS depression	Increases risk of increasing intraocular pressure	—	—	—	—
Phenothiazines	—	—	—	—	—	—	Potentiates CNS depression	—	—	—	—
Barbiturates	—	—	—	—	May have increased tolerance to barbiturates	—	—	—	—	—	—
Benzodiazepine	Decreased minimum alveolar concentration	—	—	—	—	—	—	—	—	—	—
Lithium	—	—	—	—	—	—	—	—	—	Decreased response to sympathomimetic effects of norepinephrine	Potentiates nondepolarizing NMBs, slight increase in duration of succinylcholine

*Animal study

SSRIs = selective serotonin reuptake inhibitors; MAOIs = monoamine oxidase inhibitors; CNS = central nervous system; NMBs = neuromuscular blocking agents.

Table 21-6. Interactions between Substances of Abuse and Anesthetic Agents

Substances of Abuse	Anesthetic Agents										
	Inhalational Agents	Propofol	Ketamine	Etomidate	Thiopental	Midazolam	Opioids	Anticholinergics	Local Anesthetics	Vasopressors	Muscle Relaxants
ETOH	Chronic ETOH use increases anesthetic requirements	Chronic ETOH use increases anesthetic requirements	—	—	Chronic ETOH use increases anesthetic requirements	—	—	—	—	—	Cirrhosis prolongs the duration of action of drugs dependent on hepatic elimination
Marijuana	—	Combination prolongs sleep time*	—	Potentiates ventilatory depression	—	—	—	—	—	—	—
Cocaine	Avoid: agents potentiate cocaine cardiovascular toxicity	—	Avoid: ketamine potentiates cocaine cardiovascular toxicity	—	—	—	—	—	Vasopressor interactions may precipitate hypertensive crises and myocardial ischemia	—	—
Amphetamines	Chronic use may lead to decreased MAC requirement*	—	—	—	—	—	—	—	Use direct-acting vasopressors with caution; may attenuate responses to indirect-acting vasopressors	—	—
Opiates	Anesthetic agents of choice	Potentiates CNS depression	Potentiates CNS depression	Potentiates CNS depression	Potentiates CNS depression	Difficult to predict opiate requirements due to opiate cross-tolerance	—	—	—	Potentiate respiratory depression	—

ETOH = ethanol; MAC = minimum alveolar concentration; CNS = central nervous system.

Note: Substance-abusing patients can manifest significant drug cross-tolerance, making it difficult to predict analgesic requirements.

*Animal study.

state, in which less of the substance could be used with the same subjective effect. In practice, this is often difficult to determine because patients often feel ashamed of their substance use and minimize their use under the scrutiny of others. Tolerance must therefore be assessed through an indirect approach, in which the patient and the physician agree to look at "the drinking" or "drug use" as though it were a detached third person. An interview is often best begun by asking when a person drinks or uses a particular drug, how often the substance has been used in the previous week, when substance use was at its greatest, and whether other people were present. One may begin such an interview by asking how old the patient was at the time of his or her first alcohol or other drug use, the circumstances of that use, and its subjective effect. One may continue by asking if the same effect would be obtained today or whether more substance is required to get the same effect. The goal is to document the presence of a shift in the amount required to reach the same subjective perception between an early baseline point of use and a later tolerant point of use.

When tolerance can be demonstrated, the anesthesiologist may have a clinical clue as to the person's likely response to similar nervous system agents. In the case of alcohol, for example, tolerance, once achieved, is thought to remain for long periods. Alternately, tolerance achieved may reverse for a brief period but easily resume in response to a challenge from an agent in the same drug class to which tolerance was originally acquired. Therefore, an alcoholic or sedative user whose abstinence is relatively short (e.g., a few months) may appear tolerant to sedatives compared to another person who has remained free of substance abuse for 10 years. One variation here, however, is the possibility of an innate or genetically derived tolerance to one or another agent, such as alcohol or sedatives, that may be constitutional rather than the effect of many years of excessive use.

In the case of other forms of drug abuse, such as stimulant abuse, tolerance appears to be a relatively short-lived phenomenon, and it often reverses. This is especially true in the case of cocaine. This may pose a particular danger for illegal use when, for example, a regular cocaine user has increased his or her tolerance and therefore quantity of use, stops for some period, and then resumes use, thinking that

his or her former heavy dose is the appropriate amount of drug to consume. In reality, his or her previous tolerance has reversed itself, and he or she is essentially taking an overdose of the stimulant. In street use, this may result in death. In anesthesia practice, when a central nervous system stimulant may be indicated, a history of tolerance to stimulant drugs and the timing of recent stimulant use may be critical factors in determining when or how to give such agents.

Withdrawal

After tolerance has been established, affected people usually note withdrawal symptoms on relatively abrupt cessation of use. Withdrawal symptoms may be very severe and life threatening. Alcohol withdrawal offers a particularly striking example. In most people who undergo withdrawal, evidence of sympathetic hyperactivity occurs approximately 6–12 hours after a sudden drop in the blood level of ethanol. The person may notice any or all of the following: fine tremor, nausea and vomiting, diaphoresis, and a subjective sense of "shakiness," often in association with a sense of impending disaster, as shown in anxiety states, hypertension, tachycardia, and perhaps a low-grade fever. These symptoms can be treated by giving intermediate- to long-acting benzodiazepines in sufficient dosage to control the symptoms followed by rapid reduction over a 3- to 4-day period in most cases. In the vast majority of cases, such treatment obviates further and more dangerous symptoms in the withdrawal course.

More dangerous symptoms usually occur after 2–36 hours, in which patients may begin exhibiting generalized seizure activity. The seizures, sometimes termed "rum fits," are usually not isolated events but occur in a series of three or more. They can lead to life-threatening asphyxiation and should never be regarded as self-limited or in some way undeserving of aggressive treatment, using replacement sedative doses as needed. Finally, approximately 72 or more hours after the rapid drop in blood alcohol, DTs can develop. This must always be considered a medical emergency requiring admission to an ICU. DTs is characterized by a triad of autonomic hyperactivity, marked confusion or disorientation, and hallucinations, usually visual or tactile. Left untreated, reported death rates in this condition are 10–15%. DTs requires aggressive treatment with doses of sedative agents, usually long-acting agents, such as diazepam or chlordiazepoxide. Practice trends have substituted agents of intermediate duration, such as lorazepam and oxazepam.[26] In general, these agents are reserved for people with severe liver damage, whose ability to detoxify the longer-acting agents may be impaired. Diazepam, 10 mg; chlordiazepoxide, 50 mg; or lorazepam, 2 mg, may be given intramuscularly or intravenously if the oral route is not an option. Doses should be repeated every 1–2 hours until symptoms clear or the patient is sedated. The total dosage given the first day should be administered in divided doses the second day. A gradual taper should take place over the next 5–7 days. Some have used shorter-acting benzodiazepines, such as midazolam, but these generally require more intensive clinical supervision and use of a continuous intravenous solution. Such ultrashort-acting benzodiazepines themselves run the risk of worsening the clinical course in that they may cause recrudescence of withdrawal symptoms when they are stopped. Treatment intervention should include rehydration, thiamine, and multivitamin supplements.

Patients who have experienced a number of withdrawal episodes in the past, including severe episodes, such as seizures or DTs, are very likely to encounter severe episodes in the future. This appears to be related to a kindling phenomenon, in which each episode of severe withdrawal makes subsequent episodes more easily triggered. On physical examination, the presence of marked hyperreflexia or several beats of ankle clonus may be considered clear indicators of a very irritable central nervous system with seizures and perhaps DTs likely to ensue shortly. In general, such phenomena are indicators for aggressive use of benzodiazepines.

In contrast, stimulant withdrawal generally results in a depressed central nervous system and an increased tendency to sleep, resulting in so-called stimulant crash. Such episodes rarely require medical or pharmacologic intervention. For people whose respiratory status may be already compromised, however, intervention may be needed. Most are best left in a supportive environment until the withdrawal process is complete. For some, this may be a dangerous period if the withdrawal includes profound depression of mood. Instances of this nature require psychiatric intervention and attention to safety until the withdrawal period has passed.

Similarly, opiate withdrawal, although uncomfortable, is rarely life threatening. Withdrawal may be accomplished humanely in a hospital through use of gradually decreasing doses of opiate agents. Outpatient detoxification requires the involvement of an established methadone maintenance clinic. There have been cases of patients on methadone maintenance needing a transplant who were kept on their standard maintenance dose of methadone throughout the operative procedure and the recovery phase, with few adverse effects. Analgesia is handled in such cases by adding sufficient amounts of nonmethadone opiate preparations to control pain; these are withdrawn by the end of the hospitalization in such a way that the patient is released on his or her maintenance methadone dose alone. In such cases, continuing the methadone obviates the fear of withdrawal and promotes continued successful functioning for patients who had adapted well to its use in this particular form of therapy. Intraoperatively, such patients generally are able to tolerate anesthesia well, including the addition of analgesic doses of opiate medication during the recovery. As in all cases, however, it is important to monitor the respiratory status in any person receiving opiate agents.

Patient Selection Issues

Anesthesia personnel are concerned with the preoperative evaluation, and although the potential complications of anesthesia related to alcohol or drug-dependent people are generally well known, a much more controversial role for the anesthesiologist is participating in the selection process of patients who seek a solid-organ graft. A psychiatric consultation is generally necessary for any person with a history of alcohol or substance abuse seeking a transplant, but the anesthesiologist's clinical impression is a very important part of the evaluation process.[27] The diagnosis of alcohol or substance dependence is based solely on the history of substance use, with some added information from occasional sequelae of dependency use, as with alcoholic liver disease. Prognosis for continued sobriety, and therefore continued compliance with the necessary medication regimen, similarly depends on data gathered from the clinical history. In such instances, it is critical that alcohol- or substance-dependent patients be seen several times by several different observers, who then can collate their observations to provide an informed decision about the risk of substance use relapse and whether to offer a transplant. It is important, therefore, that anesthesia personnel be attuned to the relevant issues in the evaluation that the transplant team must carry out.

The first of these issues concerns the dependent person's ability to recognize and accept the presence of his or her dependency, both as a health risk throughout the pre- and posttransplant periods and as an indication for a change in lifestyle, specifically in refraining from alcohol or substance use. The latter concern derives from longitudinal research suggesting that relapse rates are relatively high and remain a sustained risk for many years after the decision to stop using alcohol. The key to any opportunity for sustained abstinence, however, is the person's own arrival at a decision not to drink or use substances again.

Although many people speak of an alcoholic's or substance abuser's "denial" of his or her problem, a generally more accurate conception is the person's ambivalence toward use. Most people can comprehend that their use has resulted in deleterious physical sequelae, and for a time they may be able to use this information to refrain from use. Unless the ambivalence toward the pleasurable or habitual aspects of use is resolved, however, use will eventually begin again. From the point of view of assessing the likelihood of abstinence after transplant, keeping a careful ear open for this sense of ambivalence about use is important. It is most often heard in the context of the impaired control phenomenon, in which a patient may make statements such as, "I can stop whenever I want to," "I only need to cut down," or "Drinking just isn't a big problem for me." When such statements are made in the presence of a well-established diagnosis, based on criteria mentioned above, the clinician is justified in suspecting that the patient's ambivalence has not been resolved and that there is a high likelihood of relapse after transplant. Some people argue that alcohol use and prognosis are no business of the transplant team because these are personal behaviors requiring personal privacy. Although this might be true for people who do not require a transplant, the fact that few solid-organ grafts are available to the many people who need them necessitates

careful evaluation and decision-making by the transplant team to provide this procedure to those who appear most likely to benefit.

For most substance-abusing patients, the danger lies in noncompliance with the anti-immune regimen. Although many substances can injure grafted organs, the most frequent danger is rejection caused by the patient ceasing to take his or her medications properly. The clouded cognition and lack of judgment that accompanies most forms of alcohol or substance abuse can make it possible for patients to miss doses of their medications, begin the rejection reaction, and very quickly proceed to a point at which it cannot be reversed. It is primarily for this reason that preoperative dependency behavior must be assessed. It indicates a potentially bad prognosis for postoperative survival, and help must be offered when this problem has not been recognized or addressed by the patient.

Along with the need to determine whether the patient is resolving his or her ambivalence to substance use, four other prognostic factors seem to be useful in understanding recovery from a recognized alcohol or substance abuse problem. In brief, they include the following:

1. Engaging in activities that structure a person's daytime and evening hours with activities that hold his or her interest and involve other people
2. The presence of a caring other person (this is sometimes called a *rehabilitation relationship*) who both recognizes and understands the dependency problem and is willing to accept the person so long as the active dependence is in remission
3. Identification of sources of hope or improved self-esteem that can counteract the guilt that a person often feels about his or her alcohol or substance abuse
4. A negative behavioral reinforcement, constituting a painful or obnoxious result of drinking that occurs immediately and with certainty should alcohol or drug abuse resume

The first three factors involve active and beneficial change in a person's style of living. In pursuing abstinence, the person substitutes constructive activities and people who do not drink or abuse drugs at the times that were once associated with drinking alcohol or abusing substances. Some examples include time spent with family, nondrug recreational activities, and self-help group or work activities. Their importance is in structuring a person's time around activities other than alcohol or substance abuse.

A rehabilitation relationship most often involves a knowledgeable spouse who has come to understand what dependency means and begun to behave in ways that has set appropriate limits on the dependent person's ability to influence the relationship and to state very clear reasons for ceasing that relationship if dependency recurs. The person need not be a spouse, however, and may be any of a number of others, including physicians, ministers, counselors, Alcoholics Anonymous sponsors, or other family members.

The search for a source of renewed hope or self-esteem leads to questions such as "What do you look forward to in life?" or "What keeps you going in life?" Most patients can give some response about their view of the future. A problem is present when a person cannot manage any response about looking forward to the future. This is usually an indication for further psychiatric evaluation for depressive disorders.

Behavioral negative reinforcers are generally few. The reinforcement criterion of being immediate and noxious on resumption of drinking disqualifies liver disease itself, for example, which is often a very subtle process until the final stages. By contrast, acute pancreatitis or a disulfiram-alcohol reaction fulfills those criteria. It is possible to treat transplant patients with disulfiram postoperatively as well as preoperatively in some cases. Postoperatively, the patient must take immunosuppressant medicine in forms that do not contain alcohol. Large cooperative studies have shown that disulfiram alone promotes abstinence for only a brief period; a matter of only a few months or more. By contrast, longitudinal studies have shown that extended abstinence, for longer than 3 years, occurs only when people can establish any two of the four prognostic factors previously listed in their lives as a way of preventing further substance use.

Outcome data from alcoholic patients given liver transplants offer the best information on continued abstinence as well as graft survival.[25] Studies suggest no difference between alcoholic and nonalcoholic liver graft recipients in terms of 3-year graft survival. At the same time, reports from a series of centers place the likelihood of complete abstinence at the end of the first year in the range of 90–95%

for most alcoholic people who have been screened in the manner detailed earlier in this chapter. Prospective data at 3 years suggest that abstinence rates drop to approximately 75–80%. It is reasonable to suppose, therefore, that abstinence for people receiving liver grafts extends well beyond the first year after transplant. This suggests the need for continued care over the long term for people receiving organ grafts who have a dependency history.

Two other factors may bear on predicting long-term abstinence. Preliminary reports suggest that a 6-month period of abstinence before transplant is predictive of long-term abstinence after transplant.[25, 28] This idea, however, is based on an inadequately done study and has not been replicated by subsequent studies. Second, longitudinal studies have shown that people who abuse alcohol differ markedly in their natural history from those whose primary drugs of abuse are illicit substances and who have a history of antisocial behavior from childhood.[29] The former group cannot be differentiated from the general population in any prospective manner. They appear to be genetically more vulnerable toward alcoholism than those who do not develop that disorder, and their outcome is generally much better over the long term than that of the second population. In the second group of drug or poly–drug-dependent people, a pretransplant history of resolution of drug dependency is most important.

It is important to recall that in the transplant process, the care given by the transplant team itself carries a powerful and positive prognostic weight. Each of the positive prognostic factors noted in this chapter, including structured time, rehabilitation relationships, and a sense of improved hope or self-esteem, can be found in the care that the patient receives from the transplant team itself. Contact with the anesthesiologist is certainly a part of this and can be a greater or lesser part of the postoperative stage, depending on the interest of the anesthesiologist.

Conclusions

There are few procedures in medicine that evoke as much awe as organ transplantation. Since the first successful transplant, a kidney, by Murray and Hume in 1954, medical, surgical, and anesthetic advances have led to a dramatic change in survival. Despite these advances, the transplant patient and his or her family are faced with numerous psychosocial stresses in their quest to extend and improve the quality of life. Patients who were routinely excluded from transplantation consideration in the past because of a psychiatric or substance abuse disorder are now being considered. The development of newer psychotropic agents and drug combinations necessitates a close working relationship between psychiatrists and anesthesiologists to provide optimal transplant care in the future.

References

1. Howard LM, Williams R, Fahy TA. The psychiatric assessment of liver transplant patients with alcoholic disease: a review. J Psychosom Res 1994;38:643–653.

2. Kumar S, Stauber RE, Gavale JS, et al. Orthotopic liver transplantation for alcoholic liver disease. Hepatology 1990;11:159–164.

3. Surman OS. Hemodialysis and Renal Transplantation. In TP Hackett, NH Cassem (eds), Massachusetts General Handbook of General Hospital Psychiatry. St. Louis: Mosby, 1987;380–402.

4. House RM, Thompson TL. Psychiatric aspects of organ transplantation. JAMA 1988;260:535–539.

5. Levenson JL, Olbrish ME. Psychiatric aspects of heart transplantation. Psychosomatics 1993;34:114–123.

6. Sanner M. Attitude toward organ donation and transplantation: A model for understanding reactions to medical procedures after death. Soc Sci Med 1994;38:1141–1152.

7. Frazier PA, Davis-Ali SH, Dahl KE. Stressors, social support and adjustment in kidney transplant patients and their spouses. Social Work Health Care 1995;21:93–108.

8. Suszycki LH. Psychosocial aspects of hearth transplant. Soc Work 1990;33(3):205–209.

9. Dew MA, Roth LH, Schulberg HC, et al. Prevalence and predictors of depression and anxiety-related disorders during the year after heart transplantation. Gen Hosp Psychiatry 1996;18:485–615.

10. Surman OS, Casimi AB. Ethical dichotomies in organ transplantation. Gen Hosp Psychiatry 1996;18:135–195.

11. Kim WR, Therneau TM, Dickson ER, et al. Preoperative Predictors of Resource Utilization in Liver Transplantation. In PI Terasaki, JM Cecka (eds), Clinical Transplants. Los Angeles: UCLA Tissue Typing Laboratory, 1993;315–322.

12. Levy N. Psychological aspects of renal transplantation. Psychosomatics 1994;35:427–433.

13. Dixon D. Religious and Spiritual Perspective on Organ Transplantation. In J Caven, G Rodin (eds), Psychiatric Aspects of Organ Transplantation. New York: Oxford, 1992;131–141.

14. Freeman AM, Volks DG, Sokol RS. Cardiac transplantation: clinical correlates of psychiatric outcome. Psychosomatics 1988;29:47–54.

15. House RM. Transplantation Surgery. In A Stoudemire, B Fogel (eds), Psychiatric Care of the Medical Patient. New York: Oxford, 1993;803–816.

16. House RM, Dubovsky SL, Penn I. Psychiatric aspects of hepatic transplantation. Transplantation 1983;36:146–150.

17. Trzepacz PT, DiMartini A, Tringali RD. Psychopharmacological issues in organ transplantation: II. Psychopharmacologic medications. Psychosomatics 1993;34:290–298.

18. Watts D, Freeman AM, McGriffin D, et al. Psychiatric aspects of cardiac transplantation. Heart Transplant 1984;3:243–247.

19. Trzepacz PT, Maue FR, Coffman G, et al. Neuropsychiatric assessment of liver transplantation candidates: delirium and other psychiatric disorders. Int J Psychiatry Med 1987;16:101–111.

20. Trzepacz PT, Levenson JL, Tringala RA. Psychopharmacology and neuropsychiatric syndromes in organ transplantation. Gen Hosp Psychiatry 1991;13:233–245.

21. Gelfand SB, Indelicato J, Benjamin J. Using intravenous Haldol to control delirium. Hosp Commun Psychiatry 1992;43:215.

22. Kuhn WF, Davis MH, Lippman SB. Emotional adjustment to cardiac transplantation. Gen Hosp Psychiatry 1988;10:108–113.

23. Fukunishi I. Anxiety associated with kidney transplantation. Psychopathology 1993;26:24–28.

24. Bernstein L, Daviss SR. Organic anxiety disorder with symptoms of akathisia in a patient treated with the immunosuppressant FK506. Gen Hosp Psychiatry 1992;14:210–211.

25. Beresford TP, Turcotte JG, Merion R, et al. A rational approach to liver transplantation for the alcoholic patient. Psychosomatics 1990;31:241–254.

26. Naranjo CA, Sellers EM. Clinical assessment and pharmacotherapy of the alcohol withdrawal syndrome. Recent Dev Alcohol 1986;4:265–281.

27. Snyder SL, Drooker M, Strain JJ. A survey estimate of academic liver transplant teams' selection practices for alcohol-dependent applicants. Psychosomatics 1996;37:432–437.

28. Cohen C, Benjamin M. Alcoholics and liver transplantation. JAMA 1991;265:1299–1301.

29. Vaillant GE. The Alcohol-Dependent and Drug-Dependent Person. In AM Nicholi (ed), The New Harvard Guide to Psychiatry. Cambridge, MA: Harvard University Press, 1988;700–713.

Chapter 22

Overview of Solid-Organ Transplantation: Past, Present, and Future

Roy Y. Calne

Chapter Plan

Past
Present
Future
Future Ethical Dilemmas

Past

I have been involved in transplantation research and practice since 1959. At that time, organ transplantation was a "dream of crazy surgeons," an opinion supported by immunologists since Gibson and Medawar[1] showed that grafted tissue would be rejected inexorably and that the fundamental biology of the immune system was involved in this process. Surgeons, however, not being privy to this immunologic analysis, were interested in the techniques of grafting tissue and organs. Some thought that grafts were rejected only because the surgery had been done badly and that they could do it better. It took some years and repeated and consistent lack of success for surgeons to realize that long-term functioning survival of the transplanted organ could be obtained only in grafts between identical twins. This achievement at Peter Brigham Hospital by Merrill and his colleagues[2] was an outstandingly important surgical advance. Meanwhile, in Britain, Billingham et al.[3] showed that the immune system could be persuaded to accept a graft of foreign tissue if it was presented before the immune system had

developed. Thus, immunologic tolerance was achieved by intrauterine or neonatal injection of donor tissue into mice. A worry soon clarified by these workers was that the grafted tissue could react against the recipient, producing a wasting and usually lethal graft-versus-host or "runt" disease. This, of course, is of special importance in bone marrow grafting, which required destruction of the recipient's marrow by drastic total-body irradiation. When irradiation was applied to kidney grafting, the results were appalling, and another way had to be found. In 1959, Schwartz and Damashek[4] showed that the antileukemia drug 6-mercaptopurine would prevent rabbits from producing antibodies against foreign protein, and this specific inhibition of antibody response persisted even after 6-mercaptopurine was stopped. 6-Mercaptopurine was shown to prolong kidney graft survival in dogs, and a close relative of 6-mercaptopurine, azathioprine, was slightly more effective.[5, 6] The use of this compound together with corticosteroids paved the way for the first successful renal allografts. Some of the early patients transplanted with this immunosuppressive protocol are still alive, some 30 years after operation.

The next main advance in transplantation was surgical. Techniques were developed for transplanting the heart, liver, heart and lungs, lungs, and pancreas. The only significant advance in immunosuppression was the development of antilymphocyte antibodies produced in animals injected with human lymphoid cells. The early preparations were variable in efficacy and sometimes toxic, but improvement in production techniques has resulted in more reliable products.

In the late 1970s, the cyclic peptide, cyclosporine, was discovered by Borel[7] in Sandoz to have immunosuppressive properties and also to prolong skin grafts in mice. White and I found that it also prolonged experimental organ grafts.[8] When cyclosporine was introduced into clinical practice, the results of allografts of all organs improved, but an unpleasant and unexpected finding—not apparent in the animal experiments—was that cyclosporine in humans was nephrotoxic,[9] and dosage had to be adjusted very carefully for each patient.

In the intervening years, there have been many advances in the use of immunosuppressive drugs but no consensus as to exactly how agents should be used. One strategy that has been proved popular is to give relatively small, nontoxic dosage of several drugs (e.g., azathioprine, steroids, and cyclosporine). The aim was to have additive immunosuppression and to avoid the individual side effects of the different agents.

The unraveling of the genetics of the major histocompatibility complex (MHC) and the development of tissue typing as a repeatable and reliable exercise have shown that within a family, MHC matching is very important. Thus, in transplants between matched siblings, 90% of the patients have functional grafts at 10 years, although they still require immunosuppressive treatment. For half-matched transplants between parents and children or half-matched siblings, the figure falls to approximately 70% at 10 years compared with approximately 50% for grafts between unrelated individuals. The results of transplants of all organs are comparable, although liver transplants with good function after a year tend to have better long-term functional survival and less chronic rejection than other organs. Some patients have been able to stop immunosuppression for many years without rejection; this is an example of "operational tolerance" in patients with liver transplants. There have been important advances in genetics and disease association with the MHC, and the avoidance of a positive cross-match in donor-recipient combinations is essential to prevent hyperacute renal allograft rejection, which can occur in the presence of cytotoxic antibody.

Present

Currently, transplantation provides an excellent form of therapy for many patients and has now become a major surgical specialty. There is still a great deal of room for improvement, however, particularly in the management of immunosuppression, and research work has returned to the old theme of trying to induce immunologic tolerance. It would appear that all forms of tolerance require a period of immunologic engagement between donor and recipient. During this encounter, acceptance of the graft is unstable, and rejection may occur or a "tolerant" or "almost tolerant" state may result. If immunologically active donor-derived bone marrow cells have been transplanted with the graft, especially if the recipient is immunocompromised, graft-versus-host disease may occur, which is very difficult to treat and likely to prove fatal. Figure 22-1 is a schematic diagram of the relationship of the spectrum of immunologic reactivity to the patients being treated. Most patients with good allograft organ function require reasonably substantial maintenance immunosuppression. A few can do well with very small doses, and some liver patients require none.

In the laboratory, the only method of producing tolerance without using immunosuppressive drugs is the classical fetal or neonatal tolerance and tolerance that results after liver grafting in the pig and the rat between MHC-mismatched animals.[10] The livers undergo a rejection reaction with liver cell damage that recovers spontaneously. The animals then become tolerant and will accept grafts of other tissues and organs from the same donor.[11]

Other forms of tolerance require immunosuppression, antilymphocyte serum for the thymic tolerance in rodents described by Philadelphia workers,[12] and a variety of immunosuppressive protocols are used when bone marrow–derived cells are used.

Based on the hypothesis that a "window of opportunity for immunologic engagement" is necessary for tolerance induction and that this may be frustrated by aggressive T-cell reactivity from the donor or the recipient, my colleagues and I devised experiments in which MHC-mismatched pigs with renal allografts were given donor-derived bone marrow cells in the form of spleen cells or donor blood and one dose of cyclosporine. They were then left for 2–3 days without any immunosuppressive treatment, followed by six daily doses of cyclosporine and then no further treatment. More than half of the animals became long-term survivors without any evidence of chronic rejection and normal histology after a year.[13] This protocol could be adapted for clinical use, although it is likely that humans will require a different type of immunosuppressive conditioning.

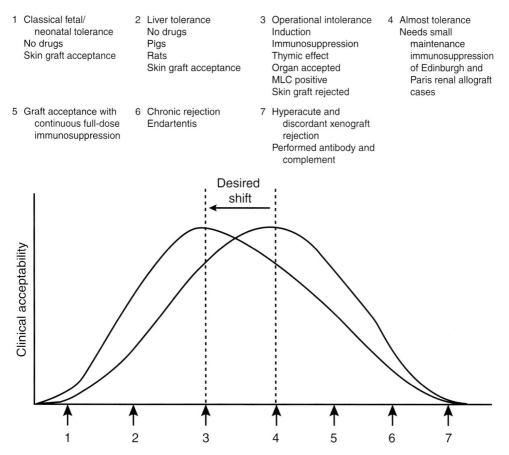

1 Classical fetal/
   neonatal tolerance
   No drugs
   Skin graft acceptance

2 Liver tolerance
   No drugs
   Pigs
   Rats
   Skin graft acceptance

3 Operational intolerance
   Induction
   Immunosuppression
   Thymic effect
   Organ accepted
   MLC positive
   Skin graft rejected

4 Almost tolerance
   Needs small
   maintenance
   immunosuppression
   of Edinburgh and
   Paris renal allograft
   cases

5 Graft acceptance with
   continuous full-dose
   immunosuppression

6 Chronic rejection
   Endartentis

7 Hyperacute and
   discordant xenograft
   rejection
   Performed antibody and
   complement

Figure 22-1. Scheme of the spectrum of immunologic engagement from tolerance to hyperacute rejection. The majority of patients with organ grafts require continuous dosage with immunosuppressive drugs. The objective would be to shift the curve to the left so that the majority of patients are operationally tolerant or almost tolerant and require only minimal immunosuppression. (MLC = mixed leukocyte concentration.) (Reprinted with permission from RY Calne. An opportunity in organ transplantation. Nat Med 1995;1:21.)

There now seems to be good evidence that some tissue mismatches are acceptable, with good long-term results expected, and that some mismatches are unacceptable.[14] I would anticipate that we will see strategies of tolerance applied to donor and recipient pairs that are either well-matched or acceptable mismatches.

Future

The imbalance of donor supply and recipient needs is becoming greater, and as the results of organ grafting improve, so this shortage of donor organs will become more acute. Even with the best type of public and medical education and encouragement of living-related donation for kidney transplants wherever possible, there still will be a shortfall, especially for patients waiting for heart and kidney grafts. Already a start has been made with living-related donation of liver and lung lobes, which raises concern about danger to the donor.

An obvious solution to the need for organs is the use of animals as donors. The most suitable donors biologically would be higher apes, but these are protected species. Other primates tend to be small, with small organs, and there is a danger of latent viral infections that could in theory be transmitted to humans. In the early 1960s, kidney transplants were performed from primates to humans; one chimpanzee kidney functioned for more than 9 months. This behavior is known as "concordant."

The Transplantation Society is the leading international society of doctors and scientists involved in the transplantation of tissues and organs. It will become proactive in promoting the monitoring and policing of transplantation activity, and in supervision of the adherence to proper principles of practice.

The Ethics Committee of the Transplantation Society will produce a document on behalf of the society, setting out guidelines on the ethical aspects of tissue and organ transplantation. This document will be promulgated through
- The World Health Organization and other international medical bodies
- The *Transplantation Society Bulletin*, thereby reaching all society members

The Transplantation Society recommends:
1. All countries should enact legislation forbidding all commercial trafficking in tissues and organs.
2. All countries should define brain death and its diagnosis and enshrine this concept in law, including the requirement that the assessors of brain death are independent and free from any direct interest in the transplant procedure.
3. All countries should ensure effective monitoring of tissue and organ transplantation through
   a. Proper regulation of mortuary activity and of tissue banks.
   b. Certification of brain death by independent assessors.
   c. Signed and dated certification by the surgeon removing the tissues and organs, stating (1) he or she has witnessed the certification of brain death and (2) which tissues and organs have been removed. Copies of this documentation must be forwarded together with all tissues and organs.
   d. Full certification by the implanting surgeon, stating that (1) he or she has inspected the retrieval documentation and deemed it satisfactory and (2) he or she has recorded the implantation of stated organs into specified individuals.
   e. Ensuring that tissues and organs not used are accounted for to relevant authorities.
   f. The introduction of methods for registering and tracking all donors.
   g. The approval and certification of transplant centers and teams by relevant government or medical professional authorities, or both.

The Transplantation Society further states that with respect to more general issues, its position remains unchanged:
1. Organs and tissues should be freely given without commercial consideration or financial profit.
2. Consent should be obtained.
3. Transplantation Society members should not be involved in obtaining or transplanting organs from executed criminals.

Figure 22-2. Adapted from the policy statement from the Ethics Committee of the Transplantation Society. (Ethics Committee of the Transplantation Society. Transplantation Society Bulletin 1995;June[3]:1–22.)

The pig is a more convenient species, given that organs can be of any size and the animals are easy to breed, but the domestic pig and humans have been separated for many millions of years of independent evolution, and all porcine proteins differ to some extent from the equivalent proteins produced by human cells. Additionally, the pig has a natural life of only approximately 15 years. There are obvious important physiologic and metabolic matters that must be studied after the major hurdle of rejec-tion has been overcome. This barrier may have a number of different stages, the first and most obvious is the immediate activation of complement, which causes destruction of capillaries in the transplanted organ and almost instantaneous failure of the organ (discordant rejection). There are a variety of ways complement activation may be prevented; probably the most attractive is to produce transgenic pigs with human anticomplement protein genes so that human complement is not activated. If this permits reasonably prolonged perfusion of organs from pigs with human blood, it will be possible to study rejection and immunosuppression to determine whether immunosuppressive agents that are effective in allografts will also control this second phase of xenograft rejection. The science of xenografting is at an early stage and holds great biological fascination. It may be some time before pig organs can be used successfully as long-term treatment for patients.

Future Ethical Dilemmas

The prospect of dying from disease affecting a vital organ is now changed so that organ grafting is a possible salvation, but because of the shortage of organs, not everybody who needs an organ graft can get one. There has been a tendency for doctors and patients in some Western countries to regard provision of organ allografts as their right, but it is really a privilege depending on the charity of donation of fellow citizens. Any abuse of the charitable gift would lead to rapid public repudiation of organ donation. It is, therefore, very important for doctors and all others involved in organ transplantation to make sure that moral and ethical standards are commensurate with the highest professional standards. There have been allegations of organs being removed from patients undergoing other operations and even of people being kidnapped or killed for removal of their organs. Not one specific case has been authenticated, but vigilance should be exercised to make sure that there is no criminal abuse of organ transplantation. Other areas are less clearly defined, such as payment or favors for living donors and more general commercialization.

The introduction of a law in the United Kingdom requiring certification of donor and recipient operations has given reassurance to both the medical profession and the public. Certificates are required by law in the same way birth and death certificates are required. The international Transplantation Society has approved a series of guidelines (Figure 22-2).

These guidelines have been adopted almost unanimously by the transplant community; it is hoped that they also will be acceptable to the entire medical profession and the public.

References

1. Gibson T, Medawar PB. The behaviour of skin homografts in man. J Anat 1943;77:299–310.
2. Merrill JP, Murray JE, Harrison, et al. Successful homotransplantation of the human kidney between identical twins. JAMA 1956;160:227–282.
3. Billingham RE, Brent L, Medawar PB. "Actively acquired tolerance" of foreign cells. Nature 1953; 172:603–606.
4. Schwartz R, Damashek W. Drug induced immunologic tolerance. Nature 1959;183:1682.
5. Calne RY. The rejection of renal homografts inhibition in dogs by 6-mercaptopurine. Surg Forum 1960;11:470–474.
6. Calne RY. Inhibition of the rejection of renal homografts in dogs by purine analogues. Transplant Bull 1961;28:445–461.
7. Borel JF. Comparative study of in vitro and in vivo drug effects on cell-mediated cytotoxicity. Immunology 1976;31:631–641.
8. Calne RY, White DJG. Cyclosporin A—a powerful immunosuppressant in dogs with renal allografts. IRCS Med Sci 1977;5:595.
9. Calne RY, White DJG, Thiru S, et al. Cyclosporin A in patients receiving renal allografts from cadaver donors. Lancet 1978;2:1323–1327.
10. Calne RY, Davies H. Organ graft tolerance: the liver effect. Lancet 1994;343:67–68.
11. Kamada N, Brons IGM, Davies H. Fully allogeneic liver grafting in rats induces a state of systemic nonreactivity to donor transplantation antigens. Transplantation 1980;29:429–431.
12. Posselt A, Barker C, Tomaszewski J, et al. Induction of donor-specific unresponsiveness by intra-thymic islet transplantation. Science 1990;249:1293–1295.
13. Calne RY, Watson CJE, Brons IGM, et al. Tolerance or porcine renal allografts induced by donor spleen cells and seven days' treatment with cyclosporine. Transplantation 1994;10:1433–1435.
14. Terasaki P, Mark MS, Takemoto S, et al. HLA Typing for Transplantation. Abstract for the Third Congress of Asian Society of Transplantation in Bangkok, December 4–6, 1993.

Index